MEDICAL RADIOLOGY

Diagnostic Imaging

Editors:
A. L. Baert, Leuven
M. Knauth, Göttingen
K. Sartor, Heidelberg

K. J. Johnson · E. Bache (Eds.)

Imaging in Pediatric Skeletal Trauma

Techniques and Applications

With Contributions by

E. Bache · K. Bradshaw · V. N. Cassar-Pullicino · S. Chapman · A. M. Davies
R. D. D. Duncan · K. Foster · P. Gibbons · P. Glithero · A. Harries · K. Hayward
D. Horton · G. J. Irwin · K. J. Johnson · R. Kanwar · R. K. Lalam · C. Lever · J. Metcalfe
K. Parkes · A. Paterson · A. Sprigg · S. Symons · J. Teh · P. N.M. Tyrrell · H. Williams

Foreword by

A. L. Baert

With 391 Figures in 627 Separate Illustrations, 19 in Color and 19 Tables

Springer

Karl J. Johnson, MD, MRCP, FRCR
Consultant Paediatric Radiologist
Department of Radiology
Birmingham Children's Hospital
Steelhouse Lane
Birmingham B4 6NH
UK

Edward Bache, FRCS (ortho)
Consultant Orthopaedic Surgeon
Birmingham Children Hospital
Steelhouse Lane
Birmingham B4 6NH
UK

Medical Radiology · Diagnostic Imaging and Radiation Oncology
Series Editors:
A. L. Baert · L. W. Brady · H.-P. Heilmann · M. Knauth · M. Molls · C. Nieder · K. Sartor

Continuation of Handbuch der medizinischen Radiologie
Encyclopedia of Medical Radiology

Library of Congress Control Number: 2007926909

ISBN 978-3-540-66196-2 Springer Berlin Heidelberg New York

Springer is part of Springer Science+Business Media

http//www.springer.com

Medical Editor: Dr. Ute Heilmann, Heidelberg
Desk Editor: Ursula N. Davis, Heidelberg
Production Editor: Kurt Teichmann, Mauer
Cover-Design and Typesetting: Verlagsservice Teichmann, Mauer

Printed on acid-free paper – 21/3180xq – 5 4 3 2 1 0

Foreword

This volume, dedicated to skeletal trauma in infants and children, is a very welcome addition to the list of titles on pediatric imaging published in the "Medical Radiology" series in recent years.

It provides a much needed update of our knowledge on and our latest insights into the role of modern radiological imaging and the optimal use of the different imaging modalities of skeletal trauma in the pediatric age group, thus ensuring optimal diagnostic and therapeutic management of these patients.

The well readable text is complemented by numerous excellent illustrations.

The editors and authors of individual chapters are well known for their particular clinical expertise and skills in pediatric skeletal trauma. I would like to thank and congratulate them most sincerely for their superb efforts which have resulted in this outstanding volume.

This book will be of great value not only for general and pediatric radiologists, but also for pediatricians and pediatric orthopedic surgeons and will provide them with state-of-the-art information on this important part of daily radiological practice.

I am confident that it will meet with the same success as the previous volumes published in this series.

Leuven

Albert L. Baert

Foreword

Preface

Imaging in acute trauma is an increasingly important and demanding part of radiological practice, the unique and specialised approach needed in pediatric trauma adds a further level of complexity. There is a need to continuously update the knowledge of radiologists, orthopaedic surgeons and others working in this field. This book aims to provide the reader with the full range of techniques available for imaging while highlighting the optimum application of these techniques on an anatomical basis. The first section of the book deals with techniques, discussing indications and correct procedures. The remaining 15 chapters look in detail at the specific types of traumatic injuries that occur in children and the best imaging approach at different anatomical sites, highlighting appropriate management pathways and typical complications.

The editors are grateful to the international panel of authors for their contributions to this book, which aims to provide a comprehensive overview of the current imaging of pediatric trauma.

Birmingham

K. J. Johnson
E. Bache

Contents

Imaging Techniques and Procedures

Paediatric Trauma Radiography

1

David Horton

CONTENTS

1.1 Introduction

Radiographs are likely to be the first imaging method used following trauma, and the first to lead to legal action if omitted or misinterpreted. Standard (plain film) radiography is the method most often relied upon in the assessment of suspected non-accidental injury of children. It is important that good quality radiographs are obtained in all circumstances and that quality is not sacrificed just because of the age and lack of cooperation of the child. It is important that all individuals interpreting radiographs in the acute trauma situation have an understanding of the normal anatomy and basic radiographic projections used.

While historically the use of radiographs has been integral to trauma management, in the future the increasing availability of CT and MRI and the use of ultrasound may alter this role.

D. Horton, MD
Consultant Paediatric Radiologist, Hull Royal Infirmary, Anlapoy Road, Hull, HU3 2JZ, UK

1.2 Paediatric Trauma

Trauma is the leading cause of death among children over the age of 1 year, more than all other causes of death combined. For every child death there are estimated to be at least 40 hospital admissions due to injury and over 1000 attendances to an emergency department. In the USA it is estimated that one in four children suffer some injury requiring attendance at an accident and emergency department each year (Nguyen et al. 2003). In the UK about 2 million children under the age of 14 suffer from accidental injury each year (RoSPA 2005). Nearly 20% of children who present with an injury have a fracture and, it is estimated, 42% of boys and 27% of girls sustain a fracture during childhood (Eiff and Hatch 2003).

The majority of injury is blunt trauma. Road accidents, either as a pedestrian, cyclist or vehicle occupant, produce many of these cases. Children aged 10 or 11 will estimate distances and gaps in traffic with similar skill to adults, but will overestimate their ability to use the available gap and so have less time to avoid danger (Plumert et al. 2004). Younger children can be completely oblivious to road dangers and small children, as pedestrians, are not easy for car drivers to see. Child passengers may be difficult to restrain unless appropriate safety devices are used and can be injured by the airbags designed to save their parents.

Children are more likely to be involved in sports than adults. The incidence of fractures of the distal forearm has increased 40% over the last 30 years, with most of the increase occurring in fractures associated with recreational activities, particularly of the distal radial metaphysis and physis (Eiff and Hatch 2003).

About 35% of severe injuries result from accidents occurring within the home, the place that is supposed to be a safe haven for children, and include falls, burns and scalds.

Penetrating injuries are much less common in children than blunt injuries, and those that do occur are usually associated with blunt trauma (such as penetrating metal fragment injuries associated with a vehicle collision). The increasing use of knives, particularly among young men, may increase the numbers of penetrating injuries in the future. Gun use by children, a significant cause of childhood trauma in some regions of the world, is thankfully still rare in most of Europe.

The attending emergency medical staff faced with such broad possibilities of aetiology of trauma in a child must have a plan of action for dealing with the situation. This plan will almost certainly include, at some point, radiography.

1.3 Paediatric Considerations

A favorite cliché of paediatric texts is that children are not small adults. True, children are usually smaller than adults, with consequences for drug dosages, blood and fluid therapies and temperature control, but the anatomical and physiological differences are not all due to the change of scale between adult and child. An understanding of the unossified cartilaginous skeleton and the normal variants of growth is vital. The faster respiratory and heart rates along with the different body fat composition provide real challenges when attempting to perform radiography, even if it is possible to keep the child still at all. The greater sensitivity to radiation of the child than the adult means that repeat examinations should be avoided where possible.

1.3.1 The Developing Skeleton

The major anatomic regions of growing bone include the epiphysis, the physis or growth plate, the metaphysis, and the diaphysis. The epiphysis is a secondary ossification centre at the end of long bones, separated from the rest of the bone by the cartilaginous growth plate. The age that ossification centres become visible on a radiograph varies according to the location, and similarly the rates of closure of the growth plates. Knowledge of the timings of these occurrences, or at least their order, can be very useful, particularly with elbow fractures and dislocations (see Chap. 18). The relative lack of ossification of many epiphyses in young children, and therefore the radiolucency of the growth plates, can make fracture identification difficult. The immature bone of the child has the ability to bow and bend rather than break in response to the forces placed on it. This leads to skeletal deformity and incomplete fracture types not seen in adults.

The attachment of the growth plate to the metaphysis is a point of decreased strength of bone and is an important site of injury after musculoskeletal trauma as damage to the growth plate can disrupt future growth at that site.

Ligaments and tendons are generally stronger than the growing bone of a child. A child is more likely to fracture a bone and an adult is more likely to tear a ligament, muscle, or tendon in response to the same amount of force. A child's periosteum is thicker, stronger, and more biologically active than that of an adult and will often remain intact following a fracture. The periosteum provides some stability across a fracture site and promotes more rapid healing than an adult, to be considered when attempting to assess when a fracture occurred.

Paediatric fractures usually heal more rapidly than adult fractures and children typically require a shorter period of immobilization. However, a malpositioned fragment may become immovable much earlier than in an adult. Fractures in children may stimulate longitudinal growth of the bone, which may make the bone longer than it would have been had it not been injured. Therefore, a degree of fragment overlap and so limb shortening is acceptable, possibly even desirable in certain fractures, to counterbalance the anticipated overgrowth.

1.4 Clinical Indications

It is important in children that any radiograph should contribute to the clinical management. The practice of performing radiographs out of habit or for poorly justified reasons is an unnecessary radiation burden to the child and is wasteful of resources. It may waste time and divert attention from more appropriate action. Departmental and institutional guidelines, such as those in the UK issued by the Royal College of Radiologists, should be developed to help the clinician in a wide variety of scenarios, including paediatric trauma. Many guidelines have been developed for head and spine injury in particular (NICE 2003; SIGN 2000).

1.5 Comparison Views

The identification of a fracture of a developing bone can be extremely difficult. A radiograph taken of the uninjured side for comparison can be a useful tool. The routine use of comparison radiographs is a more debatable practice. It is possible to find major authorities who would use comparison views liberally (Swischuk 1994) and others who point out limitations of this practice (Ozonoff 1992). Both agree that local custom and practice play a major role in the use of comparison views.

Whilst routine comparison views would encourage awareness of the normal appearance amongst emergency staff, this would be at a considerable price in terms of radiation exposure to the child and financial cost to the radiology department. Some areas lend themselves to comparison films for reasons of anatomy and possible bilateral pathology. It is common for both hips to be radiographed, for example. In other areas the use of a comparison film may actually mislead. At the ankle the presence of accessory ossicles can cause confusion when looking for evidence of fracture of the malleoli. A comparison film of the other ankle might be useful, but the ossification centre is unilateral in up to a third of cases, which can mislead the clinician into a false positive diagnosis. In one review, experienced paediatric radiologists requested comparison films in only 8% of cases, and even then there was no change of the diagnosis (McCauley et al. 1979). Reviews by others of comparison views for elbow injuries interpreted by junior and senior medical staff found no benefit in performing routine comparison views (Chacon et al. 1992; Kissoon et al. 1995).

In general, wherever possible the initial films should be viewed by an experienced paediatric radiologist before the use of comparison views. This is more cost-efficient and delivers less radiation to patients compared to obtaining them routinely.

1.6 Digital Radiography and PACS

Many centres use a digital system of radiography and have, or are developing, a PACS (picture archiving and communication system). An argument to justify the large expenditure entailed in converting to a digital system is the potential for decreasing patient dose. With the wide dynamic range of digital systems it can to some extent compensate for either under or over exposure and computerised post-processing allows manipulation of the image to optimise its appearance. This means that there is a potential for a deliberate reduction in radiation dose, below the levels needed to produce a satisfactory image with conventional film, with the ability to retrieve a diagnostic image electronically later.

This is a very attractive proposition in paediatric radiography, but it can potentially cause problems and in clinical practice considerable effort is needed to maintain standards (Willis and Slovis 2005). The equipment must be set up carefully, to optimise all of the factors under control, and these must be constantly monitored and improved. It is all too easy later on to improve poor images by increasing the radiation dose ("exposure factor creep") when other adjustments might have been effective.

The demands on image quality can vary depending on the clinical situation. The resolution required for a survey for non-accidental injury is particularly demanding of a digital system, as it is for standard film radiography, as the target lesions are small and subtle.

If automatic exposure controls become faulty or technique begins to slip, it is easy for a high radiation dose to be missed as there is little visible change to the image. The darkness or lightness of an image that traditionally was the guide to exposure is of no use when this darkness or lightness can be manipulated electronically after the image has been taken. Good quality assurance should be in place to detect this. Some method of recording actual patient dose on each film can be useful positive feedback.

Some evidence of the difficulty of establishing the optimum digital system comes from a review of European centres (Neofotistou et al. 2005). Patients' entrance surface doses were measured for three simple radiographic examinations. Doses between centres varied from 30% for lateral chest to 250% for a PA chest examination. Clearly there is work still to be done to find the optimum use of this equipment and to harmonise that standard across different institutions.

1.7 Radiation Dose and Protection

The effects of radiation on the infant and young child are greater than that on the adult. The biological effects of radiation are primarily those of damage to DNA. The faster growing tissues of children are more susceptible to this damage and they have a longer time ahead of them than an adult to express the effects of that damage. There is no known threshold below which radiation exposure is known to be safe (Slovis et al. 2002). It is prudent, and indeed in most countries a legal requirement, to reduce the radiation burden to the patient to as low a level as can be achieved to obtain the imaging information. Foremost in this is the clinical justification of the need for the radiograph in the first instance. Once the radiograph has been justified there are measures that can be taken to reduce the radiation dose.

High speed systems, high kV, short duration exposures, the use of additional filters and the avoidance of antiscatter grids are recommended. It is not always easy to do this. The alteration of equipment may need senior technical advice. If the equipment is used for both adults and children it may not be easy to quickly place and remove the antiscatter grid. This will inevitably increase the radiation dose to the paediatric patients. It is a considerable advantage if at least one room in a mixed adult and paediatric department can be adapted to optimise the radiation dose to children.

It may be acceptable in particular circumstances to obtain the necessary clinical information with a film of lower resolution and radiation dose than would normally be taken. High kV techniques and short exposure times offer a significant radiation dose reduction and an opportunity to reduce movement artefact.

Additional filtration is used to reduce the non-diagnostic soft radiation. An additional tube filter of the equivalent of 0.1 mm copper has been advised to add to equipment with 2.5 mm aluminium as standard (Cook et al. 1998).

Dose area product meters should be used routinely and the results recorded. This is an important audit tool to improve technique and radiation protection standards.

The immature gonads, the thyroid and the breast tissue are all more radiosensitive in children than adults. Haemopoietic bone marrow is also radiosensitive and is more widespread in the child than the adult. Lead rubber shielding must always be used to protect the areas near the primary beam, to reduce the dose from scattered radiation. The breast and the sternum should be protected for abdominal radiography. To reduce the skin entry dose to the developing breast the PA chest projection should be used rather than the AP projection, as soon as it becomes technically possible for the older child. Unless the shielding actually obscures the area of interest, gonad shielding should be used, obviously for new clinical presentation the area of concerns has yet to be determined and so gonadal shielding is not appropriate for a child's first pelvic radiograph.

1.8 Paediatric Service Provision

The nature of the institution to which the child has been admitted, either a dedicated paediatric hospital or an adult unit which also provides paediatric services, will affect the facilities that can be provided for the child. Most general radiographic equipment is designed for the adult patient, with the adult size, weight and body composition in mind. Children are generally smaller but also have a huge range of body size across the childhood years. Their body composition also varies with age. They are less likely than an adult to be able to cooperate in such simple matters as keeping still or holding a breath. A child who has suffered trauma may be in pain and may be frightened. They may have never been to a hospital before and feel intimidated by the crowds, the noise and the size of the equipment.

Adult patients can make decisions for themselves, and this should be respected. This is not the case for the young child, who may have strong personal reasons for not cooperating with something that the emergency staff and the parents wish to happen but will find those reasons overruled. The child may also be alone, with no parent or carer with them, or their parents may have died in the accident that they have survived. This is a particularly difficult time for everyone involved.

1.9 Issues for Paediatric Imaging

1.9.1 Pain Relief

In acute trauma one of the most important things that can be done to produce a successful radiograph is adequate pain relief for the patient. This is true in adults but particularly relevant in children. It is important that a child is not taken for their radiograph only minutes after being given their analgesia, when it has not had time to reach maximum effect. While time consuming it is important that a child does not suffer unnecessary pain while undergoing a radiological procedure.

1.9.2 Explanation

Children will be less fearful and more co-operative if they are informed according to their age and development. This does not mean that children should be told everything on every occasion since too many facts can create a greater fear. The parents are a good guide as to the appropriate level at which to pitch the information, and their cooperation is vital. The information should be given in a manner that the child can understand. Picture books are particularly useful. There are children's books that use characters familiar to children and have a hospital visit as a subject. If possible, a 'home-made' booklet illustrated with pictures of an individual department and its X-ray equipment can be very useful. Topical children's character may be incorporated into the story.

1.9.3 Play Specialist

Forming a relationship of trust with the child is important. It is seldom a good idea to lie to a child, particularly about whether something will be painful. The ideal person to form this bond of trust with the child is the play specialist, or their equivalent. They can greet the child and be with them and the parents through most of the initial trauma care. They can explain what is going on and spend the necessary time to do so, which is difficult for other staff to achieve.

1.9.4 Environment

General advice given about children in the X-ray room is to make the room "child friendly", but with little idea as to what this means in practice. What seems like a friendly room to an adult may not be through a child's perspective. It is important that care is taken to put decorations within view of the child. Bravery certificates are useful in some children, as are badges, but may be patronising to the older child and adolescent. Sweets and food need to be carefully considered, particularly as many children will be nil-by-mouth following acute trauma.

1.9.5 Supervision

It is almost always best to have the parents with the child in the X-ray room. As much time might be needed preparing them as the child, but if the end result is a good radiograph the effort is well spent. The parents or other adult carer, when properly instructed, make the best immobilisation device. Tapes, straps and blankets can be used, but in the trauma setting it may not be possible to put the limb into a position where the tape will do any immobilising, or there may not be skin to fix to. The child may be distressed by being wrapped in a blanket, though this can be useful for younger children. Good foam padding and support under and around the limb, with encouragement, are the best methods of immobilisation. The necessary projections must then be made by moving the equipment rather than the child. This requires skill and patience on the part of the radiographer or technician, who must be able to adapt to the requirements of each child. The noise of the machine can be countered by talking to the child and having them focus on a task, such as shouting when the exposure light has gone out. Distraction toys can be useful.

1.10 Radiography

There are basic principles of plain film radiography in trauma cases, whatever the age of the patient. Good quality radiography, with well centred, well collimated, well exposed images of the anatomy in question. It is no kindness to a child trauma victim to take a poor quality image of the wrong area just because it is technically easier to do so and less stressful for the child. Standard projections of each area under investigation, with views typically at 90 degrees to each other, should be used. Oblique and other projections can be used in children in the same way as with adults and these may be useful. However, if the basic AP and lateral films cannot be performed adequately due to poor technique or lack of time and care, specialised projections are likely to be no more than a radiation burden. It is much more important to do the basics well. The further projections can then be taken after review of the images.

There are excellent descriptions of the basic radiographic projections, familiar to every radiographer (Cook et al. 1998; Khon et al. 1996). These texts not only describe the projections but also discuss the radiation dose implications of them and the measures by which the quality of the image can be measured so that standards can be kept high by regular audit.

An experienced radiographer who has high standards and skills and is sensitive and adaptable to the needs of the child is a valuable resource. Such skill should be encouraged wherever possible.

1.11 Summary

Even in the emergency setting the use of ionising radiation should be justifiable.

It is an important factor in paediatric trauma radiography that good analgesia is provided for the child in pain. If possible, spend time with the child and the carer explaining what will happen in a way that the child can understand. Play specialists are extremely helpful in this. Do not lie about pain or discomfort. Gentle but firm restraint may be needed, but in trauma it may be difficult to use anything other than the hands of a volunteer. This will probably be the carer.

Good quality radiography, with well centred, well collimated, well exposed images of the anatomy in question are essential, though there might be room for some level of compromise if the clinical question permits.

An experienced clinician should examine the radiographs before repeats or comparison views are obtained.

References

Chacon D, Kissoon N, Brown T, Galpin R (1992) Use of comparison radiographs in the diagnosis of traumatic injuries of the elbow. Ann Emerg Med 21:895–899

Cook JV, Shah K, Pablot S, Kyriou J, Pettett A, Fitzgerald M (1998) X-ray imaging of children. A manual for all X-ray departments. Ian Allan, Hersham, p 5

Eiff MP, Hatch RL (2003) Boning up on common pediatric fractures. Contemporary Pediatrics 20:30 (cover article)

Kissoon N, Galpin R, Gayle M, Chacon D, Brown T (1995) Evaluation of the role of comparison radiographs in the diagnosis of traumatic elbow injuries. J Pediatr Orthop 15:449–453

Kohn MM. Moores BM, Schibilla H, Schneider K, Stender HS, Stieve FE, Teunen D, Wall B (eds) (1996) European guidelines on quality criteria for diagnostic radiographic images in paediatrics. EU 16261EN

Lally KP, Senae M, Hardin WD Jr, Haftel A, Mahour GH (1989) Utility of the cervical spine radiograph in pediatric trauma. Am J Surg 158:540–41

McCauley RG, Schwartz AM, Leonidas JC, Darling DB, Bankoff MS, Swan CS 2nd (1979) Comparison views in extremity injury in children: an efficacy study. Radiology 131:95–97

Neofotistou V, Tsapaki V, Kottou S, Schreiner-Karoussou A, Vano E (2005) Does digital imaging decrease patient dose? A pilot study and review of the literature. Radiat Prot Dosimetry 117:204–210

NICE (National Institute for Health and Clinical Excellence) (2003) Clinical guideline 4. Head injury: triage, assessment, investigation and early management of head injury in infants, children and adults. NICE, London June 2003

N Nguyen TD, Raju R, Lee S (2003) Considerations in pediatric trauma. Emedicine.com/med/topic3223.htm

Ozonoff MB (1992) Skeletal trauma. In: Ozonoff MB (ed) Pediatric orthopedic radiology, 2nd edn. WB Saunders, Philadelphia, pp 604–605

Plumert JM, Kearney JK, Cremer JF (2004) Children's perception of gap affordances: bicycling across traffic-filled intersections in an immersive virtual environment. Child Dev 75:1243–1253

RoSPA (Royal Society for the Prevention of Accidents) (2005) HASS and LASS Database. June 9 2005 www.hassandlass.org.uk/query/MainSelector.aspx

SIGN (Scottish Intercollegiate Guidelines Network) (2000) Section 5: Imaging. In: SIGN Publication No. 46, Early management of patients with a head injury. SIGN, Edinburgh, pp 8–15 (www.sign.ac.uk/guidelines/fulltext/46/section5.html)

Slovis TL, Berdon WE, Hall EJ (2002) Effects of radiation on children. Harcourt International, Florida (E Book www.harcourt-international.com/e-books/pdf/820.pdf)

Stiell IG, Clement CM, McKnight RD et al (2003) The Canadian C-spine rule versus the NEXUS low-risk criteria in patients with trauma. N Engl J Med 349:2510–2518

Swischuk LE (1994) The extremities. In: Swischuk LE (ed) Emergency imaging of the acutely ill or injured child, 3rd edn. Williams and Wilkins, Baltimore, pp 361–362

Willis CE, Slovis TL (2005) The ALARA concept in pediatric CR and DR: dose reduction in pediatric radiographic exams – a white paper conference executive summary. Radiology 34:S162–S164

Radiographic Positioning

2

Kate Parkes

CONTENTS

2.1 Preparation

Good radiographic technique depends heavily on patient preparation and the relationship formed between the radiographer, the child and their carers.

The room should be prepared in advance with lead protection, ideally with a range of sandbags and foam pads easily available. Distraction toys or projection lamps, when available, occupy the child and carers and help to provide a more relaxed environment. A few minutes spent reassuring the child and allowing them to become accustomed to the light beam diaphragm through play often results in a much smoother examination.

K. Parkes, MD
Superintendent Radiographer, Radiology Department, Birmingham Children's Hospital, Steelhouse Lane, Birmingham, B4 5NH, UK

All items of clothing should be removed from the appendicular skeleton prior to imaging to prevent artefacts due to decoration on clothing. When the trunk is imaged patient privacy must be respected, particularly in adolescent patients, and care must be taken to ensure the minimum amount of clothing covers the area under examination and that these items are also free from artefacts. Adolescent girls undergoing pelvic imaging should be sympathetically questioned as to the date of their last menstrual period and the risk of pregnancy in accordance with Departmental Protocols. To reduce the child's radiation dose grids/buckys are not routinely required for pre-school children. Lead protection should routinely be applied unless the area under examination will be obscured. A film focus distance of 100 cm is used.

The explanation of the examination to the child must be given at the appropriate level of understanding. The carers also should consent to and receive a careful explanation of any form of immobilisation that may be required to allow the examination to be completed successfully. Lead protection is always worn by the carer when supporting a child for imaging.

2.2 Pelvic Radiographs

2.2.1 Antero-posterior (AP) Pelvis/Hip

The child is encouraged to lie on the table in a supine position. The older child's mid-sagittal plane should run parallel with the long axis of the examination table if the 'bucky' is to be used. The legs should be straightened and internally rotated from the hips until both knees are supported in the AP position with the patella lying in a central position over the femoral condyles; this often results in the big toes touching. The anterior superior iliac spines should be equidistant from the film to prevent rotation of the pelvis (Fig. 2.1).

2.2.2 'Frog Lateral' Position of the Hips

From the above position the knees are flexed to form an angle of 90°, externally rotated to 45° and supported on pads (Fig. 2.2).

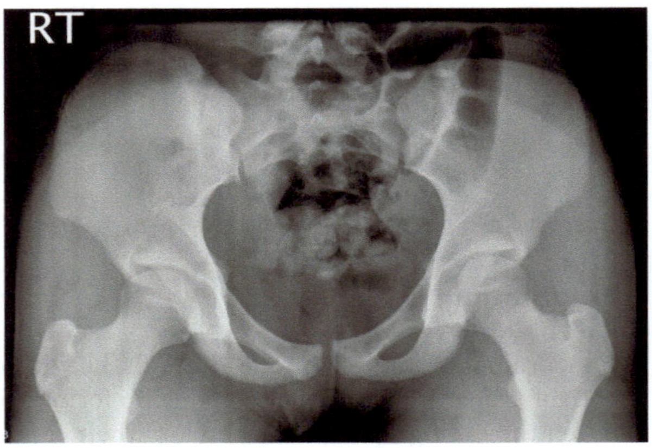

Fig. 2.1. AP pelvis and hip. *Centre.* Pelvis: Two child's fingers' width above the symphysis pubis along the mid-sagittal line. Hips: at the level of the femoral pulse along the mid-sagittal line. Hip joint: directly over the femoral pulse. *Area imaged.* Pelvis: To include the iliac crests superiorly, the full width of the pelvis and the femoral greater trochanter inferiorly. Hips: To include the anterior superior iliac spine superiorly, the full width of the pelvis and the femoral greater trochanter inferiorly. Hip: To include the anterior superior iliac spine superiorly, the symphysis pubis to the lateral wall of the pelvis and the femoral greater trochanter inferiorly

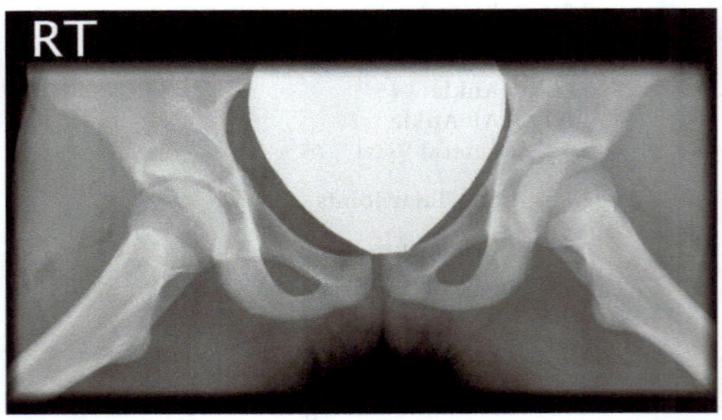

Fig. 2.2. Frog Lateral Hips. *Centre.* Pelvis: Two child's fingers' width above the symphysis pubis along the mid-sagittal line. Hips: At the level of the femoral pulse along the mid-sagittal line. Hip joint. Directly over the femoral pulse. *Area Imaged.* Bilateral hips: To include the anterior superior iliac spine superiorly, the full width of the pelvis and the femoral greater trochanter inferiorly. Hip: To include the anterior superior iliac spine superiorly, the symphysis pubis to the lateral wall of the pelvis and the femoral greater trochanter inferiorly

2.2.3 Horizontal Beam Lateral Projection

From the AP position the affected side may need to be slightly raised using a foam pad to allow the joint to be demonstrated. The unaffected leg is removed from the field of view by either; bending the unaffected leg to 90° at the hip and knee and encouraging the child to move their unaffected knee towards their head as much as possible. The leg would need supporting in this position by a carer. Alternatively the unaffected leg is abducted as much as possible and is allowed to the rest over the side of the table. The film is positioned vertically, with its long axis 45° to the mid-sagittal line with the upper border at the top of the crest. The centre of the film should be in line with the groin crease. The beam is rotated into the horizontal position and is angled so that it is perpendicular to the centre of the cassette.

2.3 Femoral Radiographs

2.3.1 AP Femora

The legs should be straightened and internally rotated from the hips until both knees are supported in the AP position with the patella lying in a central position over the femoral condyles; this often results in the big toes touching. The anterior superior iliac spines should be equidistant from the film to prevent rotation of the pelvis (Fig. 2.3).

2.3.2 'Turned Lateral' Projection

From the AP position the knees are flexed to form an angle of 90°, the leg under examination is then externally rotated until the whole of the lateral aspect of the femora is in direct contact with the film/table surface. The pelvis will often lift on the unaffected side to allow this position to be obtained. Foam pads applied under the lifted portion of the pelvis will assist in maintaining the position, as will asking the patient to keep the unaffected foot flat on the table surface. It is important to abduct the unaffected leg sufficiently to prevent the side under examination to be obscured (Fig. 2.4).

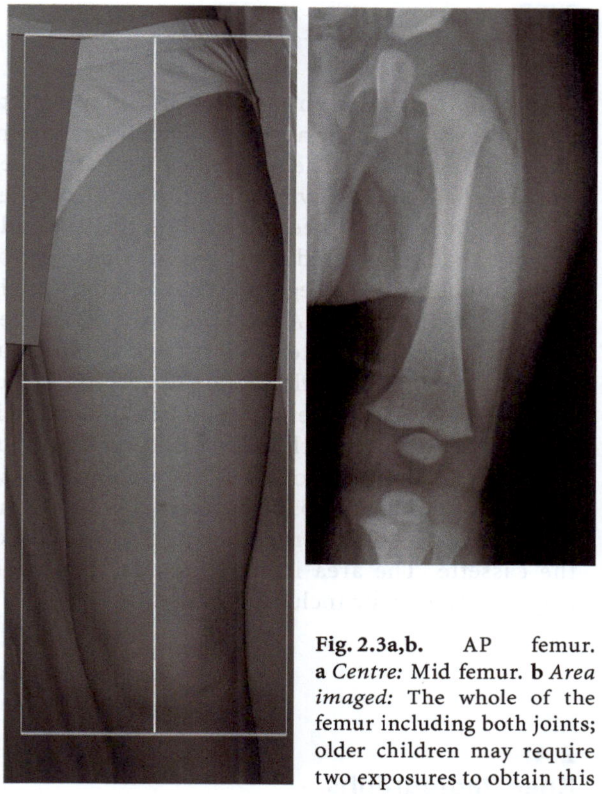

a b

Fig. 2.3a,b. AP femur. **a** *Centre:* Mid femur. **b** *Area imaged:* The whole of the femur including both joints; older children may require two exposures to obtain this

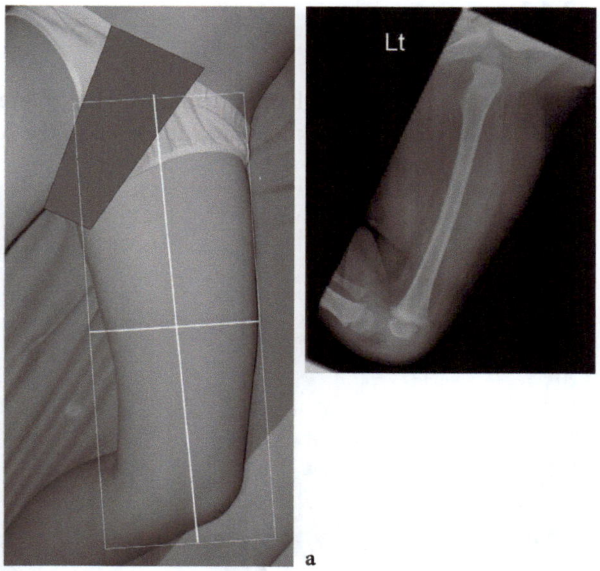

a b

Fig. 2.4a,b. Lateral femur. *Centre:* (femur): In the centre of the femur. *Centre* (hip): Directly over the femoral pulse of the side under investigation. *Area imaged* (femur): Area imaged to include the whole of the femur including both joints. *Area of coverage* (hip): To include the anterior superior iliac spine superiorly, the symphysis pubis to the lateral wall of the pelvis and the femoral greater trochanter inferiorly

2.3.3 Horizontal Beam Lateral Projection

From the AP position the affected side may need to be slightly raised using a foam pad to allow the joint to be demonstrated. The unaffected leg is removed from the field of view by bending the unaffected leg to 90° at the hip and knee and encouraging the child to move their unaffected knee towards their head as much as possible. The leg would need supporting in this position by a carer. Alternatively the unaffected leg is abducted and externally rotated as much as possible and the leg is allowed to fall over the side of the table. The beam is centred mid femur, the film is positioned vertically with its long axis parallel to the femur with the upper border at the top of the crest. The beam is rotated into the horizontal position and is angled so that it is perpendicular to the centre of the cassette. The area imaged includes the whole length of the femur including both joints.

2.4 Knee Radiographs

2.4.1 AP Knee

The legs should be straightened and internally rotated from the hips until both knees are supported in the AP position with the patella lying in a central position over the femoral condyles; this often results in the big toes touching. The anterior superior iliac spines should be equidistant from the film to prevent rotation (Fig. 2.5).

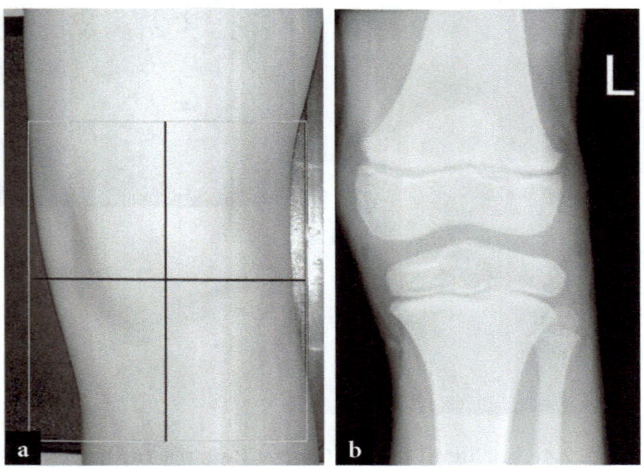

Fig. 2.5a,b. AP knee. *Centre:* Midway between the femoral condyles; the child's finger's width below the inferior aspect of the patella. *Area imaged:* The full width of the joint, including the whole of the patella and the proximal portion of the tibial tuberosity

2.4.2 'Turned Lateral' Projection

From the AP position the affected knee is flexed to form an angle of 120° and externally rotated until the whole of the lateral aspect of the femora/tibia is in direct contact with the film/table surface. The unaffected leg should be bent, raised and positioned over the side under imaging and allowed to rest on the table. Foam pads applied under the lifted portion of the pelvis will assist in maintaining the position, as will asking the patient to keep the unaffected foot flat on the table surface. It is important to rotate the child sufficiently to allow the patella to be positioned perpendicular to the table (Fig. 2.6).

2.4.3 Horizontal Beam Lateral Projection

Positioned as in the horizontal beam femur projection described in Section 2.3.3. The leg under examination should be externally rotated until the condyles are superimposed.

With the centre over either the medial or lateral condyle, the film is positioned vertically parallel to

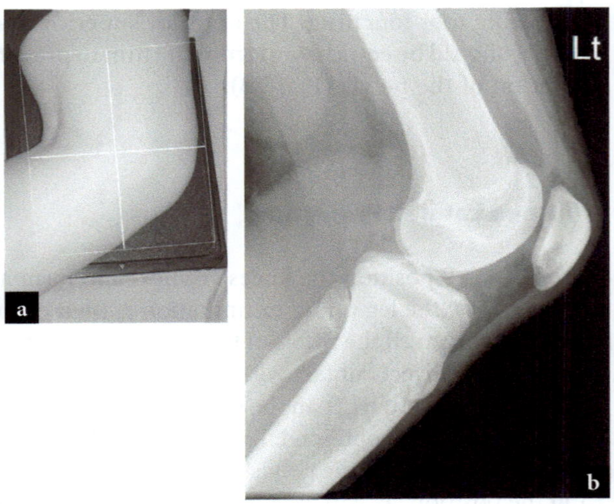

Fig. 2.6a,b. Lateral knee. *Centre:* On the medial condyle of the knee with a 3–5° cranial angulation along the femur. *Area imaged:* To include the whole of the patella and the proximal portion of the tibial tuberosity

the knee. The beam is rotated into the horizontal position and is angled so that the central ray is perpendicular to the centre of the cassette.

The area imaged should include the whole of the patella and the proximal portion of the tibial tuberosity.

2.5 Tibia and Fibula

The legs should be straightened and internally rotated from the hips until the knee is supported in the AP position with the patella lying in a central position over the femoral condyles; this often results in the leg being internally rotated from the hip. The malleoli at the ankle should be equidistant from the film to prevent rotation (Fig. 2.7). The foot should be flexed to open up the ankle joint. This position can be maintained by placing a 45° pad against the foot secured with sandbags.

2.5.1 Lateral

The child is turned onto their side until the knee lies in contact with the film and both malleoli are superimposed. The child should be encouraged to pull their toes up towards their nose and the foot may be supported in this position using foam pads and sandbags against the child's sole (Fig. 2.8).

2.5.2 Horizontal Beam Lateral

Positioned as in the horizontal beam femur projection described in Section 2.3.3, the film is positioned perpendicular to the table along either the lateral or medial surface of the lower leg. The central ray is rotated until it is perpendicular to the cassette. The centre is midway between the ankle and the knee. Both joints should be demonstrated, as well as the full width of the tibia/fibula.

2.6 Ankle

The leg is extended and all clothing is removed from the joint.

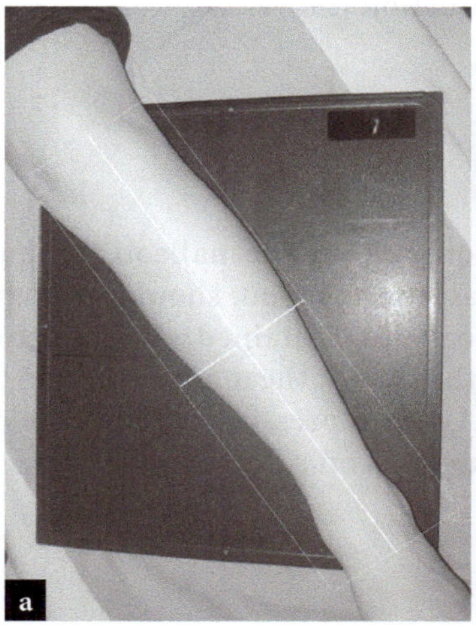

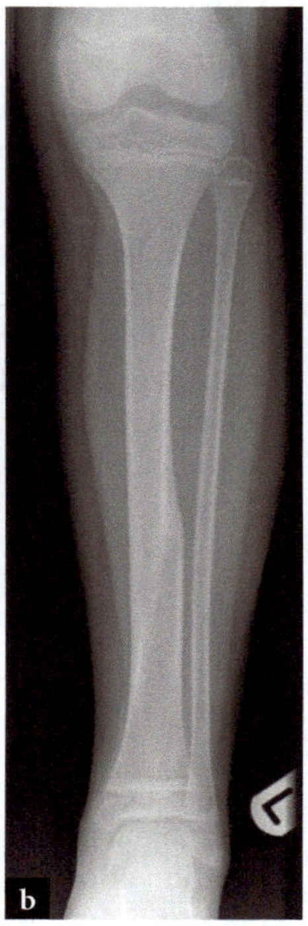

Fig. 2.7a,b. AP tibia/fibula. *Centre:* Midway between the ankle and the knee. *Area imaged* Both joints should be demonstrated, as well as the full width of the tibia/fibula

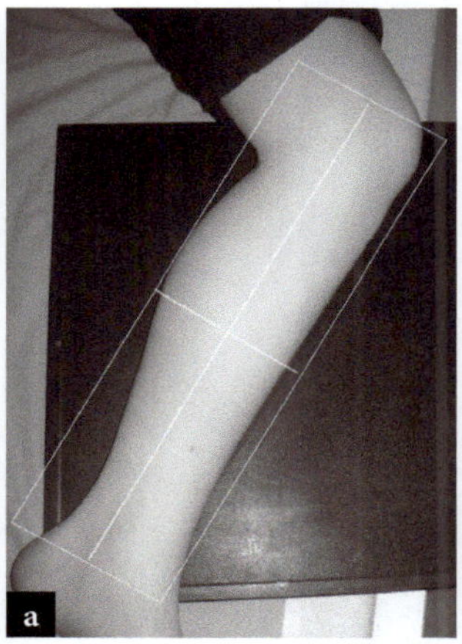

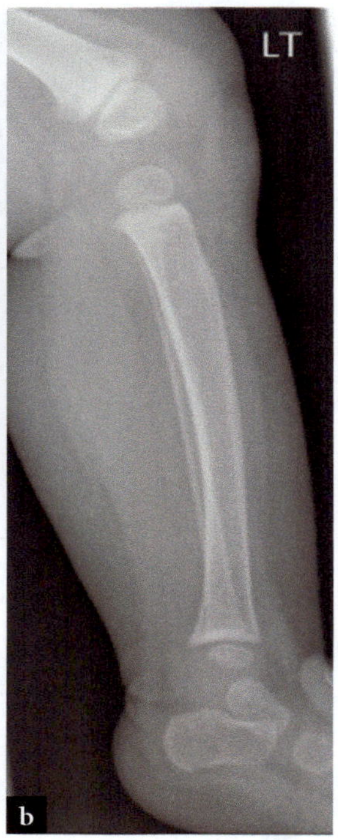

Fig. 2.8a,b. Lateral tibia/fibula. *Centre:* Midway between the ankle and the knee. *Area imaged* Both joints should be demonstrated, as well as the full width of the tibia/fibula

2.6.1 AP Ankle

The ankle joint is rotated until the malleoli are equidistant from the cassette, this often results in the leg being internally rotated from the hip. The foot should be flexed to open up the ankle joint (Fig. 2.9). This position can be maintained by placing a 45° pad against the foot secured with sandbags.

2.6.2 Lateral View

The ankle is rotated until the malleoli are superimposed. Care needs to be taken to prevent over-rotation and the use of a small pad under the 5th toe can help correct this situation (Fig. 2.10).

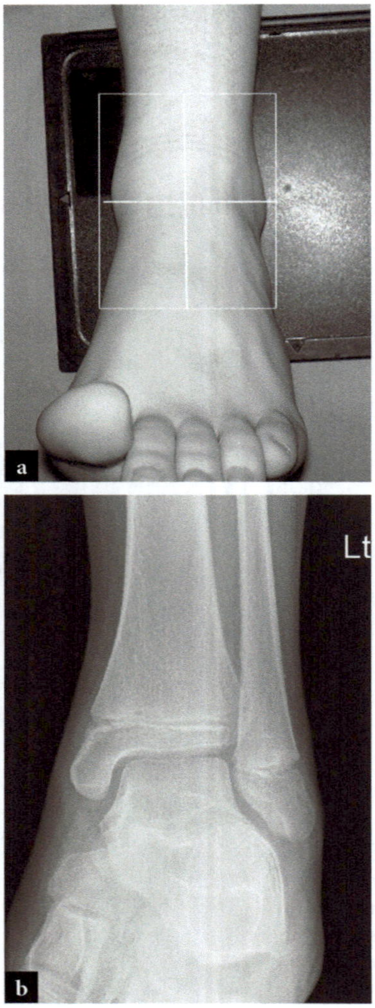

Fig. 2.9a,b. AP ankle. *Centre:* Midway between the malleoli. *Area imaged* The talus, distal tibia and fibula and soft tissue structures should be demonstrated

2.7 Sub Talar Joints

The positioning for these projections is similar to the oblique lateral malleolus projection. The foot is rotated internally 45° and the central ray angled 20°, 30° and 40° cranially and centered midway between the malleoli. The foot is then externally rotated 45° and the central ray angled 12°, 15° and 18° cranially. This examination has been replaced by CT scanning.

2.8 Calcaneum

This projection again requires the co-operation of the child to dorsi-flex the foot to allow the full length of the calcaneum to be demonstrated.

2.8.1 Lateral Projection

The ankle is rotated until the malleoli are superimposed. Care needs to be taken to prevent over-rotation and the use of a small pad under the 5th toe can help correct this situation (Fig. 2.11).

2.8.2 Axial

The ankle joint is rotated until the malleoli are equidistant from the cassette. The foot should be dorsiflexed. The flexion can be maintained with the use of a bandage around the base of the toes that is held by the child or carer. Upward pressure is then applied to the bandage 'like reins on a horse' (Fig. 2.12).

2.9 Feet

The child is seated on a pillow or small seat on the table with their socks and shoes removed. This position allows the foot to naturally fall into a dorsiplantar (DP) position.

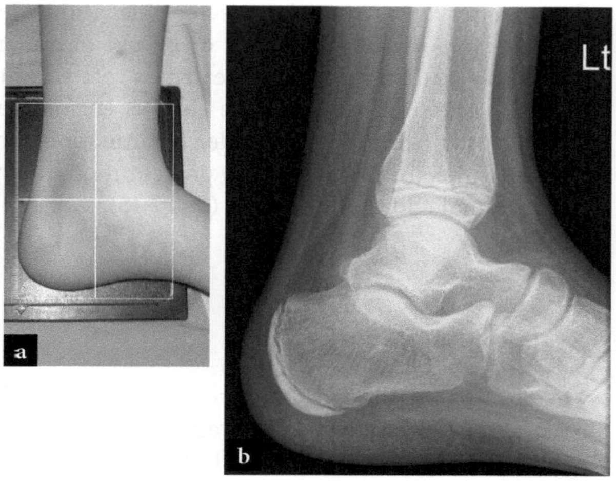

Fig. 2.10a,b. Lateral ankle. *Centre:* Directly over the medial malleoli. *Area imaged:* The calcaneum, talus, distal tibia and fibula and soft tissue structures should be demonstrated

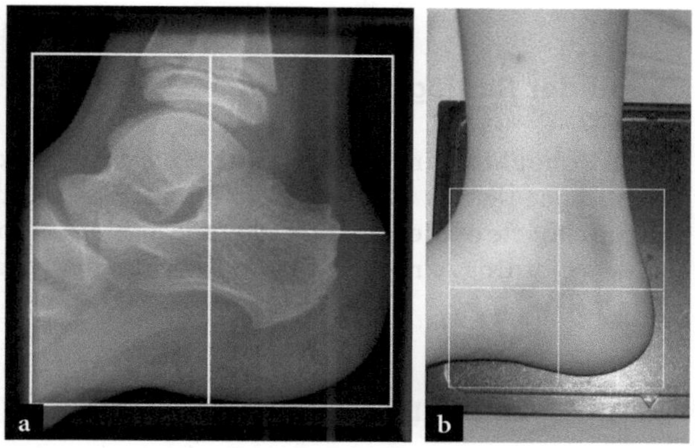

Fig. 2.11a,b. Lateral calcaneum. *Centre:* Midway between the lateral malleolus and the sole of the foot. *Area imaged:* The whole of the calcaneum and the distal tibia/fibula and talus

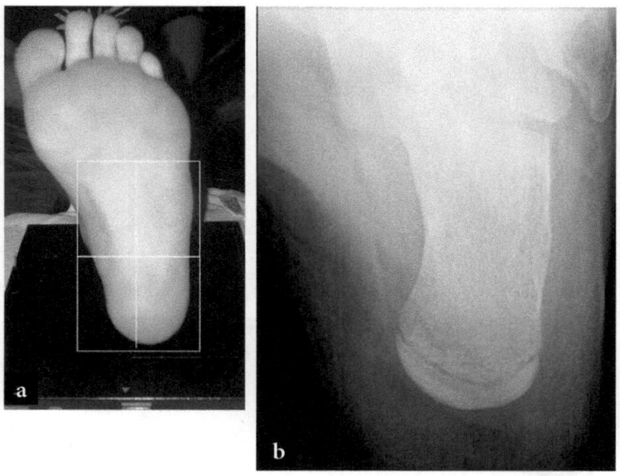

Fig. 2.12a,b. Axial calcaneum. *Centre:* In the centre of the calcaneum with a central ray angled 40° cranially. *Area imaged:* The whole of the calcaneum

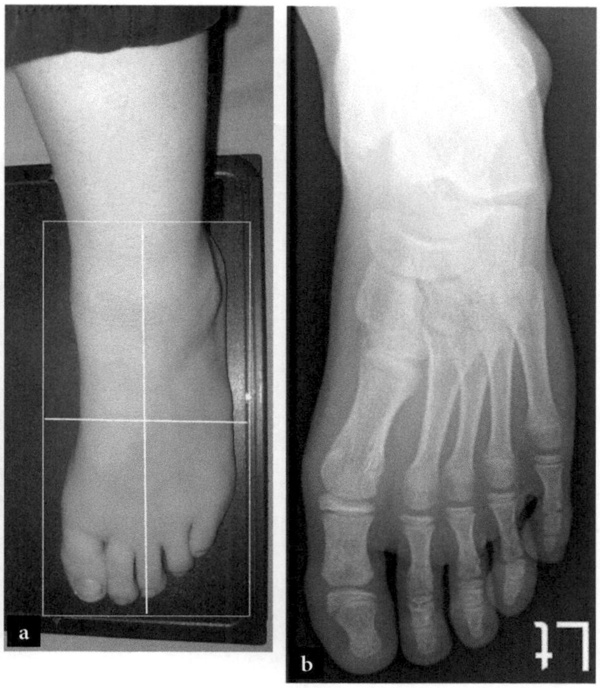

Fig. 2.13a,b. DP foot. *Centre:* In the middle of the 3rd metatarsal. *Area imaged:* The whole of the foot from the distal phalanx back to the ankle joint

With the DP projection the foot is placed directly on the cassette. The lower limb may be rotated and supported in position to maintain the DP position. The beam is centred in the middle of the 3rd metatarsal and the whole of the foot from the distal phalanx back to the ankle joint should be on the image. With the oblique projection the foot is internally rotated 30° and supported by foam pads or by the carer. With the lateral projection the foot is externally rotated until the lateral aspect rests directly on the cassette and is supported by foam pads or by the carer in this position (Figs. 2.13, 2.14).

2.10 Shoulder Radiographs

An AP shoulder girdle is often the preferred projection in paediatrics as trauma often results in injury to the clavicle of the upper third of the humerus. The child's clothing is removed from the shoulder area.

2.10.1 AP Shoulder Girdle

The child is encouraged to either stand (which is less painful for the child) or lie (the recommended method in the case of younger children) with their back against the cassette. The arm on the affected side is adducted 45° and supported by the carer or by use of a foam pad in the axilla if required. The arm is rotated until the palm faces forward and the child is encouraged to look away from the side under examination. The chin often needs to be raised to prevent it obscuring the proximal end of the clavicle (Fig. 2.15).

2.10.2 AP Shoulder Joint

The child is positioned as above but is additionally rotated approximately 45° towards the side under examination until the affected shoulder joint lies perpendicular to the cassette.

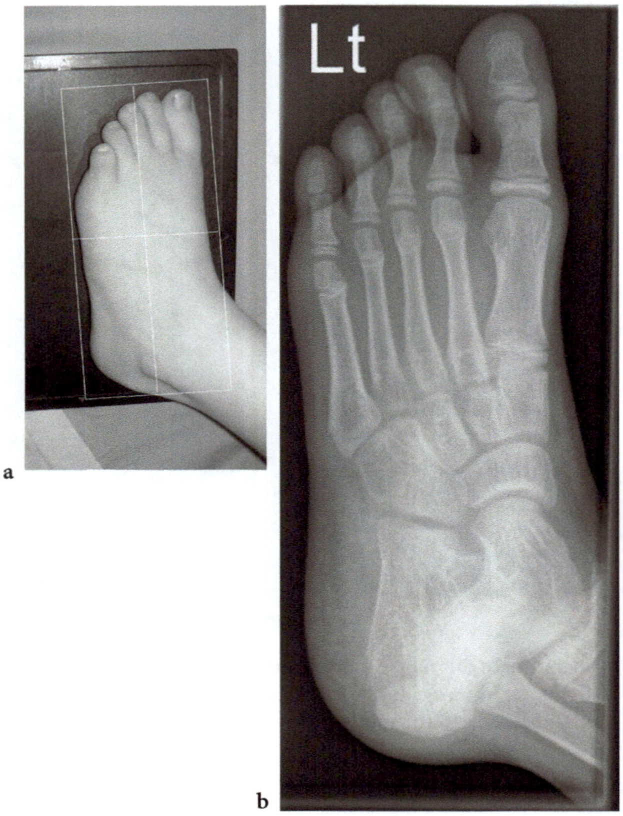

Fig. 2.14a,b. Oblique foot. *Centre:* Over the middle of the 3rd metatarsal, divergent beam may be used by centring over the head of the 5th metatarsal but in paediatrics this method is not used as it is good practice to limit the radiation field. *Area imaged:* The whole of the foot from the distal phalynx back to the ankle joint

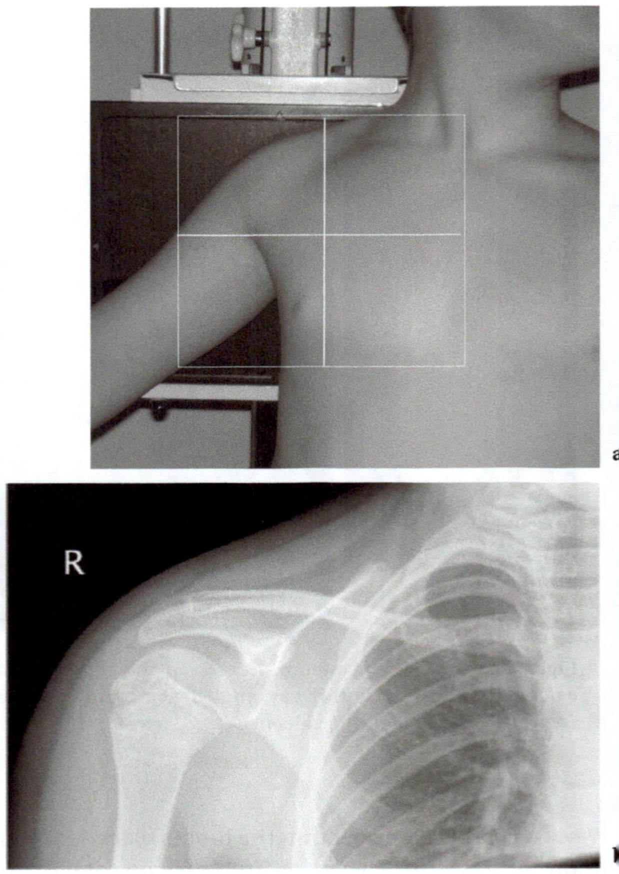

Fig. 2.15a,b. AP shoulder girdle. *Centre:* Medial to the shoulder joint making sure the full length of the clavicle and scapula is demonstrated. *Area imaged:* Full length of the clavicle, scapula, upper 1/3 of the humerus and the shoulder joint

2.10.3
Axial Shoulder
(Supero-inferior/Infero-superior Projection)

The child is seated with the affected side against a table (younger children can sit on the carers knee). The height of the table is altered until the child is comfortably able to lean across the table. The arm on the side under examination is raised over a 45° angle pad and the child is encouraged to lean across the table to allow the shoulder joint to project clear of the rib cage over a cassette. The child is then encouraged to look away from the shoulder or tilt the head forward out of the radiation beam (Fig. 2.16)

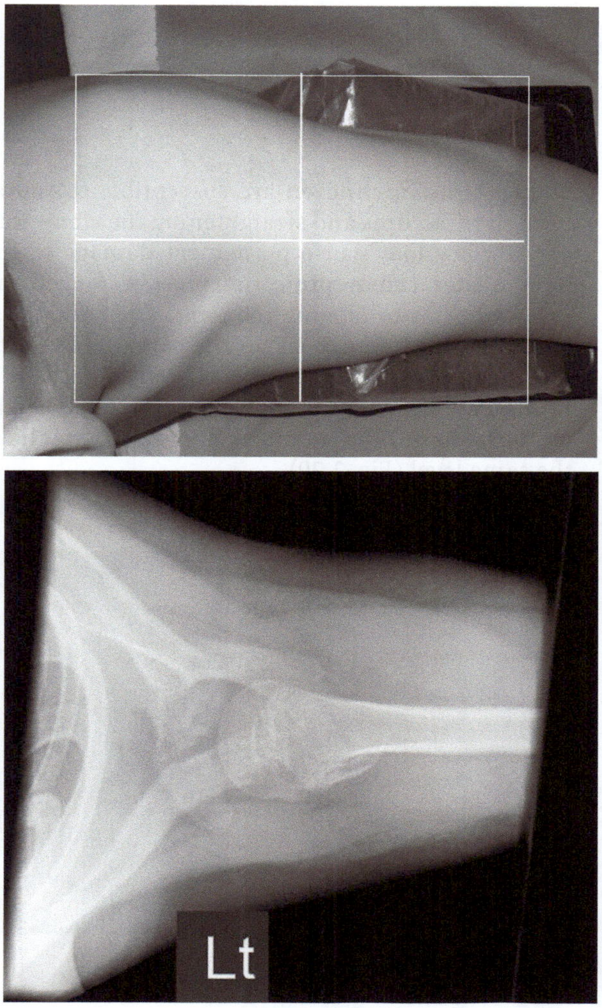

a

b

Fig. 2.16a,b. Axial shoulder. *Centre:* Directly through the shoulder joint, a 5° angle along the lateral aspect of the humeral shaft towards the hand may be used. *Area imaged:* The glenoid and proximal portion of the humerus

Alternatively a small child may be placed supine on a table with the affected arm abducted. The cassette is placed either in the axilla or resting on the superior border of the shoulder depending on the size of the child. The X-ray tube is rotated into a horizontal position and is directed through the shoulder joint in either an infero-superior or supero-inferior direction. The child will often need to be raised on a pad to allow the X-ray tube to achieve this position.

2.10.4
Lateral Scapula (Y-View)

The easiest way to achieve this position is to have the child standing facing a cassette with the affected arm held across the body holding the unaffected shoulder. The child is then rotated until the scapula lies perpendicular to the cassette.

Alternatively the child rests against the cassette in either the supine or erect position and again holds the unaffected arm across their body. Their torso is then turned until the scapula lies perpendicular to the cassette and the child needs to be supported in this position either by the carer or a 45° foam pad (Fig. 2.17).

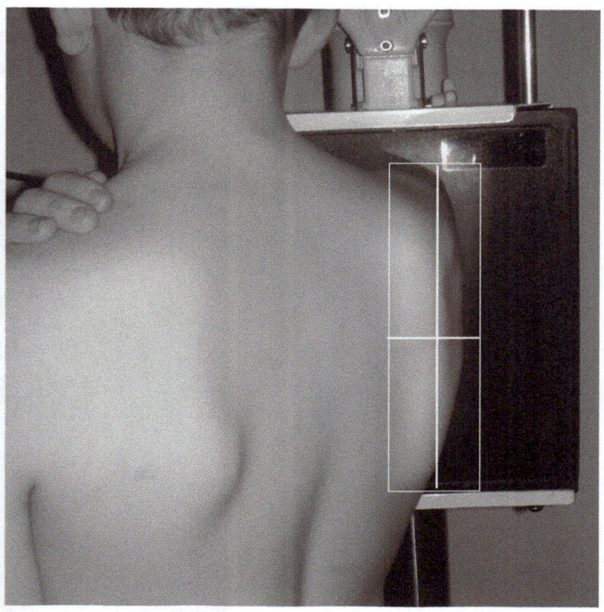

Fig. 2.17. Lateral scapula (Y-view). *Centre* (AP view): directly on the middle point of the medial surface of the scapula. *(PA view)*: midway between the inferior and superior surface of the posterior border of the scapula. The scapula, glenoid and proximal portion of the humerus

2.11 Clavicle

The child is encouraged to stand or lie directly in front of the cassette with the arm resting at the side of the body. Distraction techniques may be used to encourage the child to look away from the side imaged. Initially one AP projection is imaged and if no fracture is seen the film is repeated using a 10° cranial angle.

2.12 Humerus

The child is encouraged to either stand (or lie in the case of younger children) with their back against the cassette. The arm on the affected side is adducted 45° and supported by the carer or the use of a foam pad in the axilla if required.

2.12.1 AP Humerus

The arm is rotated until the palm faces forwards and the child is encouraged to look away from the side under examination (Fig. 2.18).

2.12.2 Lateral Humerus

From the above position the child is turned to face the cassette, the affected arm is abducted, bent at the elbow and held across the front of the body with the palm facing upward. A 45° foam pad placed between the arm and the body as illustrated in Figure 2.19 helps maintain the correct position.

Alternatively if the child remains with their back against the cassette the affected arm is abducted, bent at the elbow and held by a carer with the palm facing cranially. Foam pads are used to support the humerus parallel to the cassette.

2.13 Elbow

Elbow joints in children are susceptible to supracondylar fractures and straightening the elbow into an AP view may cause permanent damage to the joint. A lateral elbow projection *must* be imaged and assessed prior to moving the joint. The child is sat (younger children can sit on the carers knee) with the affected side against a table. The arm is carefully raised and placed on the table and the table height is adjusted until the shoulder, elbow and wrist lie at the same level (Fig. 2.20).

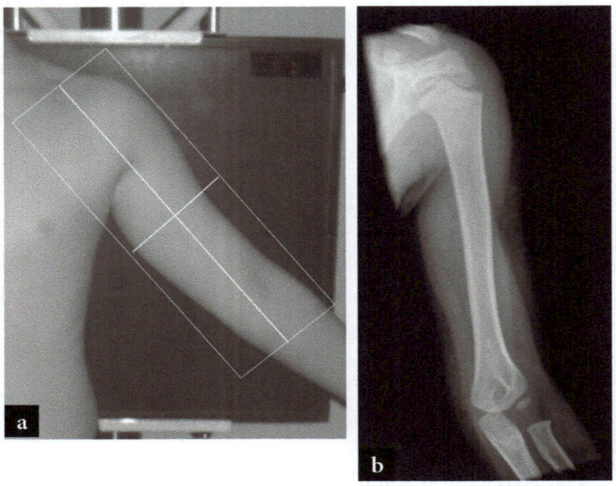

Fig. 2.18a,b. AP humerus. *Centre:* Midpoint of the humerus. *Area imaged:* Full length of the humerus including the shoulder and elbow joint

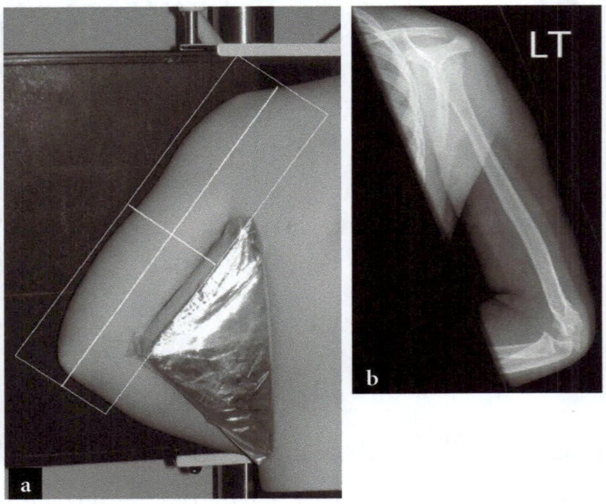

Fig. 2.19a,b. Lateral humerus. *Centre:* Midpoint of the humerus. *Area imaged:* Full length of the humerus including the shoulder and elbow joint

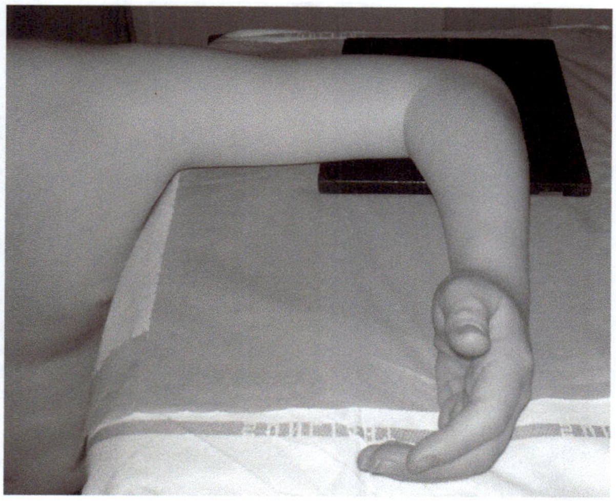

Fig. 2.20. Positioning of upper limb for imaging

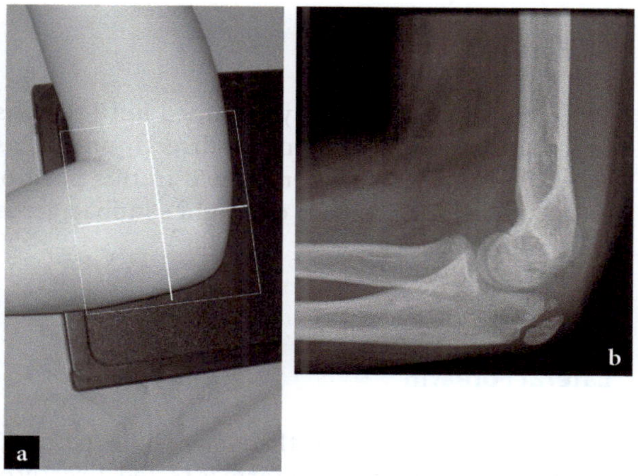

Fig. 2.21a,b. Lateral elbow. *Centre:* Directly over the lateral condyle. *Area imaged:* The distal humerus, proximal radius and ulna and surrounding soft tissue

2.13.1 Lateral Elbow

The child is positioned as stated above. The cassette is placed on the table directly beneath the elbow joint. The elbow is flexed to 90° and the wrist/hand is rotated until the styloid processes of the radius and ulna are superimposed. The position of the hand may be maintained by the use of carers/sandbags or foam pads. In the younger child the carer may also provide support by holding the middle section of the humerus (Fig. 2.21).

In cases of suspected supracondylar fracture careful handling of the joint is required. An older child may be less distressed if the lateral elbow is imaged in the same position as shown above for an erect lateral projection of the humerus.

2.13.2 AP Elbow

From the above position the arm is gently rotated externally and then carefully extended as far as the child can tolerate. The arm is then supported with foam pads and/or the carer in this position. The humerus and the forearm should be equi-angled from the cassette (Fig. 2.22).

A horizontal beam technique may also be used with the joint either held at the child's side away from the body or raised and supported on foam pads with the child in a seated position.

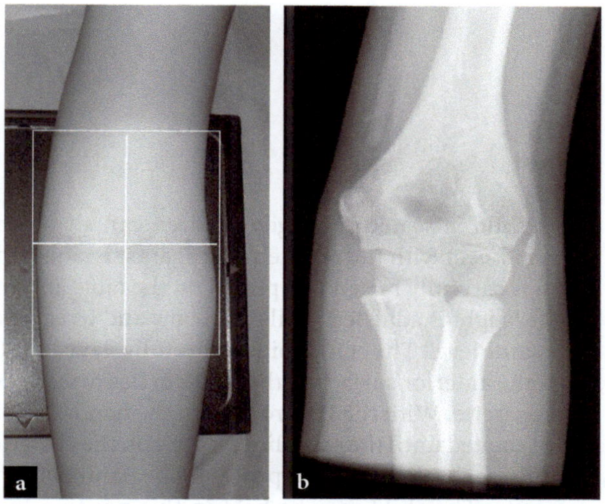

Fig. 2.22a,b. AP elbow. *Centre:* Midway between the condyles. *Area imaged:* Distal humerus, proximal radius and ulna and surrounding soft tissue

2.14 Forearm (Radius and Ulna)

The child is sat (younger children can sit on the carers knee) with the affected side against a table. The arm is carefully raised and placed on the table and the table height is adjusted until the shoulder, elbow and wrist lie at the same level.

2.14.1 AP Forearm

The elbow joint is carefully extended until the posterior surface of the forearm lies directly on the cassette. The hand may either be held in this position by a carer or with the use of a light sandbag across the palm (Fig. 2.23).

2.14.2 Lateral Forearm

From the above position the elbow is flexed to 90° and the medial aspect of the arm is rested directly on the cassette. The hand and wrist are externally rotated until both styloid processes are superimposed. Again this position may be maintained by the use of a sandbag resting against the palm or the hand held by the carer (Fig. 2.24).

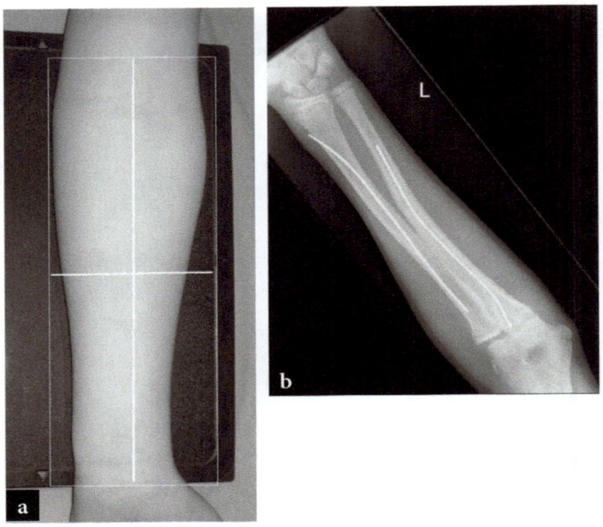

Fig. 2.23a,b. AP forearm. *Centre:* Mid forearm. *Area imaged:* Full length of the radius and ulna, including both elbow and wrist joints and the surrounding soft tissue

2.15 Wrist

The child is seated (younger children can sit on the carers knee) with the affected side against a table. The arm is carefully raised and placed on the table and the table height is adjusted until the, elbow and wrist lie at the same level. The elbow joint is carefully flexed to 90° and the anterior surface of the forearm lies directly on the cassette. With the PA projection, the hand/wrist is then rotated until the palm lies directly on the cassette. In this position the styloid processes lie parallel to the cassette. The child may be held in this position by a carer or with the use of a light sandbag across the palm. With the lateral projection the hand is rotated until the styloid processes are superimposed and lie perpendicular to the cassette. Again this position may be maintained by the use of a sandbag resting against the palm or the hand held by the carer (Figs. 2.25, 2.26).

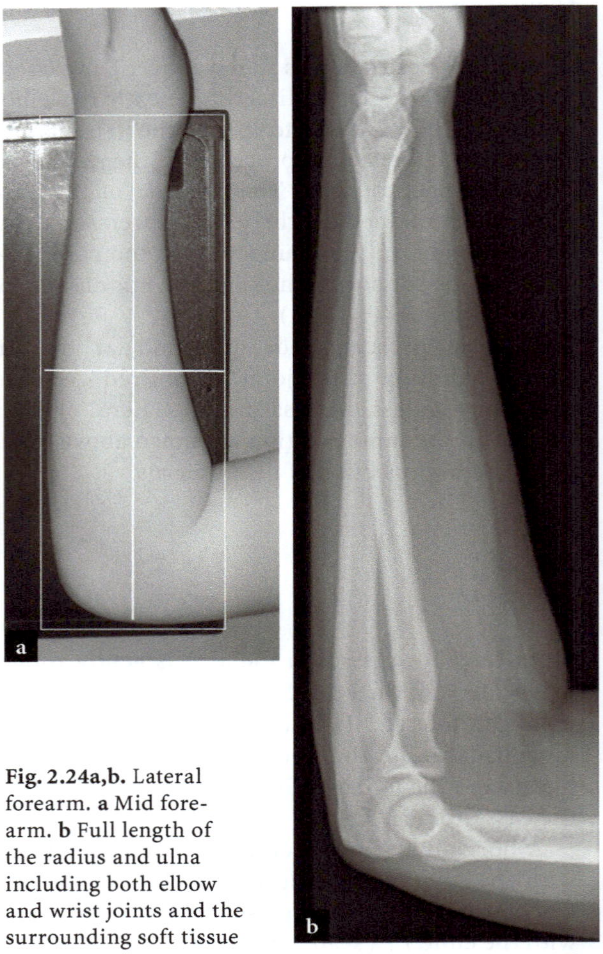

Fig. 2.24a,b. Lateral forearm. **a** Mid forearm. **b** Full length of the radius and ulna including both elbow and wrist joints and the surrounding soft tissue

2.16 Scaphoid Views

These are specialised views to demonstrate the scaphoid bone. The scaphoid bone is not ossified in

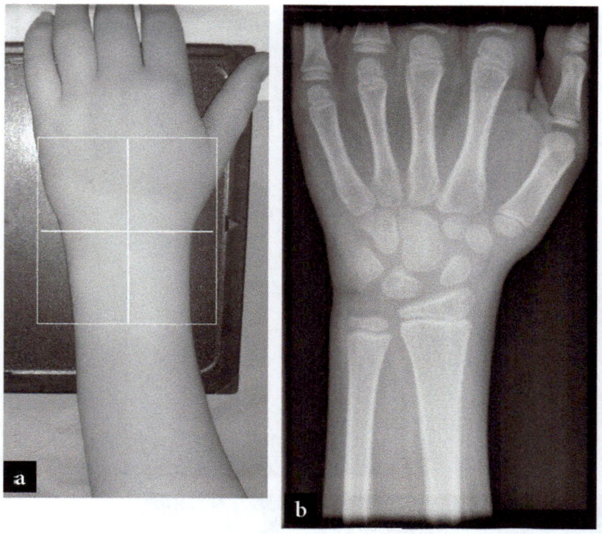

Fig. 2.25a,b. DP wrist. *Centre:* Midway between the styloid processes. *Area imaged:* Distal radius and ulna, carpel bones and proximal ends of the metacarpal bones

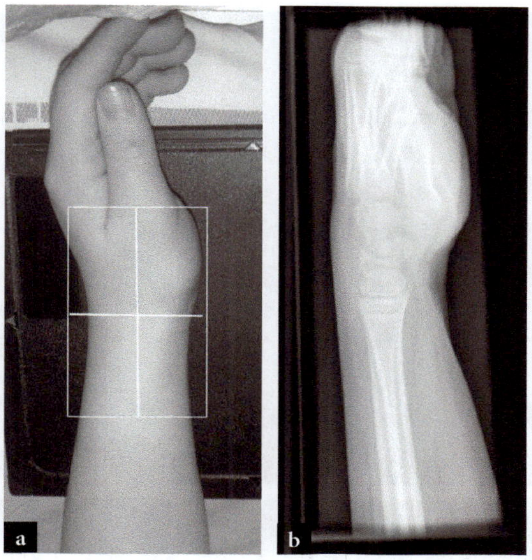

Fig. 2.26a,b. Lateral wrist. *Centre:* Directly over the medial styloid process. *Area imaged:* Distal radius and ulna, carpal bones and proximal ends of the metacarpal bones

pre-school age children and hence should not be imaged. MR imaging has replaced the delayed 10-day film often imaged if a definite fracture is not seen on the initial examination. Any casts/splints need to be removed prior to imaging. Initially the whole of the wrist is imaged on the PA and lateral projection and the oblique, 35°angled view and follow-up images are collimated to the scaphoid bone.

The child is sat (younger children can sit on the carers knee) with the affected side against a table. The arm is carefully raised and placed on the table and the table height is adjusted until the elbow and wrist lie at the same level. The elbow joint is carefully flexed to 90° and the anterior surface of the forearm lies directly on the cassette.

The examination consist of:

- PA wrist with ulna deviation.
- Lateral wrist.
- 45° Oblique view of the scaphoid bone with ulna deviation (the hand and wrist is rotated 45° from the PA position by raising its lateral aspect).
- PA wrist with ulna deviation and with 35° tube angulation along the radius towards the elbow.

Ulna deviation is achieved by moving the fingers as far as possible towards the ulna and stretching the thumb towards the radius. The 'anatomical snuff box' formed at the base of the thumb in this position indicates the position of the scaphoid bone (Fig. 2.27).

2.17 Hand

The child is seated (younger children can sit on the carers knee) with the affected side against a table. The arm is carefully raised and placed on the table and the table height is adjusted until the shoulder, elbow and wrist lie at the same level. The elbow joint is carefully flexed to 90° and the palm of the hand is placed directly on the cassette.

2.17.1 DP Hand

For the DP projection the fingers are straightened; in practical terms this is difficult to achieve in the younger age group but clear film may be used to aid immobilisation. Alternatively a carer may place their hand on the top of the child's hand and on an agreed signal from the radiographer quickly move their hand away from the child's allowing the image to be taken. With the oblique projection the child is asked to 'hold a ball', i.e. the fingers are flexed and the metacarpals form an angle of 45° from the cassette. The fingers are separated to prevent their structures overlying the adjacent finger. The same position may be achieved using a small 45° pad in the younger child (Fig. 2.28)

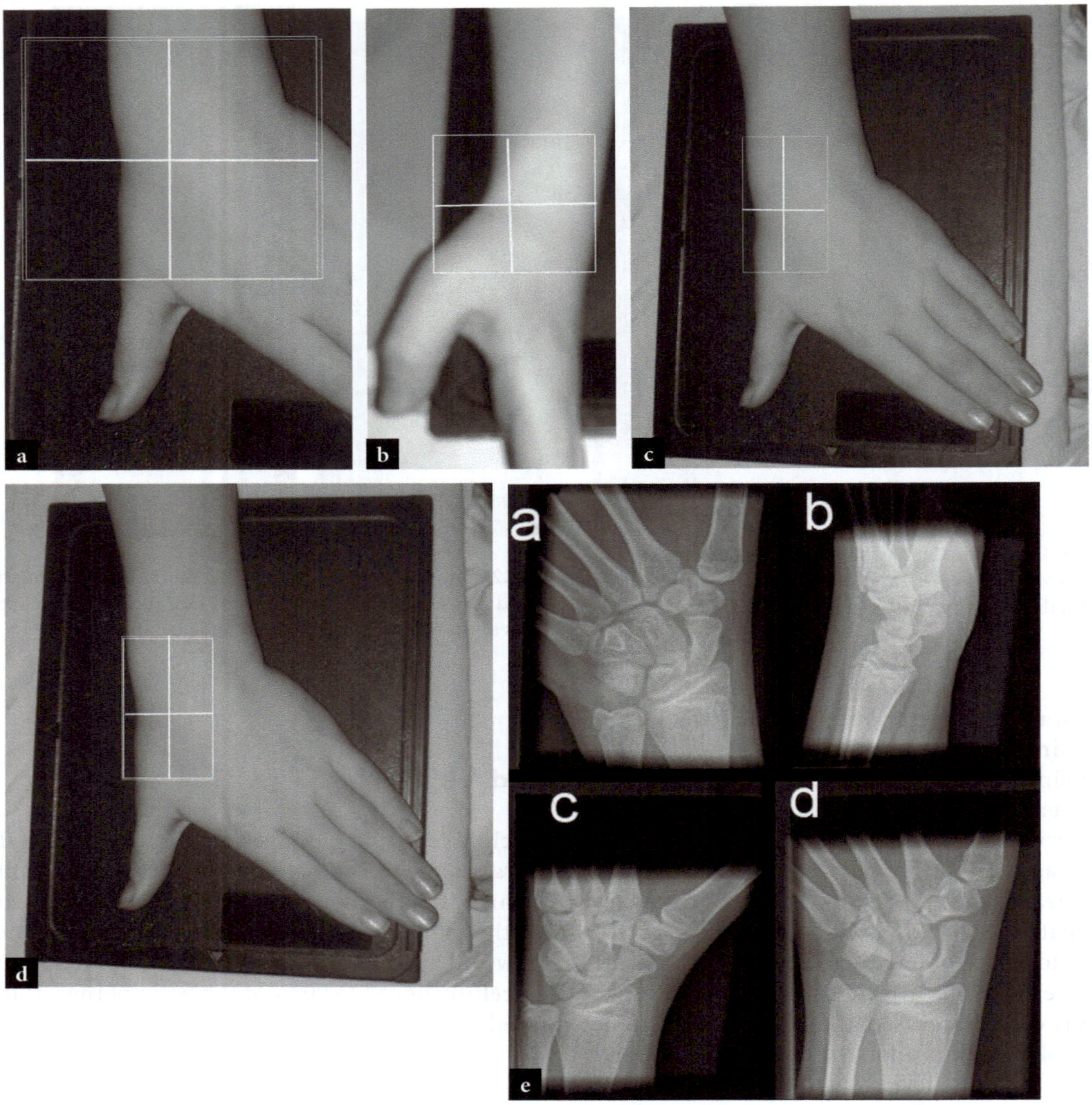

Fig. 2.27a–e. Scaphoid bone. **a** PA scaphoid with ulna deviation. **b** Lateral wrist. **c** 45° Oblique scaphoid with ulna deviation. **d** 35°angled PA scaphoid view with ulna deviation. **e** Resultant Radiographs

2.18 Spine

2.18.1 AP/PA

The child is positioned either supine or erect in front of the cassette. A bucky/grid will often need to be used for children over the age of 5. The arms should be raised above the head and if required supported by a carer. The median sagittal plane is positioned perpendicular to the cassette.

2.18.2 Lateral Projection

The child is positioned in a lateral position on the table. The knees should be bent to stabilise the position and a small foam pad may be placed between them. The arms are bent in front of the face. A carer can stand/sit at the side of the table, talk to the child at the child's eye level and gently support the arms and knees to maintain the position.

Two 45° pads placed against the child's back and tummy, held in position by placing sandbags against the pads helps prevent the child 'rocking'. A lead strip placed close to the child's back helps prevent scatter radiation and improve the image.

For spinal images the centre should be within the centre of the area under investigation such for the whole spine, midway between the chin and the symphysis pubis, and for the cervical spine midway between the external auditory canal and the head of the humerus.

For the cervical spine C7/T1 is often visualised on the initial film; however, if not, traction to the arms will improve visualisation. This needs to be applied by an experienced medical practitioner who holds the child above their elbows and gently pulls the arms towards the child's feet. Older children can be asked to stretch down to their toes to allow the cervical/thoracic junction to be demonstrated. The AP cervical spine positioning and resultant radiographs are shown in figures 2.30 and 2.31.

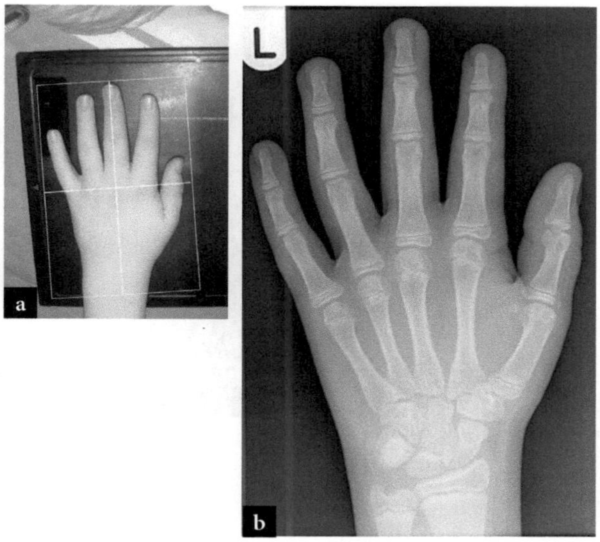

Fig. 2.28a,b. DP hand. *Centre:* Directly over the head of the distal end (knuckle) of the third metacarpal. *Area imaged:* Distal radius and ulna, carpel bones and proximal ends of the metacarpal bones

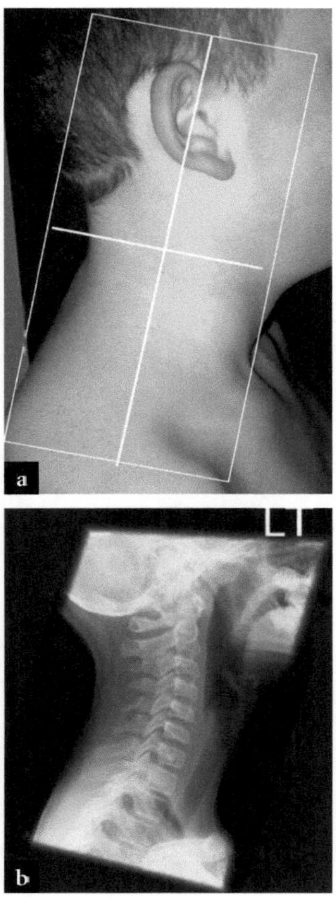

Fig. 2.29a,b. Lateral cervical spine. *Centre:* Midway between the external auditory canal and the head of the humerus. *Area imaged:* Full length of the cervical spine, 1st thoracic vertebrae and the soft tissue structures of the neck, e.g. trachea

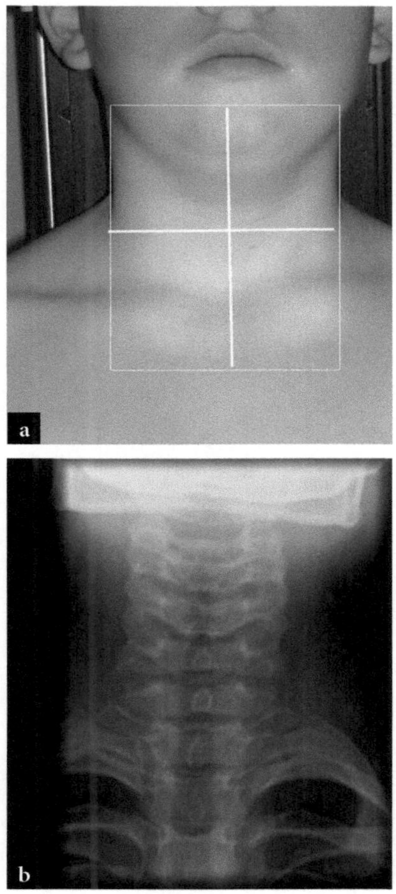

Fig. 2.30a,b. AP cervical spine. *Centre:* Midway between the chin and the sternal notch using a 15° cranial tube angle. *Area imaged:* Full width of the neck and full length of the cervical spine and the 1st thoracic vertebrae

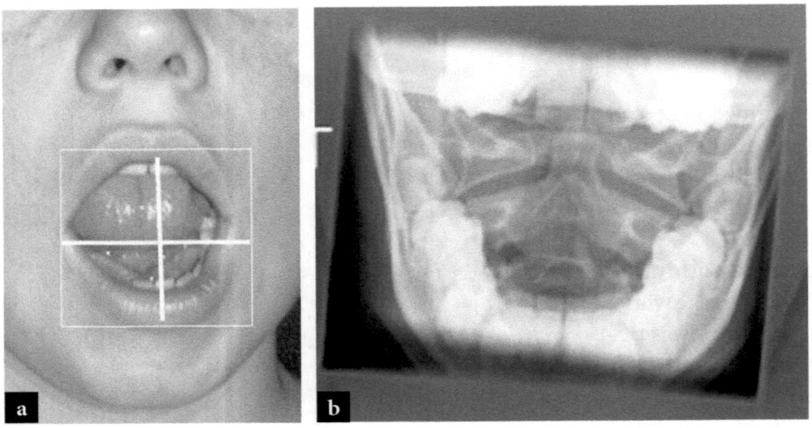

Fig. 2.31a,b. AP C1/2 (Peg) View. *Centre:* Midway between the chin and the sternal notch using a 15° cranial tube angle. *Area imaged:* Full width of the neck and full length of the cervical spine and the 1st thoracic vertebrae

CT

3

Anne Paterson

CONTENTS

3.1 Introduction

Trauma is one of the most common reasons for a child's attendance in the emergency department. Plain radiographs may remain the primary imaging modality following suspected skeletal injury, but with the advent of first single detector CT (SDCT) and now multi-detector row CT (MDCT) scanners, the role of CT in skeletal trauma has continued to develop.

In the acute situation, the speed of a CT examination and the ease with which it can be obtained, mean CT is the imaging modality of choice in cases of polytrauma. In some institutions, radiographs of the chest and pelvis are no longer obtained, if it is known the patient is due in CT (Chapman et al. 2005; Salamipour et al. 2005).

A. Paterson, MB BS, MRCP, FRCR
Consultant Paediatric Radiologist, Royal Belfast Hospital for Sick Children, 180 Falls Road, Belfast BT12 6BE, UK

Extremity CT is generally performed sub-acutely, with the presence of a fracture being noted on a radiograph and the limb then immobilized. The volume data sets obtained with SDCT and MDCT mean the patient can be positioned in the scanner comfortably and the need for scanning in more than one imaging plane (something that was common in skeletal CT in the past) is now unnecessary. Complex injuries such as those of the ankle and elbow, and tibial spine fractures (Fig. 3.1) may then require further imaging to determine the need for surgical intervention; the extent of the fracture and its relationship to the joint surface can be exquisitely displayed. In addition, the size of the fracture fragments, the presence of intra-articular loose bodies and the degree of articular surface offset or depression are accurately demonstrated (Haramati et al. 1994; Siegel and Luker 1995; Tigges and Fajman 2000; Salamipour et al. 2005; Buckwalter and Farber 2004; Buckwalter et al. 2001; Lawler et al. 2002; Falchi and Rollandi 2004; Chapman et al. 2005; Daftary et al. 2005).

CT is also helpful to follow fracture healing, particularly when mal or non-union (Fig. 3.2), myositis ossificans or pseudarthrosis development are suspected on plain radiographs. Those fractures involving the epiphyseal (growth) plates have the potential to interfere with later growth. Bone bridge formation and its consequent deformities are easy to illustrate with CT.

Finally, CT is helpful for those children whose fractures have radiologically healed, but whose limbs or joints have not regained the degree of function expected. Reformatted images may show unsuspected retained intra-articular loose bodies or bone overgrowth, which is hindering limb or joint movement.

This chapter provides an overview of skeletal CT techniques, with an emphasis on radiation risks, CT parameters affecting image quality, and viewing and manipulating axial source images. Tables with specimen paediatric CT protocols are also provided.

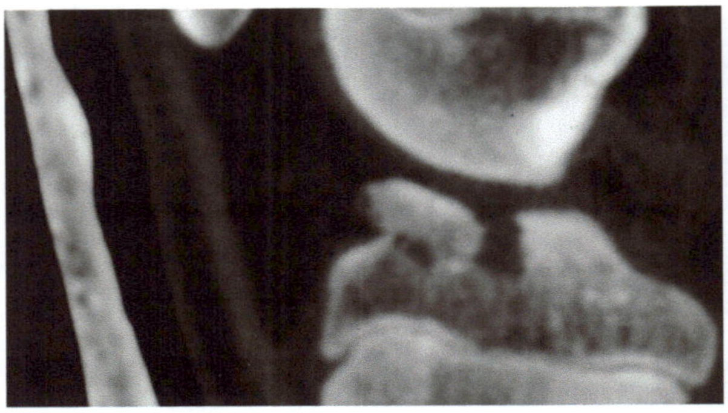

Fig. 3.1. Parasagittal MPR image showing avulsion of the anterior tibial spine. The bone fragment is angulated and displaced by 7 mm. This patient required surgery

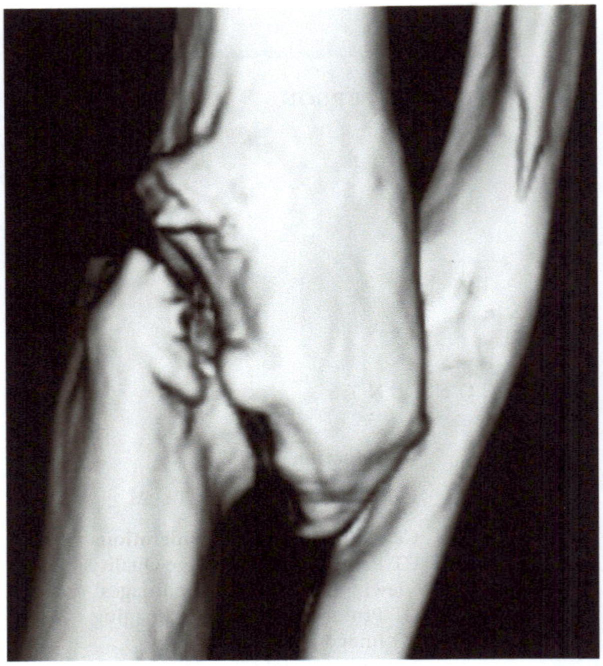

Fig. 3.2. Anterior oblique 3D VR image demonstrating non-union of a tibial diaphyseal fracture. For comparison, the adjacent fibular fracture has healed well and has started to re-model

3.2 Radiation Risks from CT

Radiation exposure from CT is an important topic to consider, with recent figures suggesting that CT now accounts for around 17% of a radiology department's workload, contributing 70%–75% of the collective population dose from medical radiation (Baker 2003; Wiest et al. 2002; Linton and Mettler 2003). At the same time, the proportion of examinations performed on children has risen; in 1999 Mettler showed 11.2% of CT studies were for paediatric patients (Mettler et al. 2000).

Such statistics are important, as it has been shown that the effective dose delivered by some CT examinations overlaps with those doses reported to increase the incidence of cancer (Brenner et al. 2001; Ron 2002). The significance of this information is more pertinent in the paediatric age group, as children's organs are more radiosensitive that those of adults (with girls being more radiosensitive than boys). In addition, children have longer lifetimes ahead of them, in which radiation induced problems may become manifest (Preston et al. 2003).

The exact risk of developing cancer from lower levels of radiation (< 30 mSv), continues to provide a much argued debate: there are some who feel such risks are speculative or perhaps even non-existent (Cohen 2002). However, whilst the absolute risk from medical radiation is not yet known, it is imperative that all radiologists weigh up the benefit to be gained from the information a CT study can provide, and balance this against the potential radiation risk incurred.

3.3 General Technical Considerations

Musculoskeletal examinations in CT encompass a broad range of patients, from the polytraumatised child in the immediate aftermath of a motor vehicle accident, to the child who is systemically well, but whose extremity is being imaged to investigate suspected complications of an injury that occurred months in the past. Regardless of the clinical situation, the preparation of any paediatric patient for a CT study includes the provision of a safe, comfortable, child-friendly environment, alongside an informed discussion with the child's carers as to the necessity for the examination and what it entails.

In the emergency situation, where the patient may be unconscious with life threatening injuries, there must be named medical staff responsible for monitoring the patient and a full resuscitation trolley available in the CT suite. It is often easier to position such patients feet-first into the gantry, as this improves access to the airway and, practically speaking, means the CT table can be used to support necessary equipment, without overstretching tubes and wires. In consultation with the accompanying medical staff, devices which may contribute to scan artefact (such as ECG leads and pulse oximeters) should be re-positioned on the patient so that they lie outside the anatomic region of interest. Unconscious patients must be assumed to have spinal injuries, and log-rolled and lifted accordingly. In a conscious trauma patient, analgesia may be required prior to the examination, as a distressed child in pain will not be able to lie still for the duration of the study.

Sedation of children for CT examinations has become less of an issue with the advent of MDCT. One early study looking at sedation rates for a 4-slice MDCT scanner versus a conventional CT scanner reported a drop in the frequency of sedation required from 18% to 3.3% (Pappas et al. 2000). This reduction in the use of sedation directly reflects the faster scanning times with MDCT.

IV contrast medium is not generally used for orthopaedic trauma CT studies, unless a combined musculoskeletal and angiographic study is required when assessing for vascular damage in the acute situation. However, IV contrast is necessary when imaging children with multiple injuries, as for example, when the spine and bony pelvis are studied along with the chest, abdomen and pelvis. Non-ionic, low or iso-osmolar contrast medium is used, the dose of which will vary depending upon the body region to be examined. In general, 2.0 ml/kg body weight are needed for abdomino-pelvic studies, whereas 1.5 ml/kg body weight will suffice for CT angiography and isolated chest CT. Given that venous catheters for younger children may be as small as 24 or 26 gauge, then warming the contrast medium will reduce its viscosity and improve the ease with which it can be injected. Larger bore catheters (22 gauge or above) can be power injected, but the smaller gauge lines, or those sited remotely in the foot or scalp veins, will need to be hand-injected. Details regarding the timing of contrast injections for different techniques are outside the scope of this chapter and the reader is referred elsewhere for details (Frush et al. 2001; Donnelly et al. 2001).

3.4.1 CT Parameters and Image Quality

Selection of appropriate imaging parameters is important not only to optimise the quality of the data obtained from the study, but also to limit the radiation dose the patient receives.

Image quality in CT is determined both by spatial resolution and contrast. It is the tube current (mA) that primarily affects spatial resolution, whilst the peak tube potential (kVp) affects both spatial and contrast resolution. Other factors influencing spatial resolution – the ability to observe small details – include in the imaging plane: the collimation (in SDCT) - or section collimation (in MDCT) and the focal spot size of the tube. The slice (section) thickness and the choice of pitch influence spatial resolution along the Z-(long) axis of the patient – thinner slices and a lower pitch leading to an improvement in spatial resolution (Huda et al. 2002).

Image contrast is related to the energy of the X-ray photons available and therefore to kVp, the inherent tube filtration and the size of the patient/anatomic regions being imaged. Increasing kVp reduces image contrast and therefore structures with higher intrinsic contrast, such as bones, can be better appreciated at lower tube voltages.

Image noise detracts from the quality of the displayed data. The amount of image noise in CT depends upon the number of photons used to generate the image and is hence related to the tube current. Less noise is present when the tube current is higher, as more photons are generated. Increasing the kVp will also reduce the image noise, as less photons will be absorbed by the patient, with more of them reaching the detector elements. Increasing the slice thickness, will also reduce the visible image noise, as more photons are used to reconstruct each slice. The wider window settings used in orthopaedic CT imaging, will also compensate for image noise to some extent (Buckwalter and Farber 2004). Image contrast must be adequate to overcome the loss of image quality that invariably occurs due to image noise.

The CT scanning parameters that can be adjusted by the radiologist include: tube current, gantry rotation time, kilovoltage, table speed and collimation (in SDCT) or detector configuration (size and number of detectors and detector rows – with respect to MDCT). Setting the scan parameters for a particular protocol not only influences image quality, but also the radiation dose to the patient and intuition tells us that you don't need as many photons (and those that you have require less energy) to image a child. Simplistically then, tube current and kilovoltage can be lower for paediatric protocols.

Current MDCT scanners have sub-second gantry rotation times. Reducing the scan rotation time from 1.0–0.5 s will halve the time taken to perform a scan (over a prescribed distance), an important consideration with children. In addition, given that there is a linear relationship between tube current (mAs) and dose, then reducing the gantry rotation time to 0.5 s will decrease the radiation dose the patient receives by 50%.

With SDCT the concept of collimation is a simple one to understand: the size of the X-ray beam is controlled by a set of collimators placed near to the X-ray tube. Collimation in SDCT is directly related to the slice (section) thickness and narrower collimation improves z-axis resolution, though requires an increase in the mAs to overcome the additional image noise.

The term "collimation" is used differently when referring to MDCT technology. "Beam collimation" is analogous to collimation as used in SDCT terminology. Depending upon the beam collimation selected by the radiologist, different parts of the detector array will be activated during each 360° gantry rotation (Rydberg et al. 2000; Dalrymple et al. 2005). Both beam collimation and table speed are parameters which are linked to affect image quality and radiation dose. The numerical values of (beam) collimation and table speed are used to calculate pitch, the rudimentary equations for which are given below:

SDCT:

$$\text{Pitch} = \frac{\text{table movement (mm)}}{\text{collimation (mm)}}$$

MDCT:

$$\text{Pitch} = \frac{\text{table movement (mm)}}{\text{beam collimation (mm)}}$$

The denominator for the latter equation can also be written as: number of detector channels × section collimation (mm) or as detector configuration (mm).

Increasing the pitch reduces the radiation dose to the patient, with pitch values of 2.0 halving the patient dose (Paterson et al. 2001). However, at pitch values of > 2.0 the spatial resolution in the z-axis is reduced noticeably due to a degradation in the section profile and increasing artefacts (Frush et al. 2003; Tack and Gevenois 2004; Kalra et al. 2004c).

The term "section collimation" in MDCT is more difficult to define. The detector bank in a MDCT scanner consists of arrays of detector elements. Depending upon the scanner manufacturer, these elements may be equal in size or have smaller elements lying centrally in a row, with wider elements lying peripherally (Rydberg et al. 2000; Buckwalter et al. 2001). The organisation of the X-ray detectors into such arrays allows the incident X-ray beam to be divided into multiple data channels (Hu 1999; Rydberg et al. 2000; Tanenbaum 2003). Section collimation relates to the way that these individual detector elements are utilized to subdivide and channel the data. The elements may be used individually or in combination with one another to produce narrow axial sections of data.

Beam collimation and table movement together (i.e. pitch) determine the volume of tissue irradiated per gantry rotation, whereas section collimation determines the minimal slice (also known as section) thickness that can be reconstructed from an examination's raw data. That is, the narrowest selected reconstructed slice thickness available will equal the selected size of the detector elements (Dalrymple et al. 2005). Section collimation may also be referred to as (effective) detector (row) thickness. The term detector configuration merely couples together the value selected for the section collimation with the number of detector elements. For example: 4 × 1.25 refers to a four-channel scanner acquiring four channels of data 1.25 mm thick. Similarly, 16 × 0.625 refers to 16 channels of data 0.625 mm thick obtained on a 16-channel scanner. From this information and the equation for pitch, it can be seen that detector configuration is numerically equal to the beam collimation (Rydberg et al. 2003; Saini 2004).

3.4.2 Viewing the Axial Source Images

The raw data collected by the detector elements is used to generate axial images. The scan acquisition parameters (as described in the previous section) define the spatial properties of the axial data and cannot subsequently be altered. Any retrospectively reconstructed axial images (altering slice thickness and interval or reconstruction algorithm) utilise this raw data from the CT scanner's hard drive; such data may not be available in the long term, depending upon image storage capabilities/arrangements (Hsieh 1996; Tanenbaum 2003). With this in mind, it is prudent for the radiologist to anticipate, which types of CT examination are likely to benefit from 3D image reformation and have a set of thin slice (section) axial images reconstructed at the time of the study (Dalrymple et al. 2005).

Before the axial data sets can be reviewed, the slice (section) thickness, reconstruction interval, display field of view and reconstruction algorithm must be selected. The slice (section) thickness is the length of the data segment of the z-axis used to calculate pixel values for the axial images (Dalrymple et al. 2005). The Hounsfield unit value for the individual pixels within an axial image is calculated from this information (Mahesh 2002). Thicker slices have reduced spatial resolution, but less image noise and are generally used to view the information from axial source images.

The reconstruction interval (also referred to as the reconstruction increment) is the distance along the z-axis from the centre of one axial "slice" (reconstruction), to the centre of the adjacent "slice". When the slice thickness and increment are numerically equal, then the axial images are referred to as contiguous slices.

The slice thickness and reconstruction interval are variable parameters, which are independent of the acquisition programme (and hence the radiation dose to the patient). If the raw data remains available, they can be altered ad infinitum.

For orthopaedic CT, when 3D reformatting is the norm, then a narrow slice thickness with an overlapping interval is selected (Tanenbaum 2003; Daftary et al. 2005). This can be used to produce images in non-axial planes, which retain a smooth contour.

3.4.3 CT Protocols for Skeletal Imaging

Paediatric patients vary considerably in size and weight, and it is important to pre-programme protocols, which take this into account into the scanner. Tables 3.1–3.3 outline specimen protocols for both SDCT and MDCT scanners. The parameters for chest and abdomino-pelvic imaging are given as they can be utilised for a polytrauma patient. In these circumstances, the slice thickness could be reduced, with an overlapping increment selected, so that the skeleton (for example the spine, bony pelvis and shoulder girdle) can be viewed in different planes, using 3D reformatting techniques.

Of course, the greater the scan length, the greater the radiation dose to the patient. However, it is imperative that the programmed scan length is sufficient to provide adequate bony landmarks to the reporting radiologist for 3D reformation work and correct interpretation of the images. Recognisable anatomical landmarks are also vital to the orthopaedic surgeons when planning operative intervention, with the aid of CT examinations.

Most manufacturers now programme paediatric protocols into their scanners and these can act as a useful starting point when tailoring an examination for an individual patient. The addition of automatic tube current modulation (ATCM) to MDCT scanners has led to a reported substantial decrease in radiation dose in CT body imaging (Greess et al. 2000, 2002, 2004; Kojima et al. 2003: Kalra et al. 2004a,b; Mastora et al. 2004; Hundt et al. 2005). With ATCM, the tube current is altered to more closely follow the patient's body contours, yet maintain a constant noise level on the images.

Angular ATCM adjusts the tube current as the X-ray tube passes around the patient's body. In regions where the cross-sectional shape of the body is non-circular (for example the upper trunk), the majority of the image noise comes from the lateral projections, where most of the incident beam is attenuated. The tube current is then reduced in the projections where beam attenuation is less. Angular ATCM can be thought of as "intra-slice" current modulation; modern CT scanners perform this function in real time (Kalra et al. 2004c; Greess et al. 2000, 2004; Hundt et al. 2005).

ACTM can also be utilized as a dose saving tool in the z-axis. When a CT protocol is selected for an examination, either the CT scanner's software or the radiologist select a desired noise level for that individual study. For orthopaedic CT, a higher noise level (index) is suggested, as the intrinsic contrast resolution of bone is high (Chapman et al. 2005). Again, the technique strives to maintain a constant noise level on the images. Some authors have likened ATCM to the auto exposure control systems used with conventional X-ray systems (Kalra et al. 2004c). With some ATCM software, minimum and maximum acceptable mA values can be programmed into the scanner, further refining the technique. Angular and z-axis ATCM can be used simultaneously for even greater reductions in patient dose.

3.4.4 3D Image Reconstruction in Musculoskeletal CT

In the acute situation, when fractures are being searched for or CT exams have been performed to further delineate fractures seen on plain ra-

Table 3.1. Guidelines for multidetector row CT parameters in children: chest[a]. [Reprinted from Donnelly and Frush (2005), with permission]

Weight (kg)	kVp	mAs[b]		Slice thickness (mm)	Pitch			Detector thickness[c] (mm)			Increment (mm)
		SDCT	MDCT		4-	8-	16-	4-	8-	16-	
5-9.5	100–120	40	30	3.75–5	0.75	0.875	0.9375	2.5	1.25	1.25	2.5
10-19.5	100–120	50	30–40	3.75–5	0.75	0.875	0.9375	2.5	1.25	1.25	2.5
20-29.5	120	60	40	5	0.75–1.5	1.35	1.375	2.5	1.25	1.25	2.5
30-39.5	120	70	50	5	1.5	1.35	1.375	2.5	1.25	1.25	2.5
40-49.5	120	80	60	5	1.5	1.35	1.375	3.75	2.5	1.25	2.5
50-75	120	100–120	70–90	5	1.5	1.35	1.75	3.75	2.5	1.25	2.5
> 75	120	120–140	≥ 110	5	1.5	1.35	1.75	3.75	2.5	1.25	2.5

Table 3.2. Guidelines for multidetector row CT parameters in children: abdomen/pelvis[a]. [Reprinted from Donnelly and Frush (2005), with permission]

Weight (kg)	kVp	mAs[b]		Slice thickness (mm)	Pitch			Detector thickness[c] (mm)			Increment (mm)
		SDCT	MDCT		4-	8-	16-	4-	8-	16-	
5-9.5	100–120	60	50	3.75–5	0.75	0.875	0.9375	2.5	1.25	1.25	2.5
10-19.5	100–120	70	60	3.75–5	0.75	0.875	0.9375	2.5	1.25	1.25	2.5
20-29.5	120	80	70	5	0.75–1.5	1.35	1.375	2.5	1.25	1.25	2.5
30-39.5	120	100	80	5	1.5	1.35	1.375	2.5	1.25	1.25	2.5
40-49.5	120	120	100	5	1.5	1.35	1.375	3.75	2.5	1.25	2.5
50-75	120	140–150	110–120	5	1.5	1.35	1.75	3.75	2.5	1.25	2.5
> 75	120	≥ 170	≥ 135	5	1.5	1.35	1.75	3.75	2.5	1.25	2.5

[a]Parameters are based on GE single and multi-detector row scanners.
[b]Use 0.5-s gantry time when an option; mA are for 4- and 8-slice MDCT; 16-slice weight-based colour-coded mA are loaded on the scanner.
[c]For anticipated multiplanar reconstructions or 3D rendering, use thinnest detector width (e.g. 0.625 mm) with 16-slice at all ages.

Table 3.3. Guidelines for multidetector row CT parameters in children: extremity skeletal examination[a]. [Reprinted from Donnelly and Frush (2005), with permission]

Weight (kg)	kVp[b]	mAs		Slice thickness (mm)	Pitch			Detector thickness (mm)		Increment (mm)
		SDCT	MDCT		4-	8-	16	4-, 8-	16-	
5-9.5	80–100	40	30	1.25–2.5	1.5	1.35	1.375	1.25	0.625	0.5–1.25
10-19.5	80–100	50	30–40	1.25–2.5	1.5	1.35	1.375	1.25	0.625	0.5–1.25
20-29.5	100	60	40	1.25–2.5	1.5	1.35	1.375	1.25	0.625	0.5–1.25
30-39.5	100	70	50	1.25–2.5	1.5	1.35	1.375	1.25	0.625	0.5–1.25
40-49.5	120	80	60	1.25–2.5	1.5	1.35	1.375	1.25	0.625	0.5–1.25
≥ 50	120	100–120	70–90	1.25–2.5	1.5	1.35	1.375	1.25	0.625	0.5–1.25

[a]Parameters are based on GE single and multi-detector row scanners. Reconstruct 0.625-mm data set at 0.5- to 1.0-mm interval to use for additional planes (e.g. sagittal and coronal). There is no need with sub-millimetre thick images for scanning in more than one plane. Protocols generally for finer detail exams such as wrists and ankles. Thicker slices and increased interval for larger regions.
[b]Consider 80–100 kVp at all ages.

diographs, axial images alone may not provide enough information. This is especially true if the fracture line(s) run in the axial plane (Pretorius and Fishman 1999). As discussed in the previous sections, a volumetric data set should be produced from the raw data, with narrow slice thickness and an overlapping interval. If this data produces voxels, which are cube shaped (i.e. symmetrical in all dimensions) rather than cuboidal (when the z-axis dimension is > axial dimension), then the data is said to be isotropic. The use of isotropic data is the key to producing high quality 3D reformatted images. In addition, when the axial data is being sent from the scanner console to the CT workstation, a standard or soft reconstruction algorithm should be selected, as this helps to minimise image noise (Buckwalter and Farber 2004).

If isotropic imaging is not possible, either due to the constraints of a SDCT scanner or because a large tissue volume is being imaged and the radiation dose delivered to the patient would be prohibitive, then the principle of obliquity can be employed to improve detail of the articular surface. The extremity should be placed in the scanner, so that the scan plane is oblique to the joint surface of interest (Buckwalter et al. 2001; Buckwalter and Farber 2004). In this manner, a large number of slices will traverse the joint surface, increasing the amount of data available (concerning its contours) to be utilised in subsequent image reformats.

Multiplanar reformations (MPR) are extensively utilised in orthopaedic CT. The data from the axial images is used to create 2D images in any plane required. Coronal, sagittal and oblique images are the most common MPR required in trauma cases; fracture lines and joint surfaces are clearly shown with this technique (Fig. 3.3). Modern CT workstations mean this type of image reformatting is now an automated process, with the radiologist being able to alter the window level and centre to view what ever structures they desire.

Surface rendering (shaded surface display, SSD) attempts to display a 3D view of the surface of an object, in a 2D image on the workstation monitor. In a semi-automated process at the workstation, the radiologist must select the object to view, either by using the electronic "scalpel" tool to separate the area of interest or by altering the CT threshold values displayed. Both methods are simple to perform; the latter is less time consuming and works well for bony structures (Dalrymple et al. 2005). SSD makes use of only a portion of the available image data – that

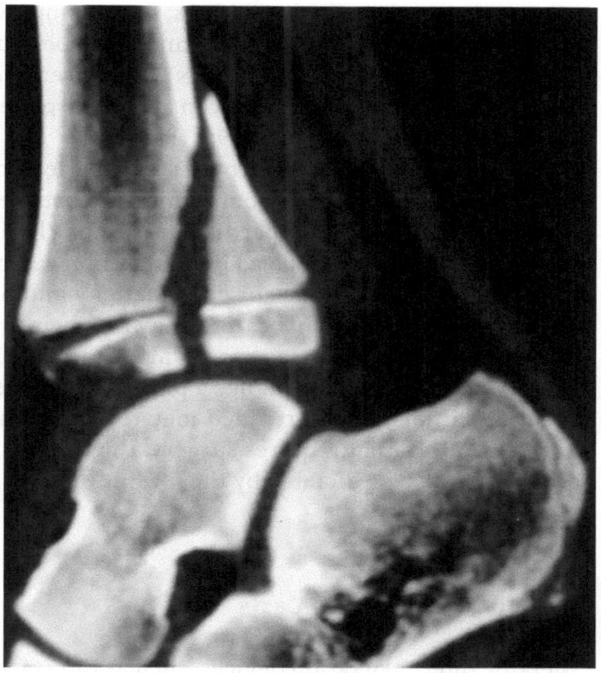

Fig. 3.3. Parasagittal MPR image showing a triplane fracture of the distal tibia. The axial component of the fracture line with widening of the growth plate is particularly well demonstrated on this view

which defines an object's surface (Fishman et al. 1987). SSD may be used to demonstrate fracture lines that have been diagnosed on MPR images (Kuszyk et al. 1996), though the technique has largely been superseded by 3D volume rendered (3D VR) images (Kuszyk et al. 1996), as "stair step" artefact can sometimes be a problem (Pretorius and Fishman 1999; Falchi and Rollandi 2004) with SSD.

VR imaging uses all of the available data in the image set (Kuszyk et al. 1996; Pretorius and Fishman 1999; Lawler et al. 2002; Dalrymple et al. 2005; Fayad et al. 2005) conveying more information than SSD (Pretorius and Fishman 1999). As more information is used to create the VR image, so too is greater computer power required. Modern CT workstations can now produce VR images in real time. In the formation of the VR image, opacity values are assigned to all voxels along a line of sight from the viewer's eye, through the complete data set (Pretorius and Fishman 1999; Dalrymple et al. 2005). Each pixel value in the displayed image must be calculated in this manner. Grey scale shadings are then applied by the software to simulate surface reflections (Levoy 1988; Drebin and Hanrahan 1988). Colour can also be applied to the opacity value histograms, further improving perceived spatial arrangements and depth perception (Dalrymple et al. 2005; Rubin 2003). Overlying structures and internal features can also be displayed on VR images (Kuszyk et al. 1996) (Fig. 3.4).

The information conveyed by 3D reformatted images can serve to improve communication between the radiologist and orthopaedic surgeon or child's carers. Information displayed in this fashion can be related more easily to the surgical anatomy and, in the case of a child and his carers, may aid their understanding of the disease process. MPR and 3D VR images may also help to change a patient's management; the information provided may reveal a more complex injury that requires surgery, the timing of which may also be dictated by the CT findings.

3.4.5 Metallic Implants and Casts

Metallic internal fixation devices, such as intramedullary rods or plates and screws, can cause considerable streak artefact on CT images. Aligning the scan plane with the long axis of the implant using a combination of patient positioning and gantry angulation can lessen this artefact. Some compensation can also be gained through the use of 3D VR techniques (Pretorius and Fishman 1999; Fishman and Kuszyk 2001; Lawler et al. 2002; Buckwalter and Farber 2004; Falchi and Rollandi 2004) (Fig. 3.5). Increasing the kVp and mA have also been reported to reduce streak artefact (Haramati et al. 1994; Buckwalter et al. 2001; Buckwalter and Farber 2004), as has the use of thin slices (Buckwalter et al. 2001; Tanenbaum 2003; Salamipour et al. 2005), though obviously these come at the expense of an increase in the radiation dose to the patient. Implants made of titanium have been shown to cause less streak artefact than other metals (Fruhwald et al. 1988; Haramati et al. 1994). Finally, at the workstation the radiologist can also increase the display window level and width, which can lessen the visible artefact (Haramati et al. 1994).

Scanning through full plaster casts or back-slabs presents no problem. Rather, the image quality may be improved, as the patient is more comfortable and they lie still for the duration of the examination.

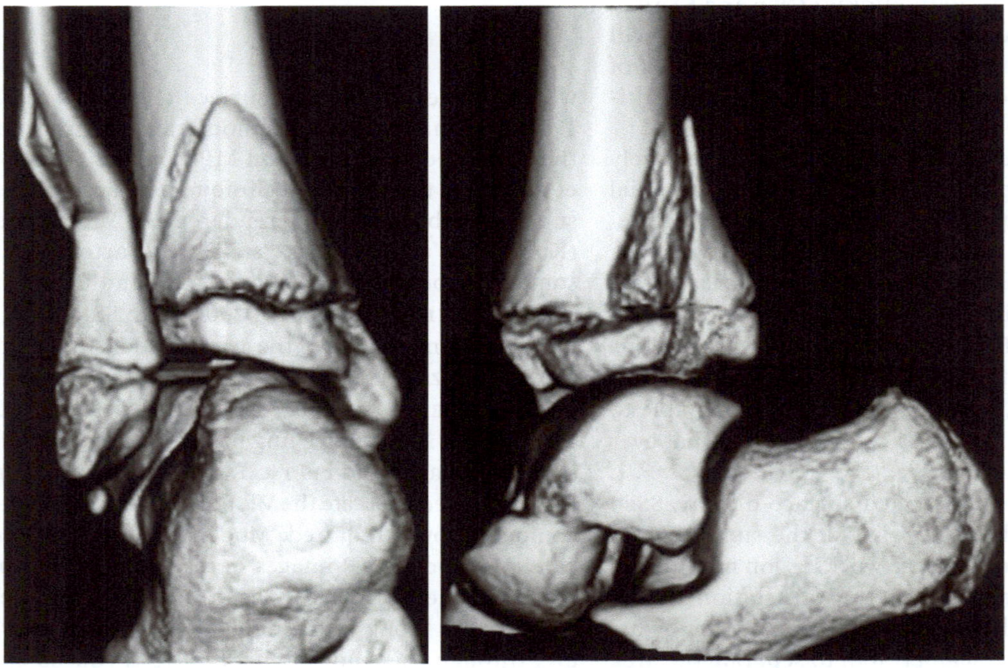

a b

Fig. 3.4. a Posterior 3D VR image of a triplane fracture (same patient as in Fig. 3.3). Involvement of the medial malleolus can also be seen on this view, along with an incomplete, angulated fibular diaphyseal fracture (**b**). The fibular has been removed from the image, using the 'scalpel' tool. The tibial component of the fracture can now be viewed on the CT workstation from all directions (lateral oblique view shown)

When MPR and 3D VR images are required, it is a simple task to "cut away" the cast using the scalpel tool at the workstation.

careful attention to technique is important, so that the maximum information possible can be extracted from the images at the lowest possible radiation dose to the patient.

3.5 Conclusion

With the advent of MDCT scanners, a continued increase in requests for CT examinations following skeletal trauma is foreseen. It is imperative that the radiologist scrutinises all such requests carefully and makes use of other imaging modalities, which do not involve ionising radiation, whenever possible. If a CT study is deemed necessary, then

References

Baker SR (2003) Musings at the beginning of the hyper-CT era. Abdom Imaging 28:110–114

Brenner DJ, Elliston CD, Hall EJ et al (2001) Estimated risks of radiation-induced fatal cancer from pediatric CT. AJR Am J Roentgenol 176:289–296

Buckwalter KA, Farber JM (2004) Application of multidetector CT in skeletal trauma. Semin Musculoskelet Radiol 8:147–156

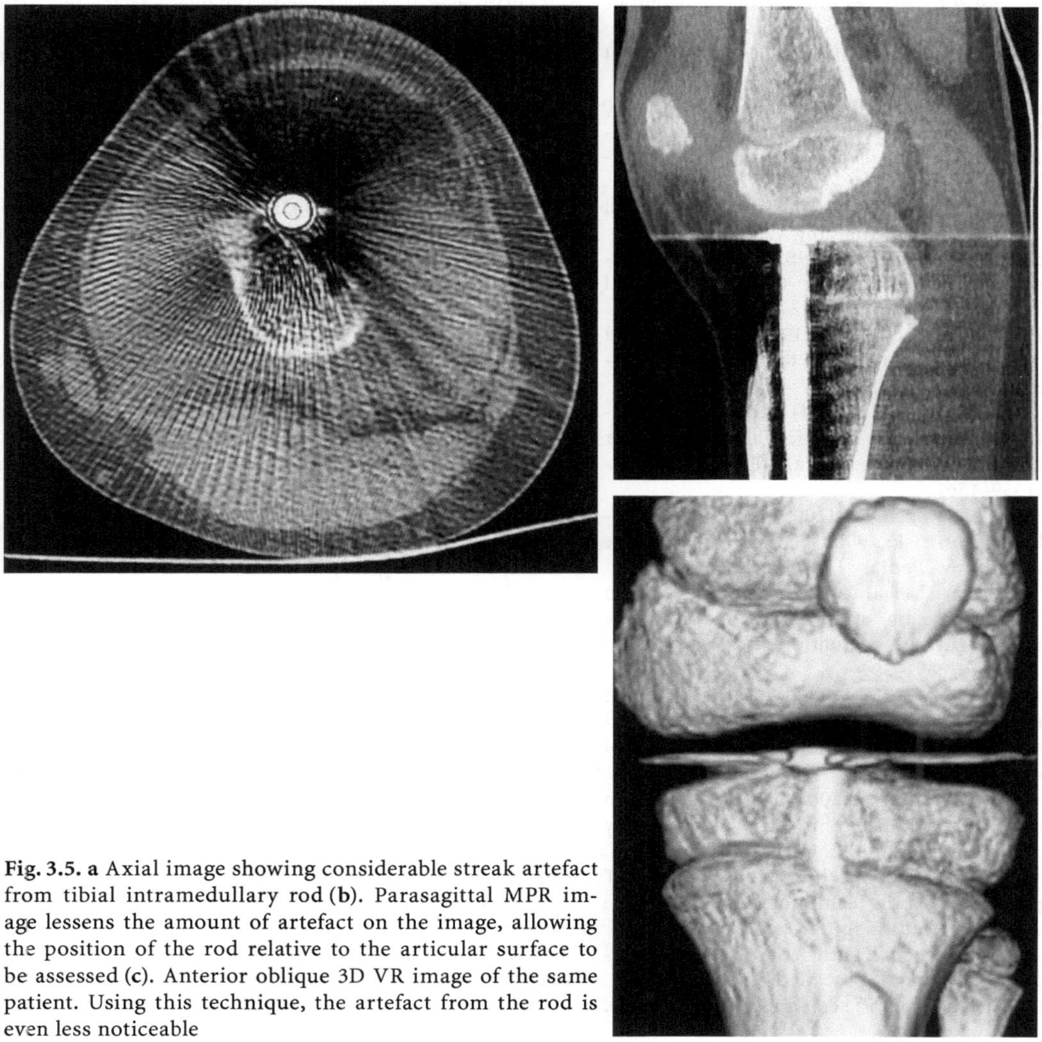

a b c

Fig. 3.5. a Axial image showing considerable streak artefact from tibial intramedullary rod (**b**). Parasagittal MPR image lessens the amount of artefact on the image, allowing the position of the rod relative to the articular surface to be assessed (**c**). Anterior oblique 3D VR image of the same patient. Using this technique, the artefact from the rod is even less noticeable

Buckwalter KA, Rydberg J, Kopecky KK et al (2001) Musculoskeletal imaging with multislice CT. AJR Am J Roentgenol 176:979–986
Chapman VM, Kalra M, Halpern E et al (2005) 16-MDCT of the posttraumatic pediatric elbow: optimum parameters and associated radiation dose. AJR Am J Roentgenol 185:516–521
Cohen BL (2002) Cancer risks from low level radiation. AJR Am J Roentgenol 179:1137–1143
Daftary A, Haims AH, Baumgaertner MR (2005) Fractures of the calcaneus: a review with emphasis on CT. Radiographics 25:1215–1226
Dalrymple NC, Prasad SR, Freckleton MW et al (2005) Informatics in radiology. Introduction to the language of three-dimensional imaging with multidetector CT. Radiographics 25:1409–1428
Donnelly LF, Frush DP (2005) Evidence based principles and protocols of pediatric body MSCT. Elsevier, p 191
Donnelly LF, Frush DP (2005) Evidence-based principles and protocols for pediatric multislice computed tomography. In: Knollman F, Croakley FV, eds. Multislice CT – Principles and Protocols. Philadelphia, PA: Elsevier, pp179–201
Drebin RA, Hanrahan P (1988) Volume rendering. Comput Graph 22:65–74
Falchi M, Rollandi GA (2004) CT of pelvic fractures. Eur J Radiol 50:96–105
Fayad LM, Johnson P, Fishman EK (2005) Multidetector CT of musculoskeletal disease in the pediatric patient: principles, techniques, and clinical applications. Radiographics 25:603–618
Fishman EK, Kuszyk B (2001) 3D imaging: musculoskeletal applications. Crit Rev Diagn Imaging 42:59–100
Fishman EK, Drebin B, Magid D et al (1987) Volumetric rendering techniques: applications for three-dimensional imaging of the hip. Radiology 163:737–738
Fruhwald F, Fellinger E, Hubsch P et al (1988) Computerized tomography analysis of cement-free total hip endoprostheses. Roentgenblatter 41:313–319
Frush DP, Donnelly LF, Bisset GS (2001) Technical innovation: effect of scan delay on hepatic enhancement for pediatric abdominal multislice helical CT. AJR Am J Roentgenol 176:1559–1561
Frush DP, Donnelly LF, Rosen NS (2003) Computed tomography and radiation risks: what pediatric health care providers should know. Pediatr 112:951–957
Greess H, Wolf H, Baum U et al (2000) Dose reduction in computed tomography by attenuation-based on-line modulation of tube current: evaluation of six anatomical regions. Eur Radiol 10:391–394
Greess H, Nömayr A, Wolf H et al (2002) Dose reduction in CT examination of children by an attenuation-based online modulation of tube current (CARE dose). Eur Radiol 12:1571–1576
Greess H, Lutze J, Nömayr A et al (2004) Dose reduction in subsecond multislice spiral CT examination of children by online tube current modulation. Eur Radiol 14:995–999
Haramati N, Staron RB, Mazel-Sperling K et al (1994) CT scans through metal scanning technique versus hardware composition. Comput Med Imaging Graph 18:429–434
Hsieh J (1996) A general approach to the reconstruction of X-ray helical computed tomography. Med Phys 23:221–229
Hu H (1999) Multi-slice helical CT: scan and reconstruction. Med Phys 26:5–18
Huda W, Ravenel JG, Scalzetti EM (2002) How do radiographic techniques affect image quality and patient doses in CT? Semin Ultrasound CT MR 23:411–422
Hundt W, Rust F, Stäbler A et al (2005) Dose reduction in multislice computed tomography. J Comput Assist Tomogr 29:140–17
John SD (1999) Trends in pediatric emergency imaging. Radiol Clin North Am 37:995–1034
Kalra MK, Maher MM, Kamath RS et al (2004a) Sixteen-detector row CT of abdomen and pelvis: study for optimization of Z-axis modulation technique performed in 153 patients. Radiology 233:241–249
Kalra MK, Maher MM, Toth TL et al (2004b) Comparison of Z-axis automatic tube current modulation technique with fixed tube current CT scanning of abdomen and pelvis. Radiology 232:347–353
Kalra MK, Maher MM, Toth TL et al (2004c) Strategies for CT radiation dose optimization. Radiology 230:619–628
Kojima M, Itoh S, Ikeda M et al (2003) Usefulness of a method for changing tube current during helical scanning in multislice CT. Radiat Med 21:193–204
Kuszyk BS, Heath DG, Bliss DF et al (1996) Skeletal 3-D CT: advantages of volume rendering over surface rendering. Skeletal Radiol 25:207–214
Lawler LP, Corl FM, Fishman EK (2002) Multi- and single detector CT with 3D volume rendering in tibial plateau fracture imaging and management. Crit Rev Comput Tomogr 43:251–282
Levoy M (1988) Display of surfaces from volume data. IEEE Comput Graph Appl 8:29–37
Linton OW, Mettler FA (2003) National conference on dose reduction in CT, with an emphasis on pediatric patients. AJR Am J Roentgenol 181:321–329
Mahesh M (2002) Search for isotropic resolution in CT from conventional through multiple-row detector. Radiographics 22:949–962
Mastora I, Remy-Jardin M, Delannoy V et al (2004) Multi-detector row spiral CT angiography of the thoracic outlet: dose reduction with anatomically adapted online tube current modulation and preset dose savings. Radiology 230:116–124
Mettler FA Jr, Wiest PW, Locken JA et al (2000) CT scanning: patterns of use and dose. J Radiol Prot 20:353–359
Pappas JN, Donnelly LF, Frush DP (2000) Reduced frequency of sedation of young children with multisection helical CT
Pärtan G, Pamberger P, Blab E et al (2003) Common tasks and problems in paediatric trauma radiology. Eur J Radiol 48:103–124
Paterson A, Frush DP, Donnelly LF (2001) Helical CT of the body: are settings adjusted for pediatric patients? AJR Am J Roentgenol 176:297–301
Preston DL, Shimizu Y, Pierce DA et al (2003) Studies of mortality of atomic bomb survivors. Report 13: solid cancer and noncancer disease mortality: 1950–1997. Radiat Res 160:381–407
Pretorius ES, Fishman EK (1999) Volume-rendered three-dimensional spiral CT: musculoskeletal applications. Radiographics 19:1143–1160
Ron E (2002) Ionizing radiation and cancer risks: evidence from epidemiology. Pediatr Radiol 32:232–237
Rubin GD (2003) 3-D imaging with MDCT. Eur J Radiol 45[Suppl 1]:S37–S41
Rydberg J, Buckwalter KA, Caldemeyer KS et al (2000) Multisection CT: scanning techniques and clinical applications. Radiographics 20:1787–1806

Rydberg J, Liang Y, Teague SD (2003) Fundamentals of multichannel CT. Radiol Clin North Am 41:465–474
Saini S (2004) Multi-detector row CT: principles and practice for abdominal applications. Radiology 233:323–327
Salamipour H, Jimenez RM, Brec SL et al (2005) Multidetector row CT in pediatric musculoskeletal imaging. Pediatr Radiol 35:555–564
Siegel MJ, Luker GD (1995) Pediatric applications of helical (spiral) CT. Radiol Clin North Am 33:997–1022
Tack D, Gevenois PA (2004) Radiation dose in computed tomography of the chest. JBR-BTR 87:281–288
Tanenbaum L (2003) Multichannel helical CT of the musculoskeletal system. Appl Radiol 32:15–24
Tigges S, Fajman WA (2000) Injuries about the knee and tibial/fibular shafts. Semin Musculoskel Radiol 4:221–239
Wiest PW, Locken JA, Heintz PH et al (2002) CT scanning: a major source of radiation exposure. Semin Ultrasound CT MR 23:402–410

Ultrasound in Paediatric Trauma

4

JAMES TEH

CONTENTS

4.1 Introduction

Investigation of paediatric skeletal trauma requires careful consideration of not only the site of injury, but the proposed mechanism of trauma and the age of the child. Ultrasound is increasingly being used to detect and delineate musculoskeletal injury, either as the primary imaging modality or as an adjunct to other modalities, particularly magnetic resonance imaging (MRI). The advent of high frequency transducers allows the musculoskeletal system to be examined in exquisite detail, giving in-plane resolution of down to 200 μm and section thicknesses of 0.5 mm, far exceeding the capability of MR-Imaging (ERICKSON 1997). Apart from the lack of ionising radiation, ultrasound has several advantages over other imaging modalities: It allows a real time dynamic assessment of musculoskeletal conditions, compared to MR-Imaging there is excellent patient tolerance without any need for sedation and it can also be used to guide interventional procedures.

Anatomical and biomechanical factors account for the difference in injury patterns encountered between children and adults. This chapter will discuss the basic concepts of ultrasound, the normal appearance of the musculoskeletal tissues and the applications of ultrasound in paediatric musculoskeletal trauma.

J. TEH, BSc, MBBS, MRCP, FRCR
Consultant Musculoskeletal Radiologist, Radiology Department, Nuffield Orthopaedic Centre, Oxford OX3 7LD, UK

4.2 Basic Concepts of Ultrasound and Techniques

4.2.1 Transducers

Transducers contain a piezo-electric crystal that vibrates when an electric current is passed through it, producing an ultrasound beam which propagates through the soft tissues. Reflection or refraction of the ultrasound beam may occur when it reaches a soft tissue interface of different acoustic impedance. The reflected ultrasound beams then return to the transducer where they are converted to electrical currents and subsequently to form an image. When there is a large difference in impedance, for example at a bone-soft tissue interface, a bright echo is produced.

Ultrasound transducers are described according to the frequency of sound produced, in units of megahertz (MHz). High frequency transducers (in the range of 10–15 MHz) allow high resolution imaging but have limited penetration of tissues. Linear array transducers allow excellent near resolution and are therefore ideal for evaluating superficial musculoskeletal structures. Curvilinear transducers allow a wider field of view to be examined and are useful for visualising deeper structures. Small foot-print transducers are usually preferable for musculoskeletal imaging as they are more easily manoeuvred around joints and allow better contact with the skin. When small structures are examined copious amounts of jelly may be necessary to maintain skin contact.

4.2.2 The General Environment

The ultrasound room and equipment may appear daunting and frightening to young children. Therefore it is essential that when young children are being examined they are placed at ease within a child-friendly environment. If possible the child should be accompanied by a parent, or else a specialist nurse or play therapist. Often the child can be examined whilst sitting on the carer's lap. There should be toys or books readily available to act as a distraction. At the end of the examination a simple reward, such as a sticker, may help to act as positive reinforcement.

4.2.3 Extended Field-Of-View Imaging

Many ultrasound machines can produce extended field-of-view (panoramic) images which allow coverage of large lesions and visualisation of adjacent structures (Cooperberg et al. 2001; Barberie et al. 1998). This facilitates measurement of large structures and allows the referring clinician to have a better understanding of the anatomy.

4.2.4 Doppler Ultrasound

Many pathological conditions affecting the musculoskeletal system result in alteration of local blood flow (Teh 2006). Following trauma, the injured tissues undergoes a repair that involves a complex series of events involving physical and chemical alterations within the tissue. As part of the repair process there is neovascularisation and increased perfusion to the area of injury. Increased blood flow on Doppler following acute muscle or tendon injury should therefore be recognised as part of a normal healing response.

There are three main problems that arise from using colour Doppler that are not encountered with power Doppler, these being background noise, aliasing and angle dependency. As a result power Doppler is preferred for musculoskeletal imaging, as there is greater sensitivity and a wider dynamic range (Rubin 1999).

4.2.5 Transducer Pressure

Certain abnormalities may not be visualised if the transducer pressure is too great. Fluid and effusions may be compressed, leading to underestimation of volume. When examining for a muscle hernia or tendon subluxation the pressure of the probe may prevent visualisation. Similarly, when assessing Doppler flow the vessels may be inadvertently compressed. The use of copious ultrasound gel is the simplest way to avoid applying excessive pressure.

4.2.6 Comparison with the Contralateral Structure

A major advantage of ultrasound is that it allows close correlation between the findings and the patient's symptoms. If there is uncertainty as to the significance of a particular finding, then comparison with the contralateral side should be made.

4.2.7 Dynamic Imaging

A major advantage of ultrasound is the ability to scan the joints, muscles and tendons in motion. This feature allows the patient to reproduce their signs and symptoms during the scan. In certain conditions such as the external snapping hip, peroneal tendon subluxation or muscle herniation the abnormality may only be visualised dynamically (Choi et al. 2002; Neustadter et al. 2004; Beggs 2003). Ultrasound can also assess the stability of a joint when the stabilising ligaments are injured (Ebrahim et al. 2006) and can aid treatment planning in tendon ruptures (Kotnis et al. 2006).

4.2.8 Examining Tendons in Relaxation and Contraction

Tendons may need to be examined in relaxed and contracted states. For example, the patella tendon may have a lax appearance and suffer from anisotropy (see Sect. 4.3 for definition) when examined with the knee extended. In the flexed position, however, when the tendon is stretched, abnormal vascularity may be underestimated due to compression of vessels. Thus, if Doppler interrogation is performed it should be with the tendon in the relaxed state.

4.3 Tendon

Tendons have the greatest tensile strength of all connective tissue due to the high collagen content of the fibres, and their closely packed parallel arrangement in the direction of force. Tendons have a hierarchical structure with individual collagen fibrils arranged into fascicles which contain blood vessels and nerve fibres enclosed by the epitendon (Benjamin and Ralphs 1997; Kannus 2000).

Tendons are classified into two types:

- Type 1 tendons are long and cross at least one joint before they attach. They may course over and around bony structures and at these locations are invariably covered by a synovial sheath comprised of visceral and parietal layers. The visceral layer is intimately attached to the tendon surface and moves with the tendon. The parietal layer is a lax covering that blends with the visceral layer at the periphery of the tendon sheath to become the mesotendon, which contains the tendon vessels. The synovial sheath has the function of decreasing the friction between the tendon and the adjacent structures allowing smooth excursion of the tendon. A small amount of fluid may be present within the tendon sheath. Certain tendon sheaths may communicate with adjacent joints, in which case excess joint fluid may result in distension of the tendon sheath. A good example of this is the flexor hallucis longus tendon, which often communicates with the tibiotalar joint.
- Type 2 tendons are thicker and have a straight course. They lack a synovial sheath and instead have a peritendon which forms a loose connective tissue envelope, lubricated by fluid that allows the tendon to glide freely. The patellar tendon and Achilles tendon are good examples.

The ultrasound appearance of tendons in children is similar to that of adults, except that in children the tendons attach to the hypoechoic cartilage surrounding the ossification centre of the bone rather than the bone itself (Fig. 4.1). Normal tendons ap-

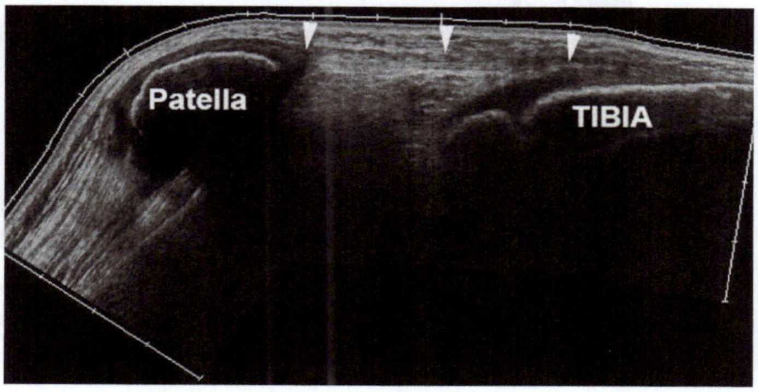

Fig. 4.1. Longitudinal extended field-of-view image demonstrating the normal patellar tendon in a 10-year-old child. Note the fibrillar echogenic texture of tendon which inserts onto low echogenicity cartilage

pear hyperechoic with a fibrillar echotexture when examined perpendicular to the beam (Fornage and Rifkin 1988). When tendon fibres are visualised oblique to the beam, there is decreased reflection of the beam and the tendon appears more hypoechoic (Fornage 1987). This phenomenon is described as anisotropy and may be misinterpreted as pathology. In practice, slight rocking of the transducer back and forth should allow differentiation of true pathology from artefact. Stretching the tendon may also improve visualisation.

4.4 Muscle

The function of muscle is to generate a force on contraction, either to maintain or change the position of a joint. There are two main types of muscle fibres: Type 1 (slow twitch), which allow sustained low energy contraction, and Type 2 (fast twitch), which allow rapid forceful contractions. Muscles are comprised of varying proportions of both types of fibres. Postural muscles are composed mainly of Type 1 fibres, with a predominantly linear arrangement of fibres, whereas non-postural muscles tend to have a higher proportion of Type 2 fibres, often within a pennate (feather-like) arrangement. Histologically muscles are composed of individual fibres that are grouped together to form fascicles which are enveloped by connective tissue referred to as endomysium. The fascicles in turn are surrounded by fibroadipose septa, known as perimysium which contains adipose tissue, vessels and nerves. Finally the entire muscle is surrounded by a fascial sheath or epimysium.

In the longitudinal plane muscle fascicles appear as multiple parallel low echogenicity lines, separated by echogenic fibroadipose connective tissue or perimysium (Fornage et al. 1983; Fornage 2000). In pennate muscle the parallel lines course obliquely to converge onto an echogenic myotendinous junction or aponeurosis. In the transverse plane the perimysium appears as multiple hyperechoic dots and short lines interspersed between the low echogenicity muscle fascicles. The septae are susceptible to anisotropy due to their linear configuration. During contraction ultrasound demonstrates changes in the muscle shape and length, with a change in the orientation of the echogenic striae representing the perimysium. The vascular supply to muscles is very rich with large variations seen in Doppler flow according to the level of exercise (Newman et al. 1997) (Figs. 4.2, 4.3).

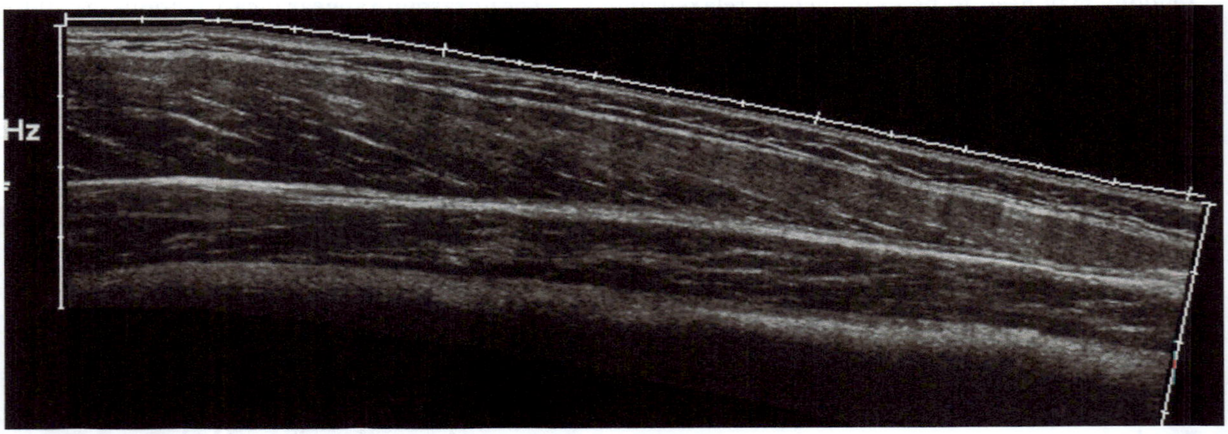

Fig. 4.2. Longitudinal extended field-of-view image demonstrating the normal quadriceps muscles in a 9-year-old child. Note the pennate appearance. The echogenic striae represent the perimysium surrounding the low echogenicity muscle fibres

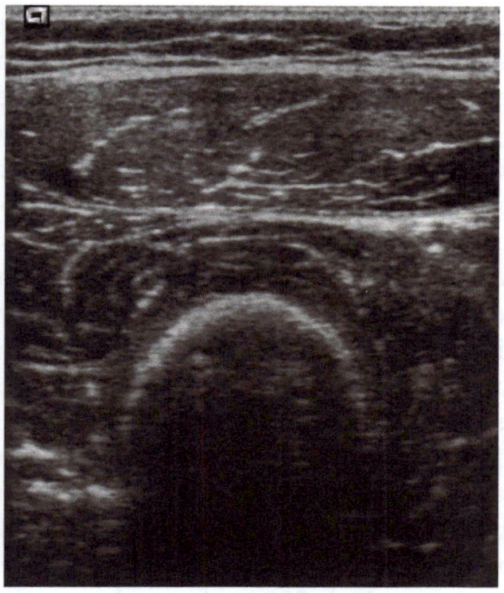

Fig. 4.3. Transverse ultrasound scan demonstrating the normal appearance of the quadriceps muscles. The perimysium appears as echogenic dots and lines

4.5 Ligament

Ligaments are cord-like or flattened peri-articular structures that join articular bone ends. They keep joints in optimal alignment during motion limiting excessive wear, and prevent excessive joint excursion, thus preventing subluxation or dislocation. Ligaments may blend in with the joint capsule or lie away from the capsule and appear as distinct structures. Ligaments may be comprised of more than one bundle, such as the anterior cruciate ligament (ACL), with the different bundles being subject to varying tension in different joint positions. The ultrasound appearance of ligaments is similar to tendons, appearing as a hyperechoic structure with a fibrillar echotexture. As with tendons, ligaments are prone to anisotropy (Fig. 4.4).

4.6 Principles of Musculoskeletal Injury

Musculoskeletal injuries in children fall into three main groups: Accidental trauma such as road traffic accidents and falls, non-accidental injury (NAI) and sport related injury. For each of these groups specific injury patterns can be recognised that are unique to the growing skeleton.

The force generated by muscle contraction is transmitted to bone by tendons, with the muscle-tendon-bone combination forming a functional unit which can be referred to as the musculoskeletal chain. There are important differences between the child, the young adult and the mature adult which account for the different injury patterns that are encountered (Harris 1981). In children, the weak links in the musculoskeletal chain are at the bone-tendon interface and at the growth plate, which accounts for the high occurrence of apophyseal avulsion injuries

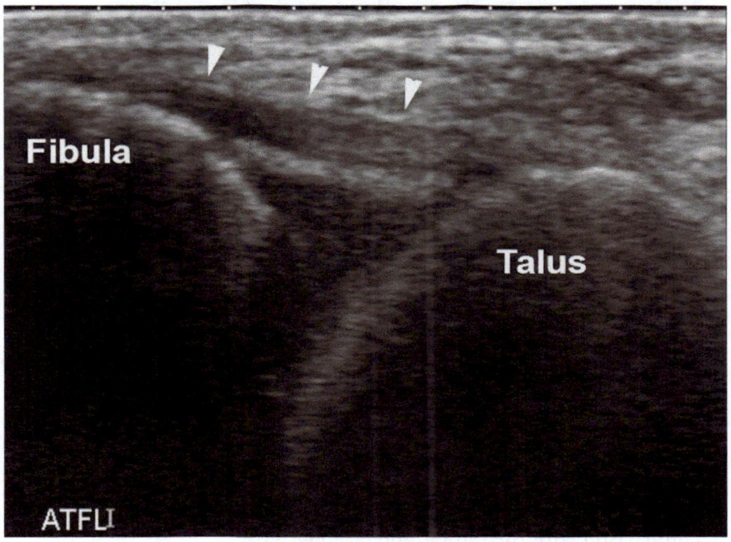

Fig. 4.4. Ultrasound of the normal anterior talo-fibular ligament. Note the fibrillar echogenic structure. The proximal portion of the ligament is of lower echogenicity due to anisotropy

and Salter-Harris type fractures. In the young adult and athletes the main region of weakness is at the myotendinous junction where the transition zone between muscle and tendon is relatively inelastic. In the mature skeleton the main weakness is within the tendon itself which is prone to degeneration.

4.7 Bony Injury

4.7.1 Diametaphyseal Injuries

Immature bone is more vascularised and less mineralised than mature bone, leading to a difference in biomechanical properties, with increased elasticity and plasticity, and the ability to deform. Immature bone may therefore buckle or bend under tension, leading to greenstick, torus or plastic bowing fractures. Radiography is the mainstay of imaging but several researchers have shown that ultrasound may be used for the detection of uncomplicated diaphyseal greenstick fractures of the long bones (Williamson et al. 2000; Hubner et al. 2000). The disadvantage of ultrasound is that it is unreliable for the detection of non-displaced Salter Harris I fractures and for detecting fracture lines of less than 1 mm in width (Hubner et al. 2000). Furthermore, ultrasound is unable to give an overview of the entire bone and adjacent joints.

Fractures in the region of the elbow can be particularly difficult to diagnose and delineate accurately. Ultrasound has been shown to be a useful adjunct to plain radiography, particularly if clinical suspicion is high and radiographs are indeterminate (Davidson et al. 1994; Markowitz et al. 1992; Vocke-Hell and Schmid 2001). With supracondylar fractures of the humerus, ultrasound may demonstrate the fracture line in association with a joint effusion and elevation of the fat pads (Figs. 4.5, 4.6).

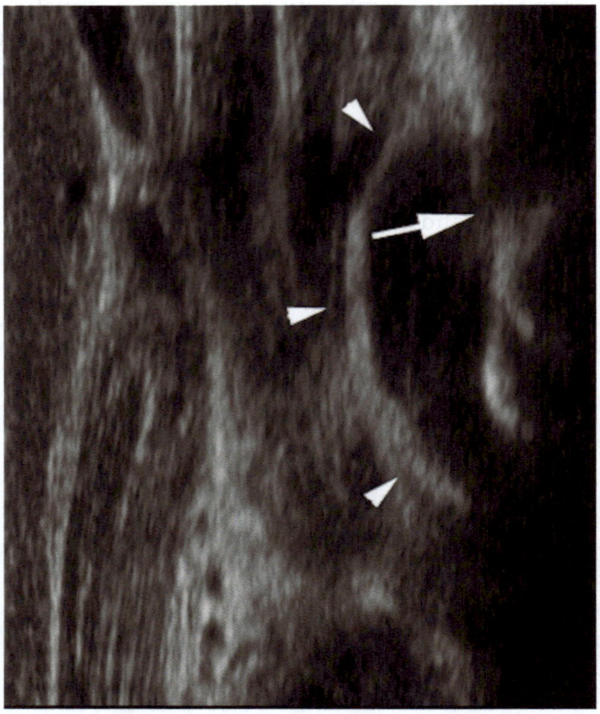

Fig. 4.5. Longitudinal image of the distal humerus in a child following trauma. There is distension of the elbow joint (*arrowheads*) with loss of cortical continuity (*arrow*) in the supracondylar region. The image has been rotated to allow comparison with the radiograph (see Fig. 4.6)

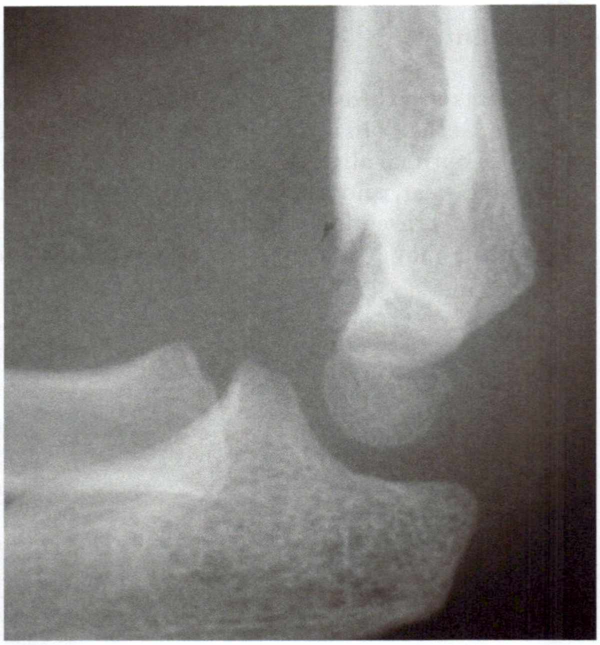

Fig. 4.6. Lateral radiograph of the elbow confirms the diagnosis of a supracondylar fracture

4.7.2 Epiphyseal Injuries

Growth plate injuries are commonest in the older child and adolescent age group, probably due to a combination of weakening of the growth plate at puberty and the increased risk of high impact trauma. The injury may lead to growth disturbance and resultant bone or joint deformity. Growth plate injuries can usually be demonstrated on plain radiographs, with epiphyseal displacement and widening of the growth plate. In young children, however, the injured unossified epiphysis may be missed on radiographs. In young children with elbow trauma, ultrasound has been shown to be helpful in the diagnosis of avulsion of the unossified medial epicondyle (Davidson et al 1994; Markowitz et al. 1992). Ultrasound has also been used to differentiate stable from unstable lateral condyle fractures of the humerus in children. If the fracture of the lateral condyle extends through the articular cartilage it is considered unstable, and requires surgical fixation (Vocke-Hell and Schmid 2001). A slipped upper femoral epiphysis may present with an effusion and hip pain, ultrasound examination of the femoral epiphyseal-metaphyseal contour may reveal a step or separation (Castriota-Scanderbeg and Orsi 1993).

4.7.3 Non-accidental Injury

Non-accidental injury (NAI) is covered in greater detail in a separate chapter. It is incumbent upon all professionals working with children to be vigilant for NAI, particularly if the history and proposed mechanism of injury does not correlate with the findings. There are certain fracture types that are more suggestive of NAI, such as rib and metaphyseal fractures, for which radiographs are the mainstay of imaging (Rao and Carty 1999). Multiple fractures of differing ages are also highly suspicious. In certain circumstances, if radiographs are equivocal ultrasound can be used to examine the suspected region of injury. Ultrasound can demonstrate displacement or injury of the perichondrial ring which is encountered in NAI (Markowitz et al. 1993). Costo-chondral dislocation has also been demonstrated on ultrasound in a case of child abuse (Smeets et al. 1990). With subacute and chronic injuries ultrasound may demonstrate a periosteal reaction (Figs. 4.7, 4.8).

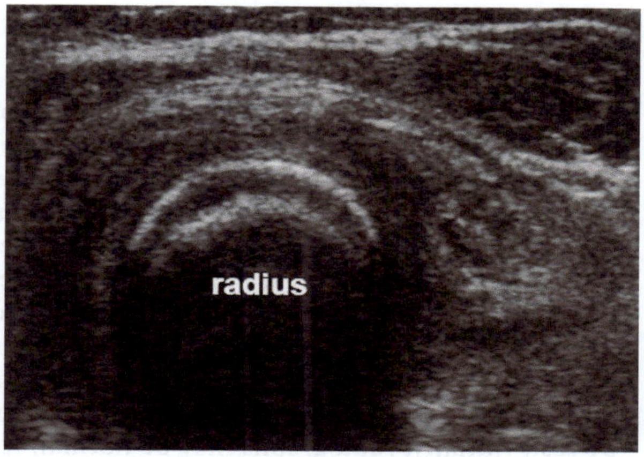

Fig. 4.7. Transverse sonogram of the radial shaft demonstrates a double cortical ring due to an established periosteal reaction in a child aged 2

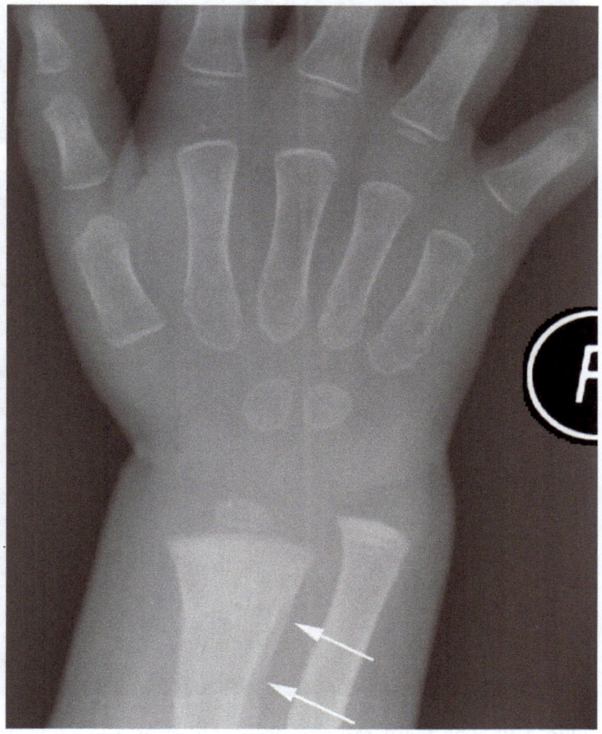

Fig. 4.8. Plain radiograph of the wrist demonstrates thep-eriosteal reaction initially detected on ultrasound

4.7.4 Stress Fractures

With the increasing demands being placed on young athletes, stress fractures are being seen more frequently. Stress fractures occur as a result of excessive mechanical loading on normal bone, mainly occurring in the lower limb between the ages of 15 to 19. Girls are more often affected than boys. Common sites of stress fractures are the tibial shaft, proximal femur and calcaneus (Sofka 2006). The typical history is of an athletic adolescent presenting with pain that is relieved by rest. Initially, radiographs may be normal. After about 2 weeks following the onset of pain a periosteal reaction and a sclerotic fracture line may be demonstrated. In some cases there is a florid periosteal reaction leading to a wide differential diagnosis including infection, osteoid osteoma and eosinophilic granuloma. If a stress fracture is suspected and the radiographs are normal, MR Imaging or an isotope bone scan are the investigations of choice. Ultrasound can, however, suggest the diagnosis as it may demonstrate a break in the cortex with associated periosteal reaction (Bodner et al. 2005). There may be an associated subperiosteal haematoma and an increase in vascularity (Figs. 4.9–4.11).

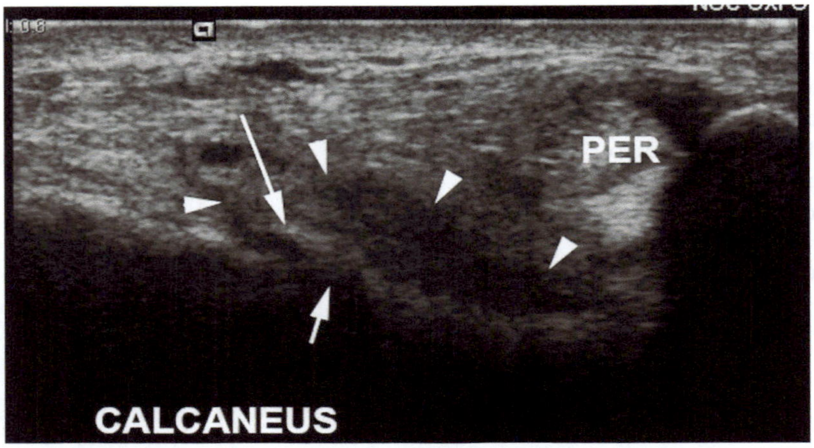

Fig. 4.9. Ultrasound of the lateral aspect of the ankle demonstrates a break in the cortical margin of the calcaneus (*short arrow*) with associated hypoechoic haematoma (*arrowheads*) and periosteal reaction (*long arrow*) in a 15-year-old athlete. The echogenic peroneal tendons (*PER*) are seen in cross-section as they course around the lateral malleolus

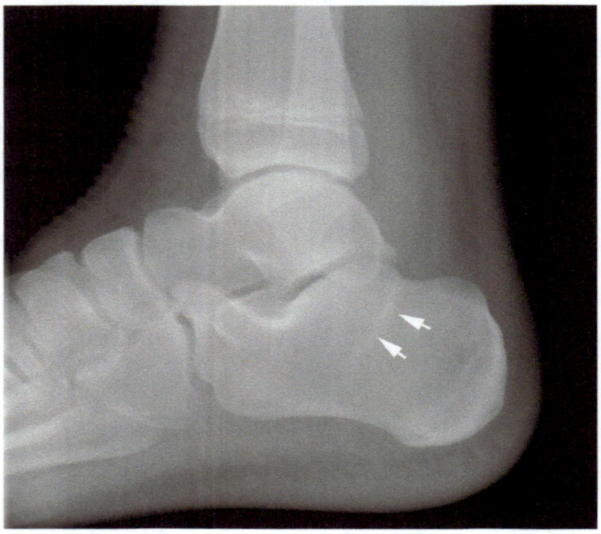

Fig. 4.10. The plain radiograph obtained on the same day as the ultrasound scan shows a sclerotic stress fracture line (*arrows*)

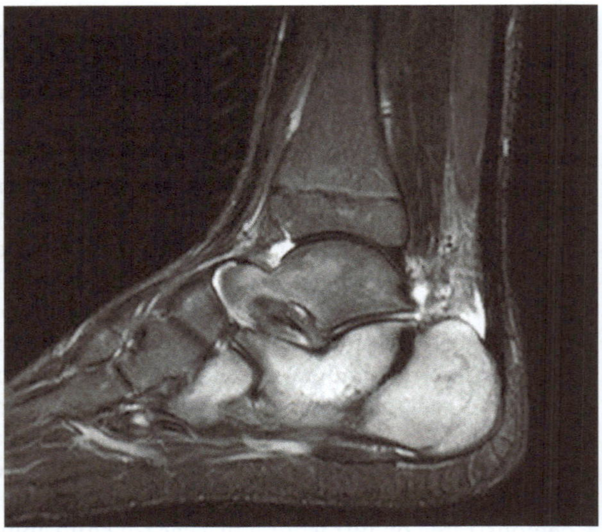

Fig. 4.11.. Subsequent MRI with a sagittal short tau inversion recovery (STIR) sequence demonstrates a calcaneal stress fracture with surrounding bone marrow oedema.

4.7.5 Acute Osteochondral Injury

Acute osteochondral injuries occur as a consequence of abnormal joint motion, leading to shearing or impaction of opposing joint surfaces. If the resulting fracture is purely chondral the fragment will not be visible on radiographs. MR Imaging (with or without arthrography) is the modality of choice for the detection and staging of osteochondral injuries as it can depict marrow oedema, assess the morphology of articular cartilage and detect loose bodies (RUBIN 1998). In young children, however, ultrasound is much better tolerated than MR Imaging. On ultrasound detached osteochondral bodies demonstrate a hypoechoic rim of cartilage that is attached to a hyperechoic bony fragment. With acute injuries there is normally an associated effusion or haemarthrosis.

The osteochondroses are a group of conditions, many with eponymous names, characterised by defective bone formation in an epiphysis or apophysis. The exact aetiology is unknown but trauma is likely to be the initial insult followed by avascular necrosis. Radiographs are sufficient for making a diagnosis; however, MR Imaging may be required to assess for stability (DE SMET et al. 1990; DE SMET et al. 1996). Ultrasound may be used to diagnose some disorders such as Legg-Calve-Perthes' (SUZUKI et al. 1987; WINGSTRAND 1999).

4.8 Tendon Injury

A broad spectrum of tendon disorders may be encountered in children, although these are less frequently seen than in adults. Because the weak link in the musculoskeletal chain in children is at the attachment of the tendon to the non-ossified cartilage, most injuries occur at this site rather than within the tendon itself. Degenerative changes and tendon ruptures are therefore rare in children.

4.8.1 Acute Apophyseal Injuries

An apophysis is a bony protuberance or growth centre where a tendon attaches to bone. Before the apophysis fuses, its cartilaginous growth plate is the point of greatest weakness in the musculoskeletal chain when a tensile force is applied. The apophysis is therefore prone to avulsion in children, particularly adolescents.

Most apophyseal avulsions occur about the pelvis (TEHRANZADEH 1987; STEVENS et al. 1999). The mechanism of avulsion injuries is a sudden, forceful contraction of a muscle or sudden, excessive stretching. In most cases, there is no direct trauma. The anterior inferior iliac spine, anterior superior iliac spine and ischial tuberosity are the commonest sites of injury (Table 4.1). The other sites include the iliac crest, lesser trochanter, greater trochanter and pubic symphysis. Acute apophyseal injuries can be visualised as well demarcated osseous fragments on plain radiography. With healing there may be mixed areas of sclerosis and lucency which may have an aggressive appearance that can be mistaken for infection or neoplasm (STEVENS et al. 1999). Abundant callus formation may occur which may eventually result in a large bony protuberance.

Ultrasound is more sensitive than radiography in the diagnosis of acute apophyseal injuries, particularly if the ossification centre is small or unossified. The spectrum of ultrasound appearances includes an irregular tendon attachment, small avulsed fragments with associated posterior acoustic shadowing, local haematoma and fissures in the cartilage (LAZOVIC et al. 1996). A key advantage of ultrasound over other imaging modalities is the ability to per-

Table 4.1.

Apophysis	Muscle attachment
Ischial tuberosity	Hamstrings
Anterior inferior iliac spine (AIIS)	Rectus femoris
Anterior superior iliac spine (ASIS)	Sartorius, tensor fascia lata
Greater trochanter (GT)	Gluteals
Lesser trochanter (LT)	Iliopsoas
Iliac crest	Abdominal obliques, Latissimus dorsi
Pubic symphysis (PS)	Adductors

form dynamic assessment to assess stability of the fragment (Figs. 4.12, 4.13).

Sleeve avulsion fractures are a particular form of avulsion injury seen in the unossified skeleton which differs from avulsions in adults because the sleeve of periosteum which is pulled off can continue to form bone if not treated. The typical location is at the lower pole of the patella, but the upper pole of the patella, the olecranon and the medial epicondyle can also be affected. Ultrasound demonstrates a sleeve of cartilage that has been avulsed usually with a small fragment of bone (Hunt and Somashekar 2005). In some cases a double cortical sign may be present, indicating elevation of a superficial layer of cortex from the underlying bone. There may be associated haemarthrosis and patella alta (Fig. 4.14).

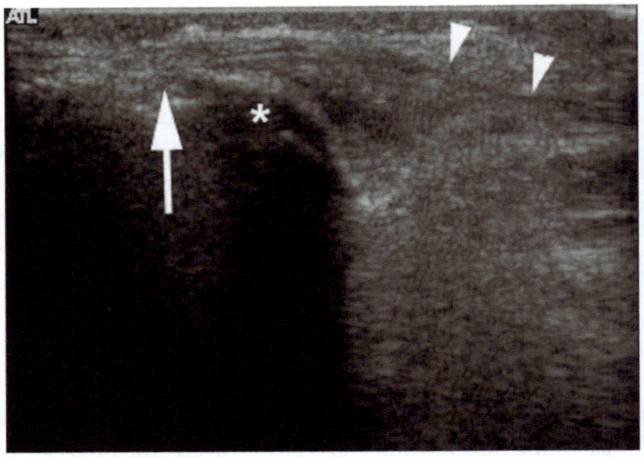

Fig. 4.12. Ultrasound demonstrating avulsion (*arrow*) of the anterior inferior iliac spine (*asterisk*) which is attached to the rectus femoris tendon (*arrowheads*)

4.8.2 Chronic Overuse Injuries

Tendons are visco-elastic structures and exhibit adaptive responses to stress. When excessive cyclical loading is applied to a tendon it may be unable to recover and adapt, leading to repeated microtrauma to the physis with avulsion of cartilaginous and bony fragments.

In children the most commonly involved sites for overuse injury are at the insertions of the patella tendon. Overuse injury to the distal patella tendon insertion results in Osgood Schlatter's disease. Boys are affected more than girls. The diagnosis is often made on clinical grounds alone, with tenderness and swelling over the tibial tuberosity. On ultrasound there is soft tissue swelling around the tibial tuberosity with swelling of the cartilage at the apophysis and thickening of the distal patella tendon (De Flaviis et al. 1989). There may be distension of the deep infra patella bursa. As the condition progresses there is bony fragmentation due to recurrent micro avulsions. Small splits in the tendon may be seen. On Doppler interrogation there is increased vascularity (Fig. 4.15). Similar appearances may be appreciated at the proximal patellar tendon insertion, with the condition referred to as Sindig-Larson-Johansen syndrome (De Flaviis et al. 1989).

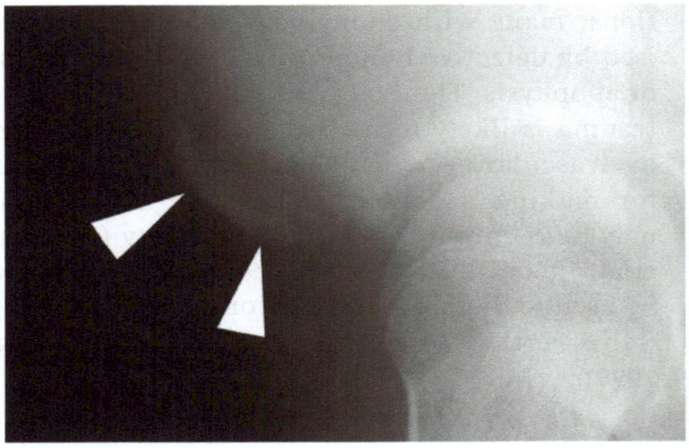

Fig. 4.13. A radiograph confirms the avulsion (*arrowheads*) seen in Figure 4.18

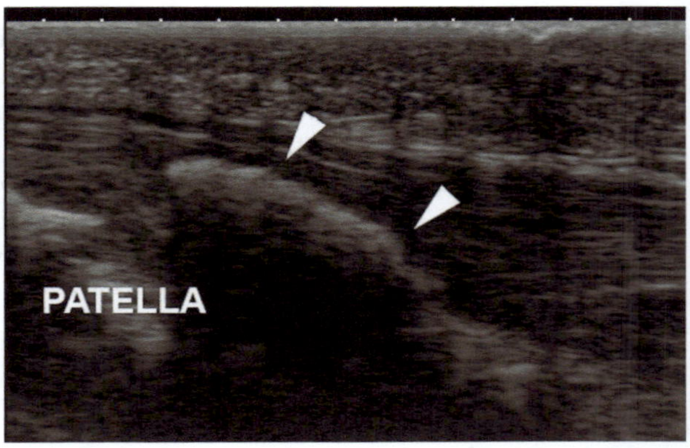

Fig. 4.14. Ultrasound demonstrating a patellar sleeve avulsion (*arrowheads*) from the inferior pole of the patella

4.8.3 Intrinsic Tendon Pathology

Unlike adult tendons which are prone to degeneration, intrinsic tendon abnormality is unusual

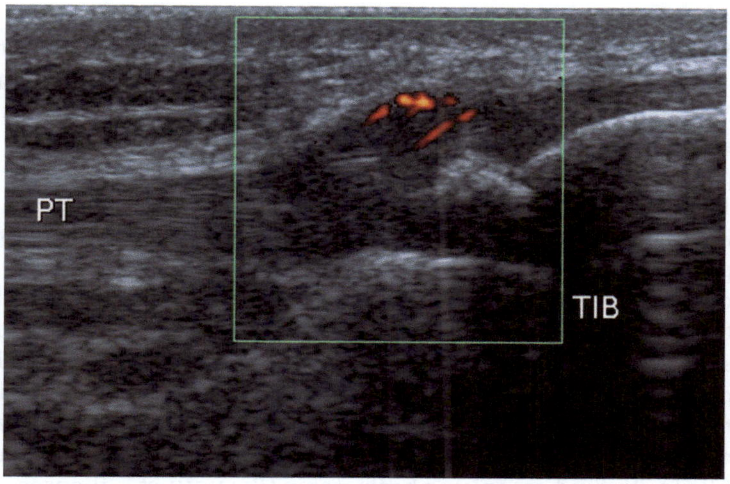

Fig. 4.15. Ultrasound demonstrating Osgood Schlatter's disease with focal swelling of the distal patellar tendon (*PT*) and increased flow on Doppler interrogation

in children. "Tendinopathy" is the generic term that is used for tendon disease, irrespective of aetiology. The term "tendonitis" implies an inflammatory aetiology, whereas "tendinosis" refers to mucoid degeneration of the tendon, normally as a result of chronic overuse, with recurrent microtears, regeneration and scarring. Inflammatory change of the synovial sheath surrounding the tendon is referred to as "tenosynovitis", whereas inflammatory change in the paratendon is called "paratendonitis".

In children, tendinosis usually occurs as a result of altered biomechanics such as a clubfoot deformity or gait disturbance. Tendinosis may also occur as a result of overuse injury, with the classic example being "jumper's knee", which is focal tendinosis of the proximal patellar tendon. The characteristic ultrasound appearance of tendinosis is thickening of the tendon with decreased echogenicity, which can be focal or diffuse (Fornage 2000; Campbell and Grainger 2001). There may be loss of the normal fibrillar echotexture in association with longitudinal splits. With Type 1 tendons, there may also be associated synovial thickening and fluid within the surrounding tendon sheath indicating associated tenosynovitis. On Doppler interrogation there is usually increased vascularity within the tendon and the adjacent tissues (Fig. 4.16).

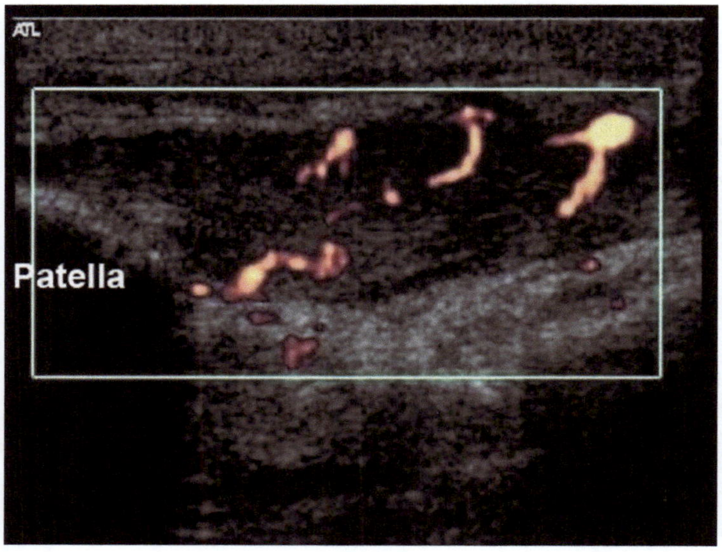

Fig. 4.16. Power Doppler ultrasound demonstrating focal swelling of the proximal patellar tendon with marked vascularity, consistent with jumper's knee

4.8.4 Tendon Rupture

Most tendon ruptures in children occur as part of an avulsion injury, but trauma, either indirect or penetrating, can result in intrinsic tendon tears. The most commonly encountered tendon ruptures in children are the finger tendons, the Achilles and patellar tendons. Predisposing conditions for tendon rupture including steroid use, diabetes, renal failure and inflammatory arthropathy. As with avulsion injuries, ultrasound has an important role in delineating the position of the tendon ends as part of treatment planning. The typical ultrasound features of tendon rupture are a gap in the tendon which is filled with fluid organising haematoma (Bianchi et al. 2005). Gentle passive flexion and extension of the adjacent joint may reveal widening of the gap in full thickness tears. It is often useful to mark the position of the tendon ends on the skin with indelible ink to help surgical planning.

4.8.5 Peroneal Tendon Subluxation

Rupture of the superior peroneal retinaculum, which extends from the lateral aspect of the distal fibular to the calcaneus, may result in peroneal tendon subluxation. Sometimes there is an associated avulsion fracture of the lateral aspect of the distal fibula. Typically, the patient will complain of painful clicking of the ankle, particularly on dorsiflexion and eversion of the foot. The diagnosis is often obvious clinically but a dynamic ultrasound may be required to confirm the diagnosis and determine if there is underlying tendinopathy (Neustadter et al. 2004; Diaz et al. 1998) (Fig. 4.17).

4.8.6 Snapping Hip

The snapping hip is a common condition affecting young athletes. The cause may be intra-articular abnormality or extra-articular. Intra-articular abnormalities, such as labral tears, usually require MR arthrography for full evaluation. However, extra-articular causes such as a snapping iliotibial band or iliopsoas tendon are particularly well evaluated by dynamic ultrasound (Choi et al. 2002). In some subjects the iliopsoas tendon does not glide smoothly over the iliopectineal eminence but rather moves with an abrupt jerk (Cardinal et al. 1996; Pelsser et al. 2001). Similarly, the iliotibial band may flip abruptly over the greater trochanter, demonstrating a change in morphology on hip flexion. There may be associated bursitis in some cases.

4.9 Muscle Injury

Muscle injuries are relatively uncommon in children. Muscle injuries may be direct (e.g. muscle contusion) or indirect (e.g. muscle strain or tear).

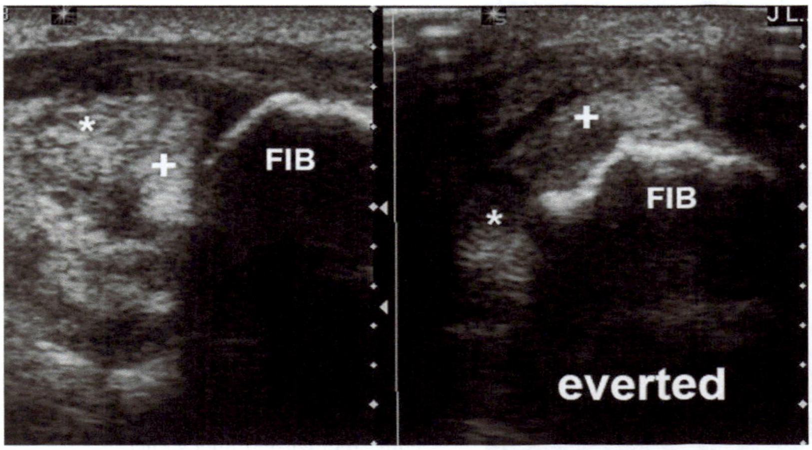

Fig. 4.17. Peroneal subluxation on dynamic ultrasound examination. The peroneus brevis (+) and peroneus longus (*) are seen to flip over the distal fibula with the foot everted

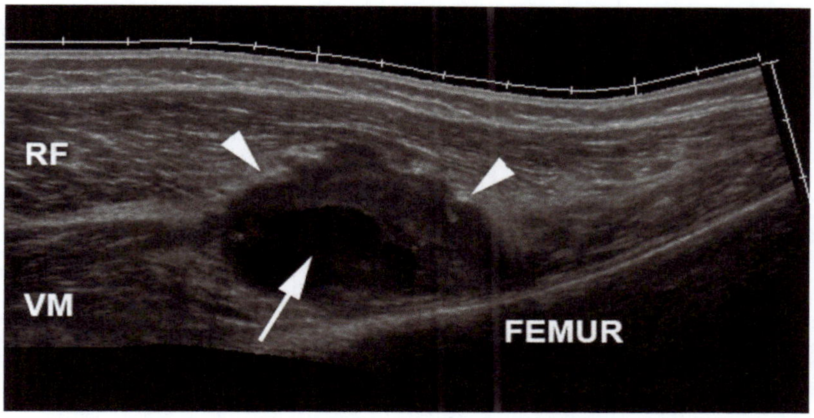

Fig. 4.18. Extended field-of-view ultrasound demonstrates a mass-like organising haematoma following contusion involving the vastus intermedius (*VM*) and rectus femoris (*RF*) muscles. The arrowheads indicate the margins of the echogenic organising haematoma which surround a fluid collection (*arrow*)

4.9.1 Direct Muscle Injury

4.9.1.1 Muscle Contusion

Muscle contusion is the result of direct compressive force upon the muscle, often during sporting activity or accidents, resulting in disruption of muscle fibres and formation of haematoma (Aspelin et al. 1992). The main pathological process is the formation of haematoma, which starts to organise at between 48–72 h. The injury can be clinically graded into mild (when joint movement is more than two thirds of the normal range), moderate (when joint movement is between a third and two thirds of normal) and severe (when joint movement is restricted to less than a third of normal). Acute contusion (within 48 h) appears as an ill defined area of muscle swelling with increased echogenicity, with loss of normal fascicular definition. At 2–3 days after the initial insult the contusion develops a better defined echogenic margin, with the haematoma appearing of low echogenicity. Over the following weeks the echogenic periphery fills in centripetally with regeneration of muscle and scarring. The haematoma can have the appearance of a complex ovoid mass with internal septations (Fig. 4.18 and Fig. 4.19).

4.9.1.2 Muscle Laceration

Muscle laceration occurs as a result of direct penetrating injury. The laceration fills with haematoma which appears of low echogenicity (Fornage 2000). There is a high risk of scar formation.

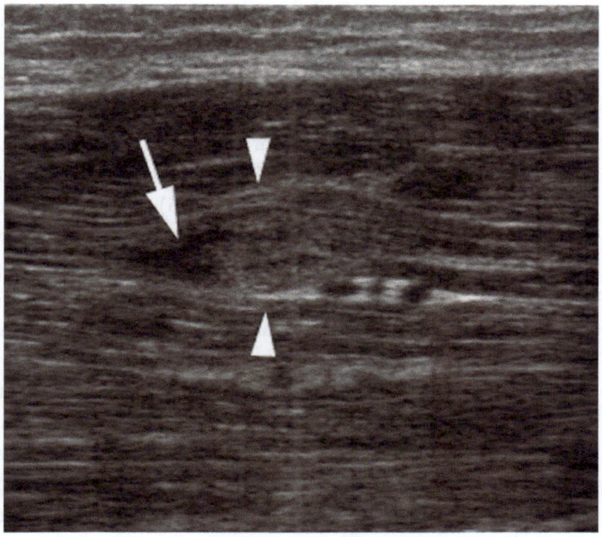

Fig. 4.19. Ultrasound demonstrates an acute grade I injury (less than 5%) of the vastus medialis (*arrow*) with minor bunching up of the muscle fibres (*arrowheads*)

4.9.2 Indirect Injury

4.9.2.1 Delayed Onset Muscle Soreness

Delayed onset muscle soreness (DOMS) usually occurs 12–24 h following strenuous unaccustomed exercise. It is thought that the cause is damage to the muscle fascicles, particularly at the myotendinous junction. The diagnosis is made on clinical grounds but imaging plays an important role in excluding significant muscle injury. On ultrasound there is usually no abnormality; however, on MR Imaging diffuse muscle oedema has been described (Evans et al. 1998). The condition is usually self-limiting, with the symptoms usually resolving by 1 week.

4.9.2.2
Muscle Tear

A muscle tear or strain occurs due to excessive tensile force being applied across the muscle. Muscles with a high proportion of Type 2 fibres are prone to this form of injury as they generate the greatest forces, with the rectus femoris and hamstring muscles being particularly affected (Noonan and Garrett 1999). The myotendinous junction is the most common region to be injured followed by the junction of the muscle fibres with the epimysium (Noonan and Garrett 1992; Takebayashi et al. 1995).

There are three grades of muscle injury on imaging (Takebayashi et al. 1995; Rybak and Torriani 2003; Rehman and Robinson 2005). On ultrasound Grade I injuries have a normal appearance or less than 5% disruption of muscle volume. Haemorrhage may lead to an area of ill defined increased echogenicity. Grade II injuries are partial tears involving greater than 5% of muscle volume. Initially there is echogenic haematoma but within 24 h oedema and inflammatory infiltrate renders the injury hypoechoic (Fornage et al. 1983; Fornage 2000). As the haematoma organises an echogenic rim forms, which gradually fills in over a number of weeks. Grade III injuries are complete tears with bunching of the muscle on stressing with complete loss of function. The "bell-clapper" sign may be apparent on stressing, referring to the contracted muscle belly surrounded by low echogenicity fluid rim tracking along the fascia (Fig. 4.20).

4.9.3
Rhabdomyolysis

Rhabdomyolysis, or muscle necrosis, is a rare consequence of trauma that leads to systemic release of injured cellular contents of affected muscles. The condition may occur as a result of prolonged pressure in an unconscious patient or be a consequence of burns, infection or crush injury. In the acute phase ultrasound may demonstrate muscle oedema and with patchy areas of heterogeneous altered echogenicity with loss of the normal architecture (Fornage 2000; Fornage and Nerot 1986). There is usually associated muscle swelling and increased vascularity. Later on the lesion may appear more hypoechoic and develop fluid filled collections.

4.9.4
Complications of Muscle Injury

4.9.4.1
Scar

Scar decreases the ability of the muscle to contract effectively. On ultrasound scar appears as linear or stellate echogenic tissue which is surrounded by relatively normal muscle (Fornage 2000). On dynamic examination there is loss of elasticity of the involved tissue which may appear tethered. Occasionally, this tethering may involve adjacent nerves resulting in referred pain.

4.9.4.2
Myositis Ossificans

Myositis ossificans occurs as a rare complication of muscle injury that is associated with a large haematoma. Typically, the lesion occurs in the adoles-

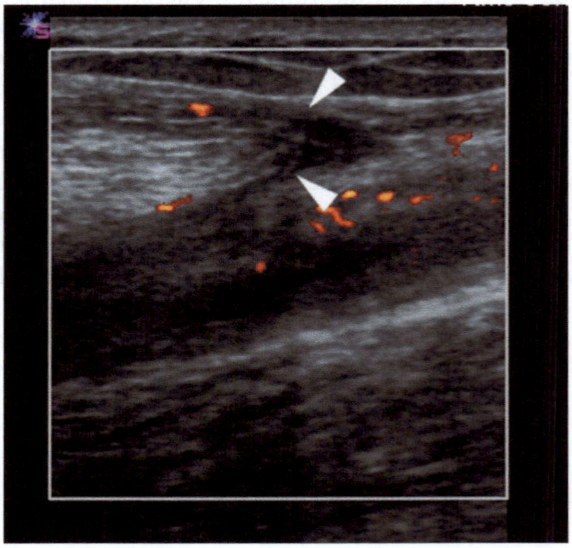

Fig. 4.20. Ultrasound demonstrates a subacute grade III (full thickness) tear of the rectus femoris muscle with retraction (arrowheads). There is increased flow on power Doppler as part of a reparative process.

cent or young adult, presenting as a painful lump following trauma. There may be no history of significant trauma. The condition is characterised by heterotopic bone formation, which is develops within the haematoma. Before the bony mineralisation develops the appearance is that of an organising haematoma with marked associated muscle oedema and swelling. On Doppler interrogation there is increased vascularity both within the lesion and in the surrounding tissues. The mass-like appearance is therefore often mistaken for a sarcoma on all imaging modalities (Shirkhoda et al. 1995). The decision to biopsy has to take into consideration the clinical and imaging features, but it should be noted that the histology of early lesions may contain immature cells and mitotic bodies that mimic malignancy. Over the next few weeks, highly specific, well defined peripheral mineralisation develops which can be detected on ultrasound before plain radiographs (Fornage 2000; Fornage and Eftekhari 1989). The mineralisation appears as hyperechoic foci with posterior acoustic shadowing, usually aligned parallel to the diaphysis. The condition usually resolves spontaneously, although mature ossification in the muscles may persist for years following resolution of symptoms (Figs. 4.21 and 4.22).

4.9.4.3
Muscle Hernia

A muscle hernia is a protrusion of muscle through a defect in the epimysium. There is often a previous history of trauma or surgery. Patients present with a palpable lump that may become more apparent and/or painful on standing or exercise. The commonest affected site is the lower leg, particularly the tibialis anterior muscle which has an intrinsic weakness in its overlying fascia due to penetrating vessels and nerves. When examining a patient for a suspected muscle hernia, particular care must be taken to avoid excessive compression with the probe which may reduce the hernia. A copious amount of jelly can be used as a standoff in this situation. It often helps to examine the limb with the patient standing or following a bout of exercise. The herniation may appear as hypoechoic lump with loss of the normal fibrillar echotexture with a hypoechoic

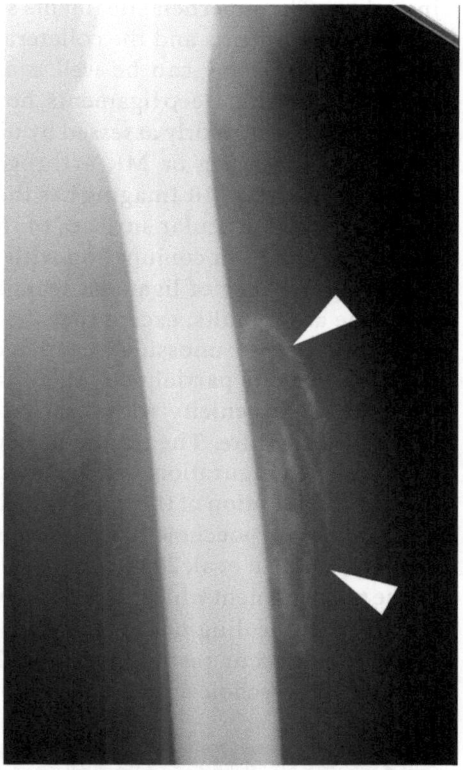

Fig. 4.22. Plain radiograph confirms the presence of myositis ossificans seen in Fig. 4.21

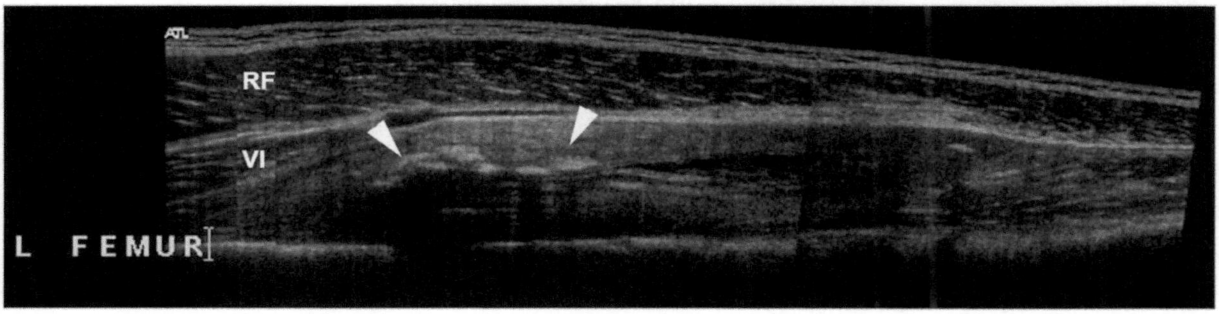

Fig. 4.21. EFOV ultrasound demonstrates well defined ossification (arrowheads) in the vastus intermedius (VI) muscle, with posterior acoustic shadowing consistent with myositis ossificans

gap seen in the echogenic epimysium (Beggs 2003) (Fig. 4.23).

4.10 Ligament Injuries

Ligament injuries affecting the immature skeleton usually occur in the adolescents as a result of sporting injury. The superficial ligaments such as the lateral ankle ligaments and the collateral ligaments of the knee and elbow can be well evaluated by dynamic ultrasound. Deep ligaments, however, such as the cruciates, are poorly assessed by ultrasound and require MR Imaging or MR arthrography for detailed assessment. MR Imaging has the advantage of visualising the articular surfaces of the joint which are often injured in conjunction with ligaments.

The appearance of ligament tears in children is the same as in adults, except that the fibres may be seen to attach to unossified cartilage rather than bone. With acute partial tears there is swelling and decreased echogenicity with loss of the normal fibrillar echotexture. The ligament, however, retains its straight configuration. With acute complete tears there is interruption of the ligament with the gap being filled by hypoechoic haematoma (Peetrons et al. 2004; Miller et al. 2004). There is loss of tension in the torn ligament which may have a wavy configuration. With healing of the ligament, scarring and fibrosis may occur resulting in a thickened hypoechoic or hyperechoic appearance. In other cases the ligament may appear thin and attenuated. Calcification may occur with ligament healing, a phenomenon that classically occurs at the proximal insertion of the medial collateral ligament (Pelligrini-Stieda lesion) (Figs. 4.24, 4.25).

Injury to the medial collateral ligament of the knee can be accurately delineated by ultrasound (Friedl and Glaser 1991; Lee et al. 1996). The normal medial collateral ligament is a thin homogeneous hypoechoic band. A sprained ligament is thickened and heterogeneously hypoechoic, with a tear appearing as a fissure traversing the ligament. Ultrasound has also been shown to be of value in assessing the medial retinacular complex following lateral patellar dislocation (O'Reilly et al. 2003). Several authors have shown that the PCL can be adequately assessed by ultrasound but MRI remains the examination of choice in evaluating the deeper ligaments of the knee. The normal PCL appears as a hypo-echoic band extending from the posterior tibial spine to the lateral aspect of the medial femoral condyle. An injured ligament appears oedematous with a heterogeneous hypoechoic echotexture, having a thicker appearance than on the contralateral side (Hsu et al. 2005; Cho et al. 2001).

Twisting injuries of the ankle in adolescents and young adults are a common cause for presentation to the Emergency Department. The ligament most prone to injury is the anterior talofibular ligament followed by the calcaneofibular ligament. Both of these structures are easily accessible by ultrasound which demonstrates intrinsic ligament injuries more frequently than physeal injuries or avulsions (Farley et al. 2001). Most acute ankle ligament

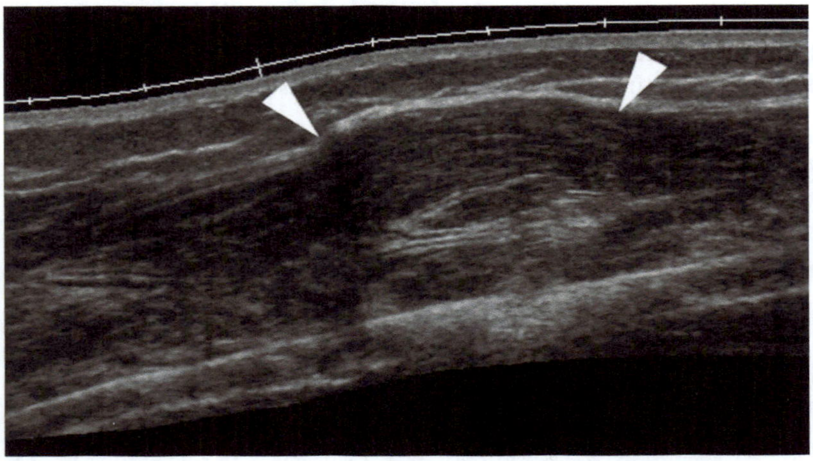

Fig. 4.23. Ultrasound demonstrating a small muscle hernia of the tibialis anterior on contraction, with a focal bulge in the normal contour (*arrowheads*)

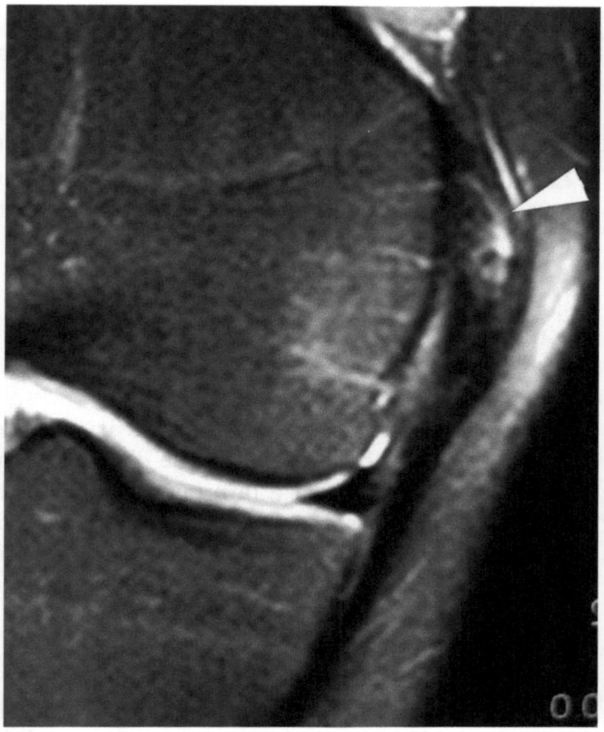

Fig. 4.24. Extended field-of-view ultrasound of the medial collateral ligament in a young adult with a Pelligrini Stieda lesion (*arrow*) following injury

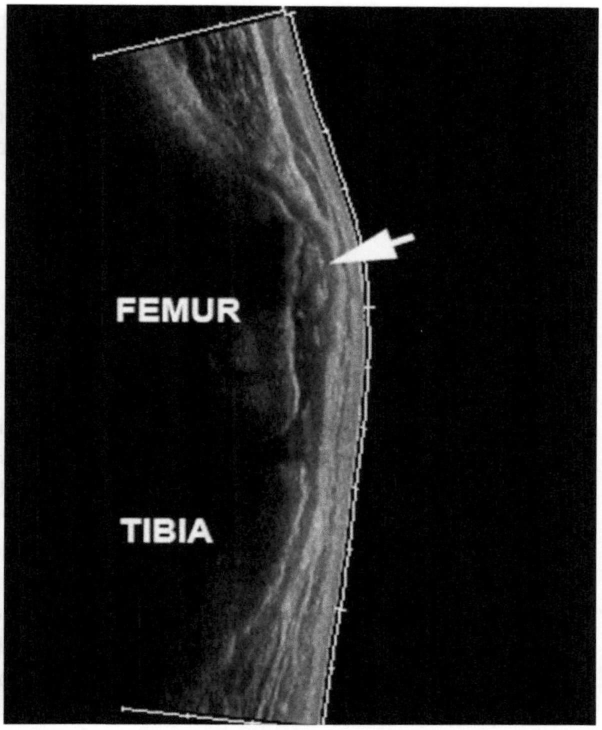

Fig. 4.25. Coronal proton density fat-saturated image demonstrating a heterogeneous swelling of the medial collateral ligament seen in Figure 4.21. Note that ultrasound demonstrates the calcification whereas MRI does not

sprains do not require imaging as the diagnosis can usually be made clinically. The decision to image the ankle ligaments is usually made on the basis of persistent pain, swelling or instability. Ultrasound can be used to detect tears of the lateral ligaments and also assess the degree of instability (Campbell et al. 1994) and exclude other causes of pain, such as anterolateral gutter impingement. MR Imaging, however, remains the investigation of choice, as it has the advantage of visualising the articular surfaces and excluding associated osteochondral lesions of the talar dome (Labovitz and Schweitzer 1998).

At the elbow, the ulnar collateral ligament complex is prone to injury in children and adolescents who undertake throwing activities, such as baseball pitchers and javelin throwers. With partial tears there is thickening and focal low echogenicity of the ligament with surrounding fluid (Miller et al. 2004). With full thickness tears there is a gap in the ligament with associated haematoma. Valgus stressing of the elbow may lead to widening of the ulno-trochlear joint (De Smet et al. 2002; Nazarian et al. 2003). Greater than 0.5 mm of opening suggests injury. Comparison with the contralateral side is extremely useful if there is uncertainty in the diagnosis. In some cases there is associated medial epicondylitis.

The pulled elbow is a common occurrence in toddlers. Classically, the child refuses to use the arm following a sudden pull, which results in the radial head slipping beneath the annular ligament. In most cases imaging is not necessary as the diagnosis can be made clinically and reduction is straightforward. If there is doubt, or there is failure to respond to manipulation, plain radiographs or ultrasound may be used to delineate the injury. Ultrasound may show an increase in the distance between the radial head and the capitellum (Kim et al. 2004; Kosuwon et al. 1993). In some cases the annular ligament may become trapped within the radiocapitellar joint and may be seen as an echogenic intra-articular structure.

Tears of the ulnar collateral ligament of the thumb, referred to as gamekeeper's or skier's thumb are frequently encountered as a result of skiing injury. The torn ligament may become interposed beneath the adductor aponeurosis resulting in the

Stener lesion, which requires surgery as healing by secondary intention will not occur. On ultrasound there is disruption of the ulnar collateral ligament with the Stener lesion appearing as a hypoechoic focal mass lying above the joint line (Ebrahim et al. 2006; O'Callaghan et al. 1994).

4.11 Foreign Bodies

Retained foreign bodies such as splinters and thorns in the extremities are a common clinical problem. The sensitivity of ultrasound has been shown to be higher than CT and MR Imaging for the detection of radio-opaque and non radio-opaque foreign bodies (Soudack et al. 2003). Foreign bodies usually appear as highly echogenic linear structures with posterior acoustic shadowing. Reverberation echoes may be present. There may be a surrounding hypo-echoic halo due to an inflammatory infiltrate or granulation tissue. On Doppler interrogation there may be increased vascularity in the tissues around the foreign body (Davae et al. 2003). If the foreign body penetrates a joint, this may lead to synovitis and effusion (Stevens et al. 2000) (Fig. 4.26).

4.12 Interventional Procedures

Ultrasound is an excellent modality for guiding interventional procedures of the musculoskeletal system as it allows real-time tracking of the needle position. In the context of musculoskeletal trauma the most common indications would be therapeutic injections for overuse injuries, aspiration of joint fluid and muscle haematomas and core biopsies to exclude sinister pathology. Specific injections are not discussed in detail here but an outline of technique is given below.

4.12.1 General Technique

A relaxed, child-friendly environment is a prerequisite. Informed consent should be obtained from the child/main carer, at a minimum outlining the risks of pain, allergy and infection. In children biopsies may require sedation or general anaesthetic, but most simple procedures are well tolerated under local anaesthetic given the right conditions. Ideally a parent should be present.

Topical anaesthetic cream can be applied over the site of entry up to 1 h before the procedure. The injection trolley should be prepared out of sight of the child and if possible the child should not see the needle, so that future needle phobia is avoided.

A 22-G needle can be used for most therapeutic injections as it can reach most superficial musculoskeletal structures in children but a larger bore needle is usually required for aspiration. For therapeutic injections, usually a mixture of depomedrone and bupivacaine 0.5% is administered, with the dose varying according to the age of the child and the region being injected.

The child should be placed in a comfortable position, preferably lying down, in case of a vaso-vagal attack. Depending on the age of the patient they may

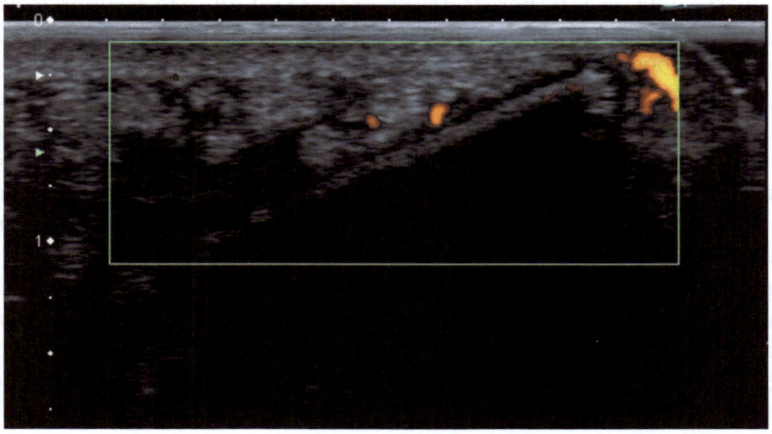

Fig. 4.26. Power Doppler ultrasound demonstrates a linear echogenic foreign body (splinter) in the sole of the foot with surrounding hyperaemia and posterior acoustic shadowing.

need to be gently restrained by a carer/parent so that sudden movements do not occur. When injecting joints or performing biopsies, a sterile probe cover should be used. The needle is best tracked when it lies parallel to the probe in the longitudinal plane, so an entry point that allows this should be chosen. The needle should enter the skin very close to the edge of the probe so that it can be tracked from the point of entry to the desired target. Distraction at the point of needle entry has been shown to be an effective way of minimising distress, for example the child can be asked to look at something interesting, blow out or take a deep breath (Fowler-Kerry and Lander 1987; French et al. 1994).

Once the procedure has been performed the dressing pack and needles should be disposed of safely as quickly as possible, to avoid the child fixating on the needle. There should be abundant praise for the child and appropriate reward.

References

Aspelin P, Ekberg O, Thorsson O, Wilhelmsson M, Westlin N (1992) Ultrasound examination of soft tissue injury of the lower limb in athletes. Am J Sports Med 20:601–603

Barberie JE, Wong AD, Cooperberg PL, Carson BW (1998) Extended field-of-view sonography in musculoskeletal disorders. AJR Am J Roentgenol 171:751–757

Beggs I (2003) Sonography of muscle hernias. AJR Am J Roentgenol 180:395–399

Benjamin M, Ralphs JR (1997) Tendons and ligaments – an overview. Histol Histopathol 12:1135–1144

Bianchi S, Martinoli C, Abdelwahab IF (2005) Ultrasound of tendon tears. Part 1: general considerations and upper extremity. Skeletal Radiol 34:500–512

Bodner G, Stockl B, Fierlinger A, Schocke M, Bernathova M (2005) Sonographic findings in stress fractures of the lower limb: preliminary findings. Eur Radiol 15:356–359

Campbell RS, Grainger AJ (2001) Current concepts in imaging of tendinopathy. Clin Radiol 56:253–267

Campbell DG, Menz A, Isaacs J (1994) Dynamic ankle ultrasonography. A new imaging technique for acute ankle ligament injuries. Am J Sports Med 22:855–858

Cardinal E, Buckwalter KA, Capello WN, Duval N (1996) US of the snapping iliopsoas tendon. Radiology 198:521–522

Castriota-Scanderbeg A, Orsi E (1993) Slipped capital femoral epiphysis: ultrasonographic findings. Skeletal Radiol 22:191–193

Cho KH, Lee DC, Chhem RK et al. (2001) Normal and acutely torn posterior cruciate ligament of the knee at US evaluation: preliminary experience. Radiology 219:375–380

Choi YS, Lee SM, Song BY, Paik SH, Yoon YK (2002) Dynamic sonography of external snapping hip syndrome. J Ultrasound Med 21:753–758

Cooperberg PL, Barberie JJ, Wong T, Fix C (2001) Extended field-of-view ultrasound. Semin Ultrasound CT MR 22:65–77

Davae KC, Sofka CM, DiCarlo E, Adler RS (2003) Value of power Doppler imaging and the hypoechoic halo in the sonographic detection of foreign bodies: correlation with histopathologic findings. J Ultrasound Med 22:1309–1313; quiz 14–6

Davidson RS, Markowitz RI, Dormans J, Drummond DS (1994) Ultrasonographic evaluation of the elbow in infants and young children after suspected trauma. J Bone Joint Surg Am 76:1804–1813

De Flaviis L, Nessi R, Scaglione P, Balconi G, Albisetti W, Derchi LE (1989) Ultrasonic diagnosis of Osgood-Schlatter and Sinding-Larsen-Johansson diseases of the knee. Skeletal Radiol 18:193–197

De Smet AA, Fisher DR, Graf BK, Lange RH (1990) Osteochondritis dissecans of the knee: value of MR imaging in determining lesion stability and the presence of articular cartilage defects. AJR Am J Roentgenol 155:549–553

De Smet AA, Ilahi OA, Graf BK (1996) Reassessment of the MR criteria for stability of osteochondritis dissecans in the knee and ankle. Skeletal Radiol 25:159–163

De Smet AA, Winter TC, Best TM, Bernhardt DT (2002) Dynamic sonography with valgus stress to assess elbow ulnar collateral ligament injury in baseball pitchers. Skeletal Radiol 31:671–676

Diaz GC, van Holsbeeck M, Jacobson JA (1998) Longitudinal split of the peroneus longus and peroneus brevis tendons with disruption of the superior peroneal retinaculum. J Ultrasound Med 17:525–529

Ebrahim FS, De Maeseneer M, Jager T, Marcelis S, Jamadar DA, Jacobson JA (2006) US diagnosis of UCL tears of the thumb and Stener lesions: technique, pattern-based approach, and differential diagnosis. Radiographics 26:1007–1020

Erickson SJ (1997) High-resolution imaging of the musculoskeletal system. Radiology 205:593–618

Evans GF, Haller RG, Wyrick PS, Parkey RW, Fleckenstein JL (1998) Submaximal delayed-onset muscle soreness: correlations between MR imaging findings and clinical measures. Radiology 208:815–820

Farley FA, Kuhns L, Jacobson JA, DiPietro M (2001) Ultrasound examination of ankle injuries in children. J Pediatr Orthop 21:604–607

Fornage BD (1987) The hypoechoic normal tendon. A pitfall. J Ultrasound Med 6:19–22

Fornage BD (2000) The case for ultrasound of muscles and tendons. Semin Musculoskelet Radiol 4:375–391

Fornage BD, Nerot C (1986) Sonographic diagnosis of rhabdomyolysis. J Clin Ultrasound 14:389–392

Fornage BD, Rifkin MD (1988) Ultrasound examination of tendons. Radiol Clin North Am 26:87–107

Fornage BD, Eftekhari F (1989) Sonographic diagnosis of myositis ossificans. J Ultrasound Med 8:463–466

Fornage BD, Touche DH, Segal P, Rifkin MD (1983) Ultrasonography in the evaluation of muscular trauma. J Ultrasound Med 2:549–554

Fowler-Kerry S, Lander JR (1987) Management of injection pain in children. Pain 30:169–175

French GM, Painter EC, Coury DL (1994) Blowing away shot pain: a technique for pain management during immunization. Pediatrics 93:384–388

Friedl W, Glaser F (1991) Dynamic sonography in the diagnosis of ligament and meniscal injuries of the knee. Arch Orthop Trauma Surg 110:132–138

Harris J (1981) The importance of the soft tissues in certain skeletal traumatic lesions. Radiol Clin North Am 19:601–624
Hsu CC, Tsai WC, Chen CP, Yeh WL, Tang SF, Kuo JK (2005) Ultrasonographic examination of the normal and injured posterior cruciate ligament. J Clin Ultrasound 33:277–282
Hubner U, Schlicht W, Outzen S, Barthel M, Halsband H (2000) Ultrasound in the diagnosis of fractures in children. J Bone Joint Surg Br 82:1170–1173
Hunt DM, Somashekar N (2005) A review of sleeve fractures of the patella in children. Knee 12:3–7
Kannus P (2000) Structure of the tendon connective tissue. Scand J Med Sci Sports 10:312–320
Kijowski R, De Smet AA (2005) MRI findings of osteochondritis dissecans of the capitellum with surgical correlation. AJR Am J Roentgenol 185:1453–1459
Kim MC, Eckhardt BP, Craig C, Kuhns LR (2004) Ultrasonography of the annular ligament partial tear and recurrent „pulled elbow". Pediatr Radiol 34:999–1004
Kobayashi K, Burton KJ, Rodner C, Smith B, Caputo AE (2004) Lateral compression injuries in the pediatric elbow: Panner's disease and osteochondritis dissecans of the capitellum. J Am Acad Orthop Surg 12:246–254
Kosuwon W, Mahaisavariya B, Saengnipanthkul S, Laupattarakasem W, Jirawipoolwon P (1993) Ultrasonography of pulled elbow. J Bone Joint Surg Br 75:421–422
Kotnis R, David S, Handley R, Willett K, Ostlere S (2006) Dynamic ultrasound as a selection tool for reducing achilles tendon reruptures. Am J Sports Med 34:1395–1400
Labovitz JM, Schweitzer ME (1998) Occult osseous injuries after ankle sprains: incidence, location, pattern, and age. Foot Ankle Int 19:661–667
Lazovic D, Wegner U, Peters G, Gosse F (1996) Ultrasound for diagnosis of apophyseal injuries. Knee Surg Sports Traumatol Arthrosc 3:234–237
Lee JI, Song IS, Jung YB et al. (1996) Medial collateral ligament injuries of the knee: ultrasonographic findings. J Ultrasound Med 15:621–625
Madden CC, Mellion MB (1996) Sever's disease and other causes of heel pain in adolescents. Am Fam Physician 54:1995–2000
Markowitz RI, Davidson RS, Harty MP, Bellah RD, Hubbard AM, Rosenberg HK (1992) Sonography of the elbow in infants and children. AJR Am J Roentgenol 159:829–833
Markowitz RI, Hubbard AM, Harty MP, Bellah RD, Kessler A, Meyer JS (1993) Sonography of the knee in normal and abused infants. Pediatr Radiol 23:264–267
Miller TT, Adler RS, Friedman L (2004) Sonography of injury of the ulnar collateral ligament of the elbow-initial experience. Skeletal Radiol 33:386–391
Nazarian LN, McShane JM, Ciccotti MG, O'Kane PL, Harwood MI (2003) Dynamic US of the anterior band of the ulnar collateral ligament of the elbow in asymptomatic major league baseball pitchers. Radiology 227:149–154
Neustadter J, Raikin SM, Nazarian LN (2004) Dynamic sonographic evaluation of peroneal tendon subluxation. AJR Am J Roentgenol 183:985–988
Newman JS, Adler RS, Rubin JM (1997) Power Doppler sonography: use in measuring alterations in muscle blood volume after exercise. AJR Am J Roentgenol 168:1525–1530
Noonan TJ, Garrett WE Jr (1992) Injuries at the myotendinous junction. Clin Sports Med 11:783–806
Noonan TJ, Garrett WE Jr (1999) Muscle strain injury: diagnosis and treatment. J Am Acad Orthop Surg 7:262–269
O'Callaghan BI, Kohut G, Hoogewoud HM (1994) Gamekeeper thumb: identification of the Stener lesion with US. Radiology 192:477–480
O'Reilly MA, O'Reilly PM, Bell J (2003) Sonographic appearances of medial retinacular complex injury in transient patellar dislocation. Clin Radiol 58:636–641
Peetrons P, Creteur V, Bacq C (2004) Sonography of ankle ligaments. J Clin Ultrasound 32:491–499
Pelsser V, Cardinal E, Hobden R, Aubin B, Lafortune M (2001) Extraarticular snapping hip: sonographic findings. AJR Am J Roentgenol 176:67–73
Rao P, Carty H (1999) Non-accidental injury: review of the radiology. Clin Radiol 54:11–24
Rehman A, Robinson P (2005) Sonographic evaluation of injuries to the pectoralis muscles. AJR Am J Roentgenol 184:1205–1211
Rubin DA (1998) Magnetic resonance imaging of chondral and osteochondral injuries. Top Magn Reson Imaging 9:348–359
Rubin JM (1999) Musculoskeletal power Doppler. Eur Radiol 9[Suppl 3]:S403–406
Rybak LD, Torriani M (2003) Magnetic resonance imaging of sports-related muscle injuries. Top Magn Reson Imaging 14:209–219
Shirkhoda A, Armin AR, Bis KG, Makris J, Irwin RB, Shetty AN (1995) MR imaging of myositis ossificans: variable patterns at different stages. J Magn Reson Imaging 5:287–292
Smeets AJ, Robben SG, Meradji M (1990) Sonographically detected costo-chondral dislocation in an abused child. A new sonographic sign to the radiological spectrum of child abuse. Pediatr Radiol 20:566–567
Sofka CM (2006) Imaging of stress fractures. Clin Sports Med 25:53–62, viii
Soudack M, Nachtigal A, Gaitini D (2003) Clinically unsuspected foreign bodies: the importance of sonography. J Ultrasound Med 22:1381–1385
Stevens KJ, Theologis T, McNally EG (2000) Imaging of plant-thorn synovitis. Skeletal Radiol 29:605–608
Stevens MA, El-Khoury GY, Kathol MH, Brandser EA, Chow S (1999) Imaging features of avulsion injuries. Radiographics 19:655–672
Stoane JM, Poplausky MR, Haller JO, Berdon WE (1995) Panner's disease: X-ray, MR imaging findings and review of the literature. Comput Med Imaging Graph 19:473–476
Suzuki S, Awaya G, Okada Y, Ikeda T, Tada H (1987) Examination by ultrasound of Legg-Calve-Perthes disease. Clin Orthop Relat Res (220):130–136
Takebayashi S, Takasawa H, Banzai Y et al. (1995) Sonographic findings in muscle strain injury: clinical and MR imaging correlation. J Ultrasound Med 14:899–905
Teh J (2006) Applications of Doppler imaging in the musculoskeletal system. Curr Probl Diagn Radiol 35:22–34
Tehranzadeh J (1987) The spectrum of avulsion and avulsion-like injuries of the musculoskeletal system. Radiographics 7:945–974
Vocke-Hell AK, Schmid A (2001) Sonographic differentiation of stable and unstable lateral condyle fractures of the humerus in children. J Pediatr Orthop B 10:138–141
Williams GA, Cowell HR (1981) Kohler's disease of the tarsal navicular. Clin Orthop Relat Res (158):53–58
Williamson D, Watura R, Cobby M (2000) Ultrasound imaging of forearm fractures in children: a viable alternative? J Accid Emerg Med 17:22–24
Wingstrand H (1999) Significance of synovitis in Legg-Calve-Perthes disease. J Pediatr Orthop B 8:156–160

Magnetic Resonance Imaging

5

Karl J. Johnson

CONTENTS

5.1 Introduction

The multiplanar ability, excellent tissue resolution and image contrast of magnetic resonance imaging (MRI) is well recognised and its use in paediatric musculoskeletal disease is firmly established. While MRI is not predominately a first line investigation for traumatic injuries, it is increasingly being used in the evaluation of the more complex cases. It is helpful in planning treatment, monitoring patient follow-up and in the detection of complications, particularly those involving the physeal growth plate (White et al. 1994; Close and Strouse 2000; Lee et al. 2005).

In the paediatric skeleton, there are a variety of cartilaginous structures including the unossified epiphysis and metaphysis for which MRI is able to provide considerably more information, when compared with any other imaging modality (White et al. 1994; Close and Strouse 2000).

K. J. Johnson, MD, MRCP, FRCR
Consultant Paediatric Radiologist, Birmingham Children's Hospital, Steelhouse Lane, Birmingham, B4 6NH, UK

In acute trauma, prompt and easy access to imaging is required and this is not always achievable in paediatric MRI units. In particular for the younger child, the use of sedation or general anaesthesia may not always be readily available. Therefore, the use of MRI in the majority of acute situations is limited; however, it has been utilised for scaphoid, knee and elbow injuries (Beltran et al. 1994; Johnson et al. 2000; Pudas et al. 2005). In the more chronic long-term conditions, it is increasingly being used to assess growth plate injuries and non-uniting fractures (Jaramillo et al. 1990a,b; Smith et al. 1994; Anupindi and Jaramillo 2002).

In some institutions, the prospect of performing an MRI examination on a child can be daunting; however, if the same principles that are applied in adults, namely, improved signal to noise ratio, appropriate sequence selection and reduction of artefacts are employed then excellent image quality can be achieved.

5.2 General Considerations

Diagnostic MRI needs appropriate sequence selection and good quality images. Sequence selection is dependent on the clinical question being asked and the possible pathological processes that may be encountered. Image quality is dependent on the signal to noise ratio, spatial resolution, image contrast and any associated artefacts.

It must be remembered that with MRI there is often a 'play-off' between signal to noise, imaging time, contrast and resolution. Altering one parameter to improve one of these factors will often result in a worsening of another parameter. Achieving an appropriate balance between imaging time, imaging resolution and signal to noise is the essence of good quality MRI.

The specific demands and requirements of paediatric imaging need to be fully considered. Paediatrics encompasses children aged between birth and 16 years, which means that a flexible and pragmatic approach to imaging needs to be adopted. Each different age category will have specific requirements to ensure satisfactory images are obtained. For each child, their age and clinical presentation should be considered individually and a patient specific approach adopted.

5.3 Specific Absorption Ratio (SAR)

The thermoregulation and associated physiological changes that the human body exhibits in response to exposure to the radiofrequency pulses used during an MR examination is dependent on the amount of energy absorbed. The term specific absorption rate (SAR) is used to describe the absorption of radiofrequency (RF) energy. It is the amount of RF energy that is absorbed per unit mass and is expressed as Watts per kilogram (Adair and Berglund 1986). The amount of RF radiation absorbed during a procedure can be characterised either in respect to the whole body averaged out or as a peak level. Various countries have different maximum SAR levels which relate to the imaging of children and consideration of these levels is important. These levels should never be exceeded. The maximum SAR level may influence the type or duration of a particular sequence (Bitar et al. 2006).

The SAR level is related to a number of variables which includes the RF frequency, the strength of the magnetic field, the repetition time, the type of RF coil used, the volume of tissue contained within the coil and the configuration of the anatomic region exposed, in particular with respect to the orientation of main magnetic field. The maximum SAR level will be greater for larger body parts and those with a greater degree of conductivity, as there is increased ability to disperse the heat energy. Consequently in children, in view of their relatively small size, the maximum allowable SAR levels will be lower.

5.4 Patient Preparation

When initially positioning the child, it is important that the area of interest should be as close to the centre of the magnetic field as possible to reduce any field inhomogeneities. This is particularly important in the smaller child, who will only occupy a small area, typically outside the centre of the magnet field.

It is vital that the patient remains relatively stationary during the sequence acquisition time as significant movement will result in reduced image quality and potentially uninterpretable images. With children, achieving this immobility can be challenging and techniques to overcome it will be influenced by the age and development of the patient. In the older child and teenager, simple explanation is usually all that is necessary to achieve good compliance and adequate immobility. In the younger child, if they have relatively good comprehension, the use of simple explanation, reassurance and encouragement may suffice. In some instances, the use of rewards will help achieve and maintain this compliance. The use of good immobilisation and distraction techniques can be useful. Typical distraction techniques include playing suitable music and if available video/digital images to the patient while within the scanner. When using immobilisation devices, it is important that the child remains comfortable as this increases the likelihood that they will remain stationary (Barnewolt and Chung 1998).

With young children, particularly those under 5 years of age and those with developmental problems, the use of either sedation or general anaesthesia is often required to achieve appropriate immobilisation.

It must be borne in mind that obtaining the child's trust and co-operation may take some extra time which needs to be considered when booking the patient schedules. As a consequence, fewer children may be imaged within the same unit of time when compared with the number of patients imaged in adult centres.

5.4.1 Sedation and Sleep Techniques

The child who is under 1 month of age, if swaddled and kept warm, may often fall asleep after a feed for a sufficient length of time to enable an MR examination to be performed. This "feed and wrap" technique relies upon the radiography staff being comfortable with the handling of small babies.

Sedation is an artificially induced decrease in conscious level that may be associated with anxiolysis and amnesia. As a child's level of consciousness falls, there is a reduction in muscle tone of the oropharynx and a risk of the airway being occluded by the tongue. With further loss of consciousness, there is loss of the glottic reflexes with a risk of aspiration and respiratory depression. To allow for adequate MR examination, a level of sedation is required that ensures the child remains asleep and stationary, during the entire image acquisition time, but they should still be able to be roused if necessary. It is important that any sedation regime does not result in a child drifting into a deep unrousable level of unconsciousness, during which they may lose control of their airway and become at risk of aspiration or asphyxiation (Sury et al. 2005).

Within any group of children, there will be an individual variation in the level of sensitivity to the sedation medication used. Any regime which is 100% successful is in effect providing a level of sedation that is sufficient to sedate the least sensitive child. This potentially puts a child who is particularly sensitive at risk of being over sedated. Consequently, a small failure rate with any sedation regime is acceptable. Regardless of the sedation regime that is being employed, it is important that it is widely distributed throughout the hospital, it is used for all children being imaged and is acceptable to the anaesthetic department. Any regime should be regularly audited with any significant complication reviewed.

Sedation is widely used in many institutions and is often a nurse-led service. A variety of different sedation regimes have been published. While the child is sedated, they should be monitored continuously by dedicated nursing or medical staff who are separate from those involved in the imaging acquisition (Sury et al. 1999, 2005). Appropriate areas within the hospital need to be available to safely administer the sedation and recover the patient at the end of the scan. MR compatible equipment is needed to monitor the patient's respiration, oxygen saturation levels and heart rate. Care must be taken with the leads to ensure they do not coil around the body and touch the sides of the MR unit to prevent any radio frequency induced burns (Kanal and Shellock 1990a,b). In cases of acute respiratory arrest, immediate medical assistance should be available.

Sedating children can be time consuming and requires sufficient resource allocation to ensure it is done safely. The timing of children falling asleep can be variable, so flexibility in the running and management of the MRI sessions is needed.

A possible alternative to sedation is the use of melatonin. This is a naturally occurring hormone that induces a natural sleep. Therefore, there are no risks of over sedating a child. The use of melatonin in MRI is less well established (Johnson et al. 2002).

5.4.2 Anaesthesia

Anaesthesia is an unrousable state associated with loss of airway reflexes and respiratory depression. The nature, route of administration and monitoring of the anaesthesia is the domain of the anaesthetist.

While anaesthesia will achieve total immobility and control of respiration, it requires a dedicated paediatric anaesthetist, paramedical staff and suitable MR compatible equipment which may not be available in all institutions.

5.5 Image Contrast

With MRI, the contrast characteristics of the tissue under investigation will depend on the chemical and physical properties of the protons within that tissue, the selection of the imaging sequences and the use of a contrast agent. The most often quoted tissue properties are the T1 recovery and T2 relaxation times of the protons and also the density of these protons in the tissue being imaged (Plewes 1994; Pipe 1999). These characteristics will determine the T1, T2 and proton density (PD) contrast within a tissue.

With conventional spin echo techniques, those features that will alter image contrast are the pulse repetition time (TR) and the echo delay time (TE). With inversion recovery sequences, it is the inversion time (TI) which has the greatest effect while with gradient echo imaging, it is the flip angle that is most important (Barnewolt and Chung 1998; Bradley 1999; Anupindi and Jaramillo 2002; Bitar et al. 2006).

5.6 Signal Localisation

Variations in the magnetic field strength (gradients) are used to localise the area of tissue that the signal is coming from. Three types of gradient are utilised one each for the x, y and z axis. There is a section selective gradient, a phase-encoding gradient and a frequency-encoding gradient.

The section selective gradient identifies the section of tissue to be imaged. The phase-encoding gradient causes a shift in the phase of the spinning proton. The frequency-encoding gradient causes a change in the frequency of the spinning proton. The frequency-encoding gradient is also called the read-out gradient. Each type of gradient can be applied in any of the three axes depending on the body part being imaged and the clinical requirements (Bitar et al. 2006).

5.7 Spin Echo Techniques

Spin echo sequences (SE) are usually part of the standard sequence selection in musculoskeletal imaging as they provide good T1, T2 and proton density (PD) contrast.

A full description of the physics of spin echo sequences is beyond the scope of this chapter (Fig. 5.1). Important parameters that are adjusted to alter image contrast are the repetition time (TR) (measured in milliseconds) which is the time between the application of one RF excitation pulse and the start of the next RF pulse. The time to echo (TE) (measured in milliseconds) is the time between the application of the RF pulse and the peak of the echo detected.

With conventional SE sequences, it is the T1 recovery and the T2 decay (relaxation) of the protons within a tissue sample that have the greatest effect on image contrast. T1 recovery is the increase in longitudinal magnetisation, while the T2 decay is the decrease in magnetisation that occurs from the dephasing of the spinning protons in the transverse plane (Plewes 1994). Both these processes occur simultaneously so by altering the TR and the TE it is possible to utilise the difference in the T1 and T2 relaxation times of tissue (Fig. 5.2 a–c).

The variation in signal intensity of different tissues on both T1 and T2 weighted spin echo sequences is shown in Table 5.1.

5.7.1 T1 Weighted Spin Echo Sequences

A T1 weighted sequence has a short TE and TR. The TE is kept as short as possible to minimise T2 signal decay and keep the T1 as pure as possible. These sequences are reasonably quick to acquire. Most tissues have relatively long T1 recovery times and so are of low signal intensity on T1 weighted images including water and muscle.

T1 weighted sequences provide good anatomical orientation, allow for the identification of acute haematoma and show those tissues which demonstrate gadolinium uptake. They are useful for evaluating bone marrow disorders, avascular necrosis, stress fractures and detecting the fatty infiltration of muscle. Fat, acute haemorrhage, proteinaceous fluids and gadolinium are some of the few substances that have short T1 times and are of high signal intensity on T1 weighted images. They are useful in showing hypointense signal in sclerosis and subchondral oedema.

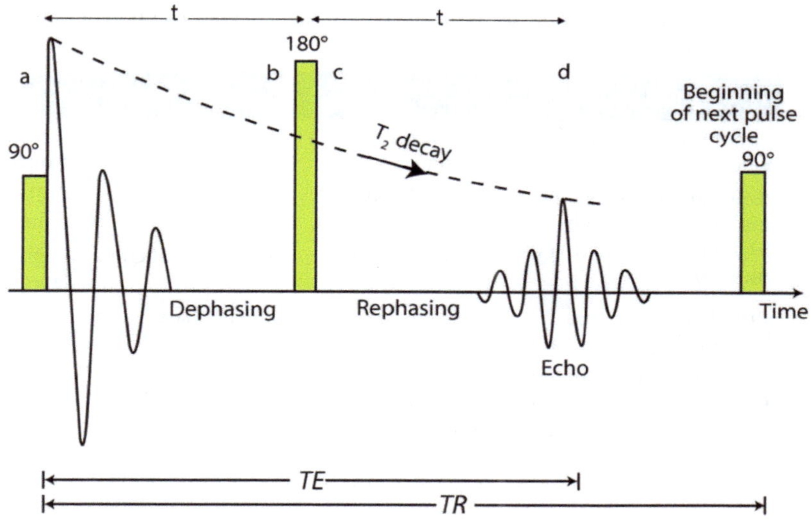

Fig. 5.1. A simplified representation of a conventional cycle of a spin echo (SE) sequence. A 90° pulse, the radiofrequency (RF) pulse, is used to rotate the magnetisation into the transverse plane. This transverse magnetisation gradually begins to dephase until 180° refocussing (or rephasing) pulse is applied which rotates the plane of this magnetisation about its axis. This 180° refocussing pulse is applied half way between the time of the initial excitation pulse and the time the echo is sampled. Step (*a*): An initial 90° RF pulse is applied. This causes all the protons to precess in the same phase. Following this, the protons begin to dephase. Step (*b*): An 180° rephasing (refocussing) pulse is applied that reverses the spin of the protons Step (*c*): The protons now begin to precess in the opposite direction and thus become more in phase. Step (*d*): The signal is sampled to produce an image. *TE*, time to echo; *TR*, time to repeat (modified from FARR 1998)

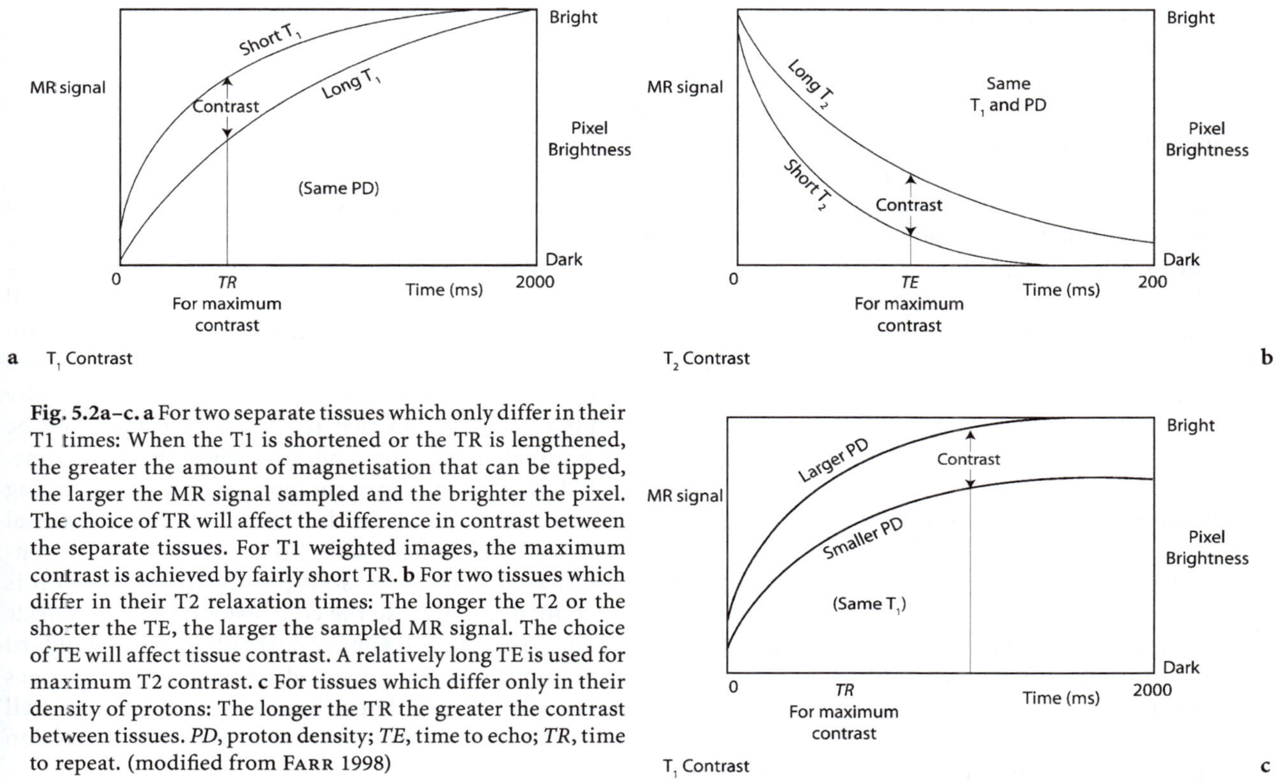

Fig. 5.2a–c. a For two separate tissues which only differ in their T1 times: When the T1 is shortened or the TR is lengthened, the greater the amount of magnetisation that can be tipped, the larger the MR signal sampled and the brighter the pixel. The choice of TR will affect the difference in contrast between the separate tissues. For T1 weighted images, the maximum contrast is achieved by fairly short TR. **b** For two tissues which differ in their T2 relaxation times: The longer the T2 or the shorter the TE, the larger the sampled MR signal. The choice of TE will affect tissue contrast. A relatively long TE is used for maximum T2 contrast. **c** For tissues which differ only in their density of protons: The longer the TR the greater the contrast between tissues. *PD*, proton density; *TE*, time to echo; *TR*, time to repeat. (modified from FARR 1998)

Table 5.1. The variation in signal intensity of different tissues on both T1 and T2 weighted sequences. (Adapted from Bitar et al. 2006)

T1 Weighted sequences	Signal intensity	T2 weighted sequences
Air, mineral rich tissue (cortical bones, calcium stones), fast flowing blood	Dark	Air, mineral rich tissue (cortical bones, calcium stones), fast flowing blood
Collagenous tissues (ligaments, tendons), high free water (kidneys, urine, bile, oedema), high bound water (liver, hyaline cartilage, muscle)	Low	Collagenous tissues (ligaments, tendons) and bone islands
	Low/intermediate	High bound water (liver, pancreas, hyaline cartilage, muscle)
Proteinaceous tissue (abscess, complex cyst, synovial fluid)	Intermediate	Fat, fatty marrow
Fat, fatty marrow, blood products (methaemoglobin), slow flowing blood, radiation changes, paramagnetic contrast agents	Bright	High free water (kidneys, urine, oedema, proteinaceous), blood products (oxyhaemoglobin, extracellular methaemoglobin)

5.7.2 T2 Weighted Spin Echo Sequences

T2 weighted spin echo sequences are obtained using a relatively long TR, to minimise the T1 saturation effect and a long TE. Most structures are of high to intermediate signal intensity on T2 weighted images. Mineralization, fibrous structures (such as menisci and ligaments), haemosiderin and high concentrations of gadolinium are of low signal intensity on T2 weighted images.

The acquisition time for T2 weighted sequences are relatively long and so they are more prone to motion artefacts. In view of this problem, fast-spin echo or gradient echo imaging is often used instead of conventional T2 SE sequences. The signal to noise ratio (SNR) of T2 weighted images is generally inferior to either proton density or T1 weighted images. The high signal intensity of water on T2 weighted sequences makes it very valuable in the detection of bone marrow oedema and other pathological processes.

5.7.3 Proton Density Imaging

Proton density weighted or intermediate weighted image (PDWI) utilise a long TR to reduce the effect of T1 contrast and a short TE is used to reduce the T2 weighting. Image contrast is then primarily due to the actual number (density) of protons within the different tissues, rather than the T1 and T2 relaxation times. The greater the density of protons within a tissue the higher the signal intensity, consequently both fat and water are relatively bright on PD images. The SNR is relatively high with proton density imaging. Conventional PDWI proton density sequences are useful in studying cartilage.

The sequences may obscure sclerosis or marrow oedema due to poor marrow fat contrast compared to T1W1 or fat saturated proton density fast spin echo (FS PD FSE) sequences.

5.7.4 Fast Spin Echo Techniques

Fast (or turbo) spin echo (FSE) techniques are a modification of conventional spin echo imaging. Essentially several echoes are generated using multiple 180° refocusing pulses during a single TR. All these echoes together are referred to as an echo train and the total number of 180° RF pulses and echoes is the echo train length. Each echo is individually phase encoded so that the multiple echoes can be summated together and so reduce the scan time. FSE images are more susceptible to image blurring and edge artefacts. With T2 weighted FSE, the signal from fat is considerably higher than with conventional SE sequences, so typically fat suppression is applied to optimise the contrast with water. Muscle and cartilage will appear darker than with standard SE sequences. Fat saturated T2 weighted FSE images are sensitive for detecting marrow oedema, as well as soft tissues pathologies such as masses, infection and acute muscle injures.

T2 or proton density fast spin echo fat suppressed (PD FSE FS) are useful for evaluating marrow oedema, articular cartilage, ligaments, tendons, synovium and meniscal morphology. They are a commonly used sequence for all appendicular joint imaging. TE values are typically less than 60 ms and TR values greater than or equal to 3000 ms. TE values are around 40–50 ms to optimise image quality.

5.8 Gradient Echo Imaging

With gradient echo (GE) imaging, instead of a 90° RF pulse to generate the transverse magnetisation, a variable flip angle of less than 90° is used. Only a proportion of the longitudinal magnetisation is therefore converted to transverse magnetisation. A large flip angle (greater than 45°) will produce T1 weighted images while T2 weighted images use a small flip angle (less than 30°) with a relatively long TR. Additional gradients as opposed to RF pulses are used to dephase (negative gradient) or rephase (positive gradient) the transverse magnetisation.

GE images have shorter scan times due to the shortened TR associated with the smaller excitation angle but are more susceptible to magnetic field inhomogeneities and susceptibility artefacts between different tissues. Artefacts associated with blood products and metallic implants can be significant. This increased susceptibility artefact is useful for imaging cartilage, and in the detection of blood products and calcification.

To reduce acquisition times and provide greater diversity in image properties, a number of advanced GE sequences have been developed. Each of the major equipment manufacturers have developed specific sequences which have a variety of acronyms (Brown and Semelka 1999).

With gradient echo imaging, there is insufficient time for all the transverse magnetisation to decay between successive TRs, so that it accumulates over time. This transverse magnetisation is unmoving and is referred to as being in a steady state. A spoiled gradient echo is where an additional RF pulse is used to nullify any residual transverse magnetisation. With steady state free precession (SSFP), this transverse magnetisation is maintained, so that it contributes to the signal obtained from subsequent echo periods. SSFP images are formed from the echo component and from the residual component. If both these echoes are acquired simultaneously, it is a dual echo in steady state (DESS). Other techniques include partially refocused (rewound) imaging which provide T2 weighted images.

All these different types of sequences allow for rapid acquisition of images, volume acquisitions and can provide a variety of contrast behaviours which are useful for image manipulation, reformatting images outside a true anatomical plane and for analysing structures that move between planes, such as ligaments and joint capsules.

GE sequences are useful in detecting meniscal pathology and cartilage. They are poor at detecting bone marrow oedema and should not be routinely used in the investigation of marrow pathology.

5.9 Acquisition Parameters

The majority of imaging strategies in MRI are designed to increase the signal from the area of interest and to decrease any unwanted noise (Bradley 1999). This signal to noise ratio (SNR) is dependent on many factors, some of which can be manipulated, some which cannot.

Non-operator dependent factors are the magnetic field strength, the density of protons within the tissue, the molecular structure of the tissue and the T1 and T2 times of the tissue's protons.

Operator dependent factors include: the time to repetition (TR), time to echo (TE), the flip angle, the number of excitations used, the type of coil employed, the sampling bandwidth and the size of the voxel. A voxel (or volume element) is the sample of tissue being imaged and is determined by the slice thickness, field of view and the matrix size (Redpath 1998). Each voxel of tissue corresponds to a pixel on the final image, with each image being made up of many pixels.

5.9.1 Magnetic Field Strength

In most institutions, the magnetic field strength is dependent on the type of MRI scanner available and is relatively fixed. A higher magnetic field strength will provide a greater signal to noise ratio, a higher spectral resolution, increased readout bandwidth (decreasing susceptibility artefacts) and faster imaging time. It is important that in children the SAR levels are not exceeded, as the absorbed energy will increase with higher strength magnets. Low magnetic field strengths will prolong imaging time but they will create fewer chemical shift artefacts, provide greater contrast resolution and less metallic artefact. With lower strength magnets, the fat and water spectral peaks are closer together and are more difficult to separate which can cause problems in obtaining frequency-selective fat saturation. Lower strength magnets may require less shielding with lower start up and running costs (Ahn et al. 1998; Rand et al. 1999; Niitsu et al. 2000).

5.9.2 Receiver Coils

Receiver coils are designed to detect the signal from within the body part being imaged. With paediatric imaging, the smallest possible coil that covers the body part under investigation should be used (Barnewolt and Chung 1998). Localised coils reduce the noise coming from non-imaged parts of the body and increase the SNR. There are many varieties of receiver coils that are currently on the market, which in simple terms can be classified as either receive-transmit or receive only coils. Receive-transmit coils improve signal homogeneity and improve the SNR, but they may be limited in their anatomical application (Schmitt et al. 1999).

It is important when dealing with children that the technicians are adaptable and versatile; for instance, it is possible to image a neonatal head or both the hands of a small child within a receive and transmit adult knee coil. Adult wrist coils are also useful for imaging the elbows and knees of children (Anupindi and Jaramillo 2002). The use of localised coils may result in relatively higher SAR levels.

5.9.3 Voxel Size

The voxel size refers to the volume of tissue of the body that absorbs the excitation pulse. In simple terms, a voxel is a sample of tissue within the body that corresponds to a specific pixel on the generated image. Each MR image is made up of a number of pixels. Hence, the larger the voxel, the larger the pixels and therefore spatial resolution is reduced.

Voxel size is dependent on slice thickness, field of view and the matrix size and is one of the most important determinants of the SNR ratio. Larger voxels have a higher SNR as they contain more protons which are producing a signal (Creasy et al. 1995). Conversely, a larger voxel will reduce the spatial resolution. The SNR is influenced by any parameter that alters the voxel size.

5.9.3.1 Slice Thickness

Slice thickness varies linearly with the SNR, thus increasing the slice thickness will increase the SNR. The use of thinner slices will improve spatial resolution by reducing the amount of volume averaging, but less tissue will be imaged and there will be a decrease in the SNR.

Slice thickness is an important consideration in the younger child since, due to the small size of the body part that may need to be imaged, thin slices are desirable. However, to maintain a satisfactory SNR, imaging times may need to be increased.

5.9.3.2 Matrix Size

The imaging matrix is the number of pixels in both the frequency- and phase-encoding directions. Typically, the phase-encoding direction is the one that is most often manipulated. Increasing the matrix size will increase the spatial resolution but this will lead to an increased scan time, as the scan time is proportional to the number of phase-encoded steps. Increasing the size of the matrix will decrease the SNR, as fewer protons will be sampled.

Doubling the matrix size, in both the phase- and frequency-encoded directions, with a fixed field of view, will reduce the SNR by a factor of $\sqrt{2}$.

Typically, in clinical practice, the phase-encoding matrix ranges from 160 to 320, and the frequency-encoding between 250 and 512. These parameters allow adequate resolution, scan times and SNR. Higher resolution matrices may be used in selective cases, when the body part is small and complex, such as the paediatric wrist or ankle (Anupindi and Jaramillo 2002).

5.9.3.3 Field of View (FOV)

The field of view (FOV) is the area of the body from which the signal is measured. The SNR varies with the square of the FOV. Decreasing the FOV will improve spatial resolution but this will lead to a decrease in pixel size and a reduction in the SNR. A reduction in the FOV from 16 cm^2 to 12 cm^2 will reduce the SNR by 44% (Anupindi and Jaramillo 2002). In paediatric imaging, it is often necessary to increase the FOV to achieve a sufficient SNR.

5.9.4 Number of Excitations (NEX)

The SNR varies with the square root of the number of excitations. Increasing the number of excitations will improve image quality but will also increase the imaging time.

5.9.5 Bandwidth

In the frequency-encoded direction, the sampling bandwidth determines the range of frequencies sampled. Reducing the bandwidth will reduce the amount of unwanted noise, while the signal will remain unaltered. Consequently, the SNR will increase with a reduction in the bandwidth. Reducing the bandwidth will decrease the number of slices possible as there is a minimum TE that can be used, as the readout time period becomes longer with a smaller bandwidth. Reducing the bandwidth will lead to an increase in the chemical shift artefact.

5.9.6 Pulse Sequences

Altering the type of pulse sequence will have an effect on SNR. With conventional spin echo sequences, all the longitudinal magnetization is converted into transverse magnetization, while with gradient echo sequences, only a proportion of this longitudinal magnetization is utilised. If all other parameters are equal, the SNR is greater for spin echo sequences.

5.9.7 SNR Summary

SNR is increased by using spin echo sequences, a larger FOV, coarse matrix, large slice thickness and an increased number of acquisitions. For each of these changes, there may be reduction in the spatial resolution or an increase in the scan time. In paediatric imaging, it is important that a balance is achieved to obtain sufficient imaging quality while not having excessively long scan times or exceeding the SAR levels. A flexible approach needs to be employed for each child to achieve this.

5.10 Imaging Time

When estimating the time for an examination, it is important that, in addition to the technical factors, the setup time is included. The setup time includes patient reassurance within the scanner room, proper positioning and immobilisation and the fitting of an appropriate coil. In paediatrics, these setup times may be considerable, as the amount of time to reassure and immobilise the child can be long. If the child is sedated or the examination is performed under general anaesthesia, there may be additional delays.

The time for each imaging sequence is dependent on the pulse repetition time (TR), the phase-encoding matrix and the number of excitations. Shortening the TR will result in shorter sequences, but will result in more T1 weighting and a reduction in the signal intensity. Consequently, reducing the TR will have an effect on image contrast resolution and will also reduce the maximum number of slices that can be acquired. Decreasing the phase-encoding matrix will reduce the imaging time and will increase the SNR, but this will reduce the spatial resolution. Reducing the number of excitations will reduce the imaging time but will also reduce the SNR.

5.11 Spatial Resolution

Resolution is the ability to distinguish between two points. Resolution improves as the voxel size reduces. Separate tissue within the same voxel cannot be discriminated but those tissues in adjacent voxels will be. If a voxel contains two or more different types of tissue then the signal intensity from that voxel is an average of the signal intensities from each of the different tissues.

Decreasing the voxel size will improve spatial resolution. If the FOV is reduced, the voxel size will also decrease, halving the FOV will reduce the voxel size by a factor of four. Decreasing the slice thickness will also reduce the voxel size.

Spatial resolution may also be improved by altering the dimensions of the FOV. The use of a rectangular FOV will increase spatial resolution without increasing scan time.

5.12 Fat Suppression Techniques

A variety of techniques can be used to reduce the signal from fat which includes opposed imaging, frequency fat selection and inversion recovery.

Opposed imaging uses in and out of phase imaging techniques. It can be used to detect a small amount of fat within a lesion and for evaluating bone marrow disease. It is a specialised technique that is not routinely used (Dixon 1984).

Selective fat saturation uses an RF pulse with the same resonant frequency as fat, which is used to dephase the entire signal from fat. With this technique, only fat is suppressed while other tissues are not affected. Selective fat saturation can be combined with any other sequence, so it is useful in post-contrast imaging. The saturation pulse requires extra time which means fewer slices can be obtained, assuming that the TR remains constant. Due to magnetic field inhomogeneities, the fat saturation may be imperfect or partial; this is worse with lower strength magnets and the removal of the fat signal also means the SNR will be reduced (Haase et al. 1985).

Inversion recovery (IR) sequences [when used for fat suppression, this is the short tau inversion recovery (STIR) sequence] utilise the difference in the T1 relaxation times of fat and water. Following an initial 180° inversion pulse, the longitudinal magnetisation of fat recovers faster than water. By applying the 90° RF pulse at the time the longitudinal magnetisation of fat reaches zero, the signal from fat will be insignificant. This technique uses the physical properties of fat and can be used on low strength magnets (Fleckenstein et al. 1991). However, this technique can only be used with spin echo and fast spin echo sequences. It does result in high contrast images, with water appearing bright. Oedema in soft tissue and bone is detected with a high level of sensitivity. The SNR is low as tissue with a similar T1 to fat is also suppressed. STIR sequences cannot be used with gadolinium (Weinberger et al. 1995).

5.13 Artefacts

Artefacts either occur from unwanted motion or as a result of the magnetic field gradient (Mirowitz 1999).

5.13.1 Motion Artefacts

Motion artefacts result from tissue movement during the period of data acquisition, which may be either voluntary or involuntary. In children, voluntary movements are not an infrequent problem because of their reduced understanding and compliance. In the young or uncooperative child, the use of sedation or general anaesthesia may be needed to achieve satisfactory immobility.

Involuntary motion artefacts can be caused by respiration, bowel peristalsis or cardiac/arterial movement. These involuntary movements cause blurring or ghosting of the image. A ghost image is when an anatomical structure is replicated in another area of the body. Reversing the phase-encoding direction may decrease the ghosting artefact (Mirowitz 1999).

Motion artefacts may be reduced by faster imaging such as GE or FSE sequences. In cooperative children, some of these sequences can be performed during breath holding if necessary.

5.13.2 Magnetic Field Gradient Artefacts

There are four types of artefacts related to the magnetic field gradients: truncation, aliasing (wrap around), chemical shift and susceptibility (Rawson and Siegel 1996).

5.13.2.1 Truncation Artefacts

Truncation artefacts occur at the interface of tissues of significant different signal intensities. This results in alternating dark and light signal bands which gradually decrease in intensity from the interface point. These artefacts are mostly marked with a low phase-encoding matrix and therefore can be limited with the use of a high resolution matrix (Turner et al. 1991).

5.13.2.2
Aliasing

Aliasing or wrap round artefacts occur when the body part being imaged is larger than the FOV and still within the receiver coil. As a consequence, the part of the body that is outside the FOV is displayed on the opposite side of the image in a different anatomical location. The aliasing occurs in the phase-encoded direction. Aliasing can be limited by increasing the FOV, using saturation bands at the edges of the FOV and by transposing the frequency and phase-encoding directions (Duerk 1999) (Fig. 5.3).

5.13.2.3
Chemical Shift

Chemical shift artefacts occur at the interface of tissues in which the protons have significantly different precession frequencies. Typically this occurs at fat-water interfaces and occurs regardless of the magnetic field strength, but is more conspicuous at high field strength. The artefact appears as a high signal intensity band on one side of an organ and low signal intensity band on the opposite side. Chemical shift artefacts occur in the frequency-encoded direction and can be reduced by reducing the bandwidth or reversing the phase- and frequency-encoded directions (Hood et al. 1999; Mirowitz 1999).

5.13.2.4
Magnetic Susceptibility

Magnetic susceptibility is a measure of the degree to which a material is magnetised when placed in the magnetic field. Magnetic susceptibility artefact results when there is dephasing of protons at the interface of tissues with different susceptibility. Magnetic susceptibility is more prominent with gradient recalled echo images as there is rapid gradient reversal rather than using a 180° refocussing pulse. Metallic artefacts are a common cause for magnetic susceptibility and this can be minimised using fast spin echo sequences, with short TE and high echo train length. A short TE minimises the time for spins to dephase (Patton 1994; Elster 1997) (Fig. 5.4).

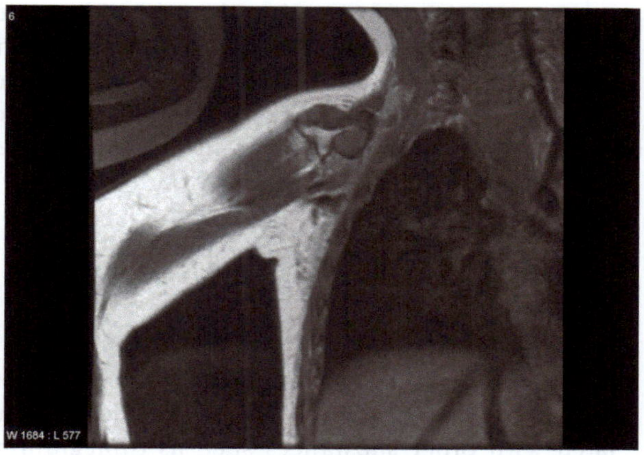

Fig. 5.3. Coronal T1 weighted images of the shoulder and upper arm in a young child. The distal arm and elbow are within the receiver coil but outside the field of view. They appear in an abnormal position on the image

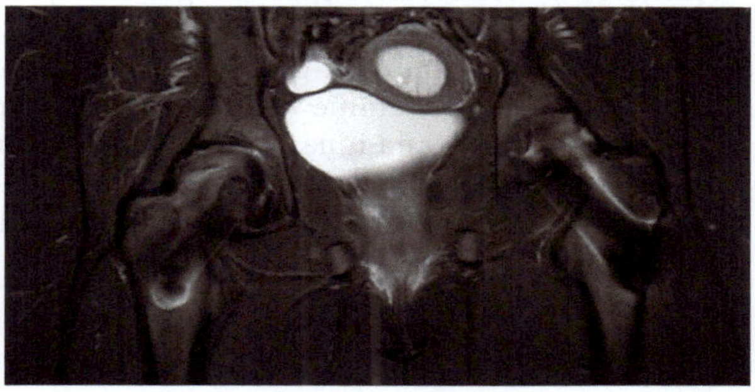

Fig. 5.4. Marked artefact and signal distortion from metallic screws inserted for bilateral slipped capital femoral epiphysis

5.13.3
Metal Objects

Metallic objects will produce their own local magnetic field and this will cause marked distortion of the MR image. This is more pronounced on gradient echo imaging.

5.13.4
Magic Angle Phenomenon

This arises in structures which are composed of parallel fibres, such as ligaments and tendons. The parallel orientation of the fibres increases the amount of T2 dephasing. However, when the fibres are placed at 55° to the main magnetic field, this increased T2 dephasing is reduced, so that a structure which is normally of low signal intensity will appear to be of increased signal intensity. The effect is increased with a short TE (Hayes and Parellada 1996; Echigo et al. 1999). This artefact may be seen with ligaments and tendons as they pass around a joint.

5.14 Contrast Enhancement

Gadolinium is a paramagnetic ion and is the most frequently used contrast agent. Gadolinium is chelated with other substances such as dimeglumine and diethylenetriaminepentaacetic acid (DTPA) before intravenous use. The usual dose for children is 0.1 mmol/kg.

Gadolinium shortens the T1 and so increases signal intensity on T1 weighted images. At higher concentrations, it can cause T2 shortening and magnetic susceptibility artefacts (Elster 1997).

The use of pre- and post-gadolinium T1 weighted imaging helps determine which tissues have increased vascularity and inflammation, as these are the areas of increased uptake. When imaging bone, the fatty marrow will often be of high signal on T1 weighted images, and the use of post-gadolinium T1 fat saturated sequences increases the image contrast by reducing the fat signal from the marrow, but there will be a reduction in the SNR.

Post-contrast images are useful when imaging for ischemia, infection, tumours and inflammatory conditions (Fig. 5.5a–c).

5.15 Applications in Paediatric Trauma

With acute paediatric trauma, standard radiographs remain the predominant imaging modality, with MRI being used as an adjunct. MRI is useful in detecting some acute injuries such as scaphoid fractures. In other circumstances it is of limited value, being relatively insensitive in detecting small ossific fragments within a joint and when there is a considerable amount of metallic hardware within the bone.

While protocols are important, each examination should be tailored to the individual patient and address the specific area of clinical concern.

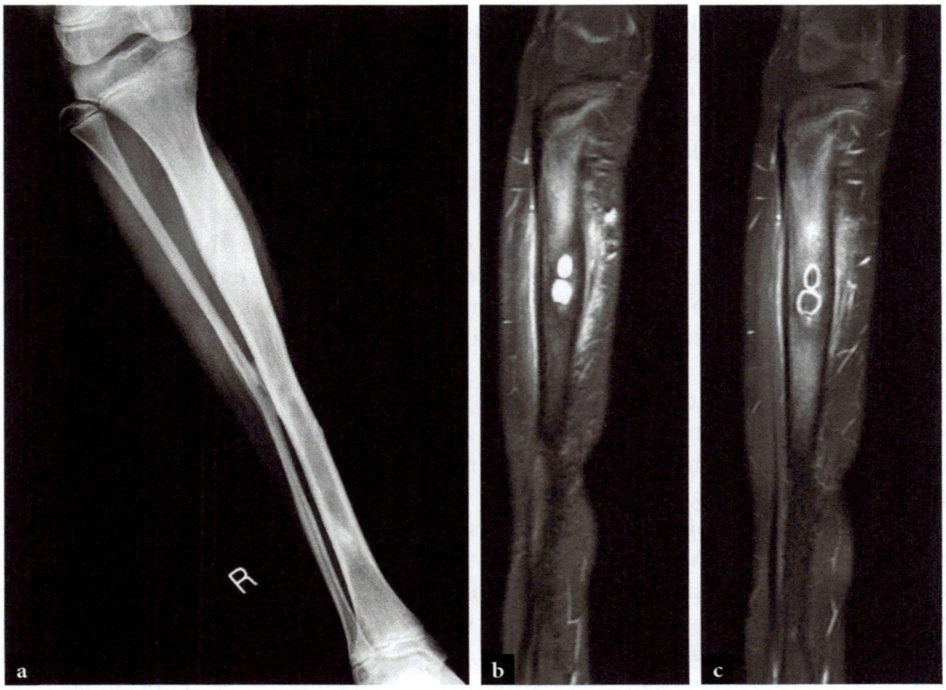

Fig. 5.5a–c. a AP radiograph of the tibia. There is a healing fracture of the proximal tibia. The child subsequently presented with pyrexia and localised swelling. **b** Coronal STIR image showing high signal fluid collections within the bone; there is surrounding high signal marrow and soft tissue oedema. **c** Coronal T1 fat saturated post-gadolinium images showing ring enhancement of the fluid collections in the proximal tibia, indicative of abscess formation. This was confirmed following surgical drainage

5.15.1 Cartilage

Problems within the cartilage of children may be congenital, developmental, post-infective or post-traumatic. Post-traumatic problems particularly affect the growth plate, causing early fusion and disrupted growth.

Proton density fast spin echo, dual echo steady state, gradient echo and multiplanar gradient recalled echo (MPGR) volume acquisition are useful when assessing cartilage. With these sequences, cartilage will appear bright (Hardy et al. 1996; Disler et al. 1997; Wang et al. 1999).

Spoilt gradient echo volume acquisitions of the cartilage allow 3D reformatting of the physeal cartilage with an assessment of the degree of any bone bridge formation across the growth plate (Jaramillo et al. 1990) (Figs. 5.6a,b and 5.7a–c).

5.15.2 Marrow

Bone marrow contains either haematopoietic cells (red marrow) or fat cells (yellow marrow) depending on the body's demand for red cell production. The fat content of the marrow will determine the signal intensity on MR imaging. Typically, fatty marrow is of higher signal intensity than surrounding muscle on T1 weighted sequences, while haematopoietic marrow is of low to intermediate signal intensity (similar to muscle).

In the newborn, the majority of marrow is haematopoietic and during life it is gradually replaced by fatty marrow, such that in the young adult, the majority of marrow is fatty. The proximal humerus and femur may contain haematopoietic marrow into adulthood. The pattern of changes goes from distal to proximal, i.e. the toe and fingers to the hip and shoulder, respectively. The epiphysis usually converts to fatty marrow before the metaphysis. In general, once the epiphyseal ossification centre has appeared (on a radiograph), the marrow will be fatty within 6 months.

Around the knee, fatty conversion may occur around adolescence and in an irregular pattern, producing a geographical type distribution and it is important that this is not confused with a malignant process (Foster et al. 2004) (Fig. 5.8).

With traumatic injuries, there will be bone marrow oedema which is easily detected as high signal

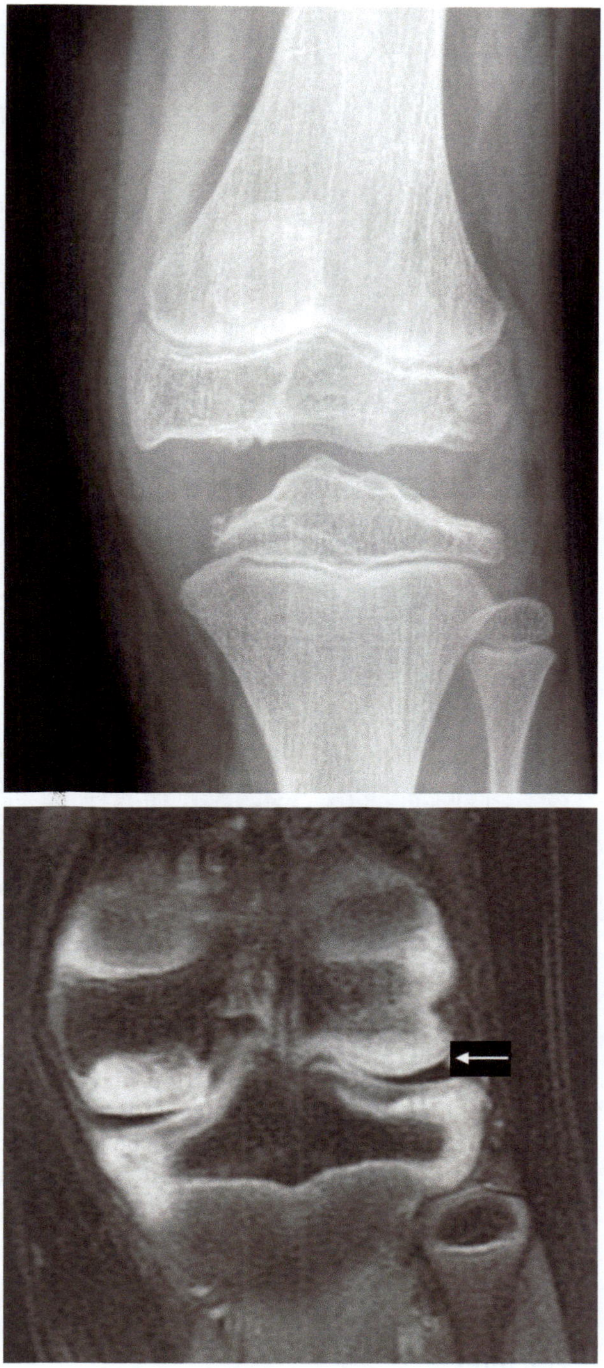

a

b

Fig. 5.6a,b. AP radiograph of the knee showing evidence of multiple epiphyseal dysplasia. There is flattening and irregularity of the distal femoral epiphysis. Coronal Proton density fast spin echo fat suppressed image of the knee. The unossified cartilage is seen as high signal around the darker ossified bone. The articular cartilage lining the joint surface is also of high signal but of a slightly different signal intensity (*arrow*)

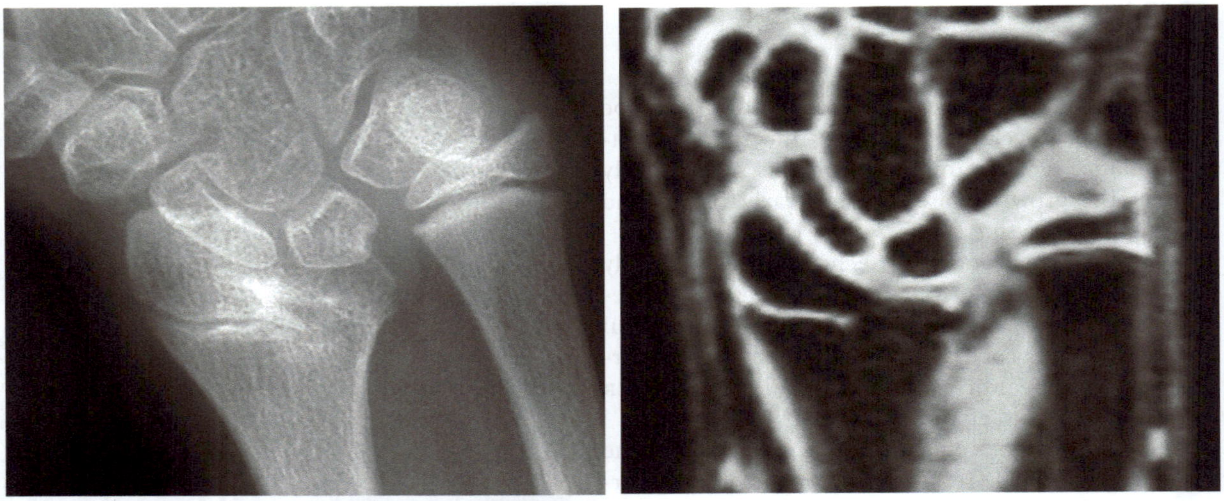

a

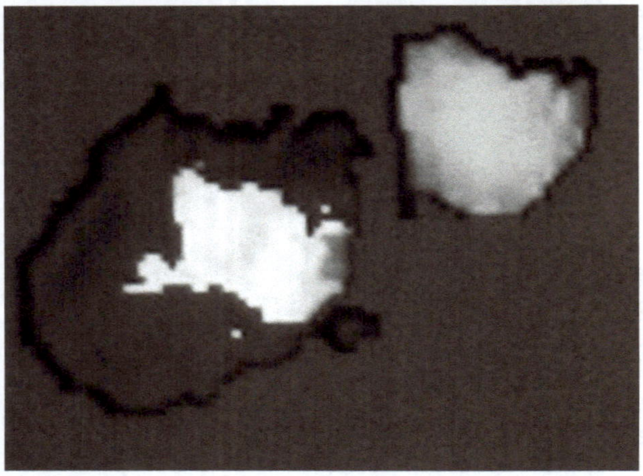

c

Fig. 5.7a–c. **a** A child has suffered a previous fracture involving the distal radial physis. This has resulted in a bone bridge across the physis with resulting growth disturbance. **b** A single slice from a spoiled gradient echo shows the dark bone bridge across the high signal physis. 3D reformatting and image manipulation shows the area of the bone bridge and can estimate the area of involvement. The white area on the right represents the area of bone bridging

on STIR or fat saturated FSE T2 weighted sequences. Malignant infiltration and infection may also give a similar high signal appearance and clinical correlation is important. Fractures often have a cortical break and/or a low signal fracture line within them. Soft tissue changes and enhancement can occur in all the pathological processes.

5.15.3 Fractures

The use of MRI is not routinely indicated in the acute setting; however, it is being increasingly utilised for scaphoid injuries (Johnson et al. 2000).

MRI is ideally suited to the assessment of avulsion injuries as it can provide detail about the marrow oedema, cartilage damage and associated soft tissue or ligament damage. Unossified cartilage is of high signal on protein density FSE fat saturated sequences. Distraction or oedema around the cartilage and apophyseal growth plate can be detected.

MRI is very sensitive in detecting the marrow oedema associated with stress fractures. The use of STIR or FSE T2 weighted fat saturated sequences will show the oedema as high signal. There may be a low signal intensity area within the marrow, corresponding to the fracture line. Periosteal new bone is seen as low signal change on all sequences.

Differentiation between ‘bone bruising’ and a fracture may be difficult. Bone contusions appear as diffuse or geographical areas of low signal intensity within fatty marrow on T1 weighted images and high signal intensity on T2 fat suppressed or STIR images. Bone bruises resolve over weeks or months. Occasionally, they may evolve into areas of sclerosis which are of low signal intensity on all sequences.

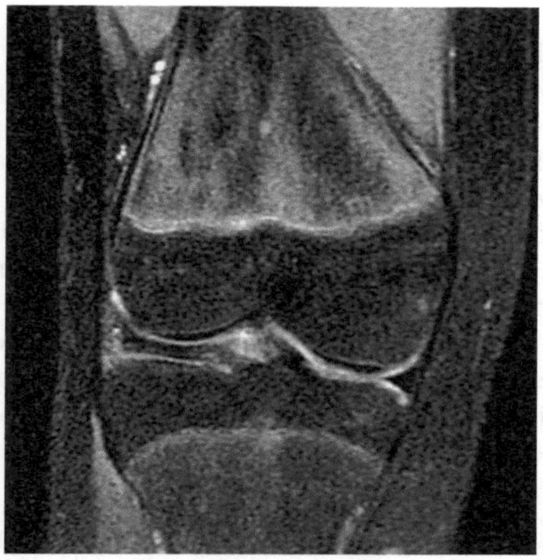

Fig. 5.8. Coronal T2 weighted fat saturated image of the knee of a teenager. There is mixed signal intensity within the distal femoral metaphysis. This is a normal feature of marrow conversion in adolescence

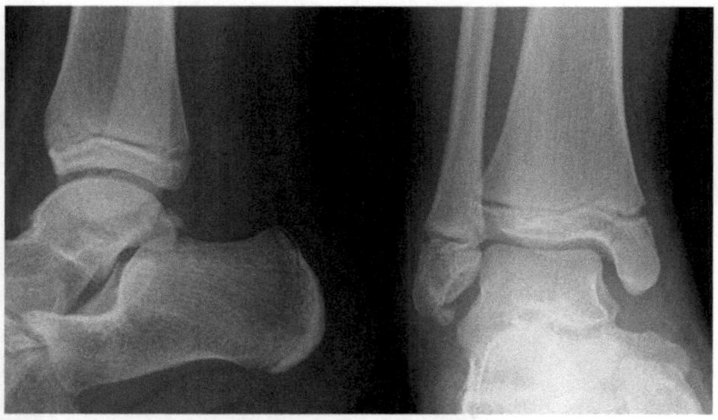

a

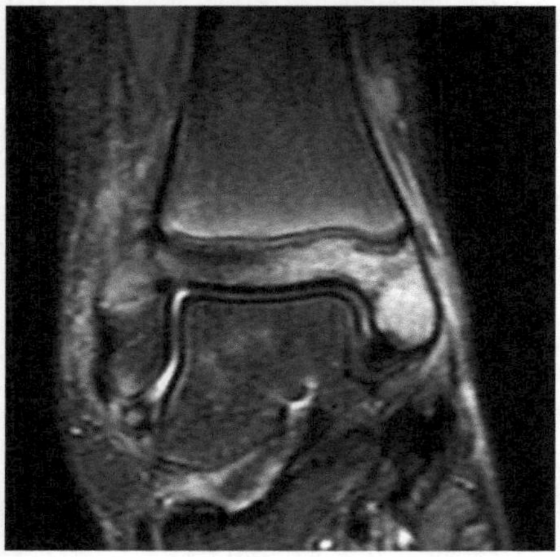

b

Fig. 5.9a,b. AP and lateral radiographs of the ankle show possible slight distortion of the medial malleolus with widening of the medial aspect of the distal tibia physis. Coronal STIR confirms the presence of a fracture involving the physis. There is extensive marrow oedema with a clearly visible low signal fracture line

With non-displaced occult fractures, the fracture line will appear as an area of low signal intensity within the oedematous marrow. Stress fracture lines are typically linear. The use of gradient echo or T1 weighted sequences to identify loss of the normal bony trabecular pattern can also be used. MRI will also allow detection of fractures through unossified portions of the skeleton. (Figs. 5.9a,b, 5.10, 5.11).

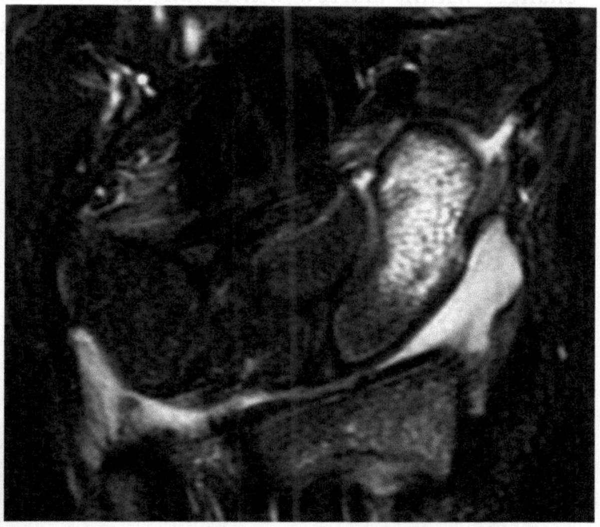

Fig. 5.10. Oblique coronal STIR image of the scaphoid. There is extensive marrow oedema with fluid around the carpal bones, features in keeping with a scaphoid fracture. Radiographs were normal.

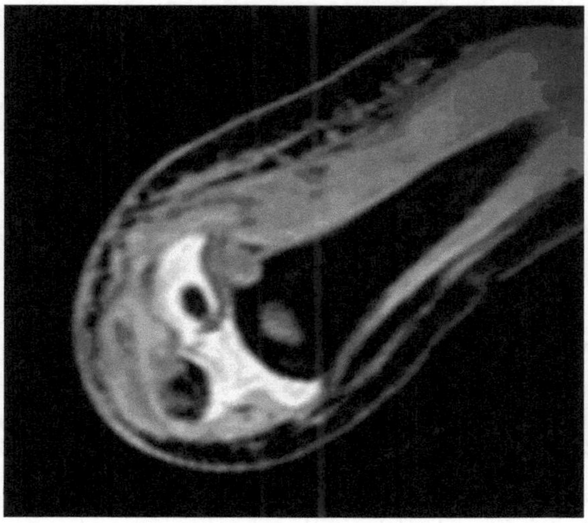

Fig. 5.11. Oblique spoiled gradient echo image of the distal humerus showing a fracture extending across the physeal growth plate and through the unossified cartilage

5.15.4 Marrow Infarction/Avascular Necrosis

Avascular necrosis can potentially complicate any fracture but is thankfully relatively rare in the younger child. In the older teenager with a scaphoid or femoral head fracture, dislocation then avascular necrosis is a more significant risk.

Marrow ischaemia will cause signal intensity changes within marrow which can lead to infarction. Transient ischaemia can occur following an acute fracture with the marrow returning to normal weeks later.

Chronic marrow infarcts are characterised by a serpiginous margin of sclerosis which is of low signal on all sequences (Fig. 5.12a,b).

In the hip, avascular necrosis (osteonecrosis) has a characteristic 'double-line sign' appearance.

The double-line sign is seen on T2 weighted or STIR images of medullary bone as a high-signal-intensity line within a parallel rim of decreased signal intensity, often with serpentine borders. Corresponding T1 weighted images demonstrate both these high and low signal intensity zones, together as a single low signal intensity band (Zurlo 1999) (Fig. 5.13a,b).

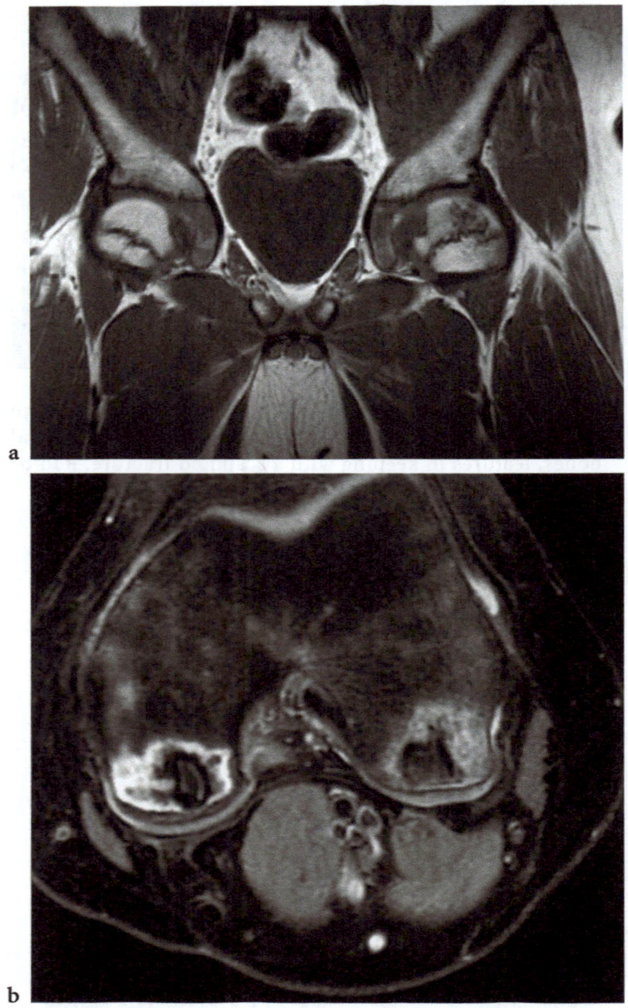

Fig. 5.12a,b. Coronal T1 weighted image of the hips. Within the left femoral epiphysis, there is a serpiginous low signal area as a result of infarcted bone marrow. Axial proton density fat saturated image through the knee in a different patient shows irregular serpiginous changes in the femoral condyles

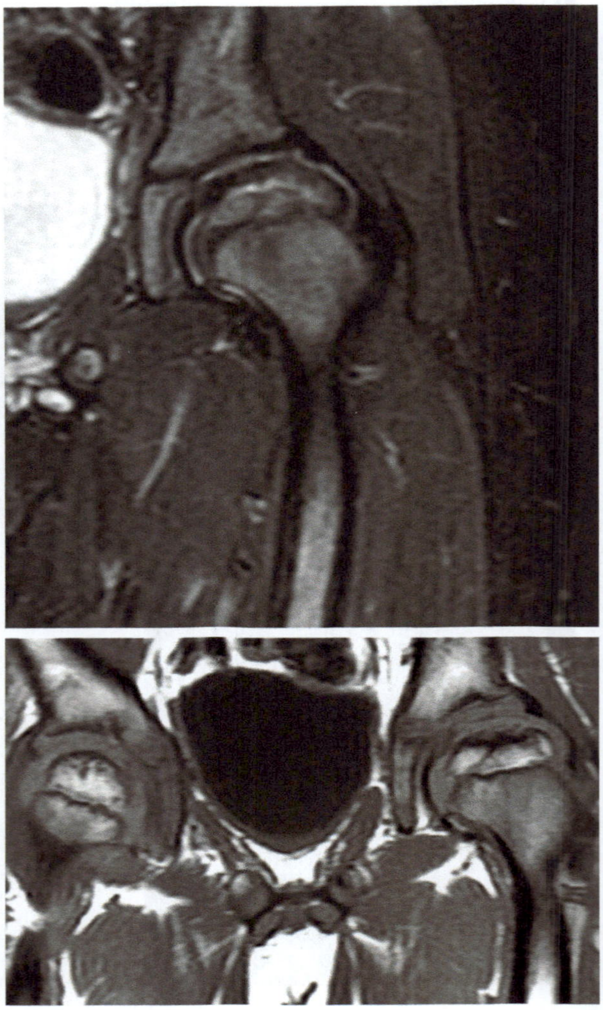

Fig. 5.13a,b. Coronal STIR image of the left femoral epiphysis (**a**) showing the central high signal intensity line with surrounding low signal areas which on the corresponding T1 image (**b**) is all low signal. Note the so called 'double line sign'

The high signal intensity inner zone represents hyperaemic granulation tissue. The low signal intensity outer zone represents adjacent sclerotic bone. Chemical shift artefact may accentuate the low signal intensity of the outer rim in some cases.

5.15.5 Ligaments

MRI is very well suited to assessing ligament injuries. In children, there is more likely to be a fracture or avulsion injury rather than a ligament tear. On both T1 and T2 weighted images, there is loss of continuity of ligament fibres. On T2 weighted images, there is high signal surrounding soft tissue oedema and fluid in the acute stages. There may be associated marrow oedema (Fig. 5.14).

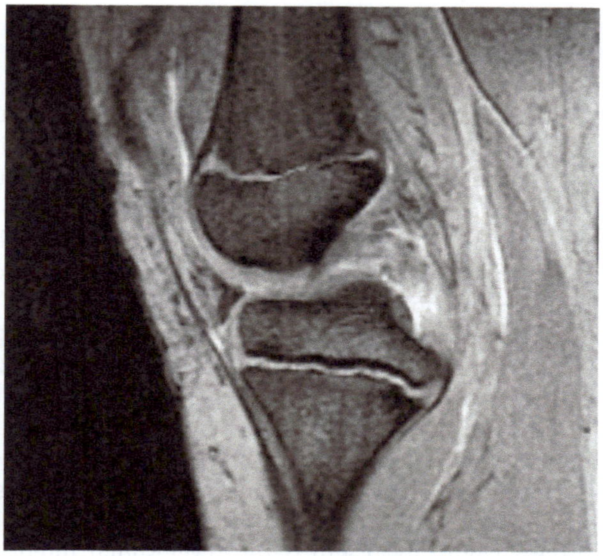

Fig. 5.14. Sagittal gradient echo image of the knee. There is rupture of the posterior cruciate ligament, with loss of continuity of ligament fibres and distortion of the surrounding soft tissues

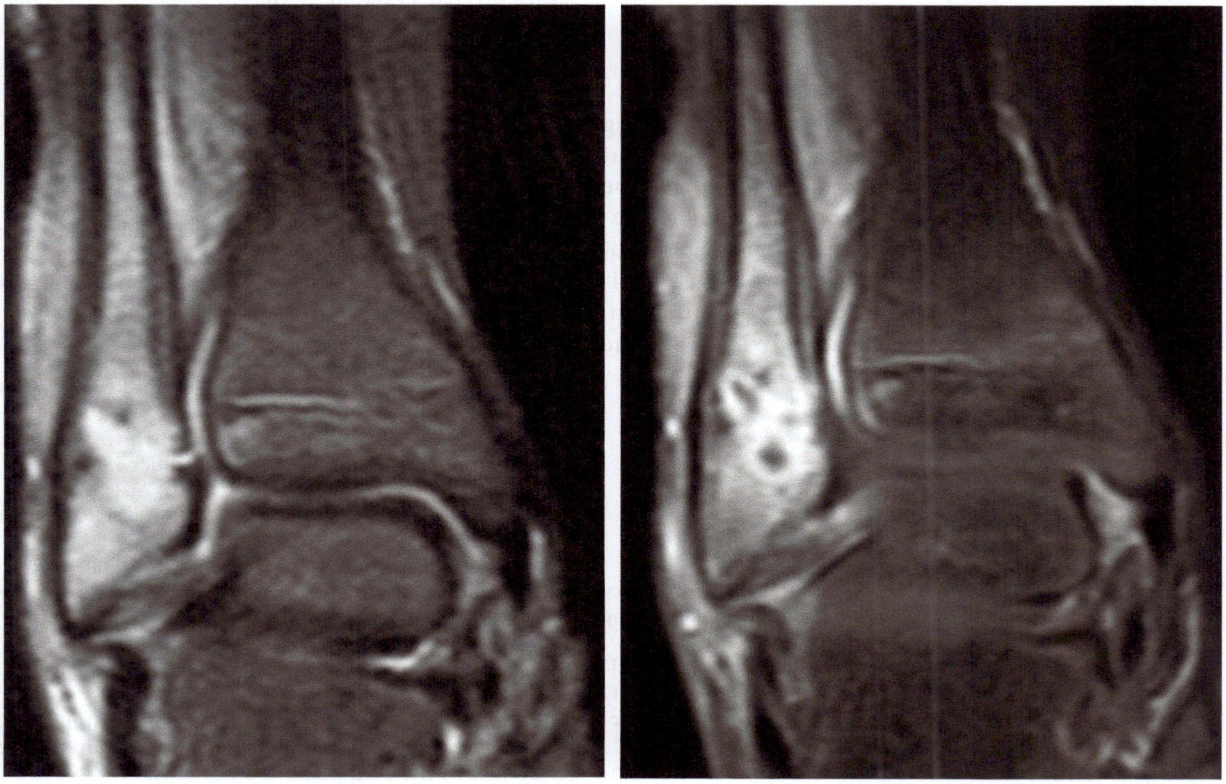

a b

Fig. 5.15a,b. Coronal STIR image of the distal fibula. There is extensive marrow oedema in the metaphysis and epiphysis. Corresponding T1 fat saturated post-gadolinium image shows multiple small abscesses in the distal fibula, which are distinct from the surrounding marrow oedema

5.15.6 Infection

Infection within the bone results in extensive marrow oedema, and typically with associated soft tissue oedema. The appearances of the oedema can be similar to that of a fracture and differentiation between infection and an undisplaced fracture may be difficult. Obviously, the clinical features and mode of presentation will often discriminate.

On T2 weighted images, there is hyperintense signal from the marrow oedema. There may be cortical thickening and cortical breaks. Differentiating abscesses from surrounding oedema may be difficult on standard T2 or STIR images. The use of gadolinium will show rim enhancement of the abscess, enhancement of the surrounding tissue but the abscess cavity itself will be of lower signal intensity (Fig. 5.15a,b). With gadolinium, there may be areas that do not enhance, suggesting areas of necrosis.

5.16 Conclusion

MRI imaging is a very valuable tool in assessing skeletal pathology in children. It is important that the patient remains safe and comfortable during the procedure, with the most appropriate sequence being performed to high standards. Optimisation of the scanning parameters will improve image quality and the diagnostic yield from the examination. Each child should be treated as an individual and the examination tailored to their clinical needs.

Reference

Adair ER, Berglund LG (1986) On the thermoregulatory consequences of NMR imaging. Magn Reson Imaging 4:321–333

Ahn JM, Kwak SM et al. (1998) Evaluation of patellar cartilage in cadavers with a low-field-strength extremity-only magnet: comparison of MR imaging sequences, with macroscopic findings as the standard. Radiology 208:57–62

Anupindi S, Jaramillo D (2002) Pediatric magnetic resonance imaging techniques. Magn Reson Imaging Clin N Am 10:189–207

Barnewolt CE, Chung T (1998) Techniques, coils, pulse sequences, and contrast enhancement in pediatric musculoskeletal MR imaging. Magn Reson Imaging Clin N Am 6: 441–453

Beltran J, Rosenberg ZS et al. (1994) Pediatric elbow fractures: MRI evaluation. Skeletal Radiol 23:277–281

Bitar R, Leung G et al. (2006) MR pulse sequences: what every radiologist wants to know but is afraid to ask. Radiographics 26:513–537

Bradley WG Jr. (1999) Optimizing lesion contrast without using contrast agents. J Magn Reson Imaging 10:442–449

Brown MA, Semelka RC (1999) MR imaging abbreviations, definitions, and descriptions: a review. Radiology 213:647–662

Close BJ, Strouse PJ (2000) MR of physeal fractures of the adolescent knee. Pediatr Radiol 30:756–762

Creasy JL, Partain CL et al. (1995) Quality of clinical MR images and the use of contrast agents. Radiographics 15:683–696

Disler DG, McCauley TR et al. (1997) In-phase and out-of-phase MR imaging of bone marrow: prediction of neoplasia based on the detection of coexistent fat and water. AJR Am J Roentgenol 169:1439–1447

Dixon WT (1984) Simple proton spectroscopic imaging. Radiology 153:189–194

Duerk JL (1999) Principles of MR image formation and reconstruction. Magn Reson Imaging Clin N Am 7:629–659

Echigo J, Yoshioka H et al. (1999) Signal intensity changes in anterior cruciate ligament autografts: relation to magnetic field orientation. Acad Radiol 6:206–210

Elster AD (1997) How much contrast is enough? Dependence of enhancement on field strength and MR pulse sequence. Eur Radiol 7[Suppl 5]:276–280

Farr RF and Allisy-Roberts PJ (1998) Physics for Medical Imaging. Saunders, London, UK

Fleckenstein JL, Archer BT et al. (1991) Fast short-tau inversion-recovery MR imaging. Radiology 179:499–504

Foster K, Chapman S et al. (2004) MRI of the marrow in the paediatric skeleton. Clin Radiol 59:651–673

Haase A, Frahm J et al. (1985) 1H NMR chemical shift selective (CHESS) imaging. Phys Med Biol 30:341–344

Hardy PA, Recht MP et al. (1996) Optimization of a dual echo in the steady state (DESS) free-precession sequence for imaging cartilage. J Magn Reson Imaging 6:329–335

Hayes CW, Parellada JA (1996) The magic angle effect in musculoskeletal MR imaging. Top Magn Reson Imaging 8:51–56

Hood MN, Ho VB et al. (1999) Chemical shift: the artifact and clinical tool revisited. Radiographics 19:357–371

Jaramillo D, Hoffer FA et al. (1990) MR imaging of fractures of the growth plate. AJR Am J Roentgenol 155:1261–1265

Jaramillo D, Shapiro F et al. (1990) Post-traumatic growth-plate abnormalities: MR imaging of bony-bridge formation in rabbits. Radiology 175:767–773

Johnson KJ, Haigh SF et al. (2000) MRI in the management of scaphoid fractures in skeletally immature patients. Pediatr Radiol 30:685–688

Johnson K, Page A et al. (2002) The use of melatonin as an alternative to sedation in uncooperative children undergoing an MRI examination. Clin Radiol 57:502–506

Kanal E, Shellock FG (1990) Burns associated with clinical MR examinations. Radiology 175:585

Kanal E, Shellock FG et al. (1990) Safety considerations in MR imaging. Radiology 176:593–606

Lee SH, Baek JR et al. (2005) Stress fractures of the femoral diaphysis in children: a report of 5 cases and review of literature. J Pediatr Orthop 25:734–738
Mirowitz SA (1999) MR imaging artifacts. Challenges and solutions. Magn Reson Imaging Clin N Am 7:717–732
Niitsu M, Nakai T et al. (2000) High-resolution MR imaging of the knee at 3 T. Acta Radiol 41:84–88
Patton JA (1994) MR imaging instrumentation and image artifacts. Radiographics 14:1083–1096; quiz 1097–1098
Pipe JG (1999) Basic spin physics. Magn Reson Imaging Clin N Am 7:607–627
Plewes DB (1994) The AAPM/RSNA physics tutorial for residents. Contrast mechanisms in spin-echo MR imaging. Radiographics 14:1389-1404; quiz 1405–1406
Pudas T, Hurme T et al. (2005) Magnetic resonance imaging in pediatric elbow fractures. Acta Radiol 46:636–644
Rand T, Ahn JM et al. (1999) Ligaments and tendons of the ankle. Evaluation with low-field (0.2 T) MR imaging. Acta Radiol 40:303–308
Rawson JV, Siegel MJ (1996) Techniques and strategies in pediatric body MR imaging. Magn Reson Imaging Clin N Am 4:589–598
Redpath TW (1998) Signal-to-noise ratio in MRI. Br J Radiol 71:704–707
Schmitt F, Dewdney A et al. (1999) Hardware considerations for MR imaging physics. Magn Reson Imaging Clin N Am 7:733–763, vi
Smith BG, Rand F et al. (1994) Early MR imaging of lower-extremity physeal fracture-separations: a preliminary report. J Pediatr Orthop 14:526–533
Sury MR, Hatch DJ et al. (1999) Development of a nurse-led sedation service for paediatric magnetic resonance imaging. Lancet 353:1667–1671
Sury MR, Harker H et al. (2005) The management of infants and children for painless imaging. Clin Radiol 60:731–741
Turner DA, Rapoport MI et al. (1991) Truncation artifact: a potential pitfall in MR imaging of the menisci of the knee. Radiology 179:629–633
Wang SF, Cheng HC et al. (1999) Fat-suppressed three-dimensional fast spoiled gradient-recalled echo imaging: a modified FS 3D SPGR technique for assessment of patellofemoral joint chondromalacia. Clin Imaging 23:177–180
Weinberger E, Shaw DW et al. (1995) Nontraumatic pediatric musculoskeletal MR imaging: comparison of conventional and fast-spin-echo short inversion time inversion-recovery technique. Radiology 194:721–726
White PG, Mah JY et al. (1994) Magnetic resonance imaging in acute physeal injuries. Skeletal Radiol 23:627–631
Zurlo JV (1999) The double-line sign. *Radiology* 212:541–542

Nuclear Medicine

6

Karen Bradshaw and Angharad Harries

CONTENTS

K. Bradshaw, MBChB, MRCP, FRCR
Consultant Radiologist, Radiology Department, Withybush Hospital, Fishguard Road, Haverfordwest, Dyfed, UK
A. Harries, MSc.
Senior Radiographer, Radiology Department Withybush Hospital, Fishguard Road, Haverfordwest, Dyfed, UK

6.1 Introduction

This chapter describes the use of bone scintigraphy in children, detailing the radiation implications and highlighting accepted indications in current practice.

6.2 Preparation of Child and Family

To produce good quality diagnostic images in nuclear medicine, care is needed for adequate preparation of both the patient and the clinical environment.

Information provided prior to the examination should be in a form which can be easily understood by both the carer and the child. If appropriate two different information forms should be used, one targeted at the carer and one at the child. The information provided should include details of what is going to happen, a list of the facilities available and details of the time delay between injection and imaging to allow consideration as to how the patient should be occupied in the interval.

In centres where 200 or more paediatric examinations are performed per year it is recommended that specific paediatric facilities be available with sessions dedicated to the imaging of children (British Nuclear Medicine Society 2001).

Bone scintigraphy involves venepuncture, a time delay following injection of the isotope and a significant subsequent period immobilised on the scanner. Topical local anaesthetic should be used prior to venepuncture. Play therapy should be utilised as the use of play specialists has been shown to reduce the need for general anaesthesia (Department of Health 2003).

Administration of the radiopharmaceutical should be performed by staff suitably trained in paediatric venepuncture and radiopharmaceutical administration (British Nuclear Medicine Society 2001).

In small children scan times can be scheduled to coincide with the child's normal daytime sleep pattern. The additional use of aids such as sandbags, Velcro straps, baby huggers and vacuum mattresses are also effective. In the older child an understanding adult to remind them about the need to remain still is usually adequate. Sedation is usually unnecessary but may need to be considered if repeated scan attempts have failed. It is recommended that an institute wide approach to paediatric sedation be adopted and followed (Mandell et al. 2003). Determination of the pregnancy status of all females of child bearing age should be performed in accordance with local or national protocols (British Nuclear Medicine Society 2001).

6.3 Image Quality

When imaging very small children it is imperative that the child remain as close as possible to the gamma camera heads. The greater the distance between the patient and the camera heads the poorer the resolution of the image and very small children or babies should be positioned directly onto the camera heads when possible. When using high energy collimators a resolution of 4–5 mm is achieved with a 0-cm subject/collimator distance, this is reduced to 17–18 mm at a distance of 30-cm subject collimator distance (O'Connor et al. 1991).

The growing metaphyses are metabolically highly active in children, necessitating the use of high-resolution techniques such as pinhole collimation to resolve subtle abnormalities.

When bones and joints are assessed individually care must be taken to image the contralateral bones or joints at exactly the same distance from the collimator surface.

6.4 Radiopharmaceutical

The most common radiopharmaceutical in clinical use for skeletal imaging is diphosphonate labelled with Technetium^{99m}. The compounds primarily used in this imaging are methylene diphosphonate (MDP), and hydroxymethylene diphosphonate (HMDP).

Technetium^{99m} is a desirable isotope for diagnostic imaging as it has a manageable half life of 6.02 h, produces a photon of energy 140 keV and it readily labels diphosphonates, producing a radiopharmaceutical which is stable over several hours. This radiopharmaceutical is susceptible to oxidation and thus care must be taken in its preparation to ensure no air is introduced to the vial. In clinical practice oxidation will result in the presence of free pertechnetate, which will result in an associated degradation of image quality due to associated uptake of the pertechnetate in soft tissue and glands (Thrall and Ziessman 2001; Haasbeek and Green 1994).

6.5 Pharmacokinetics and Localisation of Tc^{99m} Diphosphonate

Tc^{99m} radiolabelled diphosphonate is injected intravenously and is rapidly absorbed into the extracellular fluid. Although the exact mechanism of uptake of the radiopharmaceutical from the extracellular fluid into the bone is not completely understood, it is thought that both the osteoblastic activity and vascularity of the bone have roles. Following uptake the radiopharmaceutical is then adsorbed onto the surface of the inorganic crystalline bone matrix. A few hours post injection the blood level is approximately 3.5% of the injected dose and bone uptake is at 50% of the injected dose (Thrall and Ziessman 2001; Haasbeek and Green 1994).

6.6 Paediatric Doses and Radiation Burden

Any dosage of radioactive isotope in the child is subject to review and subsequent alteration. It is therefore incumbent on the staff involved in nuclear medicine that they are fully up to date with local and national procedures. At present the recommended minimum dose is 40 MBq of Tc^{99m} labelled diphosphonate and the maximum dose is 500 MBq. Paediatric doses should be scaled down according to body surface area (Hahn et al. 2000).

Radiation burden is dependent on the development of the child and decreases with age (Table 6.1).

In order to reduce the radiation burden on the patient the child is required to maintain a good level of hydration and should be encouraged to void their bladder frequently as the dose to bladder, ovary/testes depends on frequency of voiding. In children who are not toilet trained or are unable to void their bladder, consideration may need to be given as to whether catheterisation is appropriate prior to radiopharmaceutical administration The main concerns are the radiation burden to the child and the ability to acquire optimal images of the pelvis and sacrum.

Table 6.1. Radiation burden relative to age and development

Age	Effective dose equivalent (mSv)/Bq
Newborn	0.11
1 year	0.042
5 years	0.021
10 years	0.014
15 years	0.0089

(Hahn et al. 2000)

6.7 Image Acquisition

Depending upon the clinical indication for performing the bone scan, different imaging techniques may be employed in order to achieve a diagnosis.

6.7.1 Single Phase Study

Patients are injected with radioisotope and imaged after a suitable delay (usually 2–4 h). Single phase bone imaging is used to assess the skeleton by demonstrating the osteophyte activity which occurs in the interval between radiopharmaceutical administration and scan.

6.7.2 Two Phase Study

A two phase study requires imaging of the bloodpool at an interval immediately after the radioisotope has been dispersed by the arterial blood flow, thus allowing assessment of the soft tissues. Delayed imaging should occur after 2–4 h, as previously described for a single phase study.

6.7.3 Three Phase Study

Three phase bone scanning requires that the symptomatic part of the patient be positioned under the gamma camera. Dynamic images of arterial flow are commenced simultaneously with the radiopharmaceutical administration. This enables assessment of arterial blood flow to the area under investigation. Subsequently, the blood pool and skeletal phases should then be accompanied as previously discussed for a two phase study.

6.7.4 Single Photon Emission Computed Tomography (SPECT)

SPECT imaging being a tomographic technique enables the removal of overlying structures from an area of interest, and thus increases image contrast and aids localisation of a lesion. The European Association of Nuclear Medicine recommends SPECT imaging in any paediatric patient where there is unusual radiopharmaceutical uptake in the spine, pelvis and/or skull. In investigations of the spine especially, SPECT is considered to reduce the risks of misdiagnosis (Hahn et al. 2000). High resolution collimators should always be used when performing a SPECT study. Although there is a balance between count statistics and resolution, it has been demonstrated that with appropriate post processing, high resolution collimators will result in increased image contrast and require less counts than a low resolution collimators to produce the same signal to noise ratio . It is of greater benefit to have a high resolution/low count study than vice versa (O'Connor et al. 1991).

The shape of the camera orbit is also very important during SPECT. A non-circular orbit will ensure a minimum distance between the camera head and the patient. Thus the image resolution of a non-circular orbit will always be superior to that of a circular orbit (O'Connor et al. 1991). With regard to imaging of the paediatric patient consideration must be given to limiting the patient movement. Any motion will result in a reduction of resolution, physiological motion such as bladder filling is slow and is tolerated. However, extreme motion such as patient movement may result in motion artefacts being produced in the resultant processed image, rendering the acquired data useless.

6.7.5 Magnified Views

In addition to deciding which imaging technique to use, consideration should also be given to acquiring magnified views. Magnified views are especially indicated during imaging of the hands, wrists, hips and ankles. The preferential method for acquiring these views is by the use of the pinhole collimator; however, this will extend the time that the patient has to spend under investigation, as use of the pinhole collimator requires imaging of both the affected and contralateral side for comparative purposes. The main drawback to the use of the pinhole collimator is its availability as they are very large and not ideally suited for use with many modern dual headed gamma camera systems. A second problem is the distortion of the resultant image.

If no pinhole collimator is available it is possible to produce magnified images by electronic means. It is important that the magnification occurs as part of the image acquisition process as post processing magnification will result in associated degradation of the final image.

6.7.6 Delayed Imaging

Imaging of the area under investigation during the skeletal phase may be performed by either whole body imaging or static 'spot' views. It is important that wherever possible the skeleton is imaged in its entirety irrespective of the locality of the pathology. Whole body imaging is considered faster but care should be taken to ensure that the speed the patient progresses through the imaging process is accordant with their age. In general, the smaller the child the slower they will need to progress through the camera. Children under 4 years of age should always undergo 'spot' imaging (Hahn et al. 2000) (Table 6.2).

6.8 Other Imaging Techniques

6.8.1 Single Photon Emission Computed Tomography/ Computed Tomography (SPECT/CT)

SPECT/CT images may be acquired either by the use of a hybrid scanner or by fusing images from a separate gamma camera and computed tomography (CT) scanner, though a hybrid scanner will achieve better quality images (the co-registration process of fusing images from a gamma camera and a distant CT scanner introduces a significant source for error). There is a lack of clinical evidence on the use of SPECT/CT in paediatric trauma.

6.8.2 Positron Emission Tomography (PET)

PET is a useful clinical tool in the imaging of disease. The main isotope in clinical use is Fluorine-18 which is produced in a cyclotron. It is used to form a glucose analogue but unfortunately has a large radiation burden associated with its use. Due to the current lack of availability and the expense of this modality its primary clinical use is for oncology diagnosis and disease staging. The role of PET in imaging trauma patients, particularly the paediatric patient, is unrealistic at the present time.

6.9 Role of Bone scintigraphy in Paediatric Trauma

Technetium^{99m} MDP is taken up in areas of new bone formation, a fracture causes increased bone activity, the isotope is concentrated at the fracture site and the fracture is visualised on imaging with a gamma camera.

The normal epiphysis varies in appearance with the patient's age, but at all ages there is intense uptake at the level of the zone of bone growth. Other than the normal epiphysis there is homogenous uptake within the skeleton. Given good quality images, intense uptake at areas other than the epiphysis is abnormal. In addition, in normal epiphysis there should be a sharp demarcation between the epiphyseal increased uptake and the diaphysis of the bone; loss of clarity of this margin is abnormal. There are numerous aetiologies to account for this but in the correct clinical context these findings are suggestive of a fracture. Scintigraphy will show the characteristic focal areas of increased uptake after 24–48 h of injury but will remain positive for some months, a sensitive but not a specific test (Figs. 6.1 and 6.2).

Previously bone scanning was used more widely to investigate continuing symptoms in the face of negative radiography, for example in scaphoid injuries, but studies have shown magnetic resonance imaging (MRI) to be a useful diagnostic tool in the immature skeleton (Johnson et al. 2000). MRI is now superseding scintigraphy in most clinical scenarios. There are really only two residual roles for scintigraphy, one in acute trauma, namely non-accidental injury, and the second in chronic trauma, the stress fracture. There is no current role for scintigraphy for acute accidental trauma.

Table 6.2. Imaging parameters for bone scintigraphy (Hahn et al. 2000)

Image	Parameter	Setting
Arterial flow	Matrix	64×64 128×128 (Dependent on processor)
	Collimator	LEAP LEHR
	Duration	1- to 2-s frames for 60 s
Blood pool Static image	Matrix	256×256
	Collimator	LEHR
	Duration	50–100 K counts appendicular skeleton 300–500 K counts axial skeleton
Blood pool Whole body	Matrix	1024×256
	Collimator	LEHR
	Duration	Scan speed 30 cm per min
Skeletal Phase 2–4 h post injection (static spot imaging)	Matrix	256×256
	Collimator	LEHR
	Duration	50–100 K counts (hands and feet) 100–200 K counts (knees) 300 K counts (skull) 500 K counts (thorax, spine and pelvis)
Skeletal phase 2–4 h post injection (whole body images)	Matrix	1024×256
	Collimator	LEHR
	Duration	8 cm/min (4–8 years) 10 cm/min (8–12 years) 12 cm/min (12–16 years) 15 cm/min (16+ years)
Pinhole views	Matrix	256×256
	Collimator	Pinhole
	Duration	100 K counts for non-affected side and identical time for affected side to allow comparison
SPECT imaging	Matrix	128×128
	Collimator	LEHR
	Duration	20–40 s
	Number of views	60–70 views
	Orbit	Non-circular

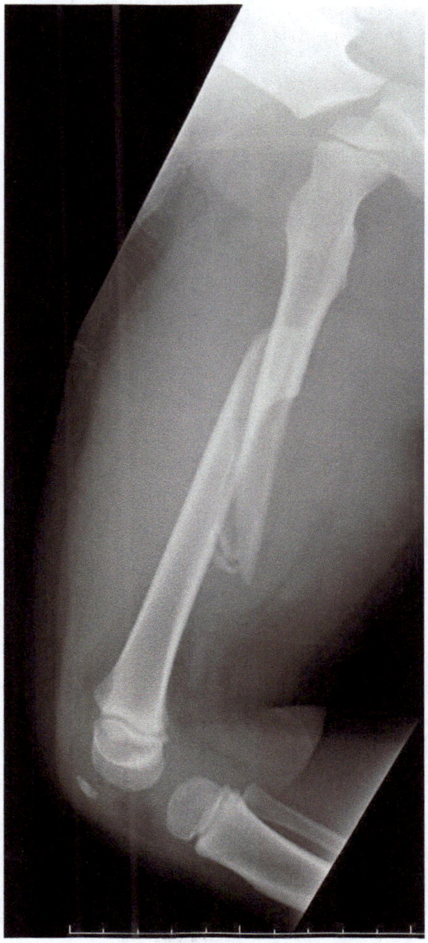

Fig. 6.1. Spiral fracture of the right femur

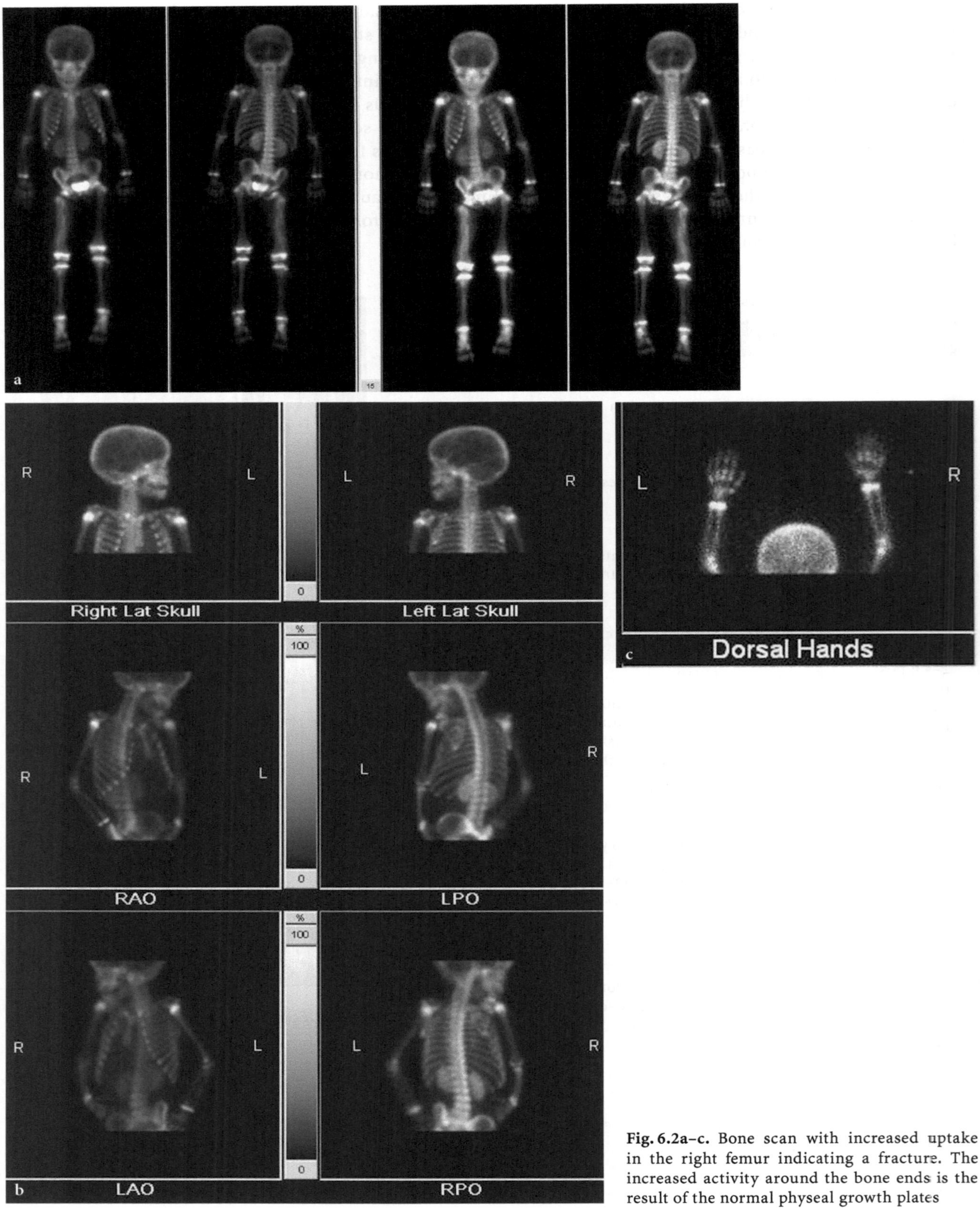

Fig. 6.2a–c. Bone scan with increased uptake in the right femur indicating a fracture. The increased activity around the bone ends is the result of the normal physeal growth plates

6.9.1 Non-accidental Injury

A skeletal survey is accepted standard practice in the investigation of non-accidental injury. Scintigraphy is more sensitive than plain films in the diagnosis of fractures, particularly in difficult areas such as the ribs. Where there is diagnostic difficulty or dispute on the findings of the radiograph which would have significant implication on either the civil or the criminal procedures, a bone scan is justified (Sty and Starshak 1983; Pickett et al. 1983; Smith et al. 1980) (Fig. 6.3).

6.9.2 Stress Fractures

Stress fractures are fractures caused by repetitive, prolonged minor trauma due to the pull of muscles upon normal bone. In children the skeleton has not yet adjusted to these forces and children are thus more prone to stress fractures than adults. Stress fractures may be difficult to detect on radiographs with the sensitivity of follow-up films possibly only reaching 50%.

6.9.2.1 Appendicular

In children common areas of appendicular stress fracture are the tibia, fibula or metatarsals and are more frequent in athletic children. Persistent pain in these areas should initially be investigated by plain film with delayed plain film in 10 days if negative. Previously, bone scan would be performed for persistent symptoms with negative radiographs but this has been largely superseded by localised MRI of the symptomatic area. If the pain is poorly localized, e.g. "whole lower limb aches" then scintigraphy can determine if there is an abnormal area and localise this area for further investigation by MRI or localised CT dependent on pathology.

Another type of injury in children is the undisplaced spiral fracture of the distal tibial shaft in children who have just begun walking, the Toddler's fracture. There is often no or minimal history of injury and children of this age poorly localise. X-rays can be normal in up to a third of patients. The radiograph can be repeated after 10 days to 2 weeks of immobilisation. Scintigraphy will demonstrate the fracture and its location usually before it is visible on an X-ray, but scintigraphy is not the accepted mechanism of investigation.

6.9.2.2 Spine

Spinal pain in children is less common than in adults. The first line in the investigation of spinal pain is a plain radiograph, AP and lateral. If the

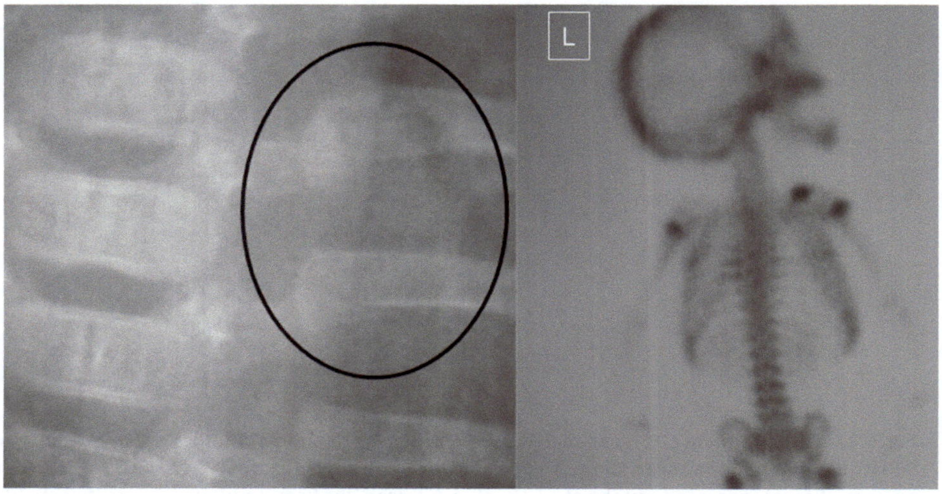

Fig. 6.3. Blown up chest radiograph and corresponding bone scan showing posterior left rib fractures. Their detection is improved by the use of the bone scan

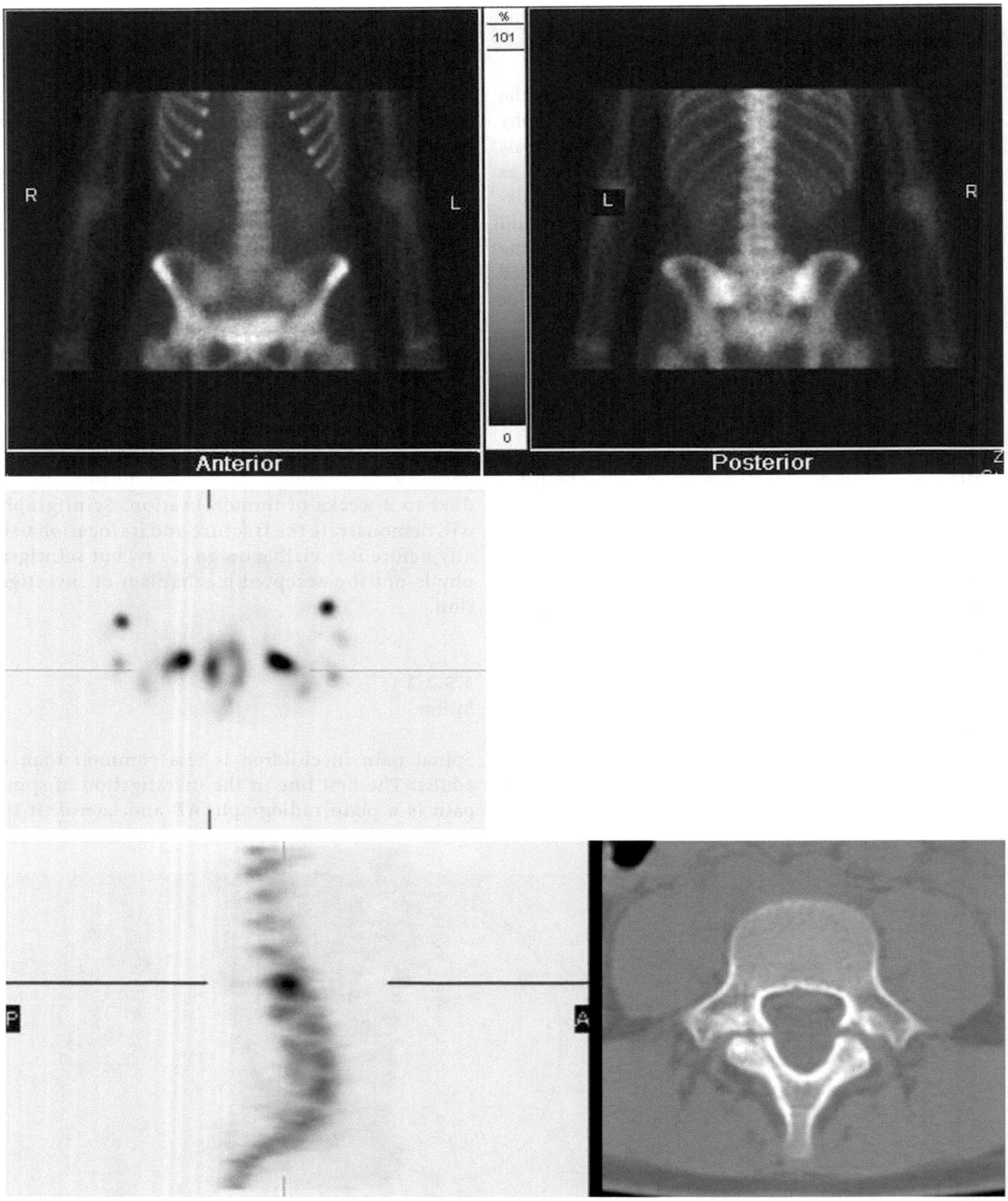

a b c

Fig. 6.4a–c. A promising 15-year-old national athlete with thoracolumbar pain and normal AP and lateral radiographs. Subsequent planar bone scan showed a possible foci of increased activity at L1 (**a**). A SPECT study demonstrates more clearly an area of focal increased uptake at L1 (**b, c**). A CT scan confirming bilateral pars defects (**d**) plain film shows a localised abnormality or the patient can accurately localise the pain, an MRI scan or localised CT are probably the second line investigation. In the context of a normal radiograph or poor localization, bone scan has a useful role for detection and localisation of pathology.

Stress injuries typically occur at the weakest part of the vertebra, the pars intra articularis, as this is relatively thin in young people. This is termed spondylolysis and is rare before the age of 5 but gradually increases to adult prevalence of 5% by age 20 (Hensinger 1995). Male Caucasians with a positive family history are recognised to have an increased risk of spondylolysis (Stewart 1953). Underlying congenital spinal anomalies, e.g. asymmetric development of the facets and transitional vertebrae may increase the risk of development . Bilateral pars defects can lead to anterior subluxation of the vertebral body on the vertebra below – spondylolisthesis. The stress is thought to be due to repetitive hyperextension of the immature spine and sports that incorporate this action lead to an increased risk (Gerbino and Micheli 1995). Spondylolysis and spondylolisthesis can be asymptomatic but an adolescent growth spurt may lead to symptoms, the pain typically radiates to the back of the thighs.

Single proton emission tomography (SPECT) detects significantly more lesions than planar scintigraphy (Mandell and Harcke 1993; Bellah et al. 1991; Collier et al. 1985; Read 1994). Radiographs and planar bone scans are insensitive to unilateral spondylolysis which occurs in 20%–25% of cases (Hensinger 1995). SPECT sequences should be routinely included in all bone scans of the paediatric spine, particularly when spondylolysis is suspected and if there is a short history of symptoms, less than 1 year (Harvey et al. 1998) (Fig. 6.4). SPECT is also of value since it demonstrates osteoblastic activity in the pars, this helps to differentiate between an actively healing lesion and a chronic non-union of the pars which may help in planning further management. SPECT can be used to assess response to treatment (Hensinger 1995). Pre-spondylotic stress reactions in the pars may be seen with SPECT and MRI. CT defines spondylolysis and provides more accurate anatomical information than MRI with acute defects being narrow with irregular edges and chronic lesions having smooth rounded margins (Hensinger 1995; Payne and Ogilvie 1996).

References

Bellah RD, Summerville DA, Treves ST, Micheli LJ (1991) Low back pain in adolescent athletes detection of stress injury to the pars intra interarticular with SPECT. Radiol 180:503–507

British Nuclear Medicine Society (2001) Quality guidelines for provision of paediatrics radionuclide imaging. British Nuclear Medicine Society

Collier BD, Johnson RP, Carrera GF, et al (1985) Painful spondylolysis or spondylolisthesis studied by radiography and single photon emission computed tomography. Radiol 154:207--211

Gerbino PG, Micheli LJ (1995) Back injuries in the young athlete. Clin Sports Med 14:571--590

Hensinger RN (1995) Acute back pain in children. Instr Course Lect 44:111--126

Hahn K, Fischer S, Colarinha P, Gordon I, Mann M, Piepssz A, Oliver P, Rune Sand VanVelzen J (2000) Guidelines for bone scintigraphy in children. European Association of Nuclear Medicine

Haasbeek JF, Green MA (1994) Adolescent stress fracture of the sacrum: 2 case reports. J Pediatr Orthop 14:336–3

Harvey CJ, Richenberg JL, Saifuddin A, Wolman RL (1998) Pictorial review; the radiological investigation of lumbar spondylolysis. Clin Radiol 53:723-728

Johnson KJ, Haigh SF, Symonds KE (2000) MRI in the management of scaphoid fractures in skeletally immature patients. Pediatr Radiol 30:685–688

Mandell GA, Harcke T (1993) Scintigraphy of spinal disorders in adolescents. Skeletal Radiol 22:393–401

Mandell A, Majid M, Shalaby-Rana E.I and Gordon I (2003) Society of Nuclear Medicine procedure guideline for paediatric sedation in nuclear medicine. Society of Nuclear Medicine, Version 3.0

National Service Framework (2003) Getting the right start national service framework for children, young people and maternity services standard for hospital services. Department of Health, 2003

O'Connor MK, Brown ML, Hung JC and Hayostek RJ (1991) The art of bone scintigraphy – technical aspects. J Nucl Med 32:2332–2341

Payne WK, Ogilvie JW (1996) Back pain in children and adolescents. Pediatr Clin North Am 43:899–917

Pickett WJ, Faleski EJ, Chacko A, Jarrett RV (1983) Comparison of radiographic and radionuclide skeletal surveys in battered children. South Med J 76:207–212

Read MTS (1994) Single photon emission computed tomography (SPECT) scanning for adolescent back pain. Br J Sports Med 28:56–57

Smith FW, Gilday DL, Ash JM, Green MD (1980) Unsuspected costo-vertebral fractures demonstrated by bone scanning in the child abuse syndrome. Pediatr Radiol 10:103–106

Stewart TD (1953) The age incidence of neuro-arch defects in Alaskan natives, considered from the standpoint of aetiology. J Bone Joint Surg Am 35:937–950

Sty JR, Starshak RJ (1983) The role of bone scintigraphy in the evaluation of the suspected abused child. Radiology 146:369–375

Thrall JH, Ziessman HA (2001) Nuclear medicine – the requisites, 2nd ed. Mosby, pp 110–114

Clinical Problems

Normal Anatomical Variants and Other Mimics of Skeletal Trauma

7

Helen Williams

CONTENTS

The effects of skeletal trauma may be simulated by normal anatomical variations during development, projection artefacts and overlap of adjacent structures. Secondary ossification centres or irregular sites of ossification that appear fragmented are often mistaken for traumatic injury. The 'mach effect' is a physiological form of edge enhancement created when there is an abrupt change from light to dark (radio-opaque to radiolucent) or vice versa at a concave or convex interface of a subject. Its presence at the interface of structures can simulate a fracture line. Similarly, overlap of normal structures such as skin or soft tissue folds can produce an identical appearance (Fig. 7.1).

7.1 Introduction

Numerous non-pathological appearances can simulate disease processes in the developing skeleton. These may be anatomical variants, related to irregular, decreased or increased mineralisation during ossification, or artefactual. Only those that simulate the effects of trauma will be covered in this chapter, which is not intended to be exhaustive. Skeletal variations that are more commonly encountered in paediatric practice are included but the reader is directed to more comprehensive texts such as Theodore Keats Atlas (Keats and Anderson 2001), which this chapter is not designed to replace as a reference text.

H. Williams, MBChB, MRCP, FRCR
Department of Radiology, Birmingham Children's Hospital, Steelhouse Lane Birmingham, B4 6NH, UK

7.2 Definitions

- *Epiphysis* – Secondary ossification centre found at the end of a long bone, which contributes to longitudinal growth of the bone. These are generally hemispheric in shape and form an articular surface, but gradually change shape as they develop joint congruity. Epiphyses are initially cartilaginous but ossify through endochondral ossification towards the end of fetal life or during childhood and fuse with the shaft during adolescence. In certain sites an epiphysis or the physeal plate may be mistaken for a fracture if visualised obliquely.
- *Apophysis* – Secondary ossification centre characteristically sited at a bony prominence which acts as the insertion site for a tendon. An apophysis is separated from the metaphysis by a physis. When it ossifies it does not contribute to longitudinal growth of the bone and these do not form articular surfaces. They are prone to acute or chronic avul-

sion secondary to tension forces from attached muscles, e.g. during exercise. A secondary ossification centre occasionally forms both an epiphysis and apophysis, e.g. proximal tibia.

- *Synchondrosis* – Primary cartilaginous joint occurring in a child's skeleton between two bones formed by endochondral ossification. This type of joint is rigid, and therefore differs from a secondary cartilaginous joint where there is an intervening fibrocartilaginous disc that allows some movement.
- *Accessory ossicle* – Small supernumerary bone found at characteristic sites as normal variants. They occur most commonly in the carpus, foot and ankle and vary in size. Typically a round, well corticated separate nodule of ossification adjacent to bone formed by the primary or secondary ossification centre. These may be mistaken for avulsion or chip fractures. Occasionally an accessory ossicle may fuse with the adjacent bone. These ossicles are usually of no clinical significance although they can occasionally cause pain. Some may be the result of previous trauma.
- *Sesamoid bone* – Ovoid nodular bones embedded within tendons, either adjacent to a joint or at sites where tendons are angled about bone surfaces. They are separated from the underlying bone by a synovium-lined bursa. Small sesamoid bones resemble sesame seeds. They are well corticated and may be bipartite. A bipartite sesamoid is larger overall than a fractured non-partite sesamoid. Sesamoids may be displaced or undergo fracture and dislocation.

7.3 Shoulder Girdle and Thoracic Cage

A companion shadow related to the upper border of the clavicle, due to overlying soft tissues is seen frequently on chest radiographs (CXR) at all ages, but is more common in older children when the bone is oriented horizontally (Fig. 7.2). This normal appearance may be incorrectly mistaken for perio-

a

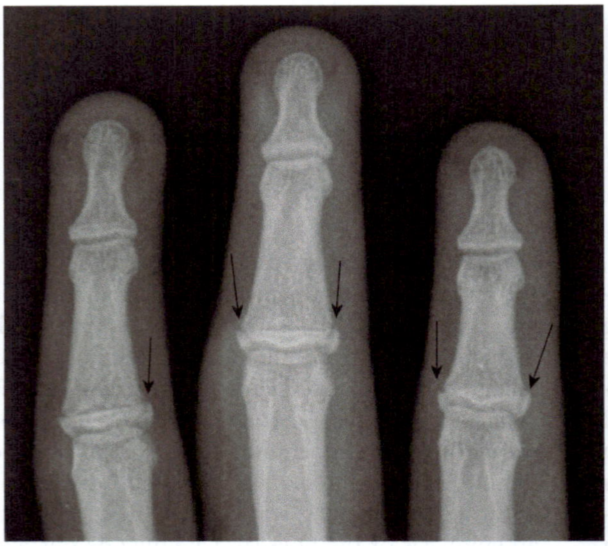

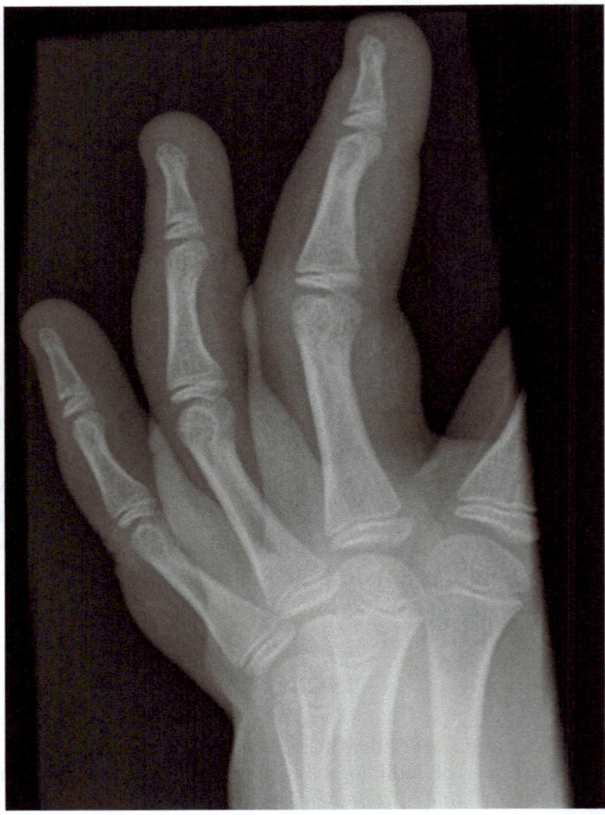

Fig. 7.1. **a** Pseudofractures of the epiphyseal ossification centres (*arrows*). The curved epiphyseal plates of the middle phalanges are superimposed on the secondary ossification centres at their bases producing an effect simulating fractures at the lateral margins. **b** Overlapping soft tissues of the fingers simulate oblique fractures in a child

steal new bone formation if not recognised. Oblique projection of the clavicle produces an apparent kink in the bone and can simulate a healing fracture with callus formation (Figs. 7.3, 7.4).

Congenital pseudoarthrosis of the clavicle may be mistaken for a fracture. This condition is almost always right sided and rarely bilateral. It usually presents with a painless, palpable prominence in the mid-portion of the clavicle. Approximately half of all patients present in the first 2 weeks of life, the others during childhood. The differential diagnosis includes cleidocranial dysostosis or a birth injury. Radiographically there is a defect in the middle segment of the clavicle, and the ends of the bones are well corticated and often bulbous and expanded, particularly the medial end of the lateral segment, whereas the lateral end of the medial segment can be tapered. The medial segment always lies higher and in front of the lateral segment, elevated by the sternocleidomastoid muscle (Fig. 7.5). Follow-up radiographs demonstrate a persistent cleft without evidence of healing (Ozonoff 1992). Overlap of the medial end of the clavicle with the transverse processes of the thoracic vertebrae may produce a lucent line simulating a fracture (Fig. 7.6).

The ossification centres for the acromion and coracoid processes may be mistaken for fractures. The acromion process may develop in two parts,

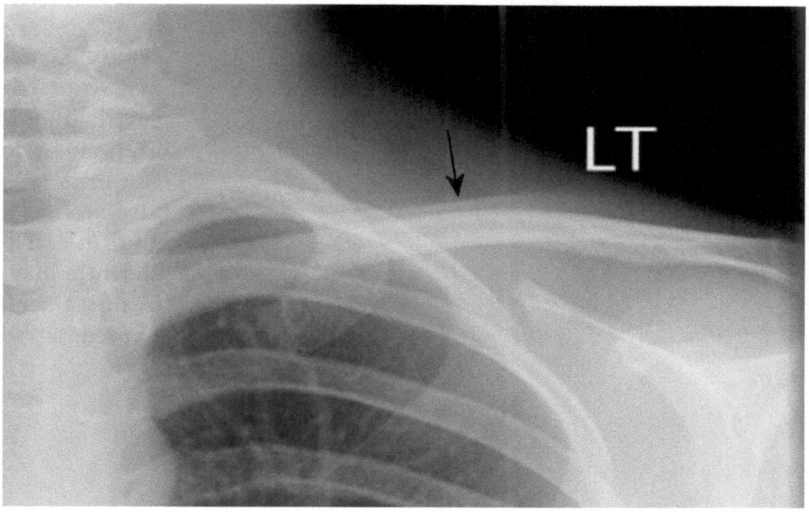

Fig. 7.2. The clavicular companion shadow, simulating periosteal new bone formation (*arrow*)

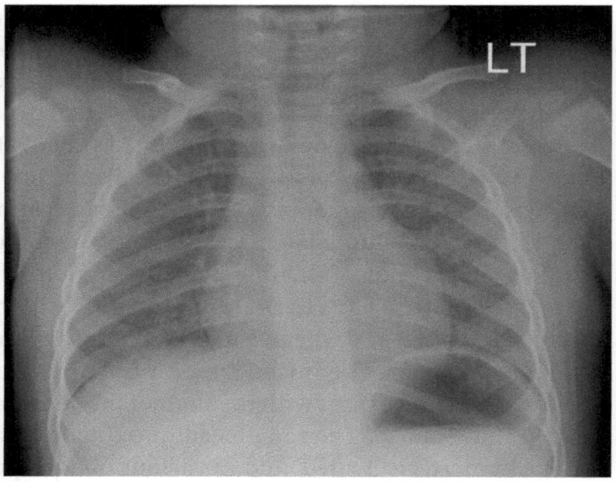

Fig. 7.3. Bilateral clavicular kink produced by oblique projection

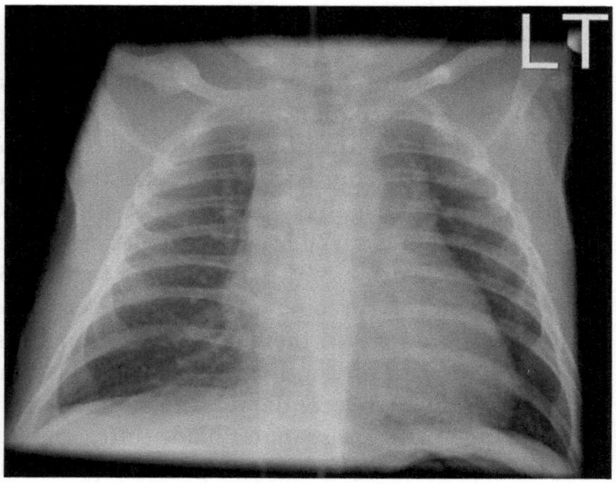

Fig. 7.4. Left sided clavicular kink artefact simulating a fracture. Compare this with the healing right clavicular fracture, the result of birth injury

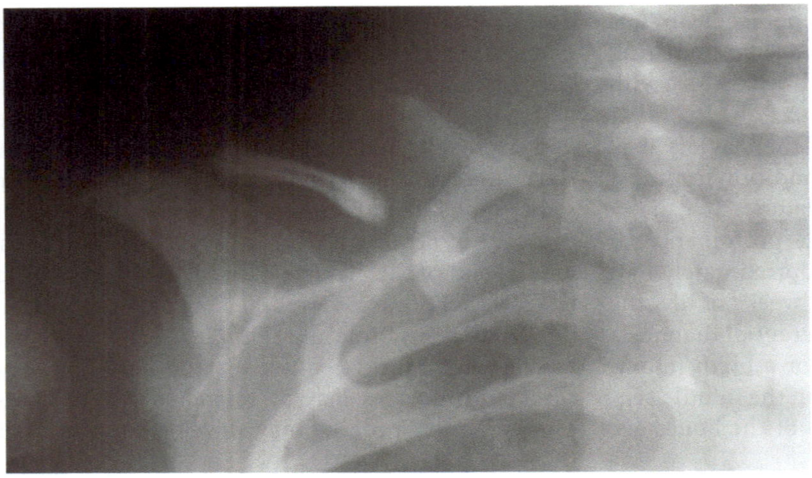

Fig. 7.5. Typical appearances of congenital pseudoarthrosis of the right clavicle in a 5-week-old infant

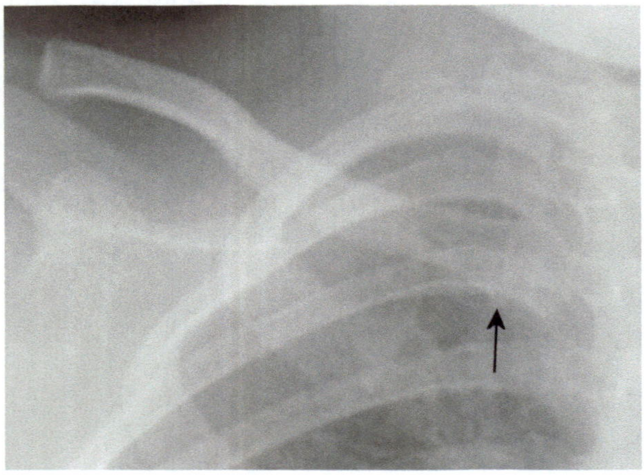

Fig. 7.6. Overlap of the medial end of the clavicle and a vertebral transverse process simulating a fracture (*arrow*)

with a separate ossification centre for the lateral half of the basiacromion that simulates a fracture highly associated with child abuse (Currarino and Prescott 1994). The secondary centre for the acromion does not usually appear until 10–12 years of age. Ossification is variable and frequently irregular (Figs. 7.7, 7.8). Fusion of the acromion occurs at 15–20 years, and the coracoid at around 20 years. Before fusion occurs or if there is persistence of these centres into adult life, both may simulate a fracture (Fig. 7.9). A further secondary ossification centre is found at the tip of the scapular blade (infrascapular bone). This normally fuses by 20 years of age (Keats and Anderson 2001) (Fig. 7.10).

Postnatal development of the sternum is highly variable. It usually forms between four and five separate cartilaginous segments or sternebrae, one or two ossification centres developing within each cartilaginous centre (O'Neil et al. 1998; Ogden et al. 1979). A double ossification centre for the manubrium is associated with Down's syndrome but is also seen as a normal variant and may persist into adult life. The separate ossification centres for the sternum may mimic healing rib fractures, and may be mistaken for signs of non-accidental injury when viewed in oblique projection (Fig. 7.11).

7.4 Upper Limb

The proximal humeral epiphysis arises from two, sometimes three separate ossification centres (Fig. 7.12). The first ossification centre develops medially at about 2 weeks of age and the second ossification centre develops in the greater tuberosity between 6–12 months of age. When the arm is internally rotated, the first appearing medial ossification centre is rotated into a lateral position and can give the false impression of shoulder joint disruption. The rare third centre occurs in the lesser tuberosity in the third year of life, and when visualised on the axillary shoulder view, may be mistaken for a fracture. This ossification centre fuses with the shaft of the humerus at 6–7 years of age. The radiolucent proximal physis of the humerus is 'tented' and in various oblique positions can be mistaken for a fracture (Fig. 7.13). The normal bicipital groove in the proximal humerus may simulate periosteal new bone formation (Fig. 7.14).

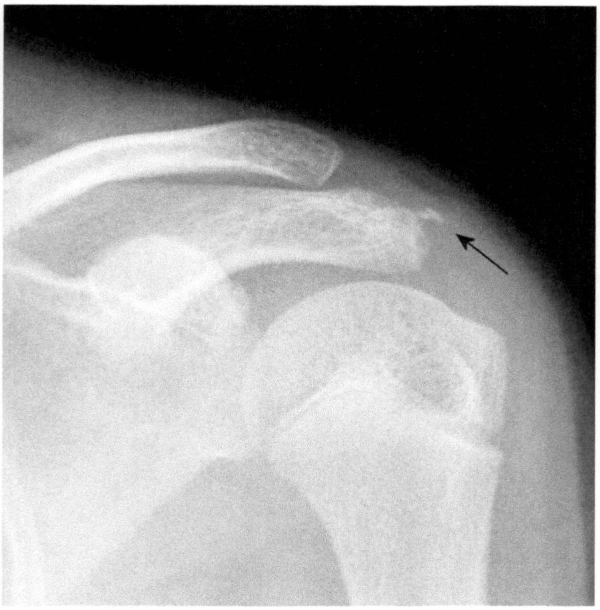

Fig. 7.7. Irregular secondary ossification centre for the acromion in a 12-year-old boy (*arrow*)

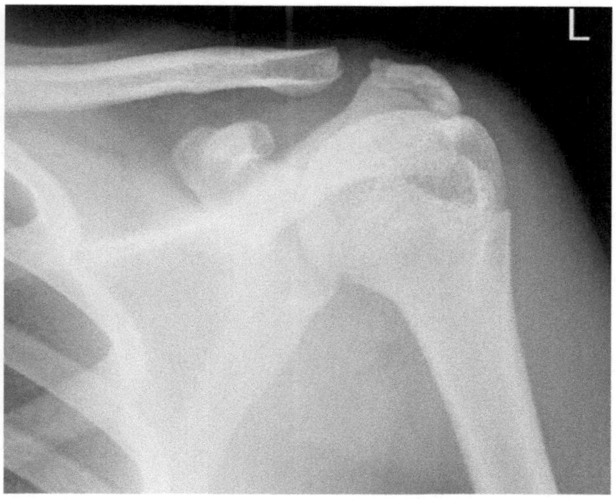

Fig. 7.8. Secondary ossification centre for the acromion in a 14-year-old boy

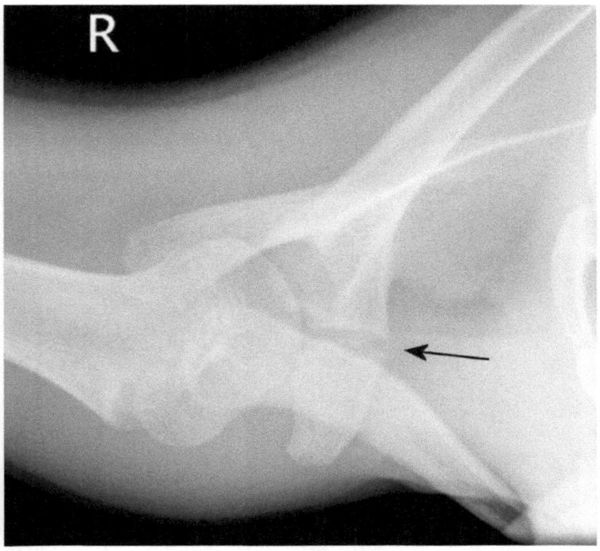

Fig. 7.9. Large, unfused ossification centre for the coracoid process in an adolescent (*arrow*)

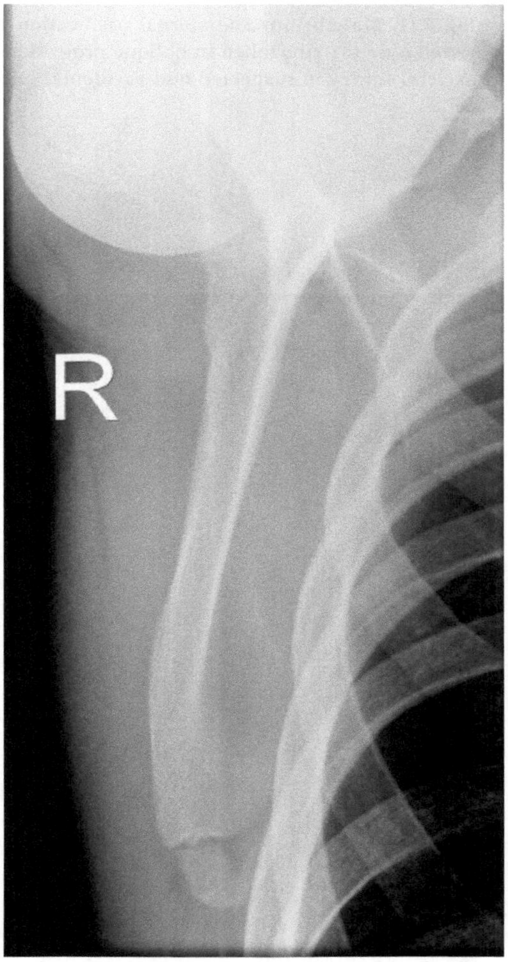

Fig. 7.10. Infrascapular bone in a 16-year-old boy

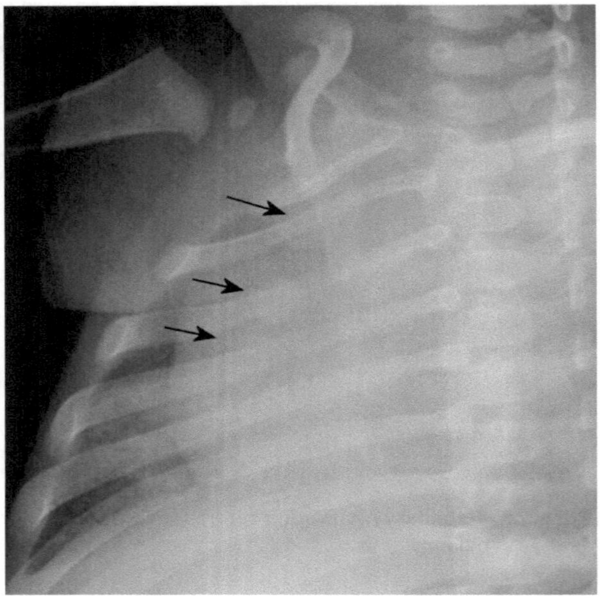

Fig. 7.11. Manubrium and sternal ossification centres projected over the ribs taken in oblique projection as part of a skeletal survey in suspected non-accidental injury (*arrows*)

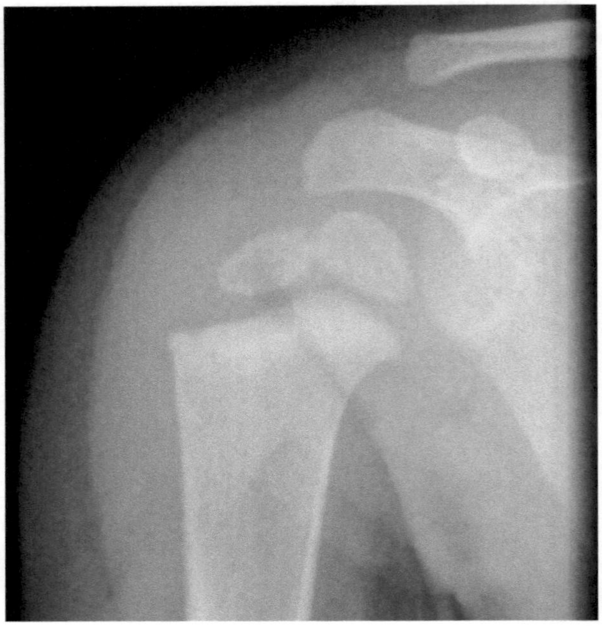

Fig. 7.12. AP radiograph right shoulder in a 14-month-old infant

a

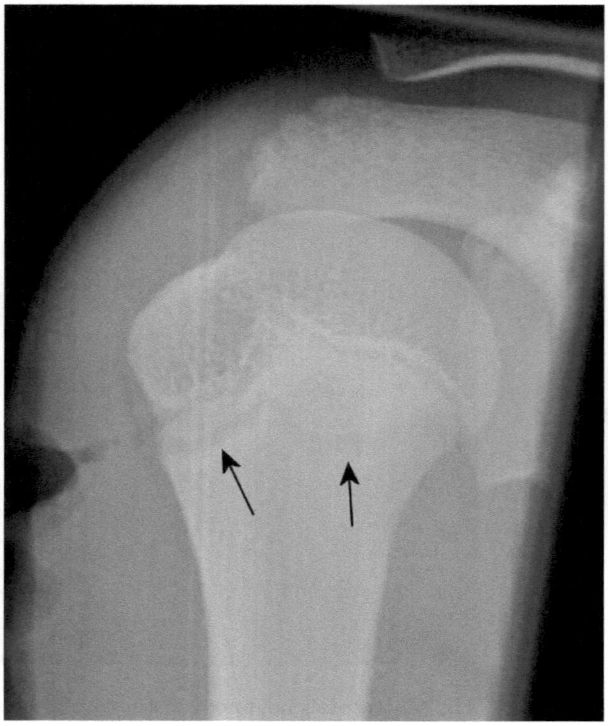

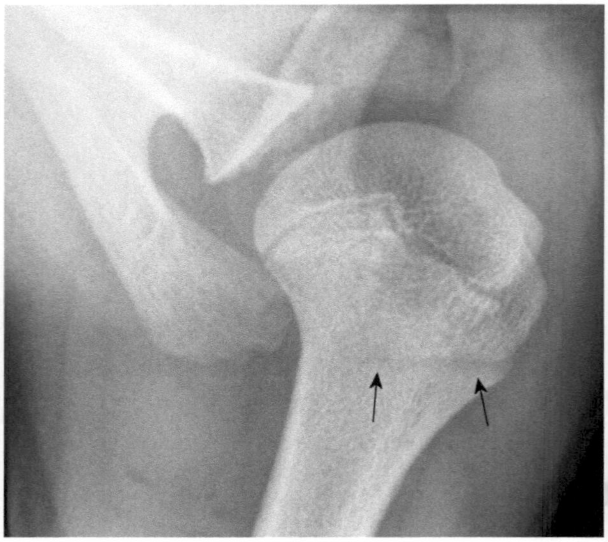

Fig. 7.13a,b. AP (**a**) and axial (**b**) views of the proximal humerus showing the normal lucent proximal humeral epiphysis, sometimes mistaken for a fracture (*arrows*)

Systematic assessment of the paediatric elbow should include a careful inspection of the ossification centres. The ossification centres for the trochlea of the distal humerus and the olecranon process of the ulna tend to be very irregular in appearance during their normal development and may simulate fractures (Figs. 7.15, 7.16). Rotation may lead to a false impression of intra-articular foreign bodies or bony fragments within the joint (Fig. 7.17a). Rotation and suboptimal radiographic positioning leads to projection of the medial epicondyle postero-inferiorly simulating avulsion injury with displacement of the apophysis (Fig. 7.17b). Compare this with the normally sited ossification centre for the medial epicondyle on lateral radiograph of the elbow (Fig. 7.18). The cartilaginous plate associated with the ossification centre for the lateral epicondyle is frequently wide in children and can look like it is separated from the humerus (Fig. 7.19). Whilst the medial epicondyle fuses directly with the humeral shaft, the lateral epicondyle fuses first with the capitellum and then both fuse with the humerus (Fig. 7.20). Un-united ossification centres may persist unfused into adult life and can simulate avulsion fractures.

Any epiphysis or apophysis may develop from multiple centres and similarly the epiphysis of the distal radius or ulna may arise from two ossification centres appearing cleft or bipartite (Fig. 7.21) (Harrison and Keats 1980). Separate ossification centres for the radial or ulna styloid processes may fuse with the main ossification centre or persist unfused as accessory ossicles into adulthood. In late adolescence or early adulthood remnants of the fusing or fused epiphysis can be mistaken for fractures. These include fine sclerotic or lucent lines and residual epiphyseal spurs (Fig. 7.22).

Accessory ossicles associated with bones in the wrist and hand can be mistaken for fracture fragments, but accessory ossicles are usually well corticated allowing them to be distinguished from fresh bony fragments resulting from recent skeletal trauma. Clinical correlation is necessary, including absence of tenderness over the area in question.

The carpal bones may appear irregular and fragmented during normal development if they develop from several ossification centres prior to coalescing into one bone mass. The pisiform is the bone most frequently affected and can be easily mistaken for a post-traumatic bony fragment or even a foreign body within the soft tissues of the palm when viewed in lat-

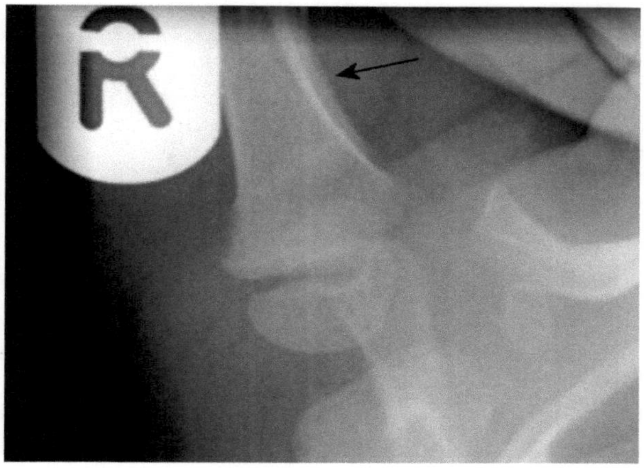

Fig. 7.14. Normal bicipital groove simulating periosteal new bone formation (*arrow*). Image taken from a chest radiograph with the upper limbs extended above the head

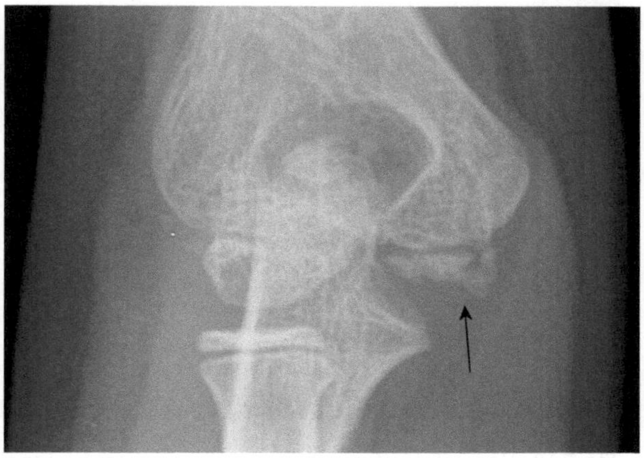

Fig. 7.15. Multiple ossification centres in the developing trochlea of the humerus in an adolescent boy (*arrow*)

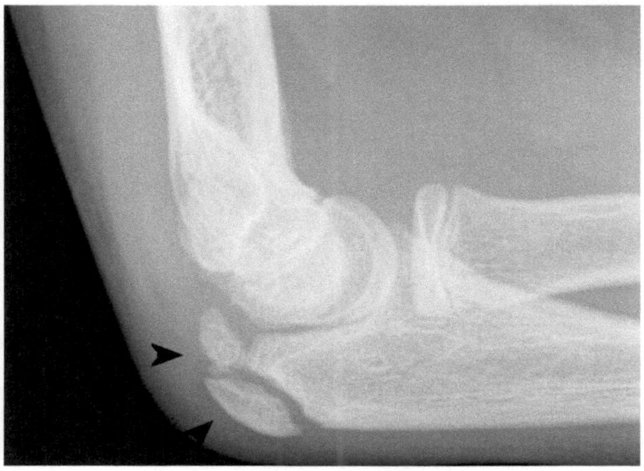

Fig. 7.16. Separate ossification centres for the olecranon in an adolescent boy (*arrowheads*)

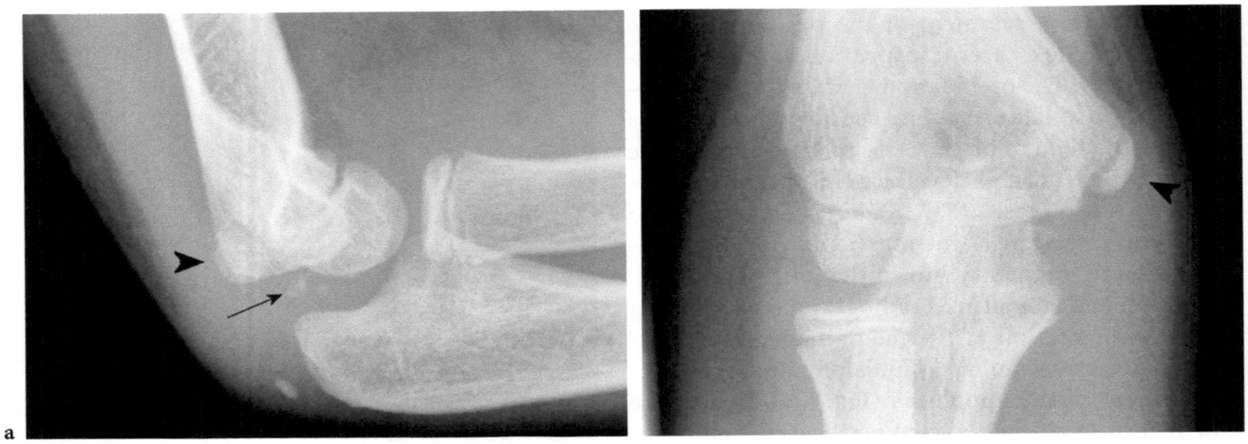

Fig. 7.17. a Irregular ossification centre for the trochlea is projected over the joint space with rotation (*arrow*). This also produces simulated dislocation of the ossification centre for the medial epicondyle (*arrowhead*), normally sited on the AP view (**b**)

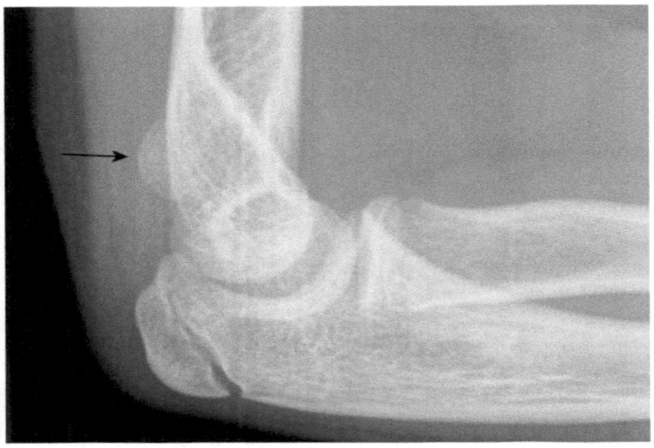

Fig. 7.18. Normal position of the ossification centre for the medial epiphysis on lateral radiograph of the elbow (*arrow*)

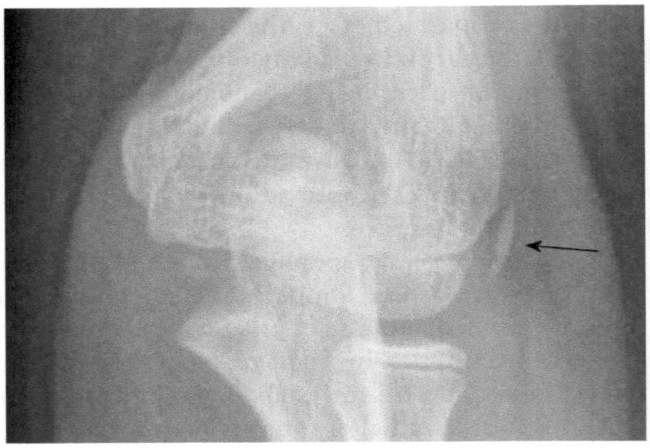

Fig. 7.19. Normal apparent separation of the ossification centre for the lateral epicondyle (*arrow*)

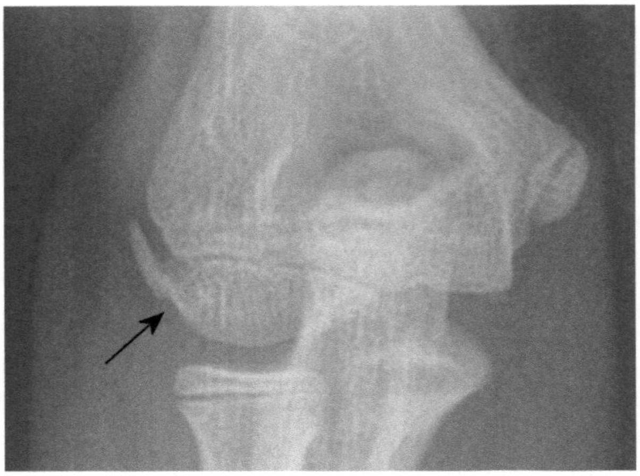

Fig. 7.20. Fusion of the ossification centre for the lateral epicondyle with the capitellum prior to closure (*arrow*)

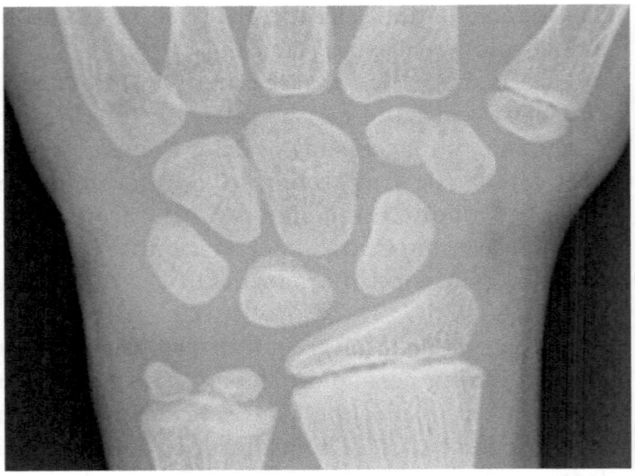

Fig. 7.21. Two separate ossification centres for the distal ulnar epiphysis

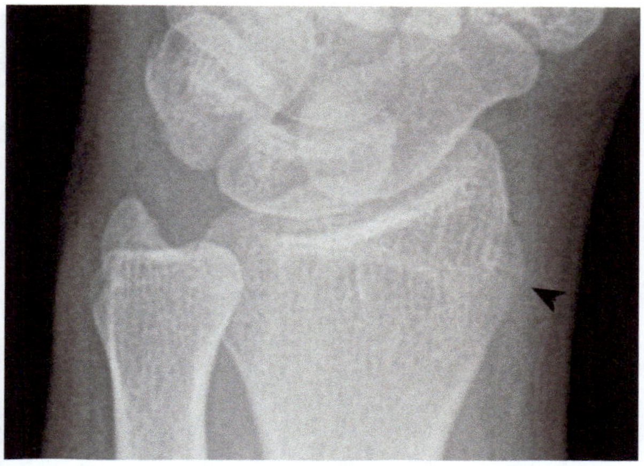

Fig. 7.22. Almost fused distal radial epiphysis (*arrowhead*)

eral projection (Fig. 7.23). A bipartite, partially cleft or notched scaphoid may simulate a fracture, but these are all normal developmental variants (Fig. 7.24).

Extra and false epiphyseal ossification centres (pseudoepiphyses) may appear in the distal cartilage of the thumb metacarpal and the proximal cartilaginous portion of the index to little finger metacarpals. These differ from true epiphyses because they arise following invasion of the cartilaginous tissue by a rod of osteogenic tissue from the shaft of the bone. The end of the rod enlarges to form the pseudoepiphysis. Unlike a true epiphysis there is bony continuity with the shaft from the beginning of their development and they contribute little to longitudinal growth (Keats 2004). The sclerotic line or small notch seen at the site of fusion with the shaft, or the cartilaginous plate itself, may be mistaken for a fracture (Fig. 7.25).

7.5 Pelvis

Various secondary ossification centres develop in the pelvis at different ages. Accessory ossification centres may develop at the tip of the ischial spine and the rim of the acetabulum between 14 and 18 years of age (Fig. 7.26). The normal apophyseal centres on the inferior border of the ischium (Fig. 7.27) should not be mistaken for avulsion injuries, although they may be separated by violent hamstring contraction. The fusing ischiopubic synchondroses may be mistaken for healing fractures, particularly

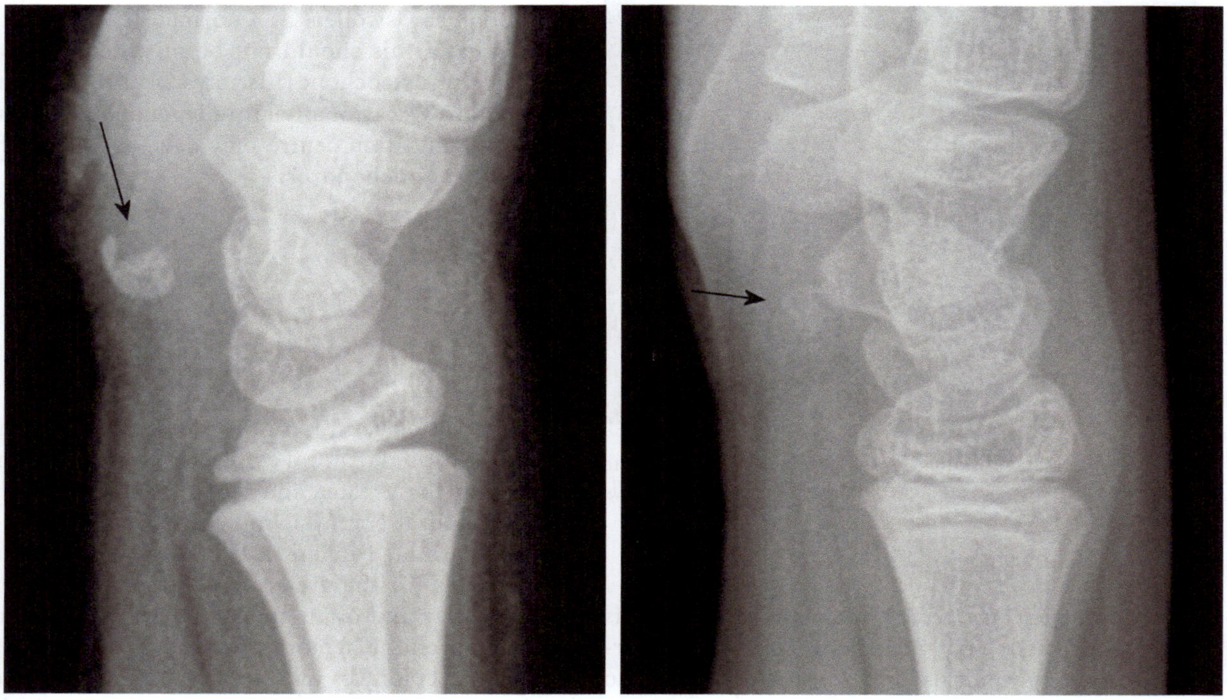

a b

Fig. 7.23a,b. Two examples of normal irregular ossification of the pisiform (*arrows*)

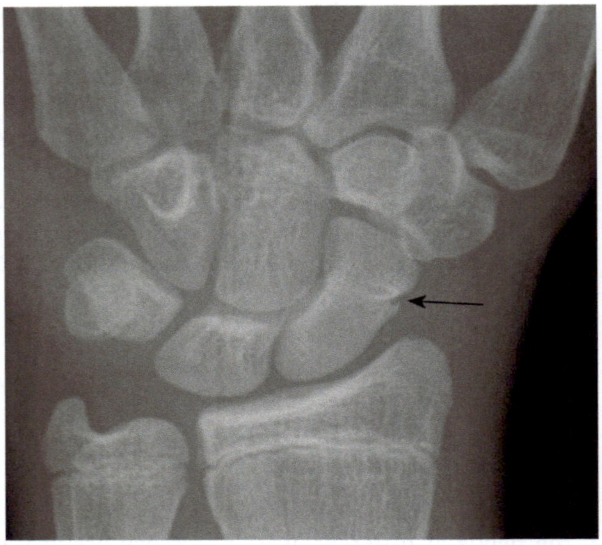

Fig. 7.24. Normal developmental notch and hook in the scaphoid (*arrow*)

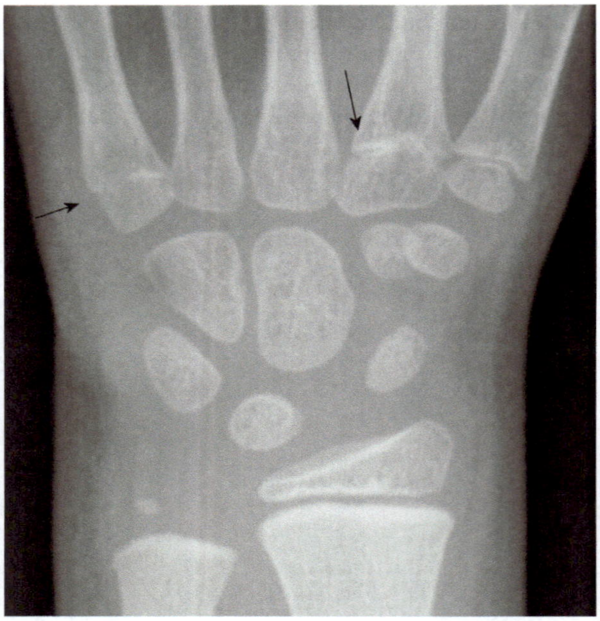

Fig. 7.25. Accessory ossification centres at the bases of the index and little finger metacarpals (*arrows*) that can simulate fractures

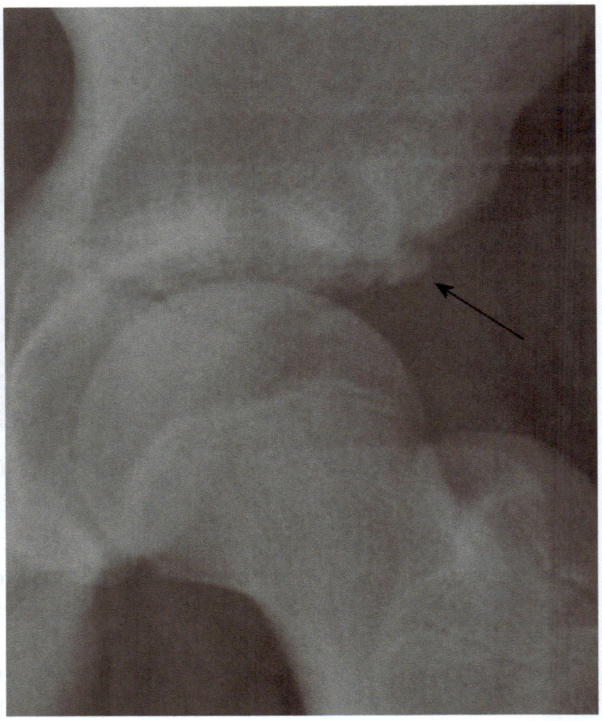

Fig. 7.26. The os acetabuli in a 13-year-old girl (*arrow*). This is an ossification centre for the acetabular rim

if asymmetric (Figs. 7.28, 7.29). Ossification of this Synchondrosis is very variable in rate and appearance. Some may be closed by 3 years, but others do not fuse until after 12 years of age (CAFFEY and ROSS 1956). Most, if not all, closing ischiopubic synchondroses appear 'swollen' as a normal developmental process, and this should not be misinterpreted as evidence of osteochondritis, or a healing fracture with callus. Occasionally an independent supernumerary ossification centre may develop within the ischiopubic synchondrosis.

7.6 Lower Limb

The ossification centres for the proximal femur consist of the capital femoral epiphysis, and ossification centres in the greater and lesser trochanters. The capital femoral epiphysis may be cleft or bifid as a normal variant. During development the ossification centres for the greater and lesser trochanters are irregular and often appear separated from the neck and proximal femoral shaft (Fig. 7.30). The distal femoral epiphysis increases rapidly in width between the second and sixth years of life. Irregularity of the lateral and medial margins of the epiphysis is

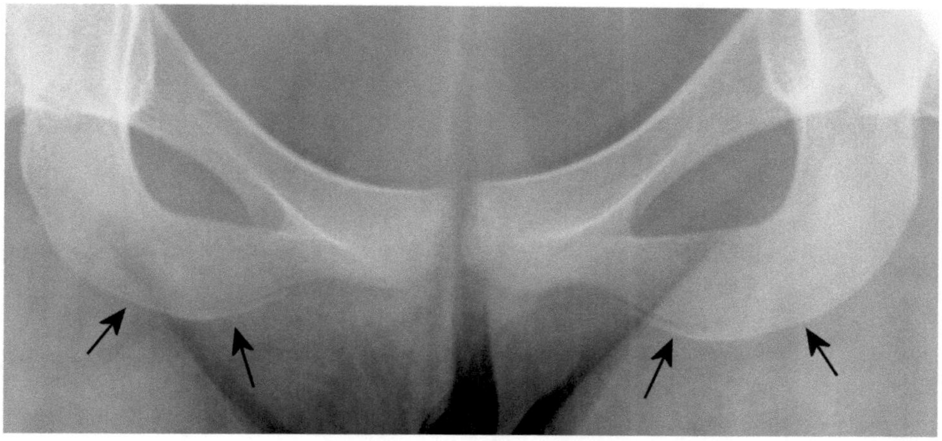

Fig. 7.27. Normal apophysis along the inferior border of the ischia in a 16-year-old girl (*arrows*)

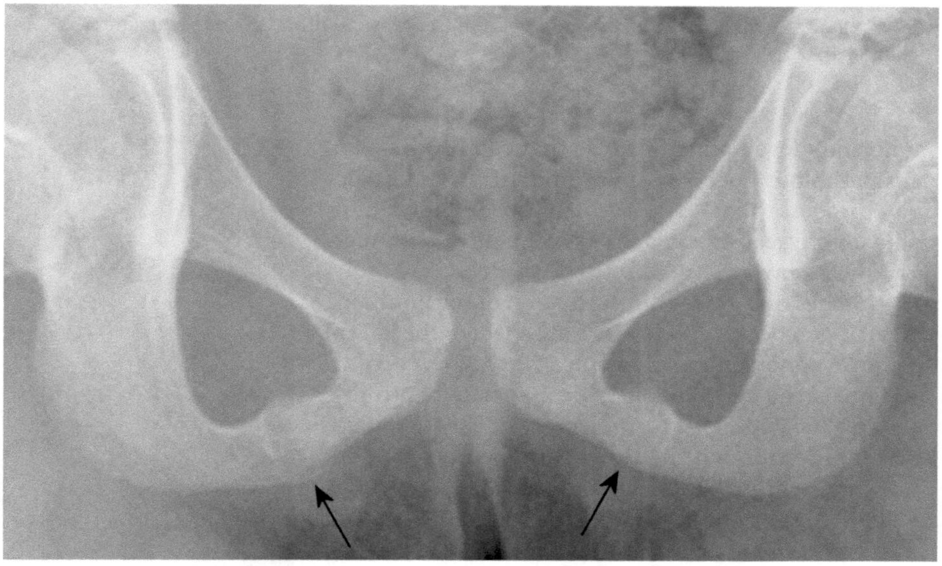

Fig. 7.28. Almost symmetrical but slightly 'swollen' appearance of the ischiopubic synchondroses in a 5-year-old boy (*arrows*)

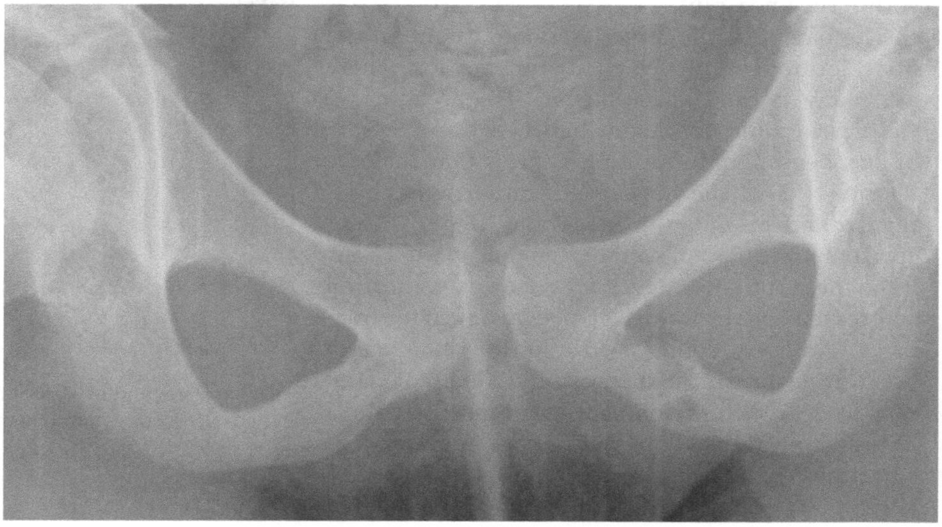

Fig. 7.29. Asymmetric ischiopubic synchondroses in a 6-year-old girl

a 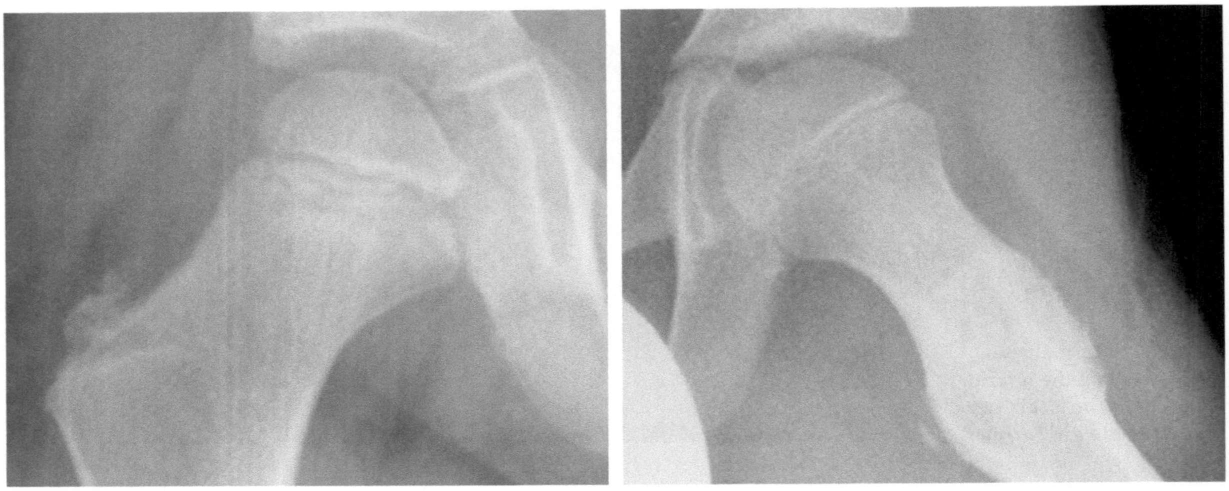

Fig. 7.30a,b. Normal irregularity and apparent 'separation' of the greater trochanter in a 5-year-old boy (**a**) and lesser trochanter in a 13-year-old boy (**b**)

a normal developmental stage that can be mistaken for pathology such as osteochondritis or a destructive process (Fig. 7.31). As in the proximal femur, this epiphyseal irregularity is frequently asymmetrical (Caffey et al. 1958).

Notches or grooves for the tendon of the popliteus muscle can be seen on the lateral aspect of the lateral femoral condyle in adolescents (Fig. 7.32). A sesamoid bone, the cyamella, may be associated with this tendon located close to the condyle. The fabella, a sesamoid bone within the gastrocnemius tendon, is seen behind the knee on lateral radiographs (Fig. 7.33). Both of these small ossicles may be bifid or irregular as normal developmental variants. They should not be mistaken for loose or foreign bodies within the knee joint.

The patella is the largest sesamoid bone in the body, located within the quadriceps tendon. There are many normal variations in its development. Ossification initially begins between 3 and 5 years of age, beginning in multiple centres that coalesce (Ogden 1984). The initial ossification may be irregular and 'granular' in appearance (Fig. 7.34) and can sometimes resemble radio-opaque foreign bodies in the soft tissues. Several secondary ossification centres may be seen which can be mistaken for fractures. The most common location of a secondary ossification centre is superolateral (Fig. 7.35) and may lead to the development of a bipartite patella if it remains unfused into adulthood. Accessory ossification centres may also be found at the upper and lower poles of the patella, and even on its medial

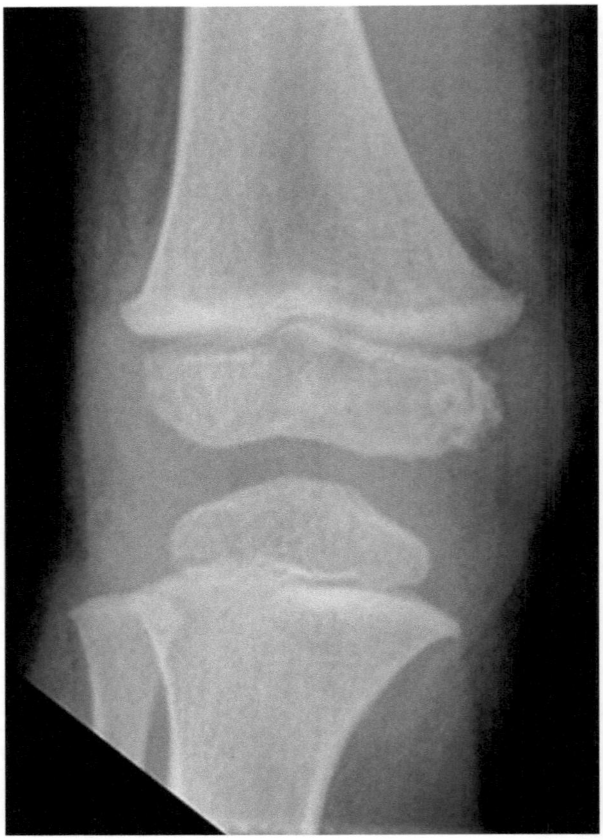

Fig. 7.31. Irregular ossification of the medial and lateral borders of the distal femoral epiphysis in a normal 2-year-old

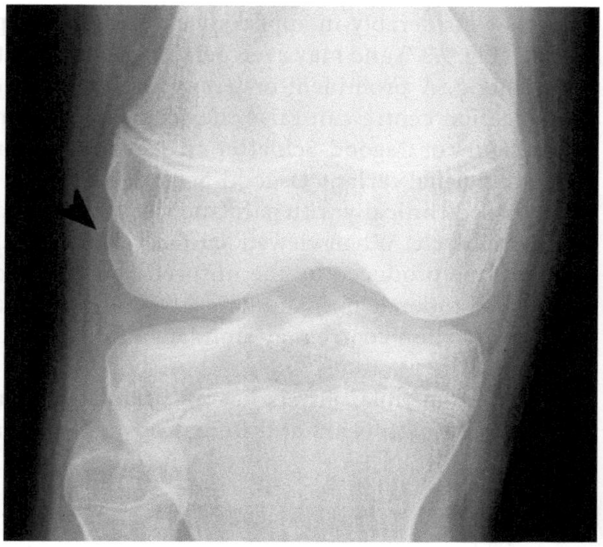

Fig. 7.32. Prominent groove in the lateral aspect of the lateral femoral condyle (*arrowhead*) for the popliteal tendon in a 15-year-old boy

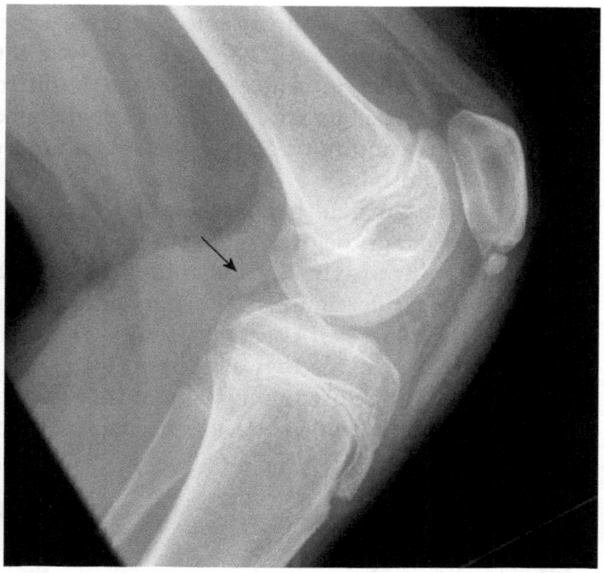

Fig. 7.33. The fabella (*arrow*) in a 15-year-old boy. There is a secondary ossification centre at the lower pole of the patella

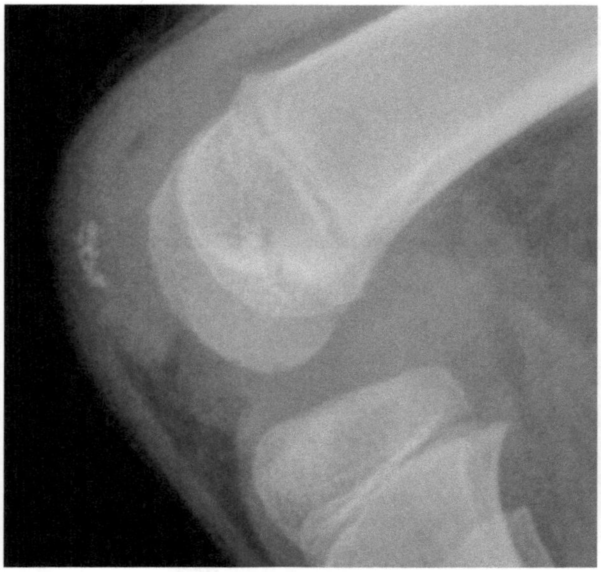

Fig. 7.34. Granular appearance of the ossifying patella in a normal 6-year-old

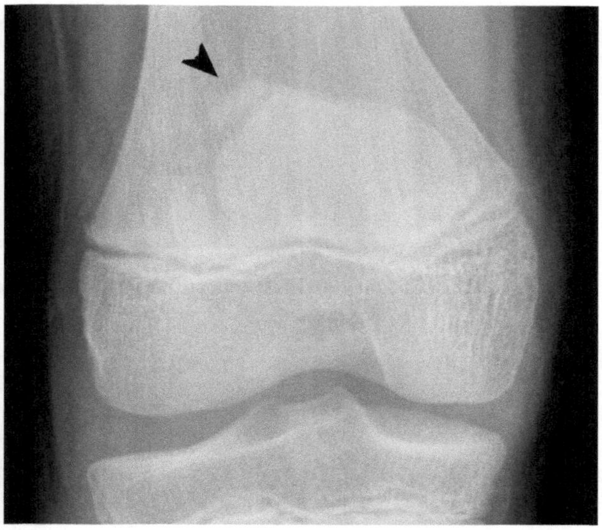

Fig. 7.35. The most common site of a secondary ossification centre for the patella (upper, outer segment) in a 13-year-old (*arrowhead*)

and lateral borders with variable and often asymmetric appearances (Figs. 7.33, 7.36). Most fuse with the main ossification centre of the patella during development. The bipartite or tripartite patella has cartilaginous continuity despite the appearance of osseous discontinuity.

The tibial tubercle begins to ossify between 7 and 9 years of age, beginning distally, and progressively enlarging proximally and anteriorly while the main tibial ossification centre expands downward towards the tubercle. A section of epiphyseal cartilage usually remains between these two ossification centers until close to physeal maturity (Ogden 1984). The ossification centre for the tibial tubercle varies considerably in appearance during development (Fig. 7.37) and may even persist un-united into adulthood. A prominent or irregular 'fragmented' ossification centre can raise the suspicion of avulsion injury or Osgood-Schlatter's disease but is more often a normal variant. Osgood-Schlatter's disease is diagnosed clinically with pain and swelling over the tibial tubercle. When viewed 'en-face' the relatively lucent line produced by the unfused apophysis for the tibial tubercle may simulate a fracture, whereas the ossification centre may simulate a foreign body (Fig. 7.38).

The distal tibial physis has an undulating contour so that it appears at different positions on ra-

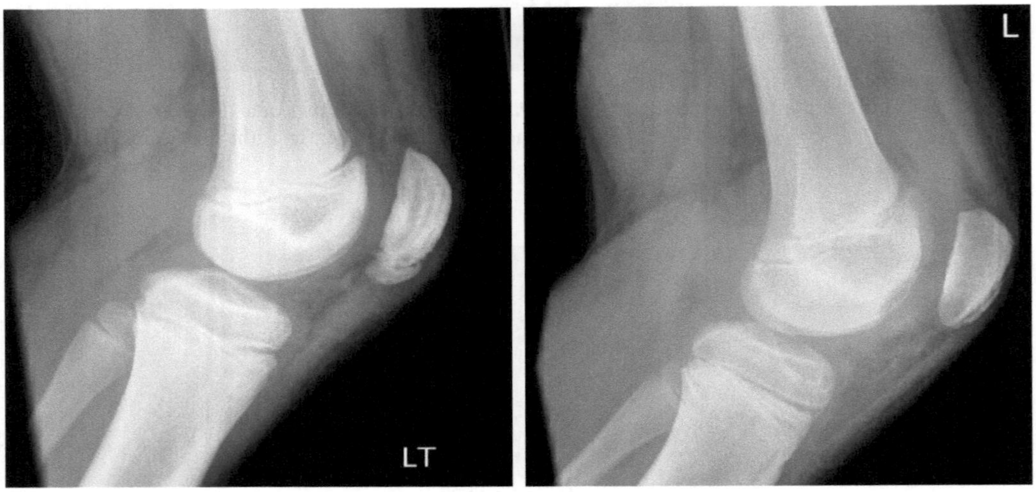

a b

Fig. 7.36a,b. Secondary ossification centres at the lower pole of the patella in adolescent boys

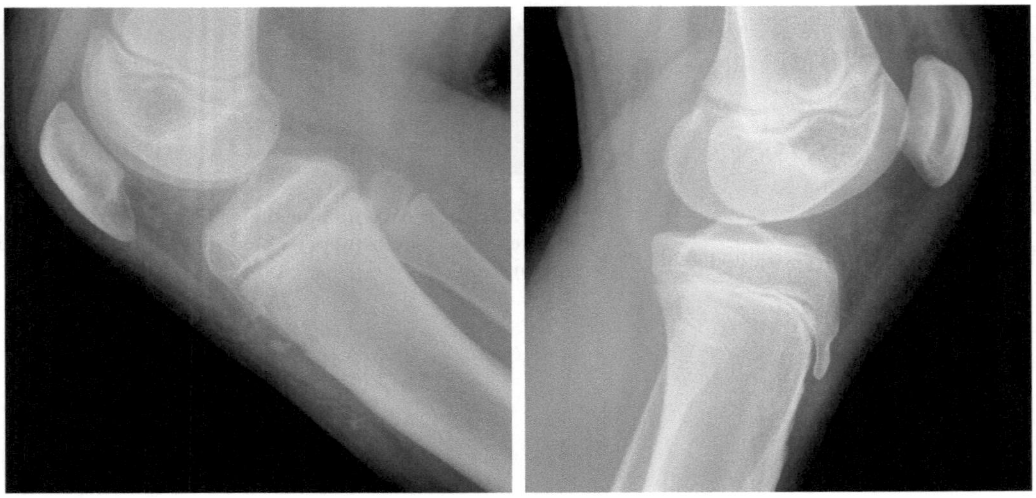

a b

Fig. 7.37a,b. Variation in appearance of the tibial tuberosity in two normal 11-year-old boys

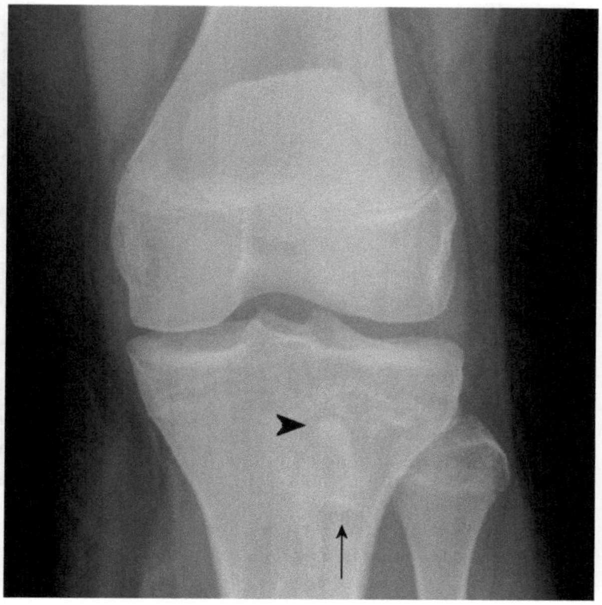

Fig. 7.38. The unfused tibial apophysis in a 13-year-old girl. Ossification simulating a foreign body (*arrowhead*) and the lucent cartilaginous portion simulating a fracture (*arrow*)

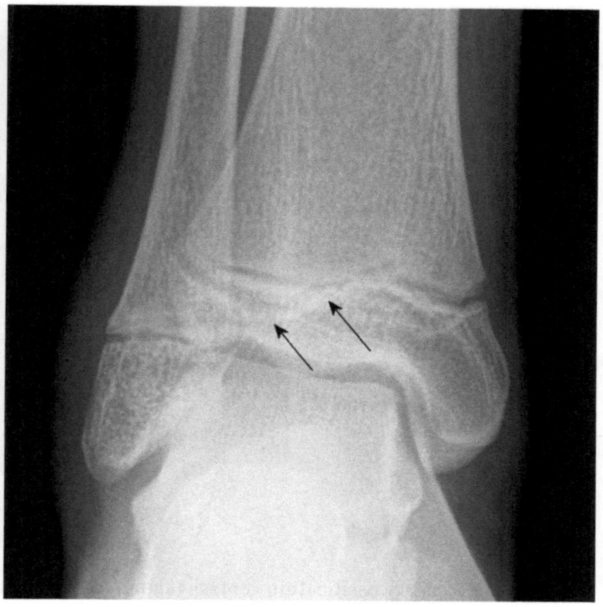

Fig. 7.39. Normal 14-year-old boy. In oblique projection the undulating distal tibial physis simulates a fracture (*arrows*)

diographs and can be mistaken for an epiphyseal fracture (Fig. 7.39) (Ogden and McCarthy 1983). Localised angulations of the distal physis causing depressions in the metaphysis or, less often, the epiphysis are normal developmental variants (Kump 1966) (Fig. 7.40). Similarly, localised angulations of the distal fibular physis causing a depression in the adjacent metaphysis can simulate a Salter Harris type I growth plate injury, especially when peripherally located. Small areas of accessory ossification, related to the epiphyses or physes should not be mistaken for fractures. Accessory ossicles may be found in association with the medial and lateral malleoli (os subtibiale and os subfibulare). They vary in size, may be single or multiple and are usually due to secondary ossification. Occasionally they may be related to previous trauma (Figs. 7.41, 7.42). Numerous accessory ossicles are found around the foot and ankle, and are named in accordance to their proximity to adjacent bones (Fig. 7.43) (Kohler and Zimmer 1968). These ossicles vary in size and shape and are usually of no clinical significance, but are important to recognise as they can simulate fractures or may occasionally be symptomatic (Figs. 7.44, 7.45). Such ossicles may be bipartite or multicentric. The os supranaviculare is an accessory ossicle that can be confused with a secondary ossification centre for

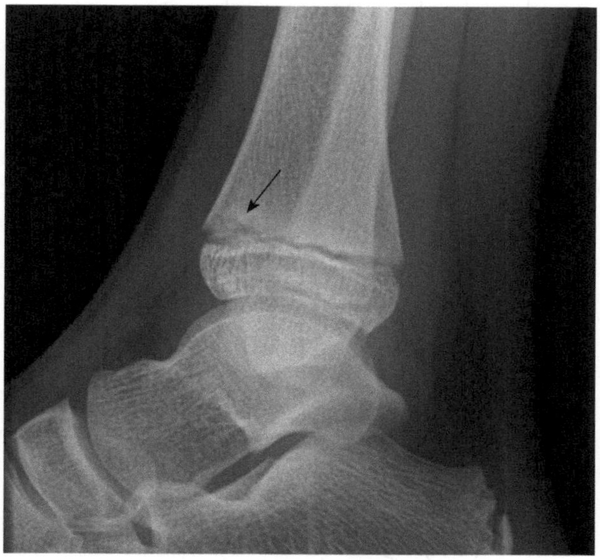

Fig. 7.40. Normal 13-year-old girl. Localised anterior angulation of the distal tibial physis causing a depression in the metaphysis (*arrow*)

the navicular and may also be mistaken for fractures. There are two variants of the os tibiale externum or accessory navicular. The first type accounts for approximately 10%–15% of cases, and is actually a sesamoid bone that lies within the tendon of the tibialis posterior muscle anatomically separate from

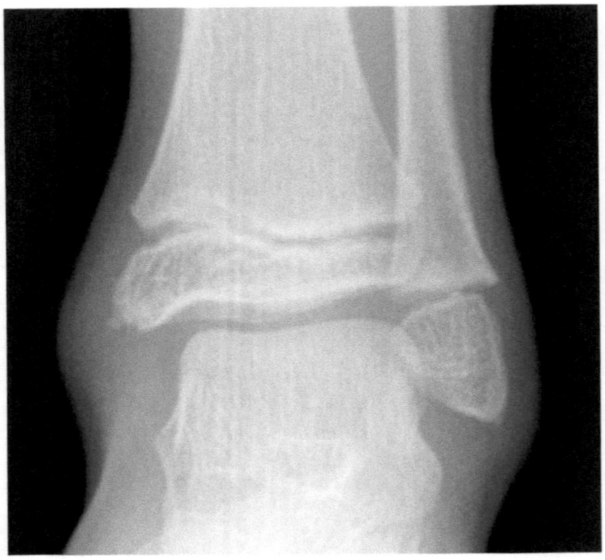

Fig. 7.41. Accessory ossification centres related to the malleoli in an 8-year-old. These can be mistaken for fractures

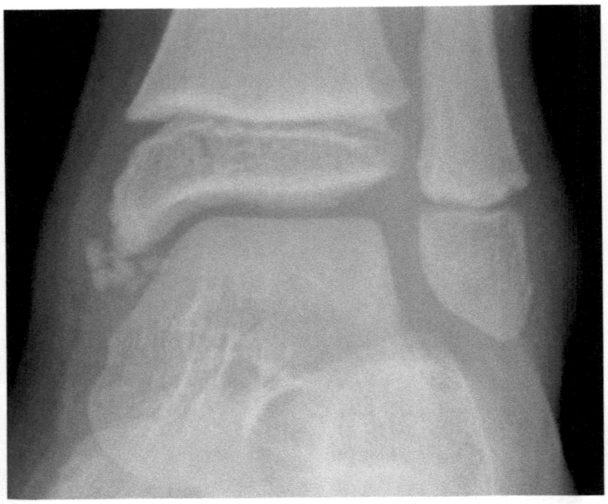

Fig. 7.42. Multiple accessory ossification centres related to the medial malleolus in a 12-year-old girl

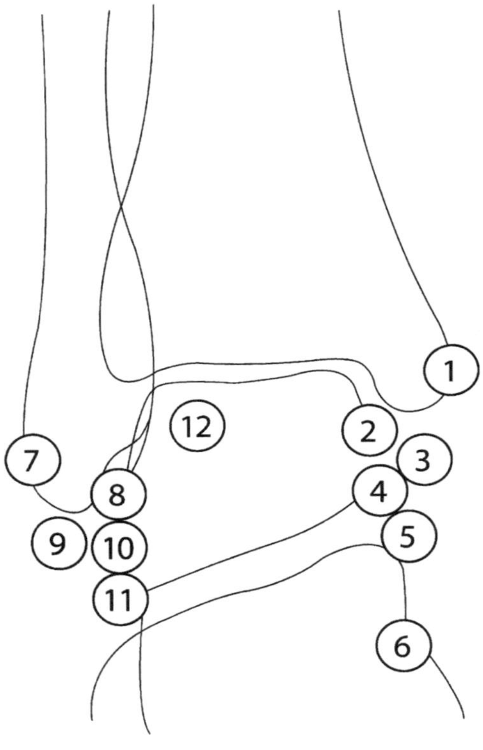

a

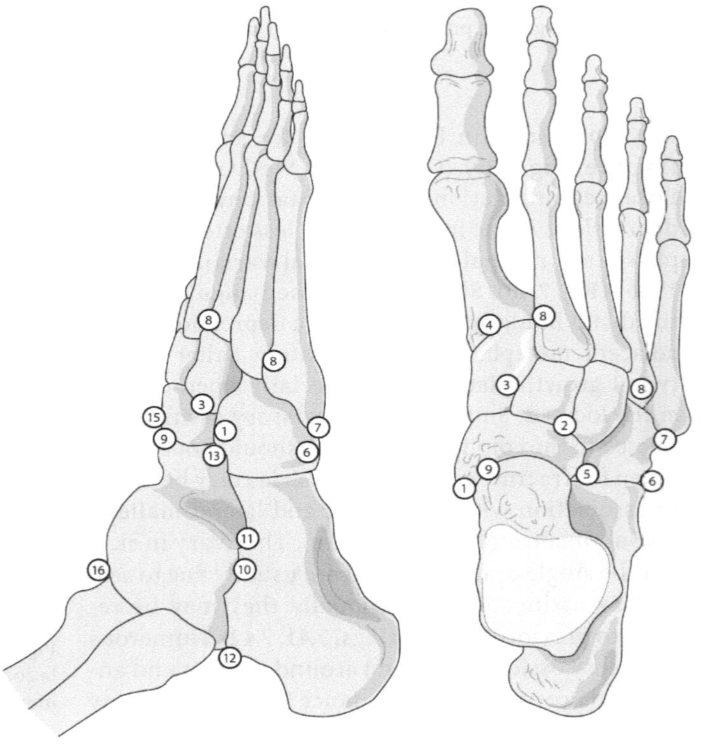

Fig. 7.43. **a** Accessory bones of the ankle as seen on an AP radiograph. (Kohler and Zimmer 1968). *1* Accompanying shadow of the medial malleolus (patella malleoli). *2* Intercalary bone or sesamoid between medial malleolus and talus. *3* Os subtibiale. *4* Talus accessorius. *5* Os sustentaculi. *6* Os tibiale externum. *7* Os retinaculi. *8* Intercalary bone or sesamoid between lateral malleolus and talus. *9* Os secundarius. *10* Talus secundarius. *11* Os trochleare calcanei. *12* Os trigonum. **b** Accessory bones of the foot. (Kohler and Zimmer 1968). *1* Os tibiale externum. *2* Processus uncinatus. *3* Os intercuneiforme. *4* Pars peronea metatarsalia. *5* Cuboides secundarium. *6* Os peroneum. *7* Os vesalianum. *8* Os intermetatarseum. *9* Os supratalare. *10* Talus accessorius. *11* Os sustentaculum. *12* Os trigonum. *13* Calcaneus secundarius. *14* Os subcalcis. *15* Os supranaviculare. *16* Os talotibiale

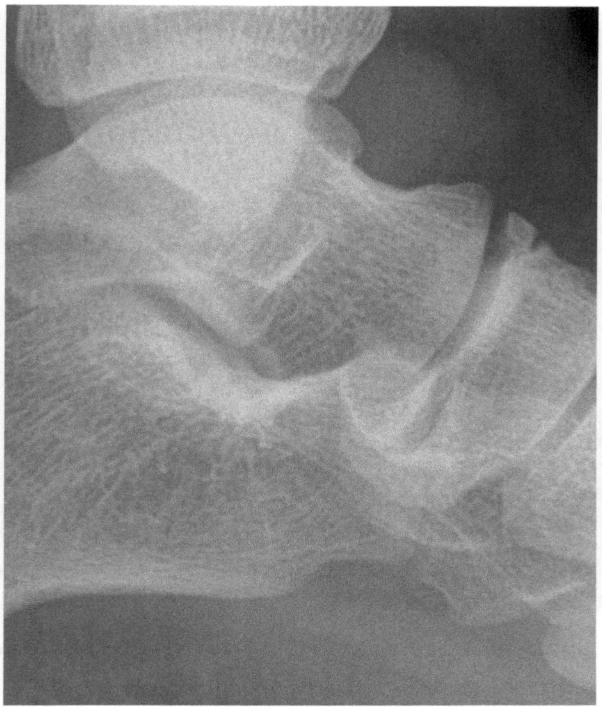

Fig. 7.44. The os supranaviculare can be mistaken for an avulsion fracture of the navicular bone

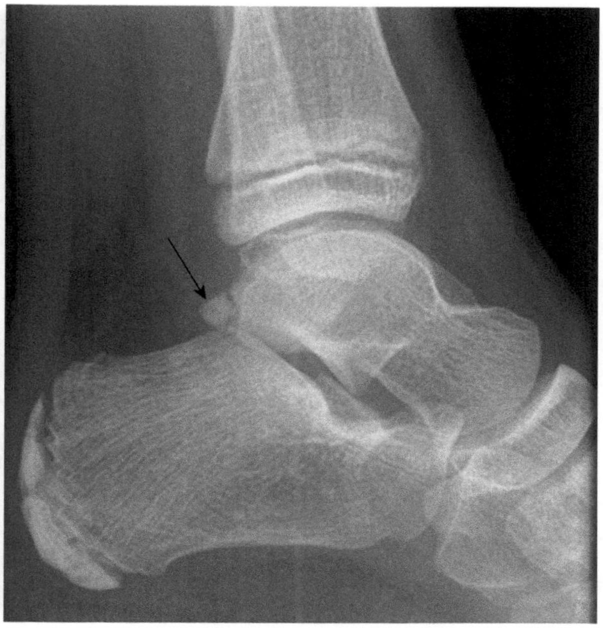

Fig. 7.45. Os trigonum simulating fracture of posterior process of the talus (*arrow*). The calcaneal apophysis appears sclerotic and fragmented but this is normal

the navicular bone. These accessory ossicles are oval or rounded in shape and rarely symptomatic. The second type is a secondary ossification centre for the tubercle of the navicular that is joined to the main bony mass by a cartilaginous or fibrocartilaginous bridge. This type is triangular in shape and has a higher incidence of symptoms such as pain and tenderness, generally developing in the second decade, more often in females than males (LAWSON et al. 1984; MOSEL et al. 2004). Bilateral ossicles are present in just over 50% of patients (Fig. 7.46).

The ossification centre for the navicular is frequently irregular and may appear fragmented simulating fracture or avascular necrosis up to approximately 5 years of age (Fig. 7.47). A bipartite or cleft navicular may be seen in older children or adults following incomplete fusion of two separate ossification centres for the navicular and may be misdiagnosed as a fracture. When radiographs are not diagnostic, computed tomography (CT) is helpful in distinguishing between a fracture and this normal anatomical variant (SHAWDON et al. 1995). The cuboid is often irregular and composed of multiple ossification centres that fuse to form a single bony mass during development. The cuneiform bones can also have a similar appearance during skeletal ossification in childhood.

The primary ossification centre for the calcaneus is present at birth. It may ossify from two or more centres, but the presence of multiple centres is associated with certain disorders including chondrodysplasia punctate (Sheffield type), GM_1 gangliosidosis and mucolipidosis type II (TAYBI and LACHMAN 1996). The centre for the calcaneal apophysis appears in the middle of the first decade and fuses with the body of the calcaneus in late adolescence. The apophysis appears irregular, fragmented or sclerotic as a normal variant before fusion (Figs. 7.45, 7.48). When viewed in oblique projection, the unfused apophysis can mimic a calcaneal fracture (Fig. 7.49). A secondary ossification centre appears at the dorsal process of the talus between 5 and 6 years of age. This either fuses with the main body of the talus between 16 and 20 years of age or persists as an accessory ossicle, the os trigonum (Fig. 7.45).

Accessory ossification centres may occur in the epiphyses of the metatarsals and phalanges of the toes. They are particularly common in the great toes (Fig. 7.50). Incompletely fused metatarsal pseudoepiphyses can be mistaken for fractures. These occur distally in the first metatarsal and proximally in the

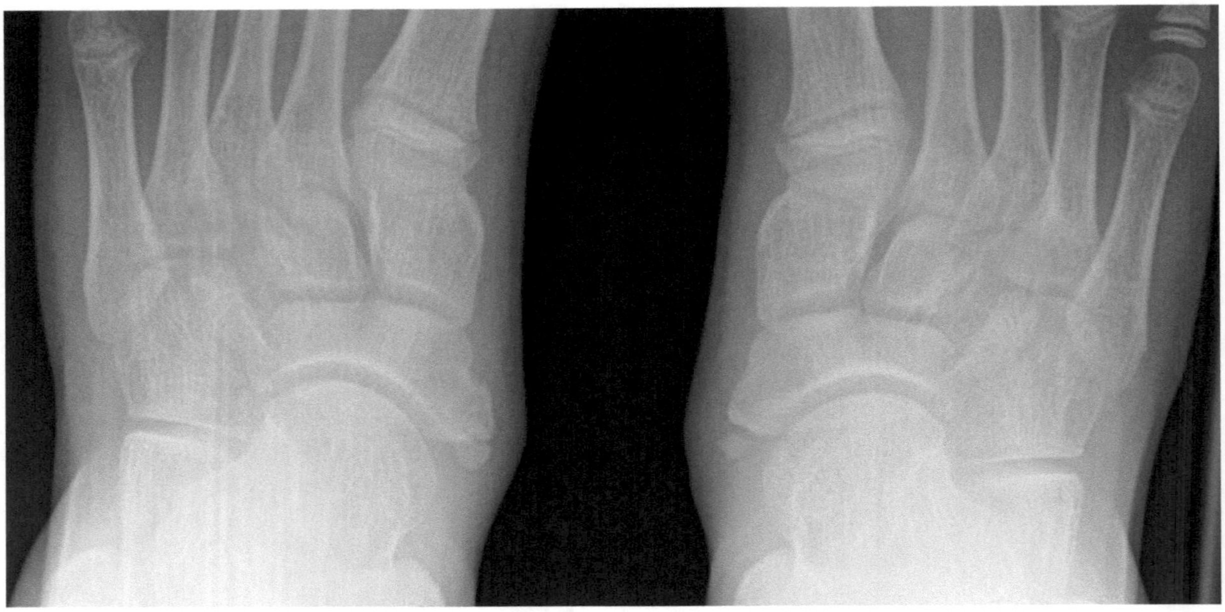

Fig. 7.46. Bilateral accessory navicular (os tibiale externum) in a 12-year-old girl with localised pain and tenderness related to these ossicles

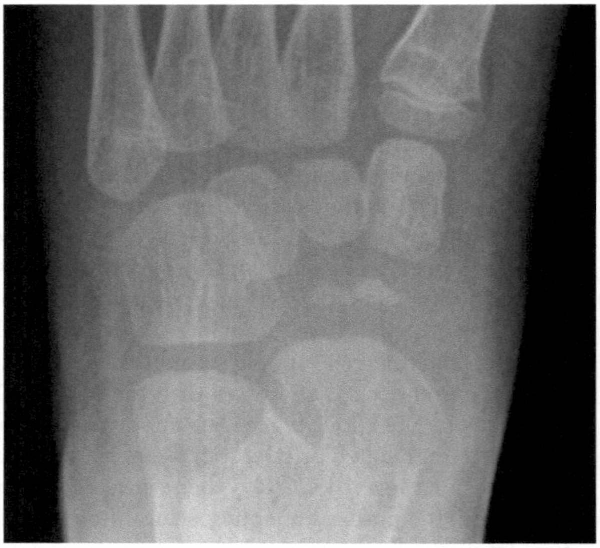

Fig. 7.47. Multicentric ossification centres for the navicular simulating avascular necrosis. This is a normal developmental variant. If the ossification centres do not fuse a bipartite navicular can be mistaken for a fracture

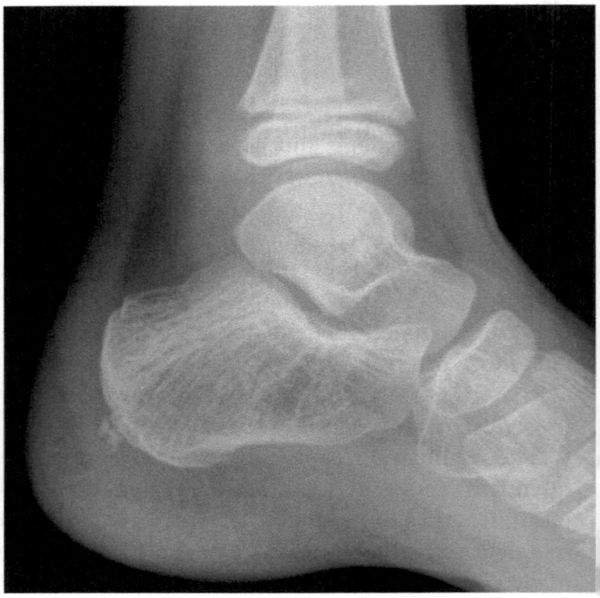

Fig. 7.48. Fragmentation of the calcaneal apophysis in a normal 8-year-old

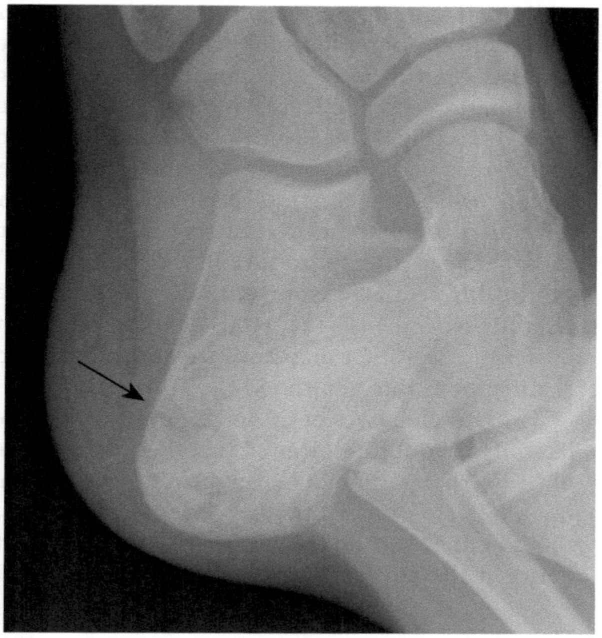

Fig. 7.49. The unfused calcaneal apophysis simulating a fracture in oblique projection (*arrow*)

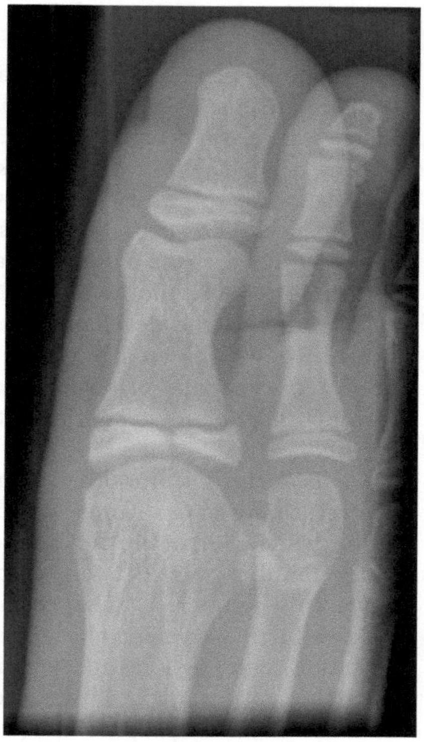

Fig. 7.50. Bifid epiphysis of the great toe proximal phalanx simulating a Salter-Harris type III injury

second to fifth metatarsals as in the metacarpals. They are variable in location and distribution is frequently asymmetric. The apophysis for the 5th metatarsal base appears during puberty and usually fuses with the shaft after a few years. Before fusion, it has variable appearances and slight separation or fragmentation can be mistaken for a fracture (Fig. 7.51), although these typically occur perpendicular to the shaft.

Sesamoid bones are found in association with tendons in the feet, as in the hands. They may be bipartite and simulate fractures, although when pain and local tenderness is present it is important to remember that a bipartite sesamoid is larger overall than a fractured non-partite sesamoid.

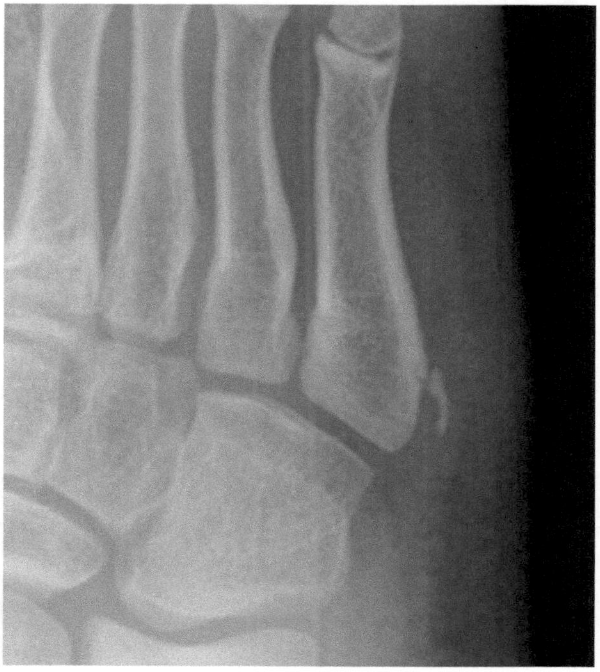

Fig. 7.51. Normal separation of the apophysis at the base of the fifth metatarsal

7.7 Skull and Spine

It is vitally important to be aware of the anatomical variants and normal developmental findings that may be present in the paediatric spine, as many of these can be confused with significant injury in the context of trauma. Imaging of the paediatric cervical spine presents a particular challenge since not only do the appearances of the spine change with age, but also the patterns of injury change with age. The anatomy of the developing paediatric cervical spine predisposes children to upper cervical spine injuries, i.e. from occiput to C2–C3 level, which are also associated with a higher risk of neurological sequelae. The spine reaches adult proportions by the time a child reaches 8–10 years of age. After the age of 10–12 years the pattern of paediatric cervical spine injuries is similar to adults. Normal anatomical variants in the developing paediatric cervical spine include epiphyseal variants, incomplete ossification of synchondrosis and hypermobility, many of which may be mistaken for pathology if unrecognised.

C1 is formed from three primary ossification centres, comprising an anterior arch and two neural arches which surround the anterior arch and fuse in the midline by 3 years of age to form the posterior arch. The anterior arch is ossified in only 20% of cases at birth and usually becomes visible as an ossification centre by 1 year of age (Fig. 7.52). The neural arches appear by the 7th fetal week and fuse with the anterior arch by 7 years of age. The presence of additional ossification centres or ossicles anteriorly results in an increased number of synchondroses compared with the most frequent arrangement of two anterior synchondroses and one posterior synchondrosis (Fig. 7.53). Prior to fusion, or if the synchondroses persist unfused, they may be mistaken for a fracture (Fig. 7.54). Occasionally there is no formation of an anterior arch (Fig. 7.55). The neural arches can attempt to fuse in the midline – this can be differentiated from a fracture because it has sclerotic margins (Baker et al. 1999). Similarly the posterior arch of C1 may not fuse and can remains cartilaginous into adulthood.

The lateral masses of C1 and C2 may be offset bilaterally in young children so that the lateral masses of C1 overhang those of C2 on the AP view, simulating a Jefferson burst fracture. This phenomenon is thought to be secondary to disparity in growth rate between the two vertebra and is most commonly

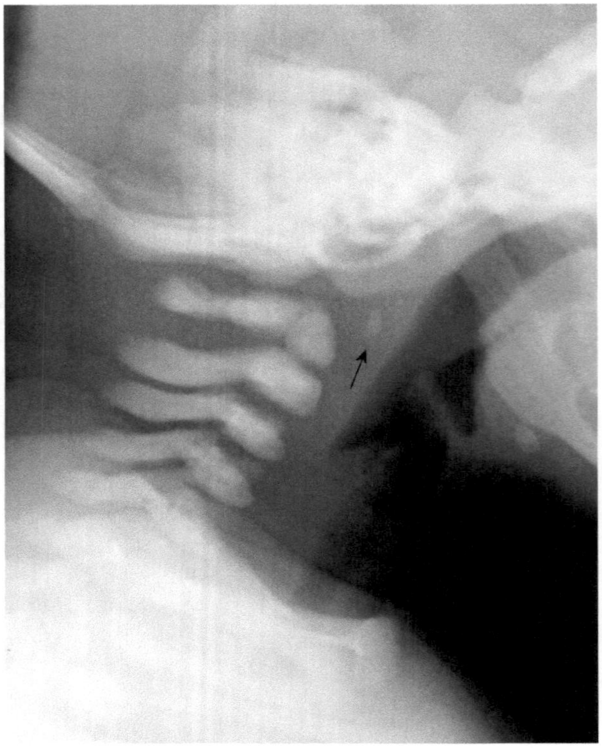

Fig. 7.52. Lateral cervical spine radiograph in a 2-week-old baby. The anterior arch of C1 is ossified (*arrow*)

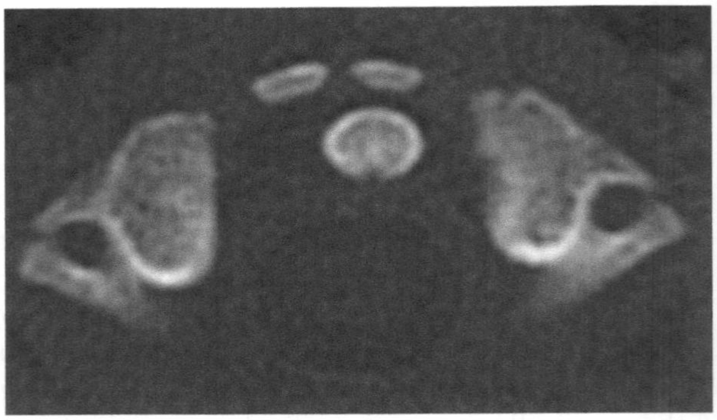

Fig. 7.53. Three synchondroses in the anterior arch of C1 due to an additional ossification centre in an 18-month-old infant. The posterior arch was normal but is not seen due to the plane of CT reconstruction

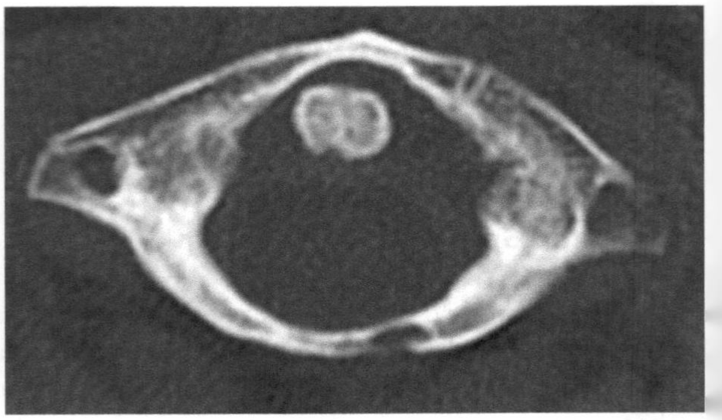

Fig. 7.54. Unfused synchondrosis between the left sided neural arch and the anterior arch in a 6-year-old

seen at around 4 years of age, but often up to 7 years of age. Up to 6 mm lateral displacement of the lateral masses of C1 relative to the odontoid is within normal limits under these circumstances (Suss et al. 1983). Offsets of C1 and C2 simulating a Jefferson fracture may also be seen in children with incomplete neural arches (Rossitch and Bohrer 1991). Unilateral offset of C1 on C2 is most often the result of rotation. In such cases the lateral mass to odontoid process distance is increased on one side and appears narrowed on the opposite side, either on radiographs or CT (Fig. 7.56). Asymmetric widening of the lateral mass to odontoid process distance without associated rotation has also been shown to be normal in some children (Wolansky et al. 1999).

C2 develops from four ossification centres at birth, one for each neural arch, one for the body and one for the odontoid process. The odontoid process itself forms from two separate ossification centres that fuse in the midline by the 7th fetal month, but occasionally can persist as a vertical lucent cleft in the odontoid (Ogden 1984). A secondary ossification centre appears at the tip of the odontoid process between 3 and 6 years of age and fuses by 12 years. This can be mistaken for an avulsion fracture (Fig. 7.57). The body of C2 fuses with the odontoid process by 2–6 years leaving a fusion line or remnant of the cartilaginous synchondrosis until 11 years of age and may be confused with a fracture either on radiographs or CT (Fig. 7.58). Pseudofractures of the odontoid process can be produced by the Mach effect by overlapping of the teeth, the posterior arch of C1, occiput or soft tissues such as the tongue (Fig. 7.59). The neural arches of C2 fuse posteriorly by 2–3 years of age and the body fuses with the neural arches by 3–6 years. Additional ossification centres may be found at the tips of the spinous

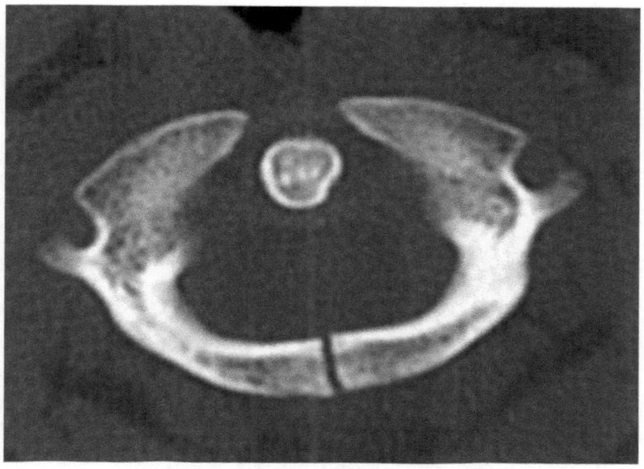

Fig. 7.55. Absent ossification centre for the anterior arch and unfused posterior synchondrosis in a 6-year-old

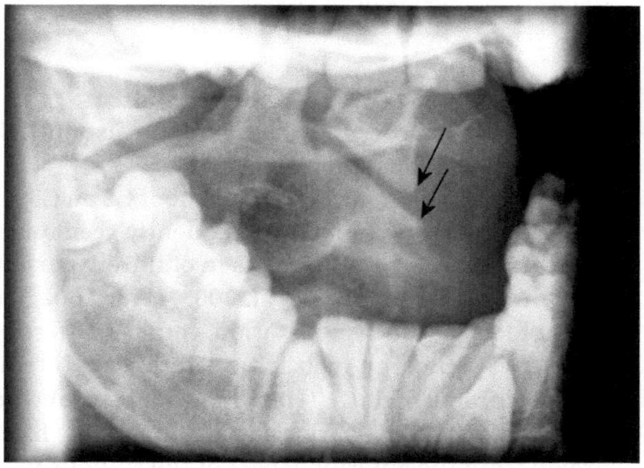

Fig. 7.56. Unilateral offset of the lateral masses of C1 and C2 (*arrows*) due to rotation. The lateral mass to odontoid process distances are unequal

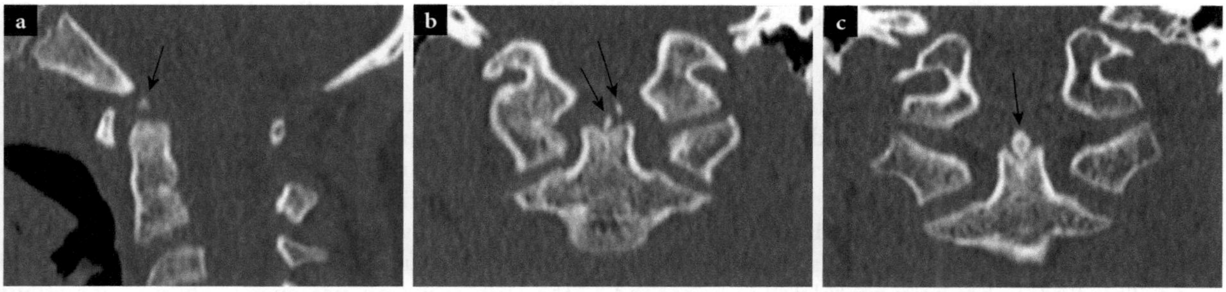

Fig. 7.57. a,b Sagittal and coronal CT reconstructions showing two foci of calcification within the ossification centre for the tip of the odontoid process in a 6-year-old. **c** Unfused, well developed ossification centre for the tip of the odontoid process in a 7-year-old

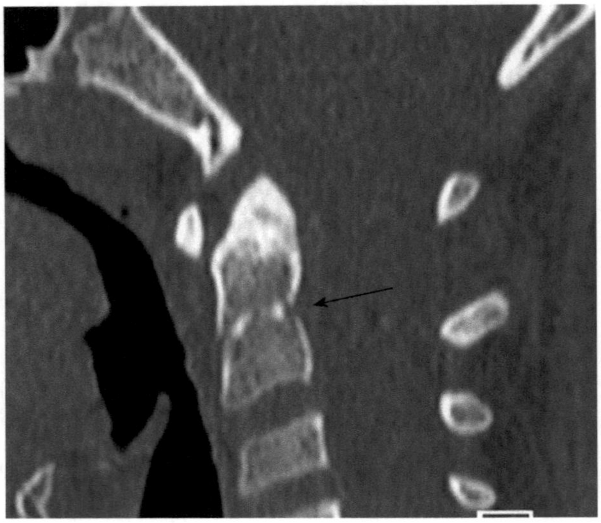

Fig. 7.58. Sagittal CT reconstruction. Almost fused synchondrosis between the body of C2 and the odontoid process simulating a fracture in an 11-year-old

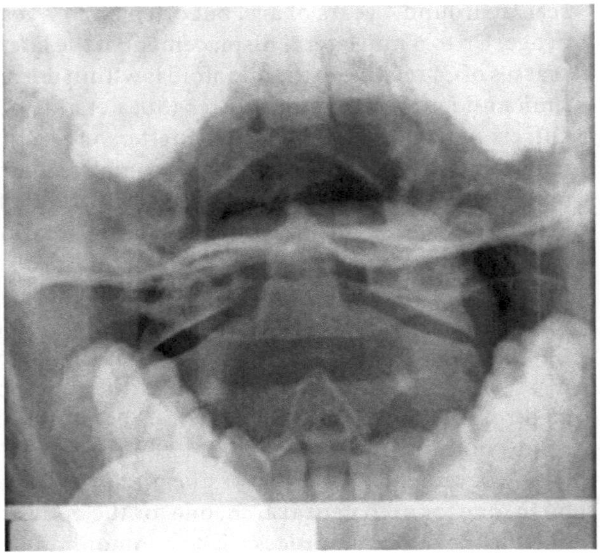

Fig. 7.59. Pseudofracture of the odontoid process produced by the Mach effect from overlapping of the posterior arch of C1 and the occiput

and transverse processes. These can persist until the third decade and simulate fractures.

Normal physiologic displacement of C2 on C3 and to a lesser extent C3 on C4 is frequently seen on lateral cervical spine radiographs in children, particularly in flexion (Lustrin et al. 2003) (Fig. 7.60). This physiologic pseudo-subluxation can be differentiated from pathology such as a bilateral pars interarticularis fracture of C2 (Hangman's fracture) when there is a normal posterior cervical line. This line is drawn from the anterior aspect of the spinous process of C1 to the anterior aspect of the spinous process of C3. The anterior edges of the spinous processes of C1, C2 and C3 should all line up within 1 mm of each other on both flexion and extension radiographs. If this line does not overlap the anterior aspect of C2 by 2 mm or more a true injury is present (Swischuk 2002).

Loss of the normal cervical lordosis can be a sign of a significant injury in adults but this is frequently seen as a normal finding in children up to 16 years of age on lateral cervical spine radiographs taken in neutral position (Lustrin et al. 2003). In children there is often an increased distance between the tips of the C1 and C2 spinous processes in flexion. This finding has been postulated to be secondary to a tight ligamentous attachment between the skull base and C1, and should not be misinterpreted as evidence of ligamentous injury (Lustrin et al. 2003). The upper cervical prevertebral soft tissues can appear abnormally wide in flexion or in expiration simulating oedema or haemorrhage secondary to a spinal fracture or ligamentous injury. This finding may require repeat radiographs in mild extension and inspiration or even cross sectional imaging if there is clinical concern (Fig. 7.61).

Anterior wedging of the upper cervical bodies particularly C3 (Fig. 7.62) is a normal developmental variant and should not be confused with a compression injury. It may be the result of relative hypermobility of the spine during childhood and resolves with increasing maturity (Swischuk et al. 1993). Secondary ossification centres ('ring' epiphyses or apophyses) appear at the superior and inferior aspects of all vertebral bodies and do not fuse with the vertebral body until early adulthood (Figs. 7.63, 7.64). These should not be mistaken for fractures, although they can be avulsed as a result of trauma (Johnsson et al. 1991).

In the infant skull accessory sutures and synchondroses can be mistaken for fractures. The most common locations for accessory sutures are intraparietal, located within the parietal bone. Intraparietal accessory sutures may be unilateral or bilateral. In the acute situation, presence or absence of overlying soft tissue swelling is helpful in differentiating between fractures and accessory sutures. Sutures also tend to have less sharply defined margins and may

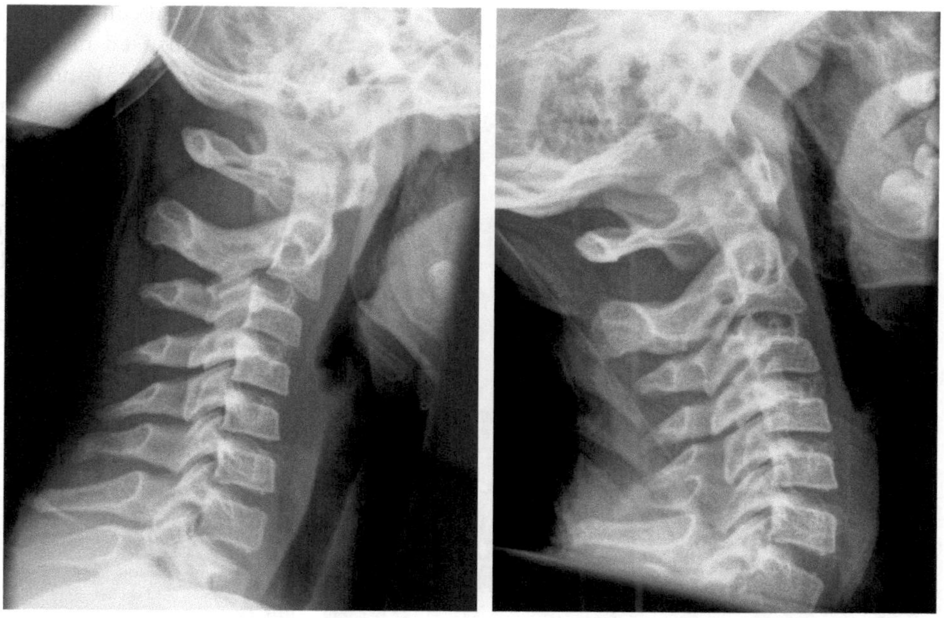

a b

Fig. 7.60a,b. Pseudosubluxation of C2 on C3 in slight flexion, the posterior cervical line is intact (**a**). Pseudosubluxation 'corrects' in extension (**b**)

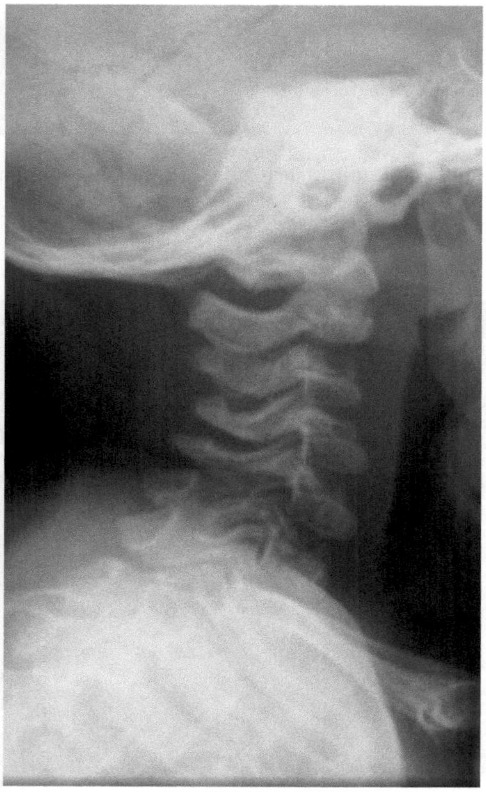

Fig. 7.61. Normal 19-month-old with widening of the upper cervical prevertebral soft tissues

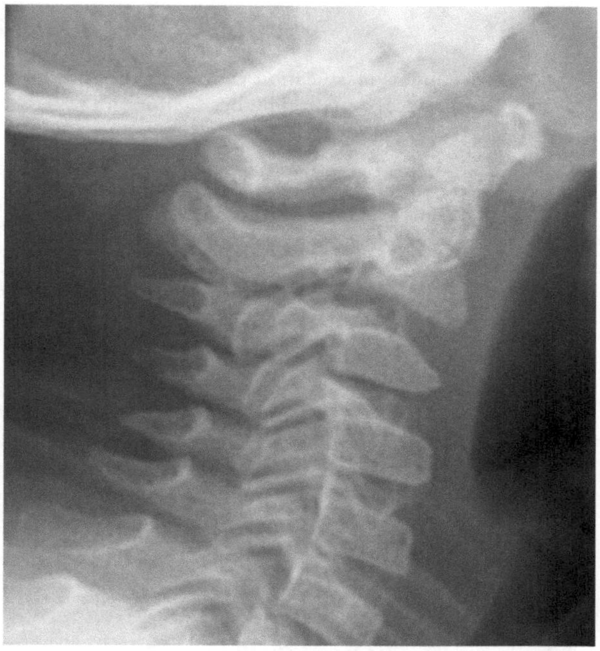

Fig. 7.62. Anterior 'wedging' of C3 in a normal 2-year-old

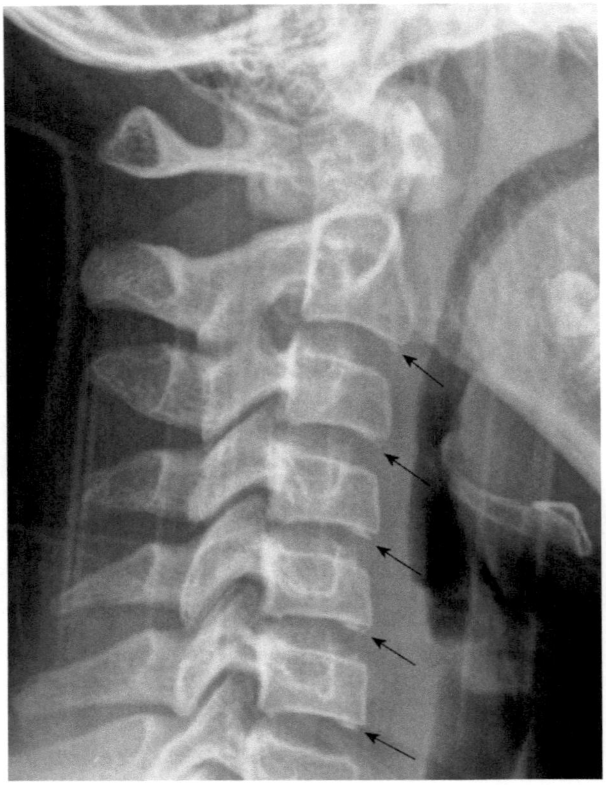

Fig. 7.63. Secondary ossification centres at the inferior aspects of the cervical vertebral bodies (*arrows*)

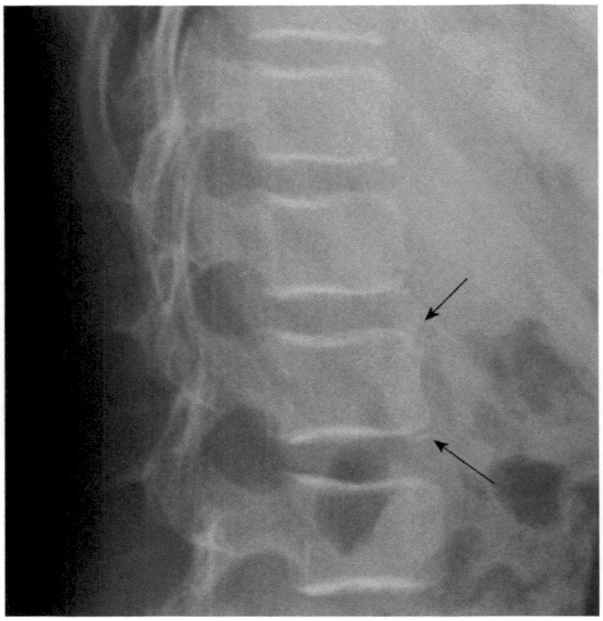

Fig. 7.64. Secondary ossification centres at the superior and inferior aspects of L2 (*arrows*) and adjacent vertebral bodies

branch, but it can be difficult to differentiate the two. Normal unfused metopic, mendosal or squamosal sutures (Fig. 7.65) and numerous other unfused synchondroses may be also mistaken for fractures and it is important to be aware of their anatomical location (Keats and Anderson 2001). Accessory bones related to the lambdoid suture, otherwise known as interparietal or Inca bones (Fig. 7.66), can be mistaken for fractures in children and may also persist into adulthood. These ossicles are variable in shape and size (Shapiro and Robinson 1976).

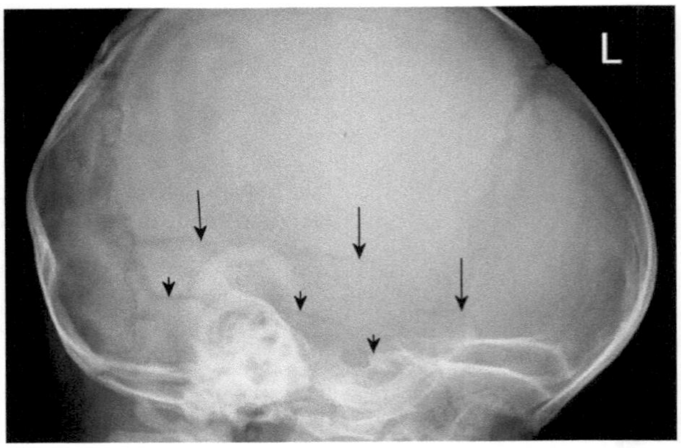

Fig. 7.65. Squamosal sutures (*arrows*) in a 6-month-old infant

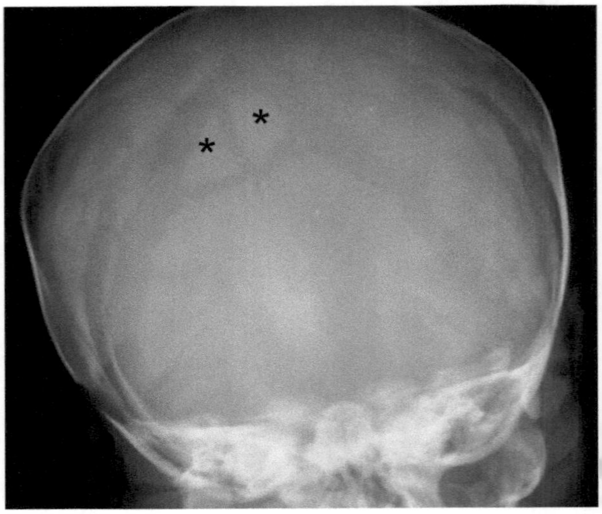

Fig. 7.66. Paired triangular interparietal bones in a 6-week-old infant (*asterisks*)

7.8 Miscellaneous and Non-site Specific Normal Variants

Subperiosteal new bone formation occurring in the long bones of infants is a well-recognised normal finding (Glaser 1949; Shopfner 1966; Hancox et al. 1951). Although the phenomenon is not completely understood, it may represent a normal physiological response of bone to growth and development, but can also be an indicator of pathology such as a metabolic disorder, malignancy, accidental or non-accidental injury (NAI). Normal physiological subperiosteal new bone formation usually occurs between 1 and 4 months of age. Its occurrence outside of these ages should prompt a search for an underlying cause. Most commonly affected sites are the tibia, femur, humerus, ulna and radius, in decreasing order of frequency (Fig. 7.67). Involvement may be unilateral or bilateral and the thickness of the subperiosteal new bone is never greater than 1.8 mm, averaging 0.7–0.9 mm (Kwon et al. 2002).

Metaphyseal ‘corner fractures’ are highly associated with non-accidental trauma and it is important not to confuse certain normal metaphyseal variants with these injuries. The normal metaphyseal variants include metaphyseal step-off, beak or spur, and proximal tibial cortical irregularity (Kleinman et al. 1991). All of these variants may be unilateral or bilateral. It is important to be familiar with their appearances in order that they are not mistaken for signs of abuse, with often devastating consequences. A metaphyseal step off is an acute, near 90 degree angulation in the extreme portion of the metaphysis adjacent to the physis (Fig. 7.68). The adjacent cortical margin may be indistinct. This variant is seen in the upper and lower limb long bones around the knee and wrist. A metaphyseal beak is a medial projection off the proximal humerus or proximal tibia. It tends to be more well-defined and dense in the humerus (Fig. 7.69). Metaphyseal spurs are discrete longitudinal projections of bone that extend beyond the metaphyseal margin but remain continuous with the cortex. It may be seen in the lateral aspect of the distal femur or distal radius, medial aspect of the distal ulna and in the metacarpals and metatarsals laterally (Fig. 7.70). Proximal tibial cortical irregularity is a focal area of irregularity in the medial aspect of the

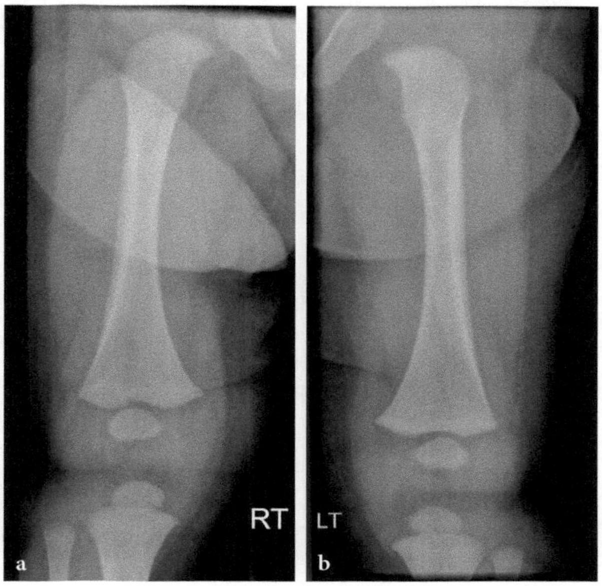

Fig. 7.67a,b. Bilateral physiological periosteal reaction along the lateral diaphysis of the femur in a normal 8-week-old infant

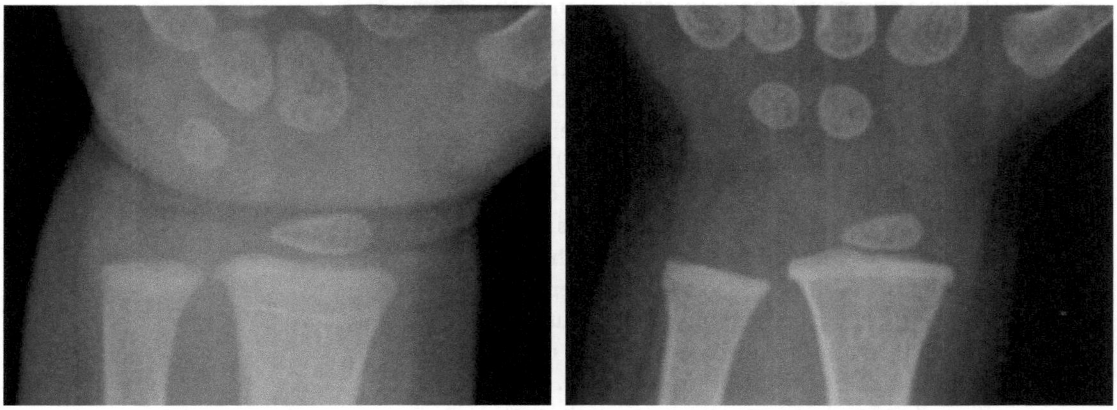

a b

Fig. 7.68a,b. Two examples of metaphyseal step off in the distal radius in normal infants aged 18 months (**a**) and 17-months (**b**)

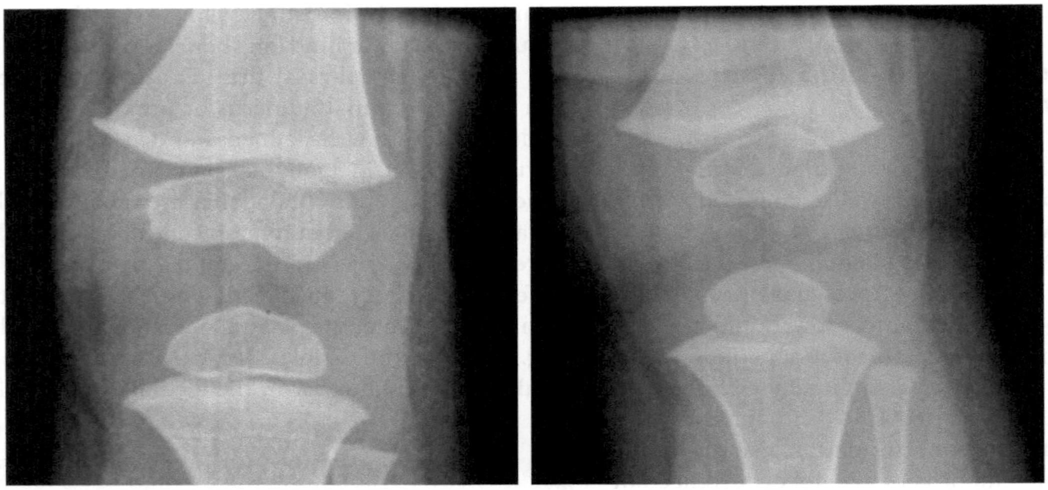

a b

Fig. 7.69a,b. A 17-month old infant with metaphyseal beak in the distal femur (a) and 9-month old infant with proximal tibial metaphyseal beak (b)

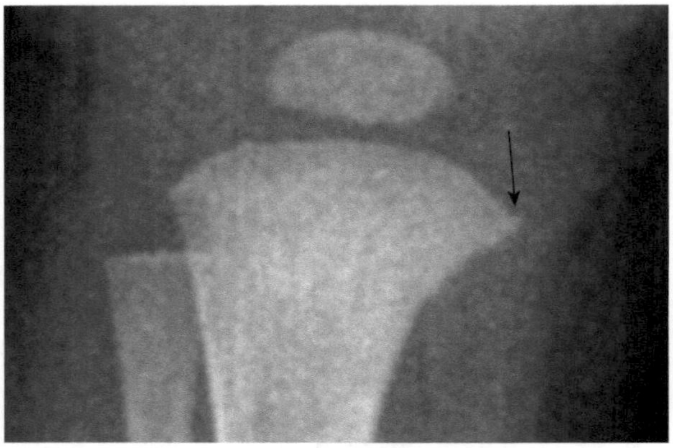

Fig. 7.70. Metaphyseal spur in a 4-week-old baby

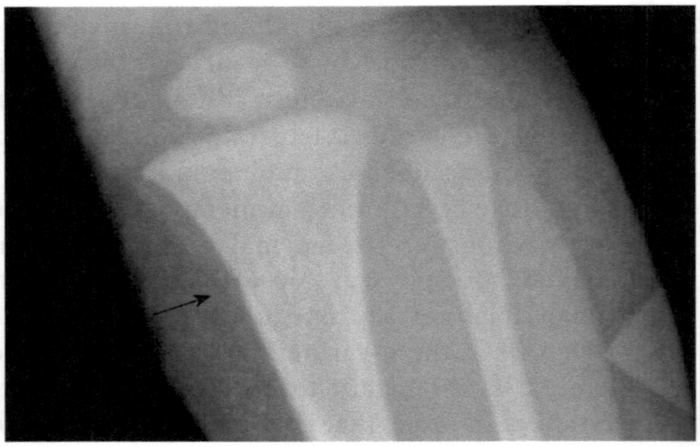

Fig. 7.71. Proximal cortical irregularity of the left tibia in a normal 8-week-old infant (*arrow*)

proximal tibial metaphysis. The appearance is seen only in the tibia and may be seen in association with physiologic new bone formation. Because of its similarity to a buckle fracture, if there is any question of NAI, further imaging, e.g. with nuclear bone scintigraphy or follow up radiographs to look for evidence of fracture healing, should be instigated (Fig. 7.71).

The fusing or almost fused epiphysis of any of the long bones can be mistaken for a fracture (Figs. 7.22, 7.72). Soft tissue injury should be considered if there is overlying soft tissue swelling and localised tenderness, which is more common than bony injury. Nutrient vessels passing through the cortex of the shaft of the long bones may also be mistaken for fractures. They are usually well defined and not associated with localised pain or overlying soft tissue swelling (Fig. 7.73).

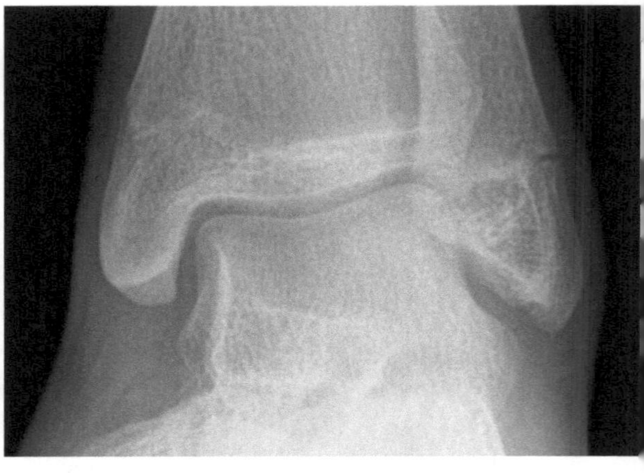

Fig. 7.72. Unfused lateral epiphysis of the distal fibula simulating a fracture

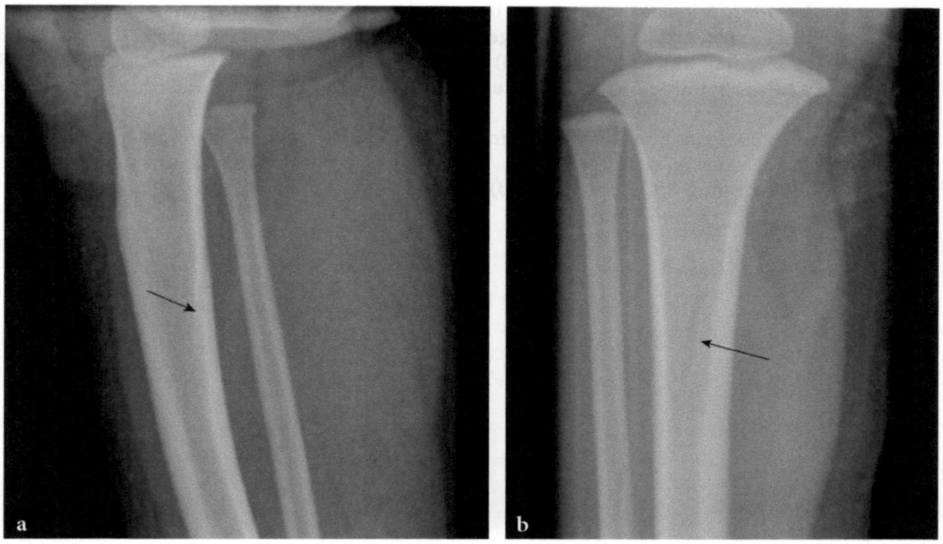

Fig. 7.73a,b. Nutrient vessel in the tibial diaphysis (*arrows*)

References

Baker C, Kadish H, Schunk JE (1999) Evaluation of pediatric cervical spine injuries. Am J Emerg Med 17:230–234

Caffey J, Madell SH, Royer C et al (1958) Ossification of the distal femoral epiphysis. J Bone Joint Surg Am 40-A:647–654

Caffey J, Ross SE (1956) The ischiopubic synchondrosis in healthy children: some normal roentgenographic findings. AJR Am J Roentgenol 76:488–494

Currarino G, Prescott P (1994) Fractures of the acromion in young children and a description of a variant in acromial ossification which may mimic a fracture. Pediatr Radiol 24:251–255

Glaser K (1949) Double contour, cupping and spurring in roentgenograms of long bones in infants. AJR Am J Roentgenol 61:482–492

Hancox NM, Hay JD, Holden WAS et al (1951) The radiological 'double contour' effect in the long bones of newly born infants. Arch Dis Child 26:543–548

Harrison RB, Keats TE (1980) Epiphyseal clefts. Skeletal Radiol 5:23–27

Johnsson K, Niklasson J, Josefsson PO (1991) Avulsion of the cervical spinal ring apophyses: acute and chronic appearance. Skeletal Radiol 20:207–210

Keats TE (2004) Chapter 2: Anatomic variants. In: Caffey's pediatric diagnostic imaging, 10th edn. Mosby, St Louis, pp 2053–2092

Keats TE, Anderson MW (2001) Atlas of normal roentgen variants that may simulate disease, 7th edn. Mosby, St Louis

Kleinman PK, Belanger PL, Karelas A et al (1991) Normal metaphyseal radiologic variants not to be confused with findings of infant abuse. Am J Roentgenol 156:781–783

Kohler A, Zimmer EA (1968) Borderlands of the normal and early pathologic findings in skeletal roentgenology, 3rd edn. Grune & Stratton, New York

Kump WL (1966) Vertical fractures of the distal tibial epiphysis. AJR Am J Roentgenol 97:676–681

Kwon DS, Spevak MR, Fletcher K et al (2002) Physiologic subperiosteal new bone formation: prevalence, distribution and thickness in neonates and infants. AJR Am J Roentgenol 179:985–988

Lawson JP, Ogden JA, Sella E et al (1984) The painful accessory navicular. Skeletal Radiol 12:250–262

Lustrin ES, Karakas SP, Ortiz AO et al (2003) Pediatric cervical spine: normal anatomy, variants and trauma. Radiographics 23:539–560

Mosel LD, Kat E, Voyvodic F (2004) Imaging of the symptomatic type II accessory navicular bone. Australas Radiol 48:267–271

O'Neal ML, Dwornik JJ, Ganey TM et al (1998) Postnatal development of the human sternum. J Pediatr Orthop 18:398–405

Ogden JA (1984) Radiology of postnatal skeletal development. X. Patella and tibial tuberosity. Skeletal Radiol 11:246–257

Ogden JA (1984) Radiology of postnatal skeletal development. XII. 2nd cervical vertebra. Skeletal Radiol 12:169–177

Ogden JA, Conlogue GJ, Bronson ML et al (1979) Radiology of postnatal skeletal development. II. The manubrium and sternum. Skeletal Radiol 4:189–195

Ogden JA, McCarthy SM (1983) Radiology of postnatal skeletal development. VIII. Distal tibia and fibula. Skeletal Radiol 10:209–220

Ozonoff MB (1992) Chapter 2: The upper extremity. In: Pediatric Orthopedic Radiology, 2nd edn. WB Saunders and Co, Philadelphia, pp 117–163

Rossitch JC, Bohrer SP (1991) Case of the month. Appl Radiology 20:56

Shapiro R, Robinson F (1976) The os incae. AJR Am J Roentgenol 127:469–471

Shawdon A, Kiss ZS, Fuller P (1995) The bipartite tarsal navicular bone: radiographic and computed tomography findings. Australas Radiol 39:192–194

Shopfner CE (1966) Periosteal bone growth in normal infants: a preliminary report. AJR Am J Roentgenol 97:154–163
Suss RA, Zimmerman RD, Leeds NE (1983) Pseudospread of the atlas: false sign of Jefferson fracture in children. AJR Am J Roentgenol 140:1079–1082
Swischuk LE (2002) Imaging of the cervical spine in children. Springer-Verlag, New York
Swischuk LE, Swischuk PN, John SD (1993) Wedging of C-3 in infants and children: usually a normal finding and not a fracture. Radiology 188:523–526
Taybi H, Lachman RS (1996) Radiology of syndromes, metabolic disorders and skeletal dysplasias, 4th edn. Mosby, St. Louis
Wolansky LJ, Rajaraman V, Seo C et al (1999) The lateral atlanto-dens interval: normal range of asymmetry. Emerg Radiol 6:290–293

Basic Science of Paediatric Fractures

8

EDWARD BACHE and KARL J. JOHNSON

CONTENTS

E. BACHE, MD
Consultant Paediatric Orthopaedic Surgeon, Birmingham Children's Hospital, Steelhouse lane, Birmingham, B4 6NH, UK
K. J. JOHNSON, MD, MRCP, FRCR
Consultant Paediatric Radiologist, Birmingham Children's Hospital, Steelhouse Lane, Birmingham, B4 6NH, UK

8.1 Introduction

Fractures account for 10%–25% of all injuries in children. Boys are affected more commonly than girls. From birth until the age of 16 years of age, a girl has a 27% chance of sustaining a fracture while this rises to 42% for boys (LANDIN 1997). The physis is the weakest part of the bone and diaphyseal long bone fractures account for approximately 10% of children's fractures. Of these, the tibial shaft is most common, followed by diaphyseal fractures of the forearm.

8.2 Fracture Types

From a radiological perspective, childhood fractures may be complete or partial (incomplete).

A complete fracture occurs when there is discontinuity between two or more bone fragments, while with incomplete fractures, a portion of the cortex remains intact. Incomplete fractures are common in children due to the increased elasticity of the bone. Greenstick and buckle fall into the group of incomplete fractures.

Fractures can also be classified as being simple, where there is a single fracture line, or comminuted, where there are several fractures. Simple fractures can be described from the appearance of the fracture line with respect to the long axis of the bone, namely transverse, oblique and spiral.

Comminuted fractures include segmental fractures and those with butterfly fragments. Open or compound fractures occur when a wound extends from the skin surface to the fracture.

A fracture may be described as displaced when there is a space between the fracture fragments.

8.3 Radiographs

For the majority of injuries, a good quality antero-posterior and lateral radiograph is the only imaging that will be required. This will allow the fracture pattern to be determined along with any shortening or angulation. Rotation is more difficult to judge, but a mismatch of the diameter of the proximal and distal fragments will imply rotational malalignment in a bone that is not circular in cross-section. An easier method is to include the joints above and below the injury on the film (Fig. 8.1). This should be standard practice and it also helps to exclude any concomitant injury to adjacent joints.

8.4 Biomechanics

Careful inspection of a fracture will allow the mechanism of injury to be determined (Fig. 8.2). This may have important implications as to the stability of a fracture and will determine how the fracture should be reduced, if this is deemed necessary.

The application of force will generate stresses within a bone. These may be either compressive, tensile or shear. Cortical bone will tolerate compressive stresses better than tensile or shear.

8.4.1 Spiral Fractures

Torsional injuries will produce a spiral fracture pattern (Fig. 8.3). The forces required to create such an injury are generally applied at the ends of the bone. An example would be a skiing injury where sudden external or internal rotation is applied to the tibia via the foot (and ski) which act as a lever. Since the point of application of the force is not directly to the tibia, there will be less trauma to the soft tissues and the prognosis for fracture healing will be better. Careful inspection will show an axial fracture line joining the two ends of the spiral. Here the periosteum will be intact and this, together with the sparing of other surrounding soft tissues, means that these fractures are quite stable. By reversing the torsional force, the fracture can be reduced and this position maintained by incorporating both the joint above and below into plaster in a position of slight flexion. Spiral fractures have a large surface area of cancellous bone in contact at the fracture site. This ensures rapid fracture healing.

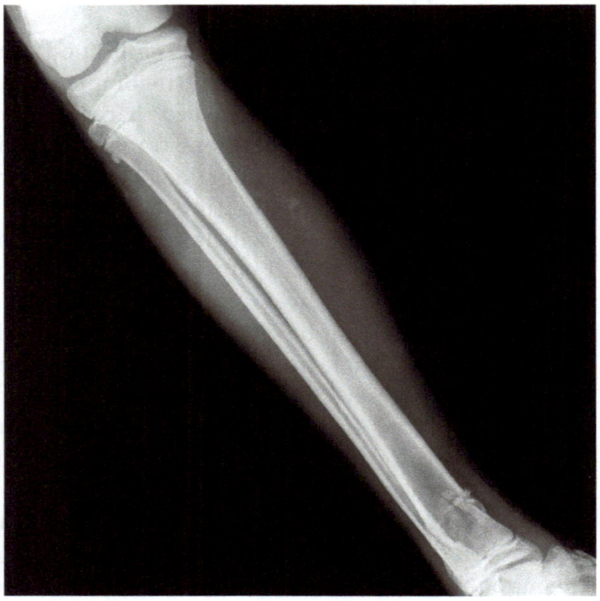

Fig. 8.1. AP radiograph of the tibia. Transverse fracture through the distal metaphysis. Acceptable angulation but note AP knee and lateral view of ankle. Malrotation of 45°

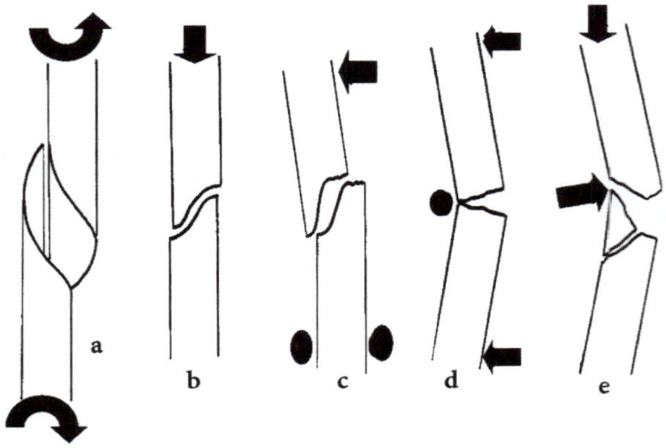

Fig. 8.2a-e. The pattern of a fracture is determined by the forces applied to produce it. **a** Spiral fracture is the result of twisting/torsional forces. **b** Oblique fracture due to compressive forces. **c** Oblique fracture (with small transverse element) due to the bone being held fast and an uneven bending force applied distal to the fracture. **d** Transverse fracture due to bending force about a fulcrum. **e-a** Butterfly fragment due to compression and bending forces

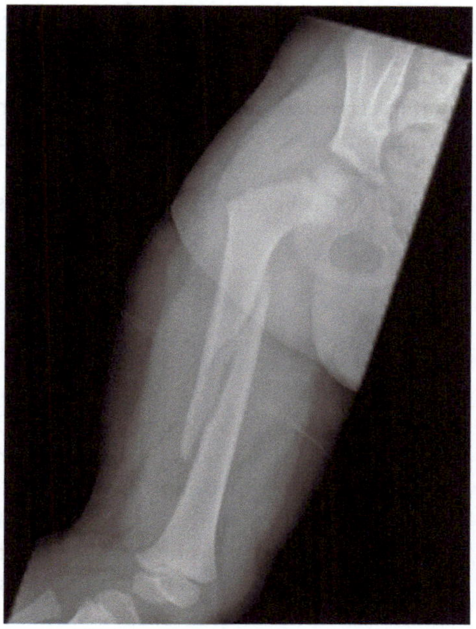

Fig. 8.3. Spiral fracture of the femoral shaft. Note AP view of hip and lateral view of knee. Fracture is rotated

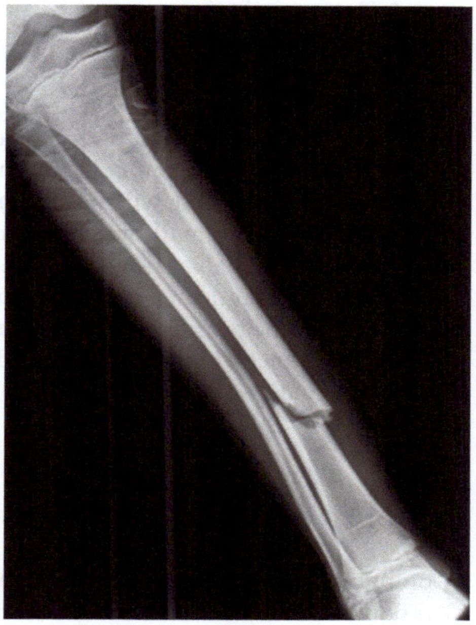

Fig. 8.4. Oblique fracture of the tibial shaft with transverse component. Plastic deformation of the fibula

8.4.2 Oblique Fractures

Oblique fractures result from shear stresses, secondary to axial loading. Pure oblique fractures, however, are rare and, more commonly, there is a minor transverse element to the fracture (Fig. 8.4). Such injuries are due to uneven bending. The middle and distal or proximal end of the bone are fixed and the free end is moved.

8.4.3 Transverse Fractures

Transverse fractures occur with pure bending forces (Fig. 8.5). The bone fails in tension with the fracture initiating at the opposite cortex where tensile forces are maximal and propagating to the fulcrum where the bending force is applied.

Transverse fractures are inherently stable if they can be reduced, since the fracture surfaces interlock. If the proximal and distal fragments are completely displaced, reduction may be difficult since one or both ends may have buttonholed through the periosteum and manipulation of the bone back through a small periosteal window may be impossible.

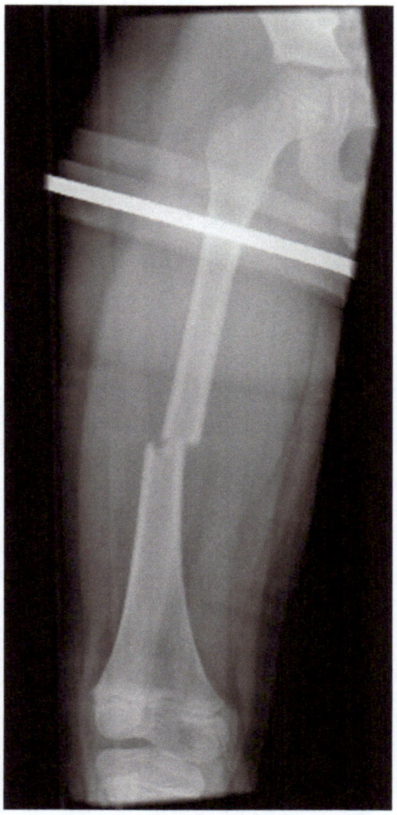

Fig. 8.5. Transverse fracture of the midshaft of the femur. Fracture reduced by traction in Thomas splint

8.4.4
Butterfly Fragment

The combination of bending plus axial compression may result in an oblique fracture with a butterfly fragment. The size of the fragment and the degree of displacement will determine the stability of the fracture. Small or undisplaced fractures may be relatively stable. However, it is important to identify these fragments since manipulation, and in particular, the passage of intramedullary devices can displace such fragments and produce a highly unstable situation (Fig. 8.2).

8.4.5
Buckle/Torus Fractures

Compressive forces in children can result in cortical bone buckling. These fractures, which are commonly also referred to as buckle or torus injuries, are incomplete and the cortex is intact (Fig. 8.6a,b). Torus is derived from the Latin meaning a protuberance or knot and typically involves both cortical surfaces, while a buckle fracture may only involve a single cortex. In practice, the terms are used interchangeably. The distal radius is the most frequently affected site, usually resulting from a fall on the outstretched hand. This injury is very stable and symptomatic treatment with a simple splint is all that is required. This is probably the most common fracture seen in children, but is much rarer in adults.

8.4.6
Greenstick Fractures

This is a descriptive term and should be reserved for those fractures which penetrate one cortex and then spreads up or down the medulla but does not cross the contralateral cortex. This fracture may be associated with some bowing of the limb. This term should not be used synonymously with torus fractures.

These fractures occur if the bone is angulated beyond its normal limits. There is complete failure on the tension side of the bone but only bending on the compression side. The cortical break occurs on the convex side of the bend (Fig. 8.7).

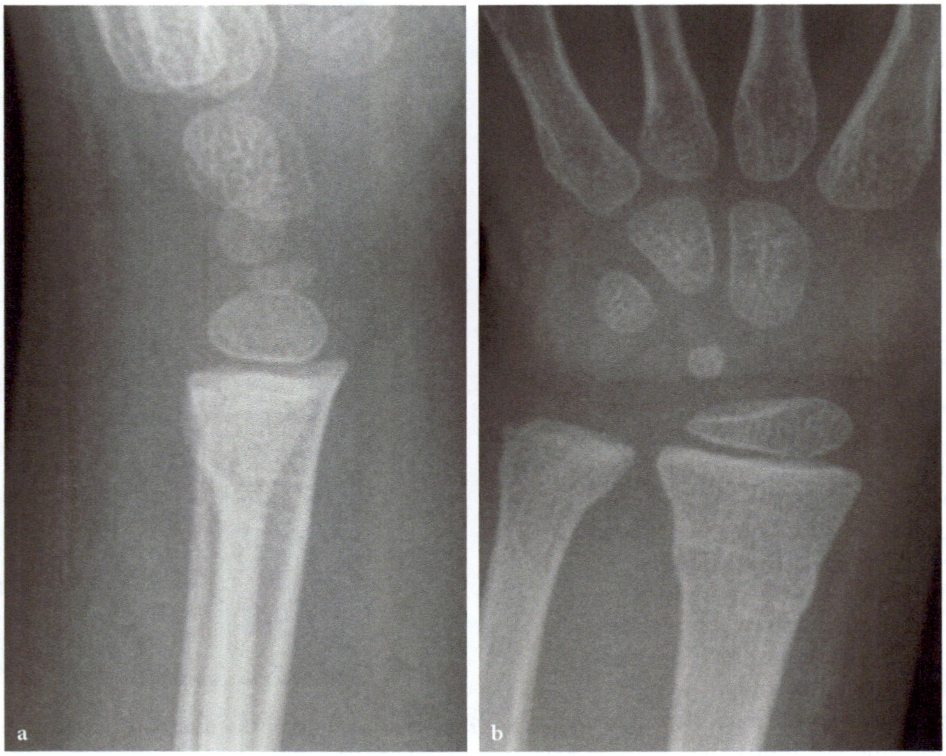

Fig. 8.6a,b. 'Torus' or 'buckle' fracture of the distal radial metaphysis

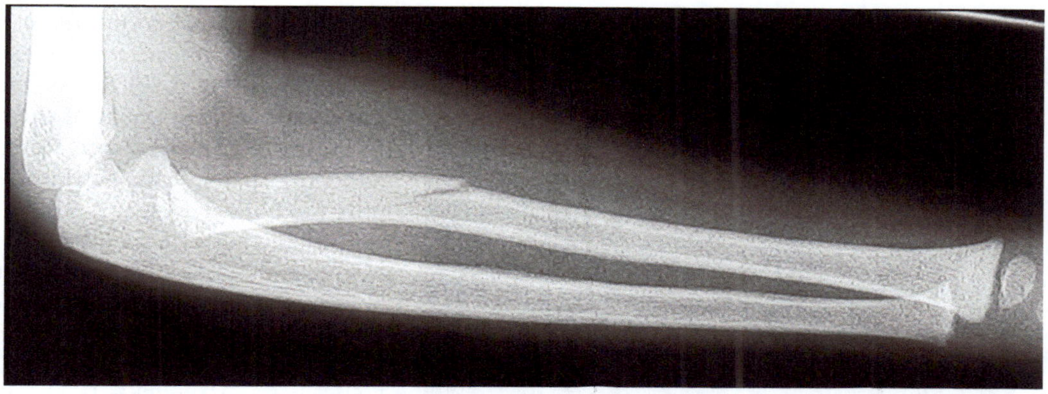

Fig. 8.7. Greenstick fracture of the radius with complete fracture of the ulna

8.4.7 Bowed Fractures

When relatively minor forces are applied, children's bones are more able to bend than those of an adult. With excess force the deformity may persist (see section 8.5.1). This is called plastic deformation. The forearm and fibula are particularly prone to plastic deformation. these injuries are often referred to as bowed fractures. they may be associated with a fracture in the adjacent bone (Fig. 8.8)

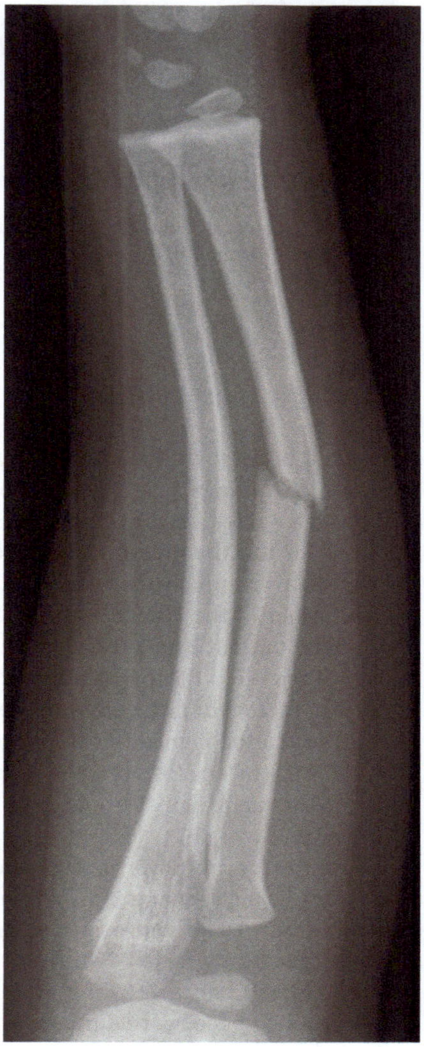

Fig. 8.8. Bowed fracture of the ulna with oblique fracture in the adjacent radius

8.5 Physiology of Bone Healing

Highly comminuted or segmental fractures may require internal fixation because of their inherent instability (Fig. 8.9). Open reduction increases the risk of complications, particularly in the case of high energy injuries with severe soft tissue injury. Further insult in the form of surgery will increase the risk of infection and delayed/non-union.

When interpreting serial radiographs of fractures, it is important to appreciate what form of healing is occurring and whether it is appropriate for the method of stabilisation being used. Fracture healing may either be primary or secondary.

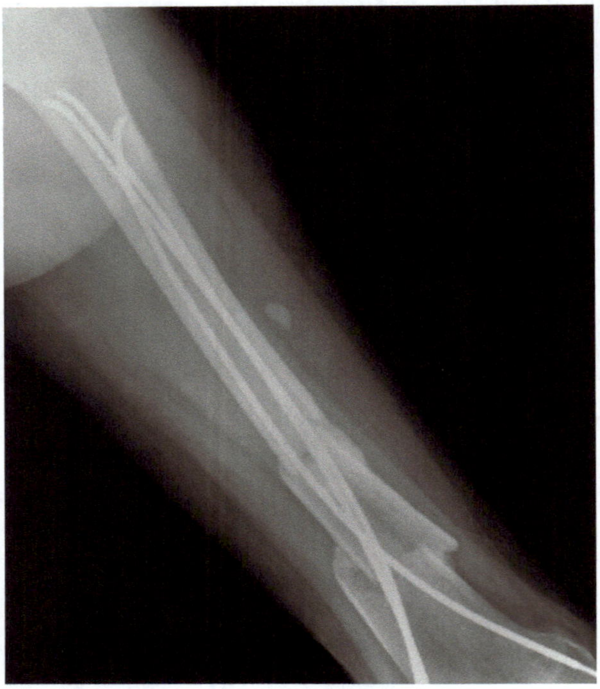

Fig. 8.9. Segmental fracture of the femur. Internal fixation with three intramedullary nails

8.5.1 Paediatric Considerations

When a body sustains a traumatic injury, the magnitude of damage sustained will be proportional to the energy released during the event and also to the rate at which the energy is released. In most cases of skeletal trauma, this relates to the kinetic energy (KE) either of the object that collides with the body or of the patient him-/herself if they hit a static object. Since $KE = ½ mv^2$, the velocity is a more important factor than the mass of the object/body. The child's skeleton is more elastic than that of an adult, so the rate of energy transfer is reduced. However, the area over which the energy is dissipated is also reduced.

High energy injuries produce more severe skeletal and soft tissue damage. This will manifest as a more severely displaced and/or increasingly comminuted fracture radiologically. Such injuries will be slower to heal, both because of the amount of bony damage and also because of damage to surrounding soft tissues.

Children's bones are more elastic than adults'. A child's forearm can be bent as far as 45° before a fracture occurs (Rang 1983). This response to trauma is best appreciated by examining a stress/strain graph (Fig. 8.10). Stress (measured along the X axis) is a measurement of the force applied and the strain produced (shown along the Y axis) is the deformity that results. As the stress increases, the more the bone deforms. A child's bone will deform more than that of an adult. When the force is removed, the bone will return to its previous state. However, at some point during bending (the yield stress), the bone enters a phase of plastic deformation. When this increased force is removed, some deformity persists. This is caused by microscopic fractures on the tensile side of the bone, but sequential radiographs will show no evidence of periosteal callus formation.

With further stresses applied to bone, it will eventually fail when its ultimate stress is reached. When the yield stress is close to the ultimate stress, as is the case in adults, there will be little plastic deformation. In the younger child, there is a significant difference between the yield and ultimate stress, so there will be greater plastic deformation.

Low energy bending injuries may produce plastic deformation (bowed fractures) or, if a cortical break is produced, it may not propagate fully across the bone. The cortex and periosteum on the compression side may be intact or undisplaced, resulting in a greenstick fracture.

8.5.2 Primary Bone Healing

Primary or cortical healing requires accurate apposition of the fracture fragments. At a microscopic level, there will be points of contact between the bones and small gaps. Cutting cones of osteoblasts and osteoclasts cross at points of contact creating new osteons. This restores mechanical continuity. The gaps fill in with blood vessels from which mesenchymal cells differentiate into osteoblasts which lay down callus which is again remodelled by the cutting cones. If there is any movement at the fracture site, this delicate healing response will be disrupted. In the clinical setting, such a pattern of healing may be observed in incomplete undisplaced fractures or in fractures that have been anatomically reduced and held under compression with screws/plates (Fig. 8.11). Such a healing response is characterised by a lack of periosteal callus on radiographs.

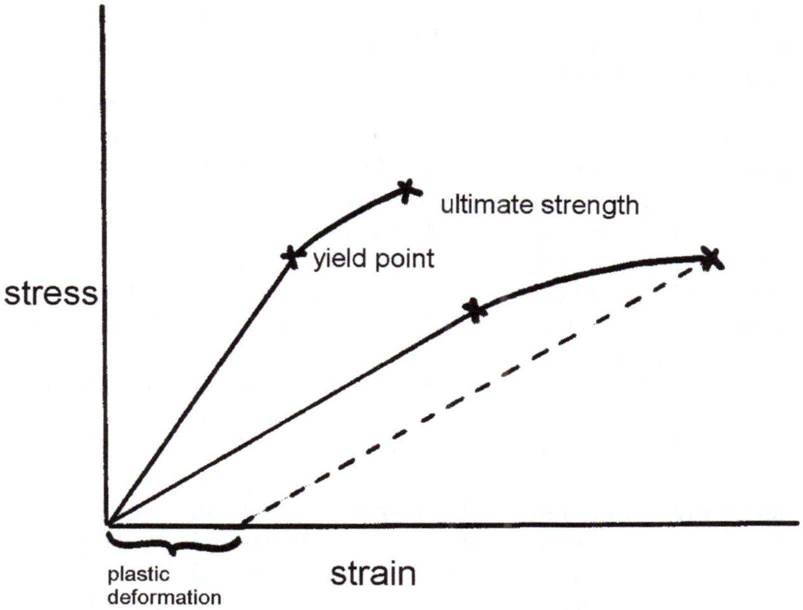

Fig. 8.10. Stress-strain curve. Deformation (*strain*) increases proportionally to the applied stress and the structure returns to its original state after removal of the stress. At the yield point, the structure enters a phase of plastic deformation. Residual deformity persists after removal of stress. The structure fails at breaking point

8.5.3 Secondary Bone Healing

The more common mode of healing is secondary. This process relies both on activity at the endosteal surface of the bone and in the periosteum. A small degree of movement encourages this pattern of healing. At the periosteum, both intramembranous and endochondral healing occur. Intramembranous healing tends to occur slightly distant from the fracture surface and results in so-called hard callus. Here, bone is laid down primarily without a cartilaginous precursor. This can usually be identified as a thin line of calcification on radiographs about 1–2 weeks post injury (Fig. 8.12). Between the bone ends, endochondral healing predominates. Here, the fracture haematoma is replaced first by cartilage to form soft callus which becomes calcified and is then replaced by woven bone.

Open reduction of the fracture will remove the haematoma and may delay the healing response. Radiologically, secondary healing is characterised by abundant periosteal callus. This form of healing is typical in displaced fractures that are treated non-operatively and when non-rigid implants such as intramedullary nails are utilised.

Around joints, an anatomical reduction of the fracture is required, since incongruity of the articular surface will cause pain and lead to degenerative change. Fixation is frequently achieved by utilising plates and

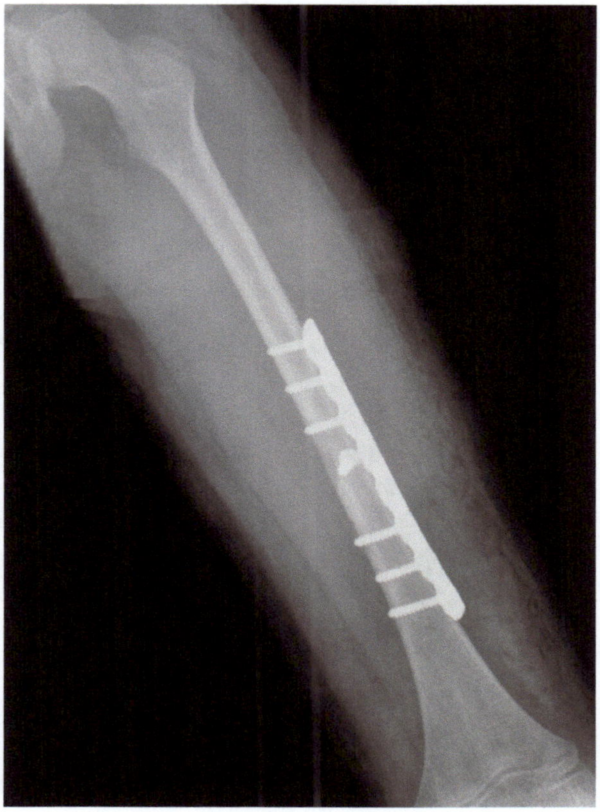

Fig. 8.11. Oblique fracture of the femur in a child with cerebral palsy stabilized with plate and screws. Medullary canal is too narrow for intramedullary implant. Fracture has united by primary healing. Note the lack of periosteal callus

screws. Diaphyseal fractures do not require such accurate reduction and overall alignment can generally be maintained with casts or intramedullary rods.

Whenever a fracture or osteotomy is stabilised with metalwork, a race is initiated. Eventually all implants will fail. The question is, will the fracture or osteotomy unite before implant failure? Obviously, the quicker the fracture heals, the less likely it is that the metalwork will fail. Radiological examination will provide early clues of impending failure. The presence of abundant periosteal callus is a good sign if an implant such as an intramedullary nail is being used, since these devices rely on secondary healing. A similar reaction around a fracture treated by rigid internal fixation with plate and screws may indicate that the implant is loose. Another sign of implant loosening is a radiolucent 'halo' around the metal. In other cases, the implant itself may fail. Plates and screws will generally bend before they break and even subtle or small angulations of such implants are significant (Fig. 8.13).

Metalwork is usually removed after the fracture has united. Stainless steel has a different elastic modulus (stiffness) than bone and this creates a stress riser at the junction between the bone and the implant which may lead to refracture. This is a particular risk for plates and screws where the screws penetrate the cortex and weaken it (Fig. 8.14).

8.6 Fracture Remodelling

Angular remodelling occurs by two mechanisms. At the fracture site, the bone remodels following Wolff's law: new bone is laid down on the compression (concave) side and resorbed on the tensile side. Angulation at any level of a bone will lead to a malalignment of the physis at each end. This causes uneven loading of the growth plate which then responds with a differential growth spurt to realign itself, so that the shaft of the bone is perpendicular to the joint reaction forces. This has been described as the Hueter–Volkmann law. It has been suggested

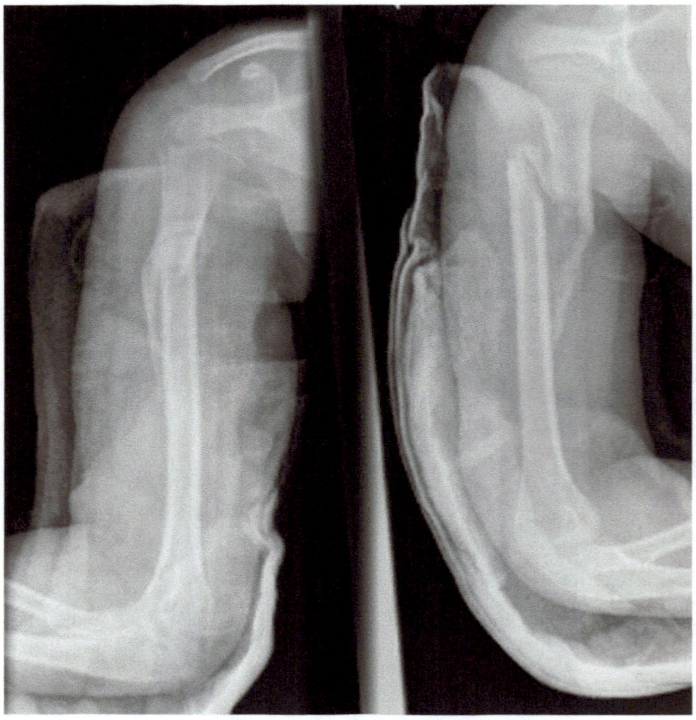

Fig. 8.12. Oblique fracture of the humerus 3 weeks post-injury. Extensive callus is visible and outlining the stripped periosteum

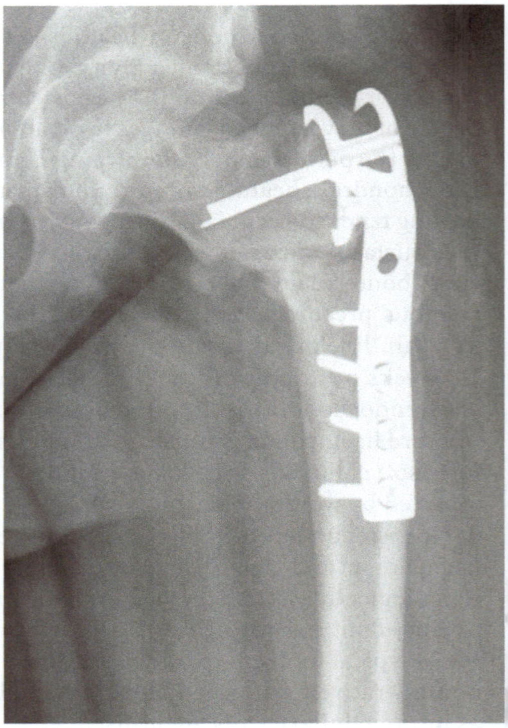

Fig. 8.13. Proximal femoral osteotomy stabilized with blade plate. There is a slight bend at the neck of plate at 6 weeks post-surgery which caused the implant to fail and the osteotomy to malunite.

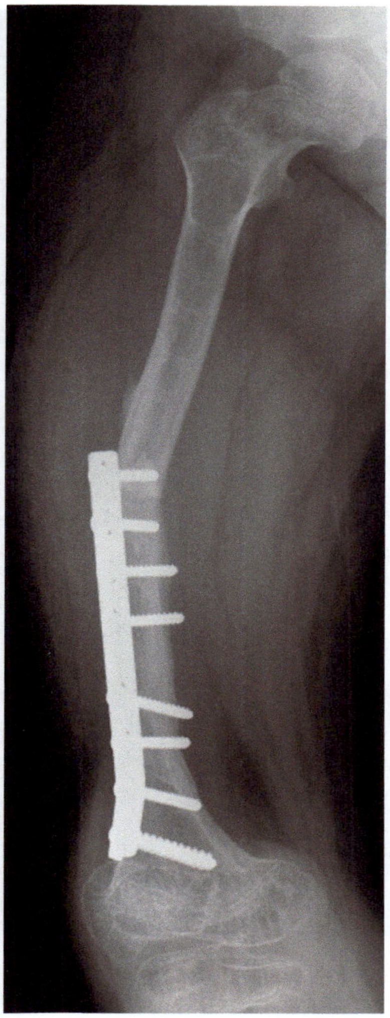

Fig. 8.14. Refracture of femur through screw hole

that the latter mechanism is responsible for as much as 75% of the correction (Wallace 1992).

Remodelling would appear to be more successful at some sites than others. Remodelling is exceptionally good around the proximal humerus and distal forearm, fair in the femur, but relatively poor in the middle third of the humerus and forearm. Remodelling is superior if the angulation is in the plane of movement of adjacent joints. The tibia is unusual that in the coronal plane, varus remodels better than valgus malunion. It is generally accepted that rotational deformity remodels poorly, although it has been suggested that there may be a limited capacity for the physis to respond by growing in a helical manner (Gasco 1997).

8.7 Fracture Non-union

Non-union is rare in children's fractures, but distinguishing delayed union from non-union may be difficult. The expected time to union of a bone will vary depending on the severity of the initial injury, the method of treatment and the age of the child. An infant's femoral fracture should be united at 4–6 weeks, whilst in children between 5 and 10 years, this will extend to 8–10 weeks. At 15 years, a similar injury may take up to 15 weeks to heal. Lack of any progression of healing on serial radiographs over several months will suggest non-union. This complication is extremely rare in children less than 10 years old (Lewallen 1985). It tends to be associated with high energy and open injuries, particularly in the presence of infection.

Non-union may be described as being either hypertrophic or atrophic, depending on the amount of callus visible on radiographs. Atrophic non-unions are related to poor local biology such as ischaemia or infection. Hypertrophic non-union have the potential for healing, but the mechanical environment is suboptimal. Generally, there is excessive movement at the fracture site. This is often addressed by bone grafting and rigid internal fixation. Preoperative planning with CT scans is very useful for determining the anatomy of the non-union (Fig. 8.15a–c). Non-union is most common in the tibia, followed by the femur and ulna.

8.8 Infection

Osteomyelitis is not uncommon in children. Bacteria may enter the bone via one of four different mechanisms:

1. Haematogenous spread
2. Spread from a contiguous source of infection.
3. Direct implantation
4. Post-operative (iatrogenic)

The last two of these are most important with respect to infection complicating trauma. A fracture haematoma provides the ideal environment for the proliferation of organisms whether it has been inoculated directly at the time of the trauma or from haematogenous spread.

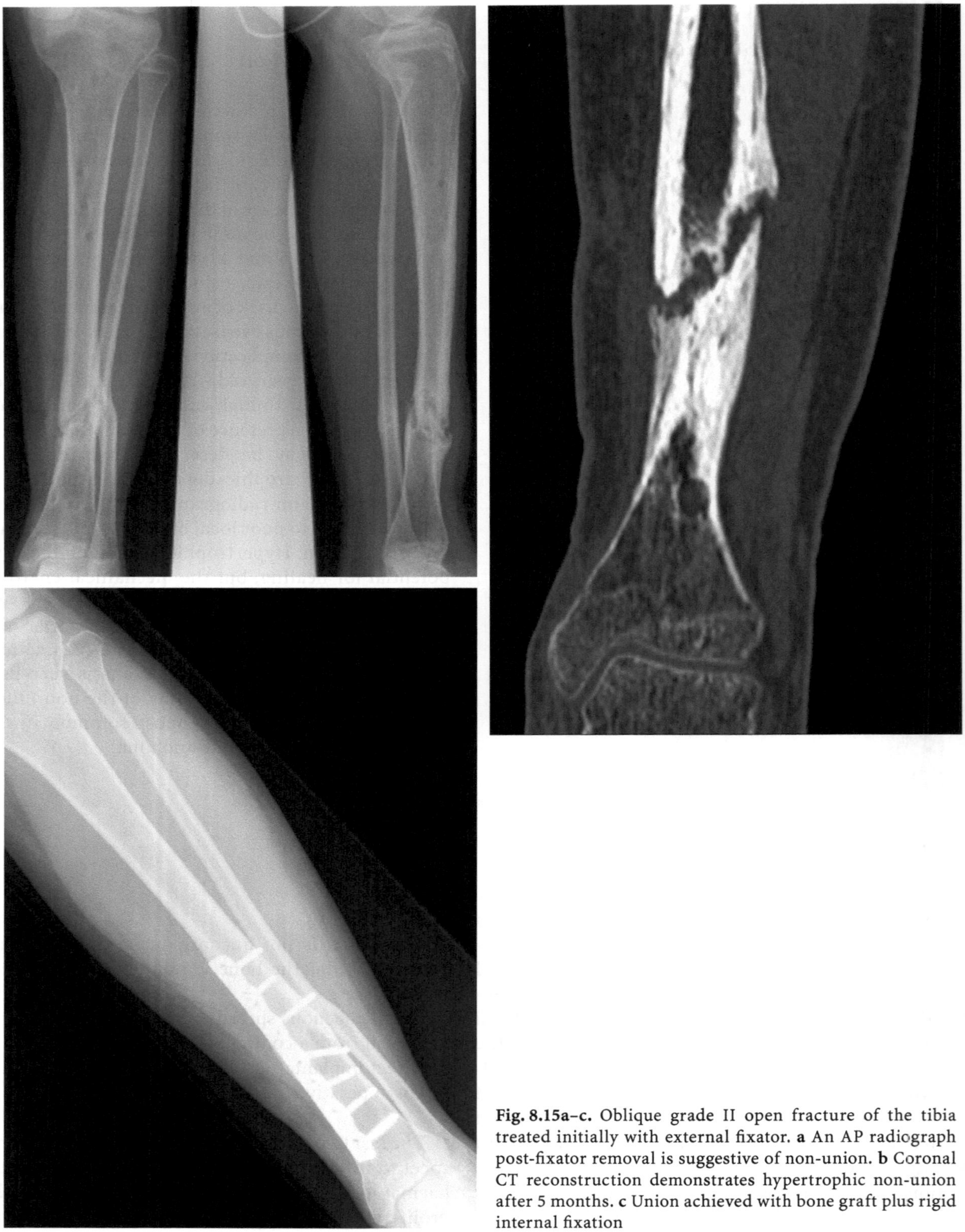

a

c

Fig. 8.15a–c. Oblique grade II open fracture of the tibia treated initially with external fixator. **a** An AP radiograph post-fixator removal is suggestive of non-union. **b** Coronal CT reconstruction demonstrates hypertrophic non-union after 5 months. **c** Union achieved with bone graft plus rigid internal fixation

8.8.1 Diagnosis of Infection

Infection can be acute, subacute or chronic, although the distinction between these is somewhat arbitrary. The clinical diagnosis of infection is not difficult if there is swelling, erythema and pus exuding from the wound. Raised inflammatory markers (ESR/CRP) may be secondary to trauma, but persistently elevated levels, particularly if the trend is upwards, would support sepsis. Ultimately, the diagnosis can only be made with certainty if bacteria are cultured.

Radiological interpretation may be difficult in the presence of trauma. Any delay in healing must arouse the suspicion of infection, but fractures may still heal under such circumstances, particularly if the infection is suppressed by antibiotics. The first radiological sign of infection is a periosteal reaction and localised osteopenia which may be present after approximately one week. It must be remembered that the fracture healing will also produce a periosteal reaction after a similar time period. With infection, the bone will then gradually show signs of poorly demarcated destruction, with permeative lytic and sclerotic changes seen on a radiograph.

The early diagnosis of acute haematogenous osteomyelitis is possible with either bone scintigraphy or magnetic resonance imaging, but in the presence of trauma, differentiation may be difficult. Wherever possible, MR imaging should be used to reduce the radiation exposure to the child

8.8.1.1 Nuclear Scintigraphy

The use of scintigraphy to diagnose infection in children should no longer be standard practice. Technetium 99^{m} labelled methylene diphosphonate is taken up by osteoblasts in areas of increased bone turnover, whether this be infection or trauma. Indium-111 labelled leukocyte scans are more specific because leukocytes are not involved in the normal bone healing response (Seabold 1991), but the radioactive dose is considerable. By combining technetium and indium labelled studies, it has been reported that sensitivity of 86% and specificity of 84% can be achieved when diagnosing infected fracture non-unions (Nepola 1993).

8.8.1.2 Magnetic Resonance Imaging (MRI)

This is highly sensitive in diagnosing infection. The involved marrow has low signal intensity on T1-weighted sequences and correspondingly of high signal on T2-weighted and short-tau inversion recovery (STIR) sequences, due to oedema. MR imaging is not specific, however, and oedema secondary to trauma will produce similar images. However, marrow oedema away from the fracture site is more suspicious of infection. The presence of soft tissue swelling and abscess formation away from the trauma site are also features of infection. It is important that post-gadolinium sequences are performed to distinguish between soft tissue oedema and abscess formation. An abscess will show as a distinct low signal area with surrounding enhancement. Image quality may be reduced in the presence of metal implants, other than those made of titanium. Caution is also required if steel implants are in situ, since the magnet field may potentially loosen them. It is important in these cases that the MR scanner suitability is determined.

MR imaging is valuable for identifying soft tissue collections, bones and abscesses and can also identify foreign material, such as wood, which will not be visible on plain radiographs (Fig. 8.16).

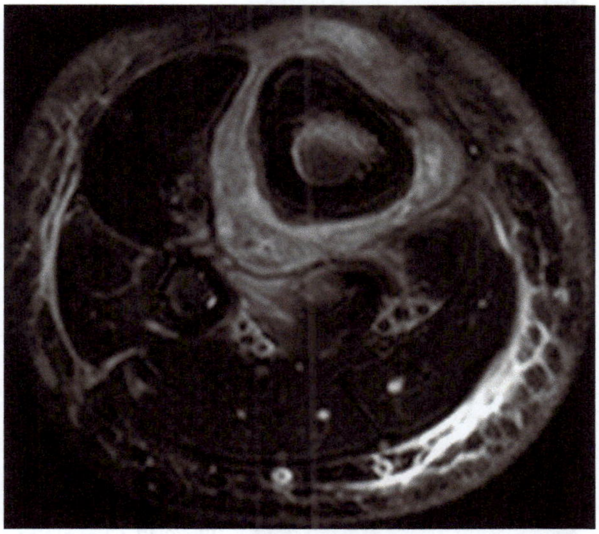

Fig. 8.16. Periostitis of the tibia. Axial T2 fast spin echo fat saturated image. The child had sustained an open injury 4 months previously when he ran into a bush. The tibia has a low signal thickened cortex. There is extensive high/intermediate signal fluid collection surrounding almost the entire circumference of the tibia, as well as extensive subcutaneous oedema. At surgery, there was shown to be a large subperiosteal abscess

8.8.2 Infected Metalwork

The diagnosis of infection is not an indication for removal of metalwork. Surgical debridement and irrigation are required along with antibiotics which are determined by the results of culture. Implants should be retained until the fracture is solid. Fractures can unite in the presence of infection but if chronic infection does develop, it may be impossible to eradicate until the implant is removed.

8.8.3 Chronic Infection

Chronic infection is generally associated with necrotic bone and this will also need to be removed if infection is to be cleared. The dead bone is referred to as 'sequestrum' and may be small or large. A large sequestrum may be surrounded by thickened new bone or 'involucrum' laid down by the periosteum. This is readily seen on radiographs (Fig. 8.17).

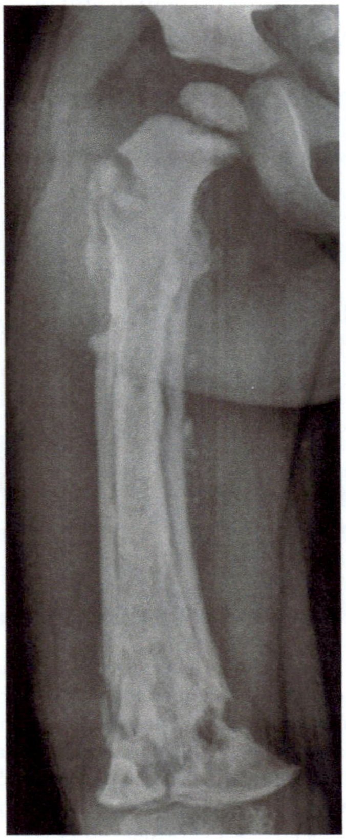

Fig. 8.17. Chronic osteomyelitis of the entire femur. The femoral shaft is necrotic and has formed a sequestrum. The periosteum has laid down new bone as an involucrum

A small sequestrum may be difficult to visualise on a radiograph and CT is useful in detecting such small necrotic pieces of bone and for the preoperative planning of their removal (Fig. 8.18).

A specific form of infection is related to the pins used as part of external fixators. These 'Shantz' screws allow percutaneous bacteria to gain access to the bone. After removal, a small persisting sinus may develop due to a small sequestrum which can develop around the screw. Such a 'ring' sequestrum has a characteristic appearance on radiographs. There is a central lucent zone created by the screw, a ring sequestrum and then another radiolucent halo due to chronic persisting infection around the dead sequestrum. The sequestrum can be removed with a curette and this will usually resolve the problem.

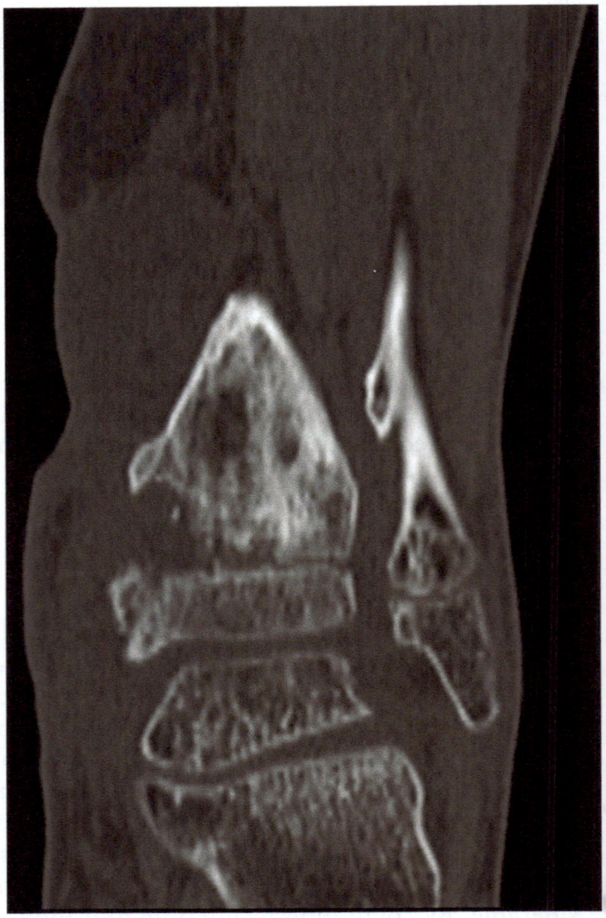

Fig. 8.18. Coronal reformatted CT scan of the distal tibia demonstrating a small sequestrum of bone and an associated defect in the cortex through which a sinus tract was found to emerge

8.9 Open Fractures

Open fractures may be classified into three major types (GUSTILO and ANDERSON 1976), with incidence of infection being related to the severity of the injury (GUSTILLO et al. 1990).

- Type I open fracture: The wound is less than 1 cm long and is relatively clean. It results from the bone puncturing the skin from the inside to the outside. The fracture is simple, transverse or oblique with minimal comminution. Infection rates are low at 0%–2%.
- Type II open fracture: The wound is more than 1 cm and there is moderate contamination and comminution of the fracture. There is not any extensive soft tissue damage. Infection rates range between 2%–7%.
- Type IIIA open fracture: This is a high velocity injury with extensive soft tissue injury but adequate coverage of the fracture. This subtype includes severely comminuted or segmental fractures regardless of the size of the wound. Infection rates are as high as 7%.
- Type IIIB open fracture: Similar to IIIA but after debridement, it is not possible to cover exposed bone without a local or free flap. Infection rates are higher at 10%–50%.
- Type IIIC open fracture: Any open injury which is associated with an arterial injury that must be repaired. Infection rates are 25%–50%.

The main principles in treating open fractures are that broad spectrum intravenous antibiotics should be administered promptly, the wound should be debrided and irrigated and the fracture should be stabilised. The use of internal fixation is indicated for most type I and II open fractures, although it is difficult for the host immune system to eradicate infection in the presence of foreign material. More severe injuries may be best managed by external fixators which provide stabilisation without having metal directly in the contaminated area.

References

Gasco J, de Pablos J (1997) Bone remodelling in malunited fractures in children. Is it reliable? J Ped Orthop (B) 6:126–132

Gustillo RB, Anderson JT (1976) Prevention of infection in the treatment of one thousand and twenty five open fractures of long bones. Retrospective and prospective analysis. J Bone and Joint Surg 58(A):453–458

Gustillo RB, Merkow RL, Templeman D (1990) The management of open fractures: current concepts. J Bone Joint Surg 72(A):299–304

Landin LA (1997) Epidemiology of children's fractures. J Ped Orthop (B) 6:79–83

Lewallen RP, Peterson HA (1985) Nonunion of long bone fractures in children. J Pediatr Orthop 5:153–142

Nepola JV, Seabold JE, Marsh JL, Kirchner PT, El-Khoury G (1993) Diagnosis of infection in ununited fractures. J Bone Joint Surg (A) 75A:1816–1822

Rang M (ed) (1983) Children's fractures. J.B. Lippencott Company, Philadelphia

Seabold JE, Nepola JV, Conrad GR, Marsh JL et al. (1991) Postoperative bone marrow alterations: potential pitfalls in the diagnosis of osteomyelitis with In-111-labelled leukocyte scintigraphy. Radiology 180:741–747

Wallace ME, Hoffman EB (1992) Remodelling of angular deformity after femoral shaft fractures in children. J Bone Joint Surg (Br) 74-B:765–769

Long Bone Fractures

9

Ed Bache

CONTENTS

E. Bache, FRCS (ortho)
Consultant Paediatric Orthopaedic Surgeon, Birmingham Children's Hospital, Steelhouse Lane, Birmingham, B4 6NH, UK

9.1 Femoral Fractures

More than 50% of femoral fractures are simple transverse, closed and non-comminuted (Rockwood 1991). The middle third is the most frequent site of fracture (70%), followed by the proximal third and lastly the distal third. Femoral fractures occurring before the child is able to walk are strongly associated with child abuse (Gross and Stranger 1983). Birth related fractures are exceedingly rare (0.13 per 1000) and usually associated with twin pregnancies, breech presentation or foetal osteoporosis (Morris et al. 2002). The majority are of spiral configuration.

It is recommended that the initial radiographs are taken before traction has been applied to the limb. The degree of shortening of the femur on this image will reflect the stability of the fracture. There is significantly more instability in those fractures that have more than 2 cm of shortening

9.1.1 Overgrowth

Overgrowth of long bones, particularly the femur, is universal post-fracture. This may be due to increased vascularity, secondary to the traumatic incident, but also possibly to release of the periosteum. It is thought that the periosteum may act as a tether or 'check rein' which slows the growth of the bone under normal circumstances. When damaged, this may allow the physis at either end of the bone to accelerate away from each other. On average, lengthening will amount to approximately 1.0 cm and is independent of age, level of fracture or position of the bone ends (Shapiro 1981). A total of 80% of overgrowth will have occurred by 18 months after the injury, although in a small number of patients, the phenomenon may continue until skeletal maturity.

9.1.2 Deformity

Angular deformity results from an unequal pull from muscles attached to the femur. This will vary depending on the level of the fracture. In the sagittal plane, an anterior bow occurs in mid and proximal fractures due to activity of the iliopsoas which inserts into the lesser trochanter proximally. (The hamstrings insert distally into the tibia; Fig. 9.1.) Significant flexion of the proximal fragment may give the false impression on an AP radiograph that the fracture is distracted. This error will be avoided if a lateral radiograph is also taken. Distal fractures will be subject to the pull of gastrocnemius inserting into the distal femur which results in a posterior bow. In the frontal plane, the adductors are attached along the length of the bone whilst the abductors insert around the greater trochanter. As a result, the majority of shaft fractures adopt a varus position. The obliquity and direction of the fracture surface will determine how likely it is to become angulated secondary to muscular forces.

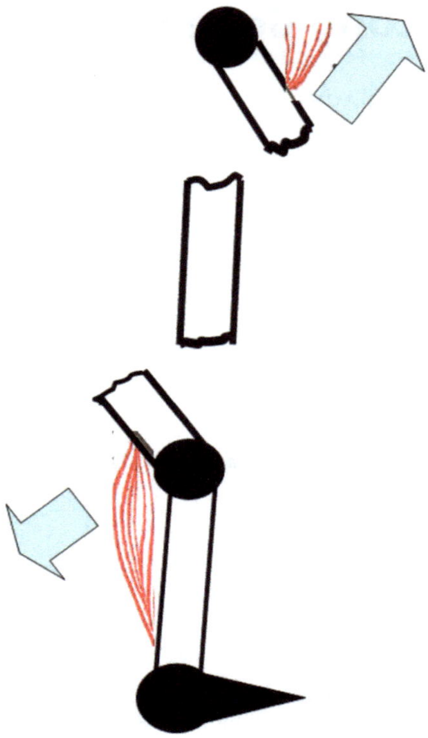

Fig. 9.1. Local muscle forces will displace fracture fragments. In the femur, the pull of iliopsoas will flex the proximal femur around the hip. Distally, gastrocnemius flexes the distal fragment at the knee.

9.1.3 Management

9.1.3.1 Non-operative

Traditionally, femoral fractures in children have been managed non-operatively. Fracture alignment can be maintained by applying traction. In infants up to 2 years of age, gallows traction utilises the patient's own weight. In older children, the Thomas splint is used. Traction is applied via adhesive tapes in smaller children but heavier limbs require skeletal traction. Intra-operative radiographs will be required to confirm that the traction pin has been inserted into the distal metaphysis and has not violated the physis. The time to fracture union will depend on various factors but frequent radiological review is recommended, so that the direction of traction can be altered if the position is deemed unacceptable. Once callus is visible across the fracture line on a radiograph (often within 2–3 weeks), the fracture is unlikely to move without the application of force. At this stage in children aged 5 years or less, traction is often substituted for a hip spica for a further 3–4 weeks until more complete bony union is achieved.

9.1.3.2 Internal Fixation

Older children are more difficult to manage non-operatively. Internal fixation reliably maintains fracture reduction and allows early mobilisation, precluding the necessity for prolonged in-patient treatment. Close evaluation of the fracture will determine the appropriate implant to be utilised. Comminuted fractures lack both axial and rotational stability. By comparison, in the reduced position, a transverse fracture will display axial stability but may remain rotationally unstable.

The most mechanically stable implant is a locked, reamed intra-medullary nail. This is the standard implant utilised in adults. The presence of cross bolts effectively removes any rotational instability. The use of such techniques in children has been controversial, since there have been reports of avascular necrosis (AVN) of the femoral head (Beaty et al. 1994). This has been attributed to damage to the middle circumflex vessels as the nail is introduced into the piriform fossa. The risk of AVN may be reduced with the newer generation of interlocking nails which can be inserted through the tip of the greater trochanter (Gordon et al. 2003). Avascular necrosis will usually present within 1 year of injury and can be detected earlier using MR imaging or bone scintigraphy. The presence of an intra-medullary device does not preclude MR imaging; however, if the nail is made from stainless steel (as are the majority of locked intra-medullary nails), the image may be of poor quality due to magnetic susceptibility artefact.

Damage to the trochanteric apophysis has not been a major issue with such devices since the majority of growth at this site is appositional. Whether such implants are appropriate will depend on careful imaging of the whole femur. If the capital femoral physis is closed, it will be safe to use this implant (Fig. 9.2). The diameter of the femoral canal must be at least 8 mm to allow passage of the nail. Undisplaced fractures elsewhere in the femur can become displaced and should be identified. Of particular importance is the undisplaced femoral neck fracture.

In 1979, a group of French surgeons in Nancy began using elastic intra-medullary nails (ESIN) (Parsch 1997). Over the last 10–15 years, Nancy nails have become the standard form of treatment for fractures of the femoral shaft in children from the age of 6 years until the capital femoral physis has closed (Fig. 9.3). Nancy nails are made from titanium and do not cause as much artefact with MR imaging.

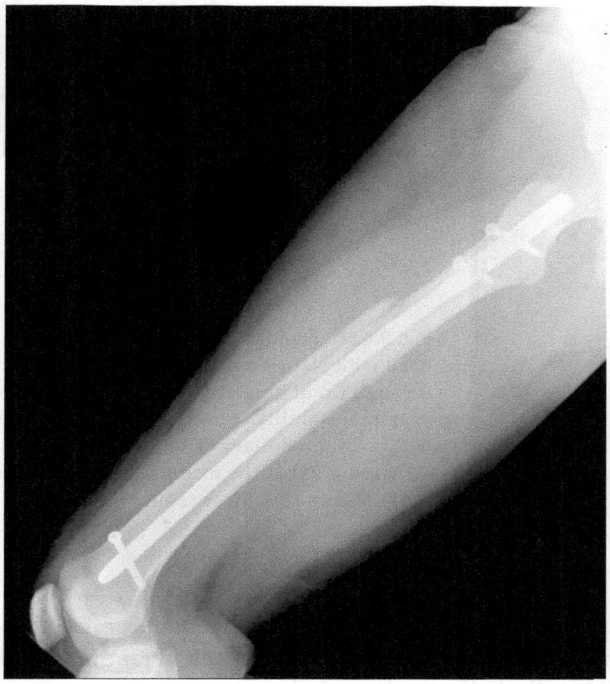
a

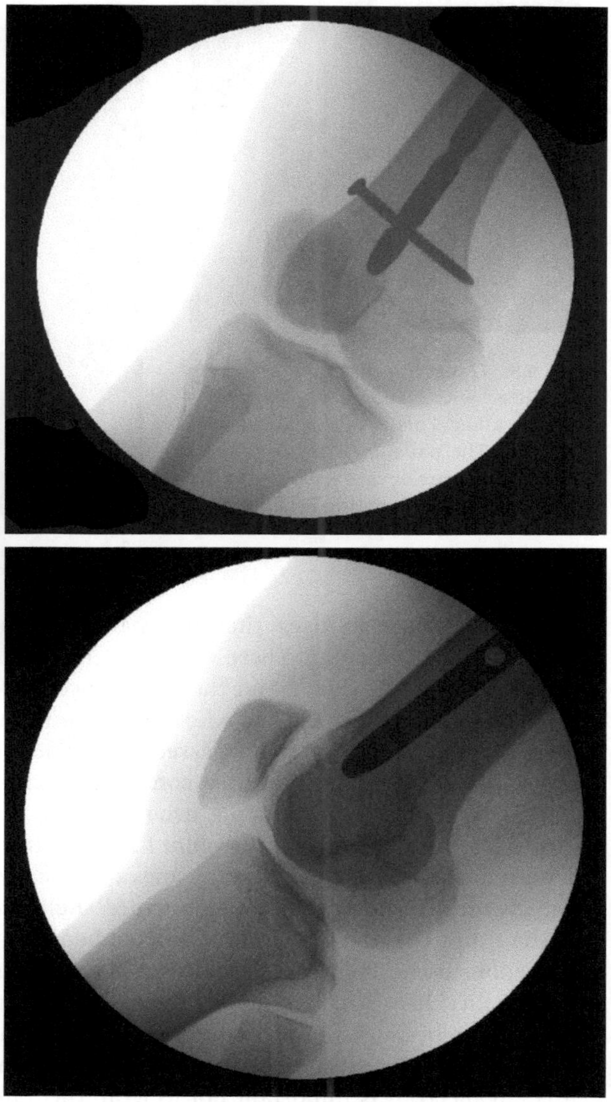
b

c

Fig. 9.2. **a** Femoral shaft fracture with large butterfly fragment. Since the proximal capital physis is closed, a locked intramedullary nail can be inserted. This nail has been introduced via the piriformis fossa. This is a very unstable fracture. **b** Image intensifier view of distal femoral locking bolt. **c** Only an accurate lateral view of the femur confirms that the locking screw has passed through the nail and not in front or behind. The screw obscures the distal hole. The more proximal distal locking hole has not been utilized.

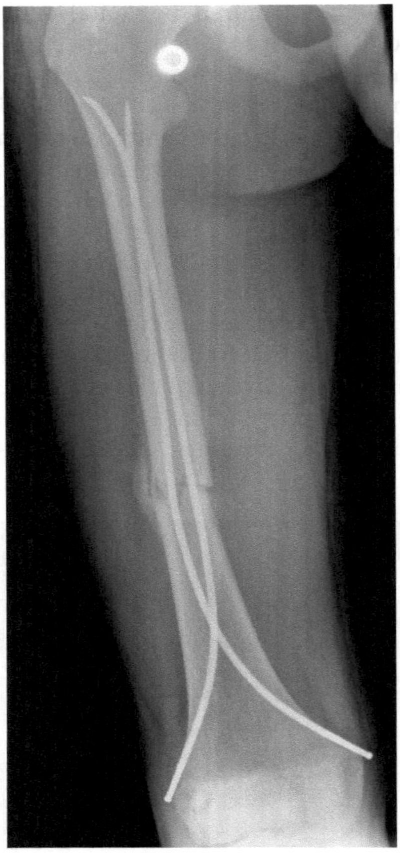

Fig. 9.3. Transverse fracture of femur stabilized with Nancy nails. Note periosteal callus. This is not rigid internal fixation. The nails cross proximal and distal to fracture but are separated at the fracture site giving optimal stability

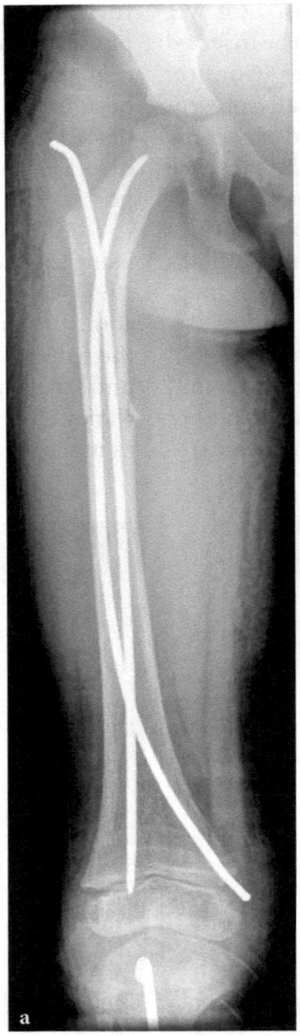

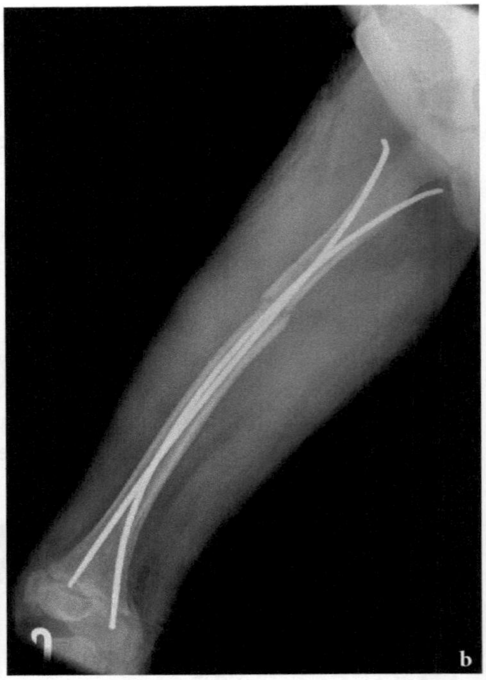

Fig. 9.4a,b. Femoral shaft fracture stabilized with Nancy nails. Lateral nail inserted through tip of greater trochanter to improve proximal stability. **a** both nails appear to be within the medullary canal on AP. **b** lateral view reveals that the medial nail has pierced the cortex in the calcar region

The technique utilises titanium nails ranging from 2–4mm diameter. These are pre-bent into a gentle curve or 'C' shape and then introduced into the femur, usually distally via a hole drilled into the metaphyseal cortex. The rod is passed up the medullary canal under image intensifier control and across the fracture site. By introducing two nails from opposite sides of the femur, three-point fixation can be achieved: at the entry point, at the apex of the curve (which ideally should be at the fracture site), and at the tip of the nail which should be embedded in cancellous bone. This provides rotational and angular stability. It is possible to alter the route that the nail passes because the tip is bent and by rotating the nail, it can be encouraged to change direction as it is advanced. It is important not to wrap the nails around each other since this will compromise 'three-point' fixation and may even result in jamming of the nails halfway through insertion. Such 'corkscrewing' should be identified per-operatively using image intensification. It is important that both nails are of equal diameter (though not necessarily equal length) and that the nails pass up opposite sides of the bone, otherwise unequal bending forces will be generated. Ideally the nails should occupy 80% of the diameter of the medullary canal on the AP radiograph. In transverse and short oblique fracture patterns, there will generally be adequate stability to allow early weight bearing but in long spiral or comminuted fractures, weight bearing should be avoided. The risk of malunion in femoral fractures managed with ESIN increases if there is comminution of more than 25%

of the fracture surface (NARAYANAN et al. 2004). Elastic intra-medullary nails are not designed to provide rigid fixation and small amounts of movement will encourage secondary healing with abundant callus visible on radiographs.

Intra-operative and post-operative imaging of fractures stabilised with intra-medullary devices requires views in at least two planes, not only to visualise the adequacy of the bone alignment but also to check the position of the implants. Elastic intra-medullary nails may appear to be within the bone in one plane but may be seen to lie outside the bone when viewed from a different angle (Fig. 9.4a,b). The nail will have either failed to traverse the fracture site (more common in long spiral fractures) or the sharp tip of the nail will have penetrated the cortex. This is particularly likely around the calcar (femoral neck) and lesser trochanter because the procurvatum of the femur tends to guide the medial nail in a dorsal direction. Imaging of the hip joint is difficult but crucial to avoid this mistake.

If it is felt that a femoral fracture merits internal fixation but the medullary canal is too narrow to accommodate two Nancy nails (generally, 6 mm), plate and screw fixation remains a viable alternative.

9.1.4 Malalignment

Whether the position of a fracture is acceptable or not will depend not only on the magnitude of deformity, but also the plane in which it lies and the age of the child. Malunion of the femur is less noticeable than similar degrees of deformity in the tibia because the femur has a larger muscle bulk surrounding it.

Angulation in the same plane as adjacent joints will be compensated for by altering the range of movement of the joint. Anterior and posterior bowing of the femur is better tolerated than varus or valgus malunion. The amount of angulation deemed acceptable varies in the literature. Most authors would suggest that in the sagittal plane, 20° will remodel in children less than 10 years of age (up to 30° if <2 years), but only 15° in older children (GASCO and DE PABLOS 1997) (Fig. 9.5a,b). In the coronal plane (varus/valgus), these values should be reduced by 5°. Remodelling may continue for up to 5 years but the majority will have occurred in the first 12 months. When assessing malalignment, long limb radiographs are extremely useful for deformity in the coronal plane. A straight line drawn from the centre of the femo-

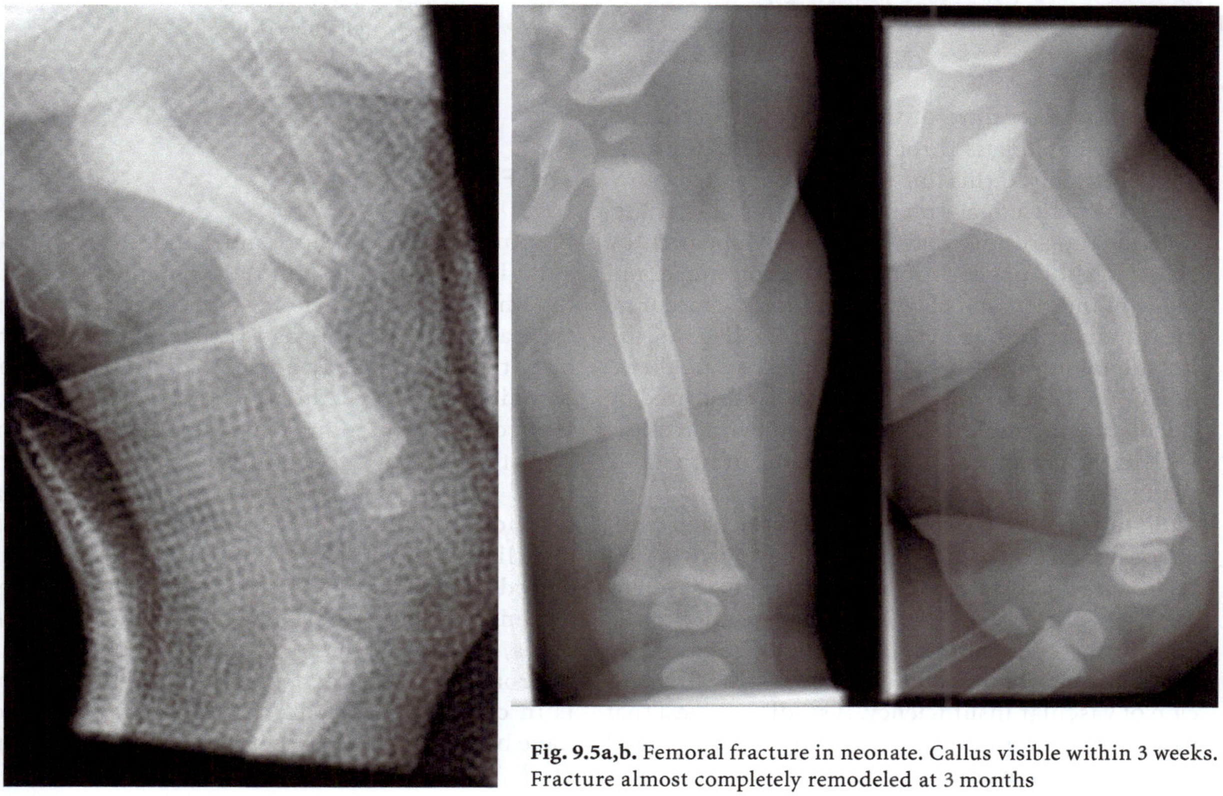

a b

Fig. 9.5a,b. Femoral fracture in neonate. Callus visible within 3 weeks. Fracture almost completely remodeled at 3 months

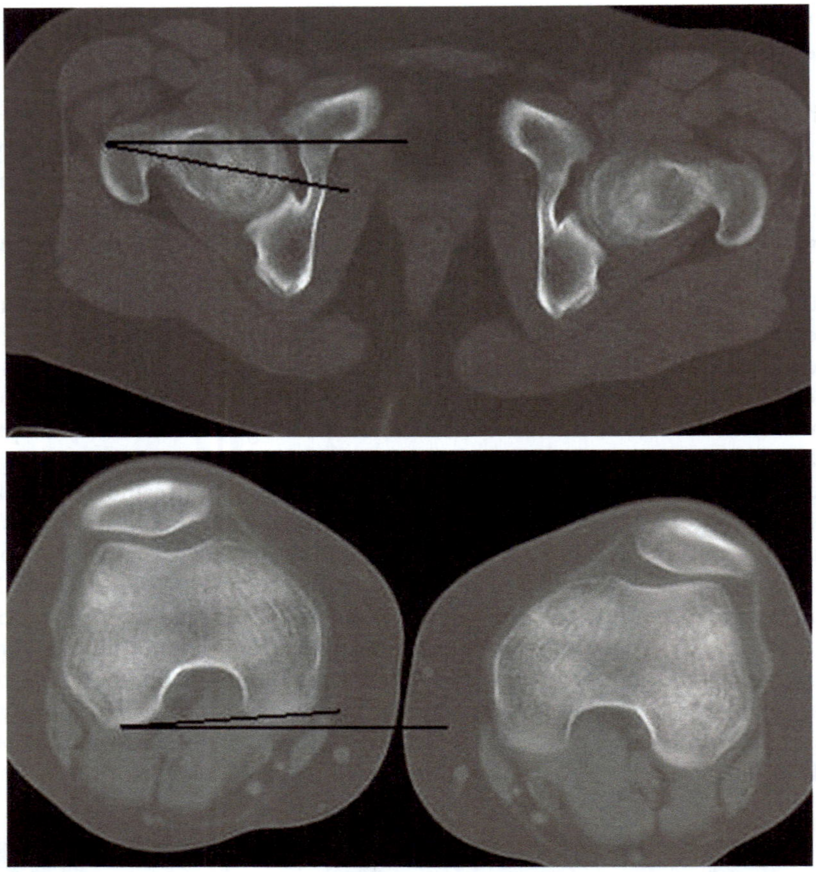

Fig. 9.6a,b. Femoral anteversion: CT measurement. Axial image at the level of the femoral necks: A line is drawn through the femoral neck and also along the horizontal plane. An angle ('femoral neck') is formed by the intersection of these two lines. Axial image of the distal femur: a line is drawn along the posterior femoral condyles and also along the same horizontal plane as used for the femoral neck. A second angle ('knee') is formed by these two lines. If the knee is externally rotated, the 'knee angle' is subtracted from the 'femoral neck angle' to obtain an angle of anteversion. If the knee is internally rotated, the 'knee' and 'femoral neck' angles are added together to obtain an angle of anteversion

ral head to the centre of the ankle joint (mechanical axis) should pass through the centre of the knee joint. Certainly, if this line passes outside the central third, the patient may run into problems in later life. Rotational deformity may be clinically apparent by observing the patient's foot progression angle and range of internal and external rotation. An accurate measurement can be obtained with CT (Fig. 9.6a,b). Rotational malalignment will manifest as an alteration of the femoral anteversion. This is measured by calculating the angle between a line drawn across the back of the femoral condyles and a line drawn along the axis of the femoral neck.

Significant blood loss may be associated with femoral fractures, but direct vascular injury is rare (1%) except in distal third fractures. Here, the femoral artery is at risk as it is in close proximity to the bone as it passes through the adductor canal. Arteriography may be valuable if there is a clinical suspicion of vascular insufficiency. If studies suggest that vascular repair is indicated, this should be preceded by skeletal stabilisation.

9.2 The Floating Knee

Fractures of both the femur and the tibia results in an unstable middle segment, the 'floating knee'. These injuries are fortunately rare and typically result from road traffic accidents. One or both fractures may be open and there is often associated head or thoracic trauma. Healing is slow due to the significant soft tissue trauma and it is difficult to maintain alignment of the limb. In view of this, it is recommended that at least one of the fractures should be surgically stabilised. The advent of ESIN which can be inserted with minimal soft tissue trauma has seen a trend towards internal fixation of both fractures, providing the local anatomy allows. This approach is precluded if one or other fracture is in close proximity to the joint. The fractures have been classified by Letts and Vincent (Letts et al. 1986).

9.3 Tibia

Half of tibial fractures occur in the distal third. The middle third is the next most frequent location and the proximal third only accounts for 10%–15% of injuries (Shannak 1988).

9.3.1 Stress Fractures

Stress fractures occur when normal bone is subjected to excessive forces. In children, the tibia is the most frequently affected bone followed by the fibula. The fracture is generally located in the proximal third of the tibia in children between 10 and 15 years and the distal third of the fibula in the 2- to 8-year age range (Devas 1963). It may be difficult to identify stress fractures on plain radiographs, although subtle signs such as endosteal cortical thickening and subperiosteal new bone may be visible after about a week. MR imaging and bone scintigraphy are much more sensitive in the detection of stress fractures (Fig. 9.7).

Bone scintigraphy will show an area of increased uptake around the postero-medial aspect of the tibia within a few days of the onset of symptoms. Whilst being sensitive, it will not rule out other differential diagnoses including infection and bone tumour and involves a relatively high radiation dose.

MR imaging is more specific and should be capable of ruling out infection. Low signal intra-medullary bands continuous with the cortex are characteristic (Tyrell and Davies 1994). There will be associated extensive marrow oedema and periosteal thickening. If there is extensive marrow oedema and soft tissue changes then a tumour should be suspect and close follow-up and possible biopsy are indicated.

9.3.2 Proximal Metaphyseal Fractures

Minimally displaced fractures of the proximal tibial metaphysis without concomitant fibular injury would appear to be relatively benign at first inspection. However, the development of genu valgum after 1 or 2 years is well reported even in fractures that have healed in an anatomical position. One theory is that the trauma produces hyperaemia around the medial side of the proximal tibial physis, resulting in asymmetrical overgrowth (Jordan et al. 1987). Alternatively, the fracture may disrupt the attachment of the Pes Anserinus over the medial side of the tibia. This may act as a 'check rein' in the same way as the fibular collateral ligament on the lateral aspect of the knee. Its release may allow overgrowth and thus the development of genu valgum. If radiographs show opening of the medial side of the fracture, this may imply that the Pes Anserinus may be trapped in the fracture. This would be further supported if the gap does not close on stressing the fracture under image intensifier control. Surgical exploration of the fracture would then be indicated. The genu valgum tends to increase over a period of approximately 18 months and then slowly resolves in most instances. Hemi epiphysiodesis or osteotomy may be considered in adolescence if the deformity has not corrected.

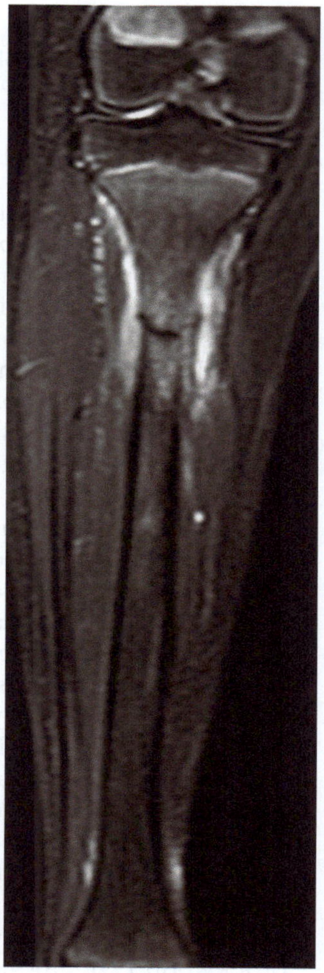

Fig. 9.7. Stress fracture of proximal tibia. With MR imaging, a coronal STIR sequence demonstrates a demarcated fracture line with bone and soft tissue oedema

9.3.3 Toddlers' Fracture

Spiral tibial fractures are common in children less than 3 years of age. The fracture can occur at any level of the tibial shaft, although it is most commonly in the distal third. The diagnosis may be difficult if the fracture is undisplaced and the child presents with a limp and no obvious history of trauma. Initial radiographs are often normal as the fracture line is very faint and there is no periosteal new bone formation. In most cases with an appropriate clinical history, no further investigations are needed and symptoms will usually resolve within days.

If required, follow-up radiographs after 1–2 weeks will show a more obvious fracture line and periosteal new bone. As for stress fractures, both bone scintigraphy and MR imaging are more sensitive investigations.

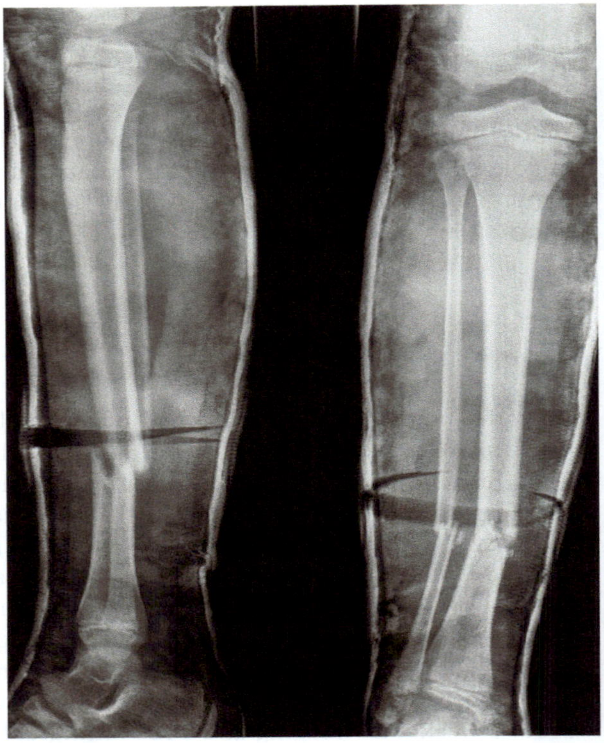

Fig. 9.8. Diaphyseal fracture of tibia and fibula. Despite wedging of the plaster cast, there is valgus alignment

9.3.4 Fractures of the Tibial Shaft

The tibia and fibula are surrounded by four muscular compartments. Anterolaterally, the ankle and foot dorsiflexors (tibialis anterior, extensor hallucis longus, extensor digitorum, peroneus tertius) are located. The lateral compartment contains the peronei. Posteriorly, there are two compartments. The deep compartment contains tibialis posterior, flexor hallucis longus and flexor digitorum whilst the superficial compartment encloses soleus and gastrocnemius. These fascial compartments are relatively unyielding and fractures of the lower leg are more prone to develop compartment syndrome than other long bones.

The arrangement of the muscular compartments is such that the anteromedial face of the tibia is subcutaneous and therefore also more likely to sustain open or compound fractures than other long bones. Because the major muscle bulk in the lower leg is lateral and posterior to the skeletal structures, there is also a tendency for diaphyseal midshaft fractures of both bones to develop valgus angulation (Fig. 9.8).

When the tibial fracture is an isolated injury, it will tend to drift into varus due to the pull of the long flexors attempting to shorten the fractured bone in the presence of an intact fibula (Fig. 9.9).

Approximately 70% of tibial fractures are isolated whilst in the remainder, the fibula is also fractured (Rockwood 1991; Shannak 1988). The tibia shows

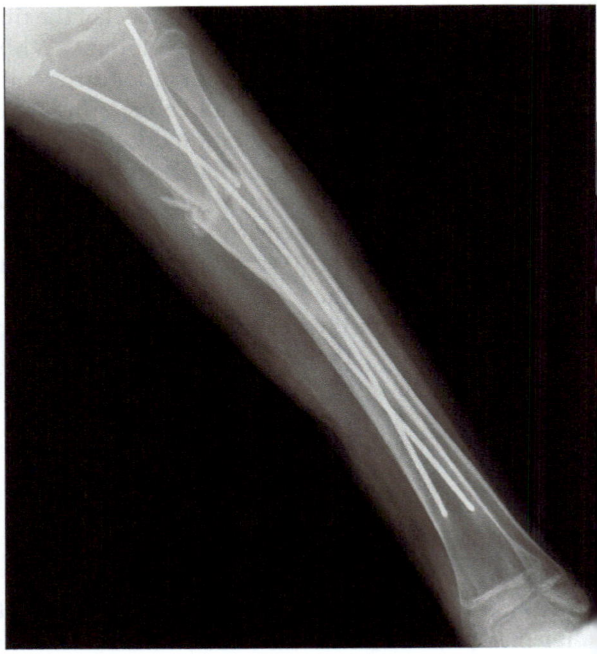

Fig. 9.9. Segmental fracture of tibia with intact fibula. Tibia remains in varus despite internal fixation. ESIN may not provide sufficient axial stability in unstable comminuted or segmental injuries

reduced tendency to remodel when compared with other long bones, particularly fractures with valgus or posterior malunion. As with the femur, there is a tendency for overgrowth following injury, although more than 5 mm is unusual.

Isolated fibula fractures are rare in children and usually result from direct blows. In adolescents however, one must be careful not to miss the 'Maisoneuve' fracture. This is a primary ankle injury where the tibio-fibular diastasis has been torn and the injury propagated proximally to exit often in the upper or middle third of the fibula. Radiographs of the ankle will demonstrate talar shift or fracture of the medial maleollus. Imaging of the entire fibula is required to identify the associated proximal fracture.

9.3.4.1 Management

The majority of tibial fractures can be managed by closed means using immobilisation in a plaster cast. One of the guiding principles of this form of treatment is that to adequately stabilise the fracture, both the joint above and the joint below should be included within the cast. Only by doing this can rotational control be obtained. In the case of femoral fractures, the hip can only be immobilised with the use of a hip spica cast which is cumbersome and poorly tolerated by older children. The tibia can be controlled much more easily using a long leg cast which extends from the toes to the thigh. By including the knee in a position of 30°–40° of flexion, this effectively controls rotation.

Malrotation of the tibia leads to an unequal foot progression angle which is cosmetically often unacceptable. Whilst malrotation of the femur can be accommodated by the hip which is a 'ball and socket' joint, this is not feasible in the knee which is a 'hinge' joint. In addition, external rotation in particular has functional implications because in this position, there is excessive pressure on the medial side of the foot, leading to pes planus (flat foot) and also the development of anterior knee pain.

9.3.5 Congenital Pseudarthrosis

Congenital pseudarthrosis of the tibia is a rare condition occurring in one in 190,000 live births (Hefti et al. 2000). A total of 50% of cases occur in association with neurofibromatosis (NF) type I. The condition however only affects 5% of patients with NF. The cause is unknown but the bone is dysplastic and there is a failure of new bone formation with segmental weakening. This results clinically in anterolateral bowing of the bone and eventually fracture (Fig. 9.10). The fracture fills with hamartomatous tissue and fails to heal, leading to pseudarthrosis. The lesion occurs most commonly in the distal third of the tibia and fibula, followed by the middle third and very rarely (<5%) the proximal third. Theoretically, the condition is not congenital. The fracture is not present at birth but usually occurs during the first decade. Crawford has classified the condition into four types, with the higher grades having the worst prognosis.

- Type I: Anterolateral bow with dense medullary canal.
- Type II: Anterolateral bow with increased medullary canal and tabulation defect (sclerotic)
- Type III: Anterolateral bow with cystic lesion (pre-fracture)
- Type IV: Anterolateral bow with fracture, cysts or frank pseudarthrosis (dysplastic)

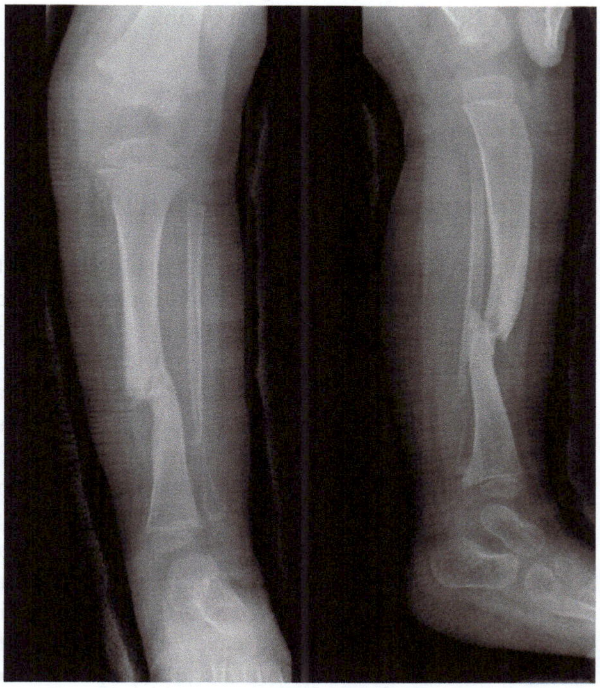

Fig. 9.10. Congenital pseudarthrosis of the tibia. The leg has developed an anterolateral bow and the dysplastic segment has fractured. There is a similar lesion in the fibula

Various methods of treatment have been advocated including bone grafting, intra-medullary rodding and free vascularised fibular grafting. The highest rates of union (75%) have been obtained with lesion excision and bone transport using circular frames (Grill et al. 2000). These techniques were introduced in Russia by Ilizarov (Ilizarov and Deviatov 1969). The bone is transfixed by wires under tension (90–130 kg) which are fixed to circular metal rings. The rings are connected to each other by threaded rods. By stacking several rings and increasing the number of wires, the construct can be made very stable. The technique is highly versatile. It was originally introduced to treat severe open fractures because it required minimal disruption of the tissues. Healing of fractures could be accelerated because the fracture could be gradually compressed by twisting the threaded rods between the rings. However, it was also noted that by slowly distracting the fracture (1 mm per day), new bone could be seen to fill the gap. This means that limbs can be lengthened and also allows excision of diseased segments of bone (pseudarthrosis, infection, tumour) which can then be replaced by bone transport. Regular radiological review is mandatory. If the quality of the new bone (regenerate) is poor, the rate of distraction should be slowed. However, if distracted too slowly, the regenerate may consolidate, making further distraction impossible.

9.4 Radius and Ulna

The elbow and wrist differ from most other joints in that certain movements (pronation/supination) are inextricably linked. This is accomplished by the mobile radius rotating around the static ulna. Proximally, the radial head articulates with the radial notch on the lateral aspect of the coronoid process of the ulna. Distally, the ulnar notch of the radius rotates around the head of the ulna. In addition, the shafts of the bones are linked by the interosseous membrane. Damage to any of these structures may restrict pronation or supination. In adults, angulation or malrotation of more than 10° can result in restricted rotation of the forearm. For this reason, adult fractures are usually managed by open reduction and internal fixation. In children, the potential for remodelling is good around the wrist and more deformity can be accepted.

9.4.1 Mechanism of Injury

The most frequent mechanism of forearm fracture is a fall on the outstretched hand. In this position, the arm is usually pronated and when the arm fractures, the distal segment is usually driven into supination. The posture of the proximal fragment depends on the level of the fracture. Injuries above the insertion of pronator teres invariably lead to supination of the proximal fragments because of the unapposed pull of supinator and biceps. In order to avoid rotational malunion, it is important that casts are applied correctly. It is not possible to alter the alignment of the proximal fragment by closed means but if its position can be ascertained, the distal fragment can then be brought into alignment with it. Distal injuries may require pronation whilst supination is the rule for proximal fractures. This can be assessed more accurately with plain radiographs (Fig. 9.11).

There are three points to consider:

1. In the supinated position, on an AP radiograph, the bicipital tuberosity should be visible in profile

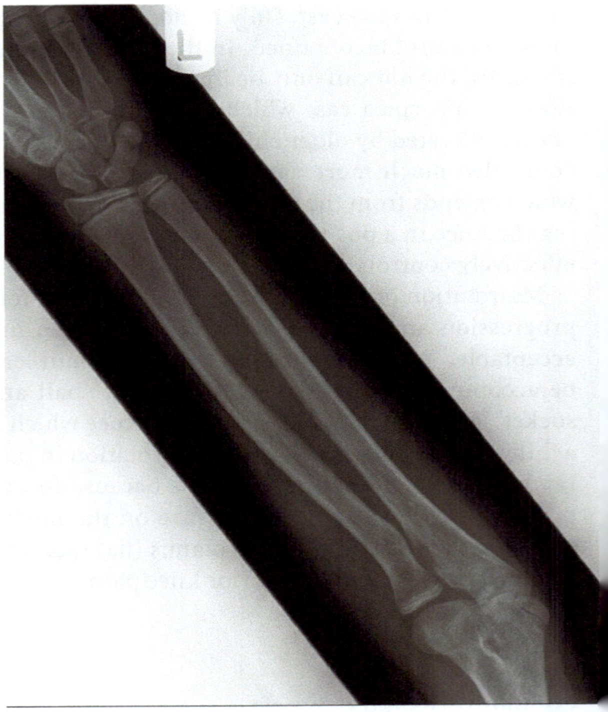

Fig. 9.11. Anteroposterior radiograph of forearm. In the supinated position, the bicipital tuberosity of the radius points towards the ulna. The convexity of the bowed radius points away from the ulna

on the medial surface of the radius. By contrast in the pronated position, the profile of the bicipital tuberosity should be on the lateral aspect (Evans 1951).
2. The radius naturally has a convex lateral bow and if this is lost, malrotation/angulation is implied.
3. In cross-section, the radius is not circular. The diameter is greater in the coronal plane than in the sagittal. As a result, if there is rotational malalignment, the diameter of the fragments immediately proximal and distal to the fracture will not be equal.

Inclusion of the wrist and elbow in radiographs of forearm fractures is mandatory to exclude associated injuries to these joints (see Monteggia/Galeazzi). One pitfall in interpreting forearm radiographs is to misdiagnose the nutrient artery as an undisplaced fracture. This vessel may be visualised on the AP radiograph at the junction of the proximal and middle third of the radius. It has a distal entrance point and runs obliquely in a proximal direction.

9.4.2 Management

Midshaft forearm fractures can only be controlled by closed means if the cast extends above the elbow. By doing this and flexing the elbow, pronation and supination are prevented. However, there may be a tendency for proximal ulnar fractures to sag in such casts, particularly if the arm is chubby or short as in young children. Such malunions may be cosmetically unacceptable.

Swelling following midshaft fractures is generally modest and compartment syndrome rare in children. To avoid displacement within the cast, it must be applied with minimal padding and must be well moulded. The cast index can be determined on radiographs. This is the ratio of the inside diameter of the plaster in the lateral view to the diameter on the AP view. A cast index of >0.8 is associated with a higher risk of losing position within the cast (Chess et al. 1994).

Midshaft diaphyseal fractures of the forearm unite more slowly than diaphyseal injuries. Nevertheless, most fractures will be solid by 6 weeks. Whilst the presence of periosteal callus around metaphyseal fractures usually indicates that the bone will be stable, this is not the case with midshaft injuries. Here, the bones may still move within the cast for 3 or 4 weeks. Weekly or fortnightly radiological evaluation is recommended until this point, since if an unacceptable position is developing, remanipulation will still be feasible.

In adults, isolated single bone forearm fractures are well reported. The 'Nightstick' fracture of the ulna results from a sharp blow, usually with a blunt instrument. Such direct injuries are rare in children where the mechanism of injury is usually a bending or torsional force. Such forces may result in single bone fractures, both bone fractures or plastic deformation. Adult fractures are invariably complete and plastic deformation exceedingly rare. Differentiating complete from greenstick fractures is very important for the orthopaedic surgeon who may be contemplating surgical fixation of the fracture. The closed passage of an intra-medullary implant requires partial reduction of the fracture. With care, this should be possible if there is an intact periosteal hinge. In the case of a completly displaced fracture of the radius, closed reduction to allow passage of the implant is often impossible. In such instances, open reduction of the fracture is invariably required.

9.4.2.1 Internal Fixation

Although the majority of forearm fractures can be managed by closed means, internal fixation has become increasingly popular over recent years. Relative indications are open fractures, fractures requiring vascular repair (rare), multiple injuries. One might also consider internal fixation for older children where limited angulation is acceptable. Open reduction of the ulna is easy because of its subcutaneous position but the approach to the diaphysis of the radius is more hazardous. Insertion of elastic intra-medullary nails (ESIN) is attractive, although complete fractures of the radius usually have to be opened at the fracture site to allow the fracture to be reduced so that the nails can be passed from one fragment to the next. The radial nail is inserted under image intensifier control. The entry point is distal in the metaphysis, close to, but not violating, the physis. The ulnar wire is passed in the opposite direction, the entry point being on the radial aspect of the bone just distal to the ulnar apophysis. The nails should be prebent into a gentle curve and inserted with the convexity of the curve of each wire facing away from its partner (Fig. 8.12). By doing this, the tension in the interosseous membrane is maintained. Other causes for poor results include selection of the wrong sized wires (Fig. 9.12). Of paramount importance is selecting the same diameter wire for each bone. The ideal width is a wire which occupies 60% of the medullary canal of the bone (SLONGO 2005). Careful inspection of radiographs should also confirm that the nails are passed as far as possible across the fracture site but not across the physis at the opposite end of the bone.

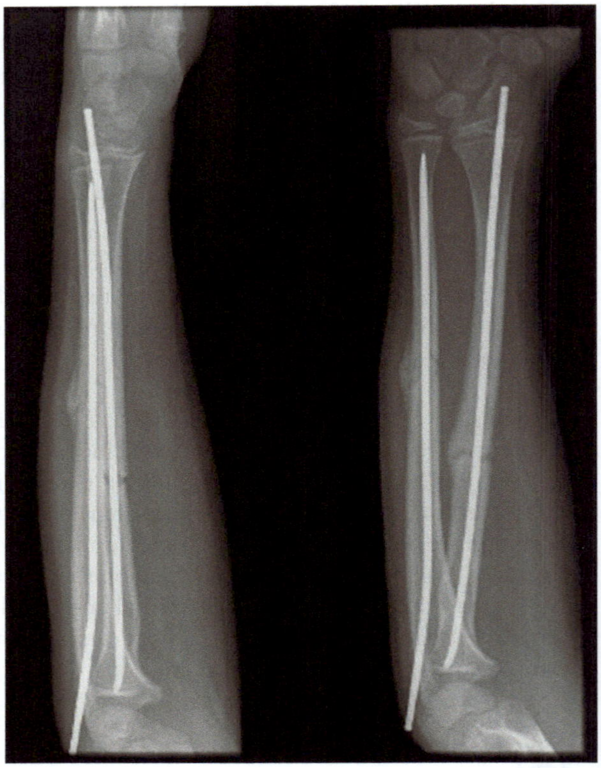

Fig. 9.12. ESIN fixation of both bone forearm fractures. Nails are of optimum diameter but the radial nail is too long. The tip of the nail abuts the physis and whilst the proximal end has avoided the growth plate, it will limit dorsiflexion of the wrist. These nails should be removed early once the fracture is solid

9.4.3 Malunion

Midshaft forearm fractures have less remodelling potential, particularly in children more than 10 years of age. However, the functional consequences of malunion are not entirely clear. Generally, up to 20° can be accepted in young children but no more than 15° in teenagers (ZIONTS et al. 2005). In the radius, the further the fracture is from the distal physis, the less the remodelling potential and the worse the functional result. When the apex of angulation of a fracture of either the ulna or radius is towards the interosseous membrane, this will tend to limit supination. Anterior angulation of the radius can lead to a bony block limiting pronation (DARUWALLA 1979). Once the arm has been mobilised out of cast, it is possible to assess the range of movement. If the rotation is less than 50% of the normal range (180 degrees), it can be anticipated that the eventual result will not be satisfactory and this may be an indication for osteotomy (RANG 1983). This decision may be aided by preliminary arthrogram. This may confirm that rotation is limited and that further attempted rotation leads to subluxation of the joint. In this situation, remodelling is unlikely (Fig. 9.13). Not infrequently, intervention is on the basis of cosmetic rather than functional grounds.

Bayonet apposition may appear alarming on plain radiographs, but healing is rapid and a good clinical result is the rule. Modest shortening of one or both bones does not seem to cause functional problems.

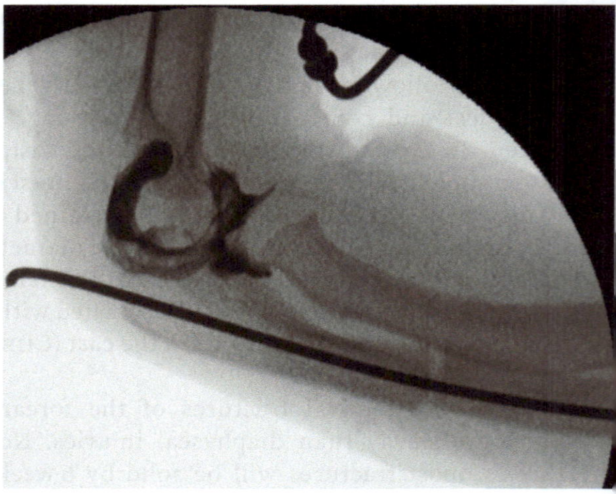

Fig. 9.13. Both the forearm bones are malunited following fracturing in a 3-year-old child initially treated by osteotomy of the ulna. Arthrogram shows that the radial head is still subluxed and radial osteotomy is required

9.4.4 Synostosis

A rare but serious complication of forearm fractures is cross-union (synostosis) of the bones. This occurs more frequently in high energy injuries where both bones are fractured. There is also an increased incidence if open reduction of both bone fractures is attempted through the same incision. The proximal third of the forearm is most commonly affected, followed by the diaphysis and very rarely, the distal metaphyseal region (Vince and Miller 1987). Clinically this will present with restricted pronation/supination and the synostosis should be visible on plain radiographs. Surgical excision has an unpredictable outcome but if it is considered, computerised tomography will help in accurately defining the anatomy of the cross-union. Delaying excision until the formation of callus has ceased may reduce the risk of recurrence.

9.5 Humeral Fractures

The radiological interpretation of humeral shaft fractures is usually uncomplicated in comparison to shoulder and elbow injuries. Fractures of the humeral shaft only account for approximately 25% of total injuries to the bone.

Transverse fractures result from direct blows. Twisting injuries produce the more common spiral fracture. In infants, this injury should always rouse suspicion of child abuse. The position of the bony fragments will be determined by the pull of adjacent muscles. For proximal metaphyseal fractures, the rotator cuff abducts the proximal fragment while the distal fragment is adducted by the pectoralis muscle.

9.5.1 Management

The standard treatment for humeral shaft fractures is non-operative. Gravity can be utilised both to splint the fracture and maintain it in a satisfactory position. A heavy hanging cast applied from just below the shoulder to the hand will apply traction to the injured limb. The muscles of the anterior and posterior compartments of the arm will be stretched and this will align and splint the limb (Fig. 9.12).

The radial nerve is closely applied to the humeral shaft in its middle and distal thirds. If, following manipulation of mid to lower third displaced fractures, a radial nerve palsy develops in association with soft tissue interposition on radiographs, surgical exploration should be considered. Entrapment of the radial nerve at this site is well documented (Holstein and Lewis 1963). Surgical stabilisation may be considered for lower third fractures even in the absence of neurological deficit, since these injuries have a tendency to develop varus malalignment (Fig. 9.14). Elastic intra-medullary nails inserted distally through the epicondyles and up the medial and lateral columns provide good stabilisation. Alternatively, rigid internal fixation with plate plus screws may be considered, although this necessitates a much larger exposure with risk of damage to soft tissues.

9.5.2 Malunion

Malunion of humeral fractures has greater significance the further the fracture is from the shoulder.

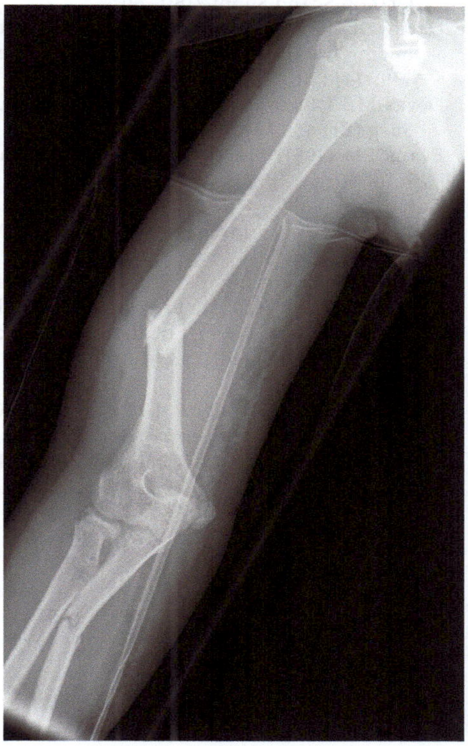

Fig. 9.14. Fractures at the junction of the mid and distal third of the humerus can unite in a varus position which is not cosmetically acceptable. The radial nerve is also in close proximity at this level and its function must be carefully assessed in such cases

Approximately 80% of humeral growth occurs at the proximal physis, so remodelling at this end is greater. In addition, the shoulder is a ball and socket joint and has a greater range of movement than any other limb joint. As a result, a malunion of the proximal end of the humerus is easily compensated in a functional sense. Shortening of the upper limb is less noticeable than the leg where it will result in a limp.

Reference

Beaty JH, Austin SM, Warner WC et al. (1994) Interlocking intra-medullary nailing of femoral shaft fractures in adolescents: preliminary results and complications. J Ped Ortho 14:178–183

Chess G, Hyndman JC, Leahey JL et al. (1994) Short arm cast for distal pediatric forearm fractures. J Pediatr Orthop 14:211–213

Crawford AH (1986) Neurofibromatosis in children. Acta Orthop Scand Suppl 218:1–60

Daruwalla JS (1979) A study of radio-ulnar movements following fractures of the forearm in children. Clin Orthop 139:114–120

Devas MB (1963) Stress fractures in children. J Bone Joint Surg (Br) 45:528–541

Evans EM (1951) Fractures of the radius and ulna. J Bone Joint Surg. 33B:548

Gasco J, de Pablos J (1997) Bone remodelling in malunited fractures in children. Is it reliable? J Ped Orthop (B) 6:126–132

Gordon JE, Swenning TA, Burd TA, Szymanski DA, Schoenecker PL (2003) Proximal femoral radiographic changes after lateral transtrochanteric intra-medullary nail placement in children. J Bone Joint Surg (A) 85A:1295–1301

Grill F, Bollini G, Dungl P, Hefti F et al. (2000) Treatment approaches for congenital pseudarthrosis of tibia: results of the EPOS Multicentre Study. J Pediatr Orthop 8(B):75–89

Gross RH, Stranger M (1983) Causative factors responsible for femoral fractures in infants and young children. J Pediatr Orthp 3:341–343

Hefti F, Bollini G, Dungl P, Fixen J et al. (2000) Congenital pseudarthrosis of the tibia: history, etiology, classification, and epidemiologic data. J Pediatr Orthop 8(B):11–15

Holstein A, Lewis GB (1963) Fractures of the humerus with radial nerve palsy. J Bone Joint Surg (A) 45(A):1382

Ilizarov GA,Deviatov M (1969) Operative elongation of the leg with simultaneous correction of the deformities. Ortop Travmatol Protez 30:32–37

Jordan SE, Alonso JE, Cook FF (1987) The etiology of valgus angulation after metaphyseal fractures of the tibia in children. J Pediatr Orthop 7:450

Letts M, Vincent N, Gaouw G (1986) The 'floating knee' in children. J. Bone Joint Surg 68(B):442

Morris SM, Cassidy N, Stephens M et al. (2002) Birth-associated femoral fractures: incidence and outcome. J Ped Orthop 22:27–30

Narayanan UG, Hyman JE, Wainwright AM, Rang M, Alman BA (2004) Complications of elastic stable intramedullary nail fixation of pediatric femoral fractures, and how to avoid them. J Ped Ortho 24:363–369

Parsch KD (1997) Modern trends in internal fixation of femoral shaft fractures in children. A critical review. J Ped Orthop (B) 6:117–125

Rang M (1983) Children's fractures. J.B. Lippincott Company, Philadelphia

Shannack AO (1988) Tibial fractures in children: follow up study. J Pediatr Orthop 8:306–310

Shapiro F (1981) Fractures of the femoral shaft in children. Acta Orthop Scand 52:649–655

Slongo TF (2005) Complications and failures of the ESIN technique. Injury 36:S-A78–S-A85

Tyrell PNM, Davies AM (1994) Magnetic resonance imaging appearances of fatigue fractures of the long bones of the lower limb. Br J Radiol 67:332–338

Vince KG, Miller JE (1987) Cross-union complicating fracture of the forearm. J Bone Joint Surg 69(A):654–660

Wallace ME, Hoffman EB (1992) Remodelling of angular deformity after femoral shaft fractures in children. J Bone Joint Surg (Br) 74-B:765–769

Zionts LE, Zalavras CG, Gerhardt MB (2005) Closed treatment of displaced diaphyseal both – bone forearm fractures in older children and adolescents. J Pediatr Orthop 25:507–512

Growth Plate (Physeal) Injuries

10

Katharine Foster

CONTENTS

10.1 Development

The paediatric skeleton is very different in composition to that of an adult. The bones are more elastic and there is the presence an unfused physeal growth plate (the physis) meaning that the paediatric skeleton will respond differently to trauma. This chapter will review the injuries that occur around the physis or growth plate and their potential complications. To understand the role of the growth plate it is important to have an understanding of normal bone growth and maturation.

K. Foster, MD
Consultant Radiologist, Department of Radiology, Birmingham Children's Hospital, Steelhouse Lane, Birmingham, B4 6NH, UK

There are two processes of bone formation. Intramembranous bone formation; the transformation of mesenchymal tissue into bone, and endochondral bone formation; indirect conversion via an intermediate cartilage model. The skull and facial bones develop from intramembranous ossification, the long bones develop by endochondral ossification. The initial sites of bone formation in the long bones (cartilaginous model) are the primary centres of ossification within the diaphysis of the bone. From the centre of the bone, ossification proceeds towards the ends of the bone. Secondary centres of ossification form at the ends of the bone, in the epiphyses. Additional ossification centres may occur within apophysis. An epiphysis is a secondary centre of ossification that adds to longitudinal growth while an apophysis does not result in bone lengthening but rather serves as a point of attachment for a musculotendinous unit. The epiphyses are typically sphere shaped cartilage structures that contain an ossification nucleus, which enlarges with time, and gradually the epiphyseal cartilage is converted to bone. A thin peripheral layer of cartilage persists, which becomes the articular cartilage. Separating the epiphysis from the metaphysis is the growth plate or physis; it is here that longitudinal growth takes place.

The growth plate consists of three main structures. The growth cartilage, the perichondral structures, and the chondro-osseous junction; this includes the zone of provisional calcification: the transitional region between cartilage and newly formed metaphyseal bone. The perichondral region is also called the "groove of Ranvier". It consists of osteoblasts, chondrogenic and fibrous cells, and forms a circumferential depression around the physis. Adjacent to the physis and lower metaphysis is a thin ring of bone: the bony ring of Lacroix. These tissue provide structural support to the growth plate and upper metaphysis.

The growth plate consists of columns of chondrocytes that multiply and become invaded by osteoblasts and vessels from the metaphysis. The growth cartilage has three distinct zones: the reserve, or germinal zone, the hypertrophic zone and a proliferative zone (Fig. 10.1). The reserve zone lies next to the epiphysis and consists mainly of matrix and a poorly organised chondrocytes. The proliferative zone is the area that contributes to increasing bone length. Here the cells are flattened, and organised in columns. These cells divide rapidly and produce matrix which contributes to bone strength. In the hypertrophic zone, adjacent to the metaphysis, cells mature and increase in size by up to ten times. At the zone of provisional calcification, the longitudinal columns of matrix, between the hypertrophic chondrocytes, become progressively mineralised, forming dense but fragile metaphyseal bone. Most epiphyseal fractures occur at this junction.

The growth plate and epiphysis both consist of hyaline cartilage rich in glycosaminoglycans. These are very hydrophilic, and hence the cartilage behaves like a sponge: releasing water when pressure is applied, and reabsorbing the water when pressure is released. Collagen fibres (mainly type II) extend from the epiphysis into the growth plate to provide strength.

With age, the growth plate becomes thinner, and eventually disappears, allowing fusion of the diaphysis and epiphyseal ossification centres. In this way, the composition of bone converts from being complete cartilage prenatally to complete bone in adulthood, apart from the articular surface (Jaramillo and Shapiro 1998a).

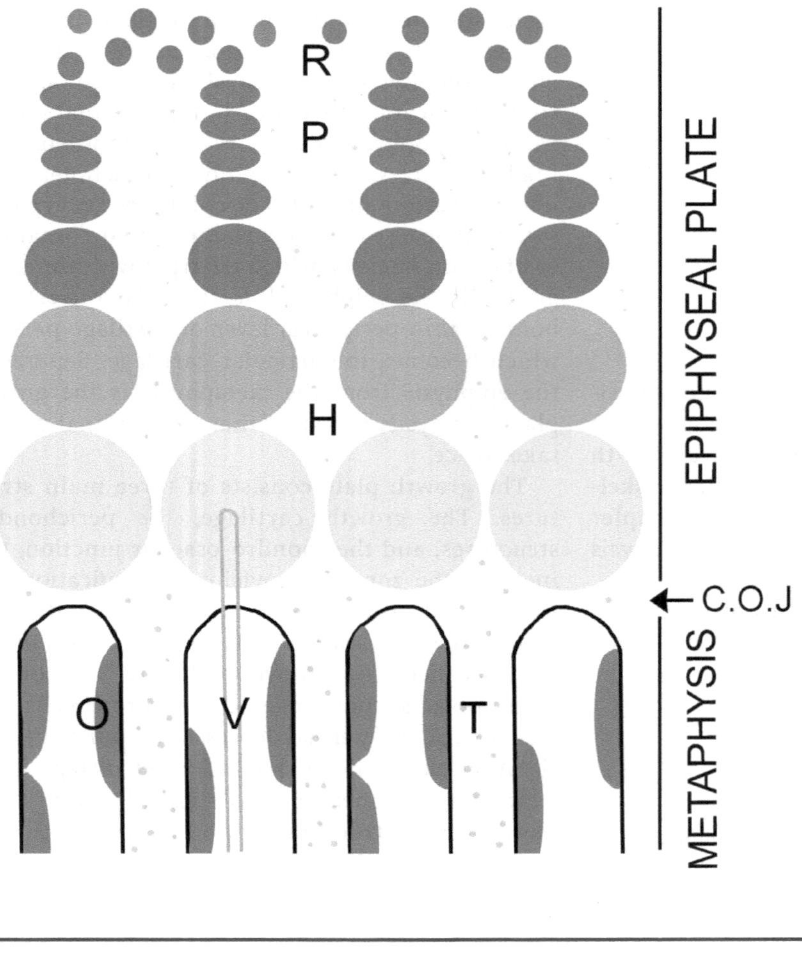

Fig. 10.1. The cellular structure of the growth plate. The physeal plate consists of well layers of chondrocytes arranged in columns in three zones: resting (*R*), proliferating (*P*) and hypertrophied (*H*). The resting zone contains abundant matrix and poorly organized cells. In the proliferative zone, the chondrocytes become flattened, undergo rapid division and synthesize matrix. The hypertrophied chondrocytes eventually become invaded by vessels (*V*) from the metaphysis. The adjacent matrix becomes progressively mineralized. Osteoblasts (*O*) line the trabeculae (*T*) and produce extracellular matrix of bone. The layer between the hypertrophied chondrocytes and the metaphysis, the chondro-osseous junction (*COJ*) where only a few mineralized cartilage spikes provide strength, is the site through which growth plate fractures occur

10.2 Normal Appearances

10.2.1 Radiographs

Cartilage is radiolucent. The diaphyses are visible in the newborn, but the epiphyses only become visible once they have started to ossify. The distal femoral epiphysis is exceptional in that it is usually present at birth. The epiphyses ossify in a predictable pattern. It is important to be aware of the normal sequence (Table 10.1). The growth plate is seen as a radiolucent line between the epiphysis and the metaphysis. As the growth plate fuses, it becomes progressively narrower.

10.2.2 Ultrasound

The articular cartilage appears as a smooth anechoic area. The non-ossified cartilaginous epiphysis is hypoechoic relative to the surrounding muscles and usually contains fine echogenic speckles. The central ossification centre is hyperechoic. The cortex of bone appears as a highly echogenic structure, with distal acoustic shadowing (as nearly all the sound waves are reflected off the bone surface) (Fig. 10.2). Ultrasound can be used to detect epiphyseal separation and displacement but is not routinely used to asses the growth plate.

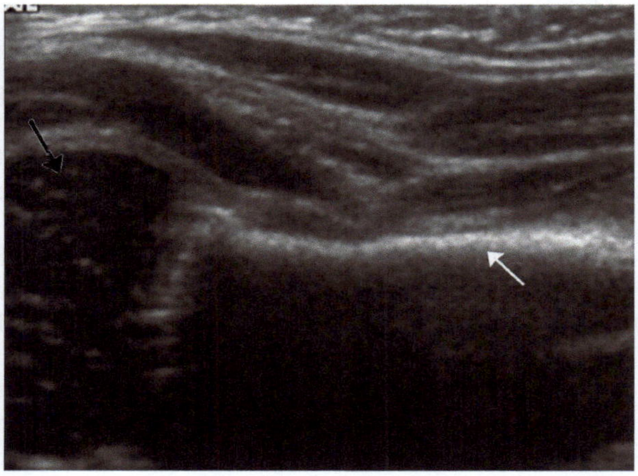

Fig. 10.2. Sagittal ultrasound of the hip of a 2-month-old child. The cortex of the femur is highly echogenic (*white arrow*), and the cartilaginous epiphysis has a speckled appearance (*black arrow*)

Table 10.1. Table of the timing of appearance of ossification centres on plain radiographs (Weir et al. 1998)

Site	Appears	Fused
Femur		
Head	4–6 months	14–18 years
Greater trochanter	2–4 years	14–18 years
Lesser trochanter	10–12 years	14-18 years
Tibia		
Tuberosity	10–12 years	12-14 years
Distal epiphysis	4 months–1 year	15–17 years
Proximal epiphysis	Present at birth	16–18 years
Patella (1–3 centres)	3–5 years	Puberty
Fibula		
Proximal epiphysis	2–4 years	17–19 years
Distal epiphysis	6 months–1 year	15–17 years
Foot		
Calcaneus	Birth	14–16 years
Talus	Birth	
Cuboid	Birth	
Navicular	3 years	
Cuneiform lateral	6 months–1 year	
Cuneiform intermediate	2–3 years	
Cuneiform medial	1–2 years	
Humerus		
Proximal epiphysis	1–6 months	15–20 years
Capitulum	4 months–1 year	13–16 years
Medial epicondyle	3–6 years	13–16 years
Trochlear	10 years	14–16 years
Lateral epicondyle	9–12 years	13–16 years
Radius		
Proximal epiphysis	4–6 years	13–16 years
Distal epiphysis	1 year	16–18 years
Ulna		
Proximal epiphysis	8–10 years	13–15 years
Distal epiphysis	5–7 years	16–18 years
Hand		
Capitate	1–3 months	
Hamate	2–4 months	
Triquetral, lunate	2–4 years	
Scaphoid, trapezium trapezoid	4–6 years	
Pisiform	8–12 years	
Metacarpal: head	1–2 years	14–19 years
Phalanges: base	1–3 years	14–18 years

10.3.3
Normal MR Imaging Appearances

The epiphysis and the physis both consist of hyaline cartilage. While hyaline cartilage is about 70% water, the T1 and T2 relaxation times are shortened as a consequence of the water being bound to large molecules (glycosaminoglycans bound to a core protein). These large molecules are more plentiful in the epiphysis compared to the growth plate, which may explain why the epiphysis is hypointense relative to the physis on T2 weighted images (Jaramillo et al. 1998). Gradient-recalled echo proton density sequences depict cartilage well, with excellent differentiation from bone (but differentiate less well between epiphysis and the growth plate). The differentiation from bone can be maximized by using fat saturation, suppressing signal from the marrow fat in the adjacent bone (Fig. 10.3). Differentiation between the zones of the cartilage can be more clearly seen on gadolinium enhanced sequences. This is because the physis and the articular cartilage enhance more than the epiphyseal cartilage which is relatively hypovascular. The growing cartilage enhances by diffusion from the vascular canals which are largely situated in the germinal layer of the physis. It has been shown that the number of vascular channels, as well as the degree of epiphyseal enhancement decreases with age (Jaramillo et al. 2004).

The physis is smooth and flat at birth, The thickness of the growth plate remains constant, until skeletal maturity. With age it undulates, and physeal closure usually occurs first at the areas of greatest undulation (Fig. 10.4). It is interesting that the position of the physis relative to the bone varies, for example with age the distal fibula epiphysis becomes more distal than the distal tibial epiphysis (Ogden and McCarthy 1983). The provisional zone of calcification, on the metaphyseal side of the growth plate, has a high mineral content resulting in low signal on virtually all sequences. However, it may appear bright on T1 sequences, relative to the haematopoetic bone marrow of newborns due to very active mineralization. MR imaging can be used to assess growth arrest due to bony bridging that may complicate fractures which have damaged the growth plate.

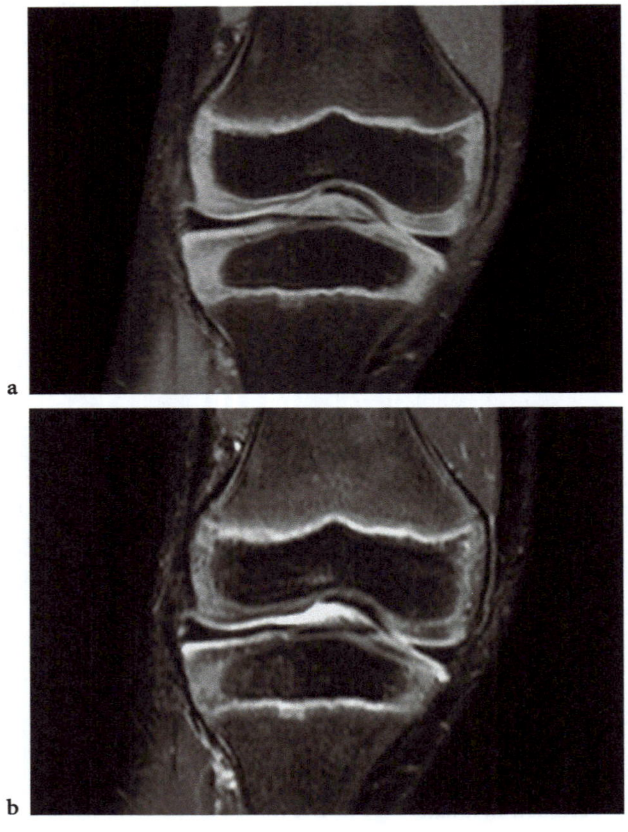

Fig. 10.3. a Coronal fat saturated proton density MR of a the knee of a 6-year-old child. The cartilage is bright compared to the surrounding bone. **b** Coronal fat saturated T2 MR of the same patient. The growth plate cartilage is of higher signal than the articular cartilage surrounding the primary ossification centres

10.4
Physeal Injuries

The transitional zone between the physeal cartilage and bone, "the zone of provisional calcification", is the weakest point in the growing skeleton. Up to 15% of fractures of the tubular bones in children affect the growth plate. The physeal cartilage is weaker than bone, which is in turn weaker than the surrounding ligaments, therefore injuries that may cause ligamentous tear, or dislocation in an adult, are more likely to cause injury to the growth plate in a child (Rogers 1970). The majority of fractures are due to shearing or avulsion. Compressive and "splitting" injuries are less common. In children the periosteum is thicker, but more loosely attached to the underlying bone. It is easily stripped away from the bone in trauma. The periosteum lays down bone and aids with stability during healing.

10.4.1 Classification

The classification system of Salter and Harris which separates fractures into five main types is most widely used (Salter and Harris 1963) (Fig. 10.5). Other fracture types have since been added to the original classification (Ogden 1981; Rang 1983). In a further classification Peterson added additional categories (Peterson et al. 1994) while including type I to IV Salter Harris injuries, type V is deleted and two new types of fractures: metaphyseal fractures with linear injuries that pass into the growth plate, and major trauma that results in destruction of part of the physis.

A useful rule of thumb is that the higher the grades of injuries, the greater likelihood that the growth plate will be damaged, which can result in long term complications. Types I, II and III have a relatively good prognosis, whereas type V has a poorer prognosis due to damage to the growth plate. Complications of growth plate injuries include malunion, premature fusion resulting in growth impairment and avascular necrosis. The latter is most likely in fractures of the femoral and radial neck.

Type I: The fracture is isolated to the growth plate and causes epiphyseal separation, without adjacent bone fracture. The fracture line passes through the hypertrophic layer of the physis. Diagnosis can be difficult, particularly when there is spontaneous reduction of the fracture. This is most commonly seen in the mostly unossified epiphyses of newborns and infants.

Type II: This the most common growth plate fracture. It is usually seen in children between the ages of 10 and 16. As a result of shearing or avulsive force, the fracture splits the growth plate, and then passes into the metaphysis, separating a small fragment of bone. This type of fracture is commonly seen in injuries of the distal radius and phalanges. This type of injury has does not commonly cause long term complications (Fig. 10.6).

Type III: In this injury, the fracture line passes through the epiphysis, and then horizontally across the growth plate. This is most commonly seen in children age 10–15, at the distal tibia. It is less frequently seen at the proximal tibia and distal femur (Fig. 10.7).

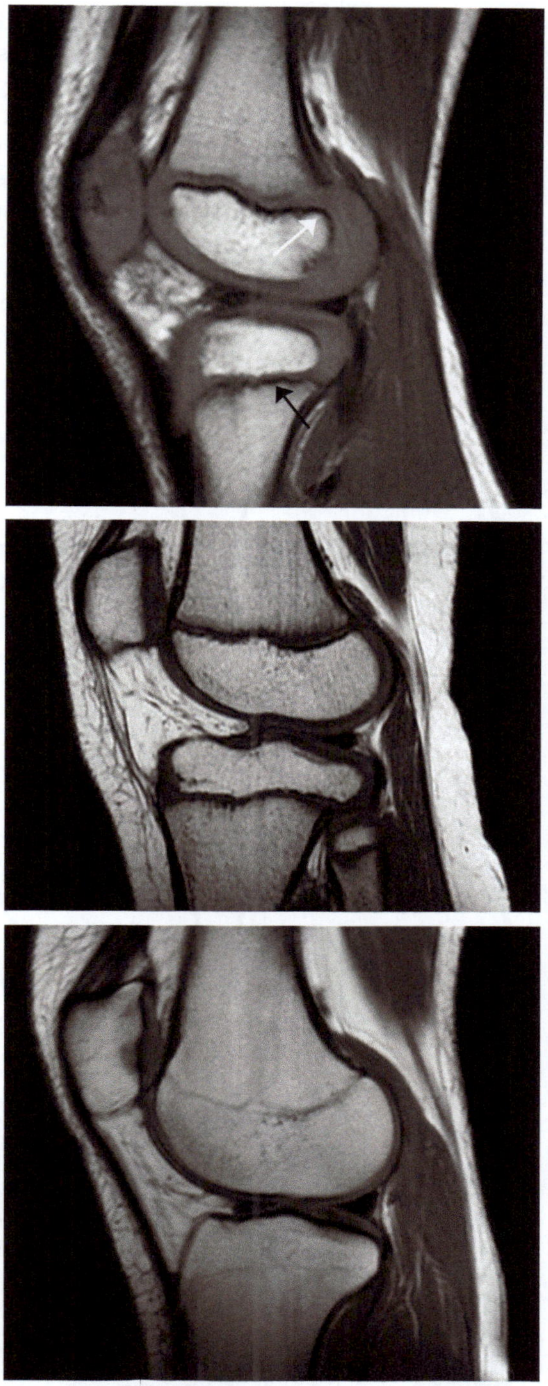

a

b

c

Fig. 10.4. **a** Sagittal T1 MR of the knee in a 6-year-old child. The zone of provisional calcification of the primary ossification centre (*white arrow*) and of the secondary ossification centre (*black arrow*) are clearly seen as linear areas of low signal. **b** Sagittal T1 MR of the knee in an 11-year-old child. **c** Sagittal T1 MR of the knee in a 15-year-old. The growth plates have fused and the primary ossification centres now have only a thin surrounding rim of articular cartilage

Type IV: This is a vertically orientated fracture, involving both the epiphysis and the metaphysis, crossing the growth plate (Fig. 10.8). This is most commonly seen in the distal humerus and tibia. As type III and IV fractures pass across the articular cartilage into the joint space, there is a higher incidence of degenerative joint disease if the fracture is not anatomically reduced.

CT can be useful, particularly for planning treatment of more complex fractures. CT is excellent at depicting bony anatomy. Images can be acquired axially and then reconstructed in any plane required. 3D surface rendering reconstructions can also be very helpful. However, as it uses a high X-ray dose, use should be restricted to more complex cases (Fig. 10.9).

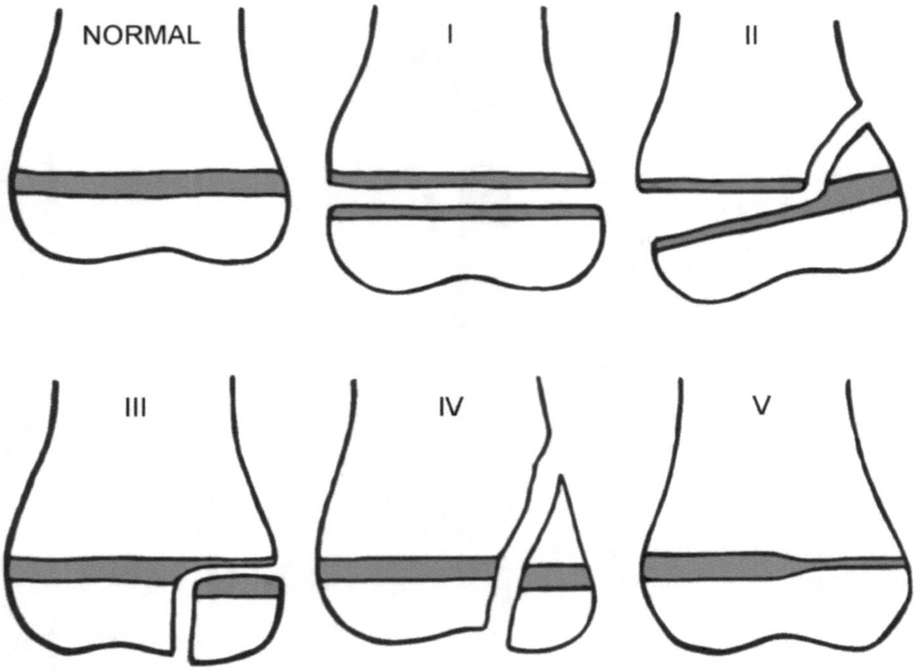

Fig. 10.5. Salter Harris classification of growth plate fractures

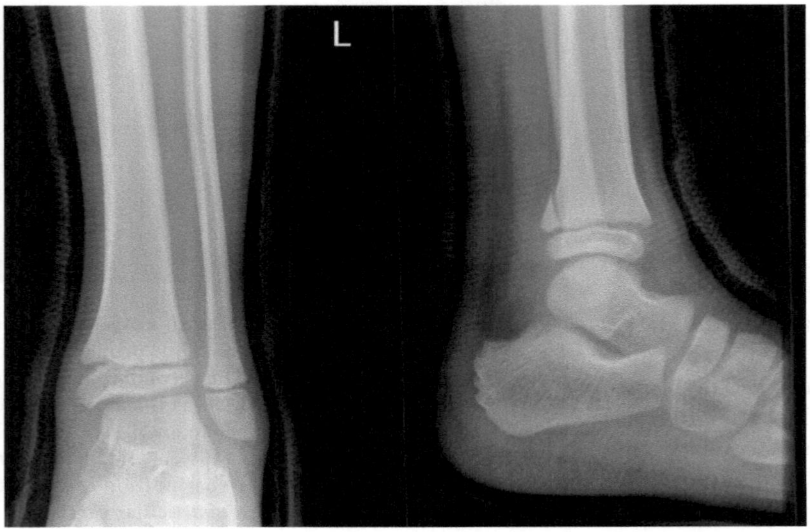

Fig. 10.6. Salter II fracture of the dista tibia

Type V: This is quite a rare fracture, resulting from compressive force, crushing the growth plate. Damage to the growth plate can cause subsequent deformity. The distal femur and tibia are the most commonly involved sites. The diagnosis is often made retrospectively when growth arrest is discovered at a later date.

10.4.2 Avulsion Injuries

Commonly a muscle will insert into an apophysis which in children is the weakest point of the of bone, tendon and muscle junction. Consequently traction on the muscle will result in avulsion of a boney fragment. Avulsion injuries are common sports injuries in children. They are most commonly seen at muscle insertion sites around the pelvis and elbow.

In children repetitive traction forces can result in microtrauma to the apophysis, for example injury to the physis of the internal epicondyle of the elbow. This occurs in gymnasts and in activities with repetitive throwing: giving it the name "little leaguers' elbow".

In adolescents complete avulsion is more likely, which if not treated correctly can result in non-union. Usually radiographs are sufficient to diagnose avulsion injuries provided the avulsed fragment is ossified. MR imaging can be helpful in difficult cases; STIR images are useful to highlight oedema within the avulsed fragment and the adjacent parent bone.

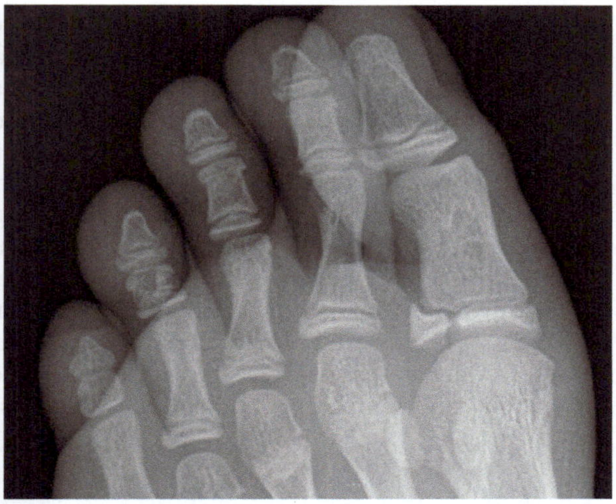

Fig. 10.7. Salter III fracture of the proximal phalanx of the left big toe

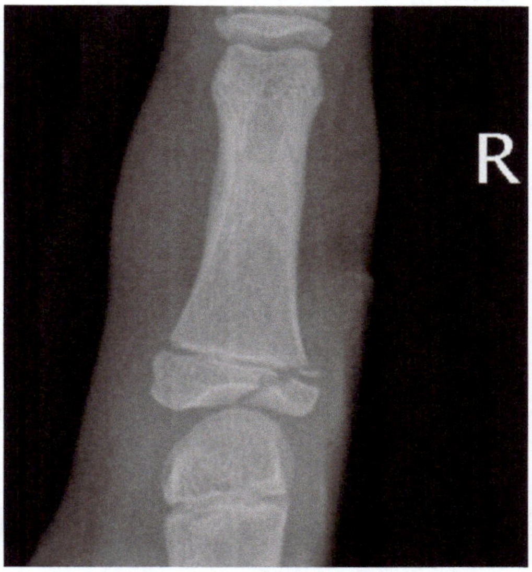

Fig. 10.8. Salter IV fracture through the base of the middle phalanx of the right index finger

a

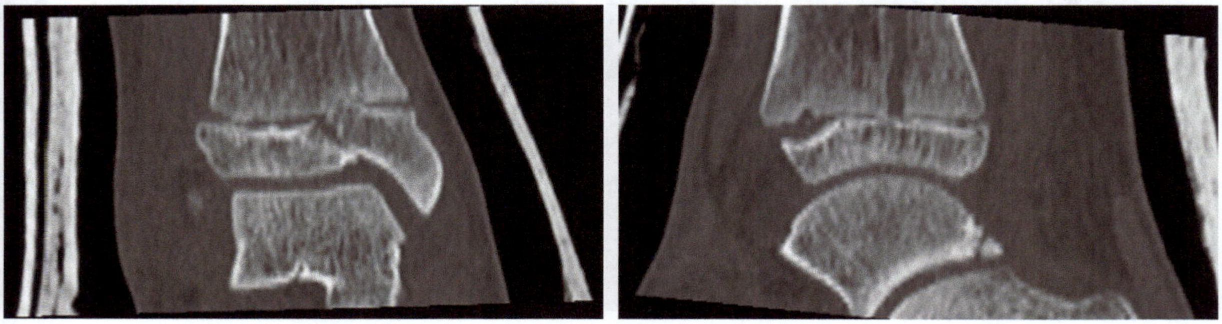

b

Fig. 10.9. a Coronal reconstruction CT image of a Salter IV fracture showing the fracture through the distal epiphysis of the tibia. **b** Sagittal reconstruction CT of the same patient showing the fracture passing though the distal tibial metaphysis

10.4.3 Chronic Growth Plate Injuries

Repeated sports activities may damage the physis. For example preadolescent gymnasts may damage the distal radial physis. Patients with insensitivity to pain, are also at risk of repeated trauma. MR imaging will show focal areas of thickening of the growth plate, bone bridging, physeal widening, intraphyseal clefts and loss of clarity of the zone of provisional calcification. Chronic injury can result in premature closure of the growth plate.

10.4.4 Metaphyseal Fractures

Metaphyseal fractures occur in the plane of the physis and extend into the primary spongiosa of the metaphysis. They typically have the appearance of a "corner fracture" (Caffey 1957) or of a "bucket handle". These appearances are due to the shape of the fracture fragment, which is made up of epiphysis, physis and a thin layer of metaphyseal bone. The peripheral margin of this thin disc of bone is relatively thick and produces the corner and bucket handle appearance, depending on the radiographic projection. An angulated projection results in a curvilinear bone density (bucket handle appearance), whereas if the long axis of the metaphysis is at right angles to the radiographic projection a triangular fragment or corner fracture is seen. These injuries are believed to be the result of twisting, pulling or shearing injuries and have an association with inflicted, non-accidental trauma (Kleinman 1990). If there is no clear history to explain these injuries, it is important that the imaging findings in such cases are fully discussed with the referring clinicians (Fig. 10.10).

10.5 Complications of Fractures

10.5.1 Growth Arrest

Damage to the growth plate after a fracture can result in the formation of a section of bone or fibrous tissue that extends from the epiphysis to the metaphysis, across the physis. This so-called bony bar or bridge can act as a tethering point. If the tethering point is peripheral, this results in angular deformity, with the point of tethering being at the apex. Damage to the center of the growth plate results in growth arrest. This complication is most commonly seen following Salter Harris type IV injuries. Type I and II fractures rarely result in growth arrest because the fracture does not transgress the germinal layer of the physis. Shortening or cupping of the metaphysis

a

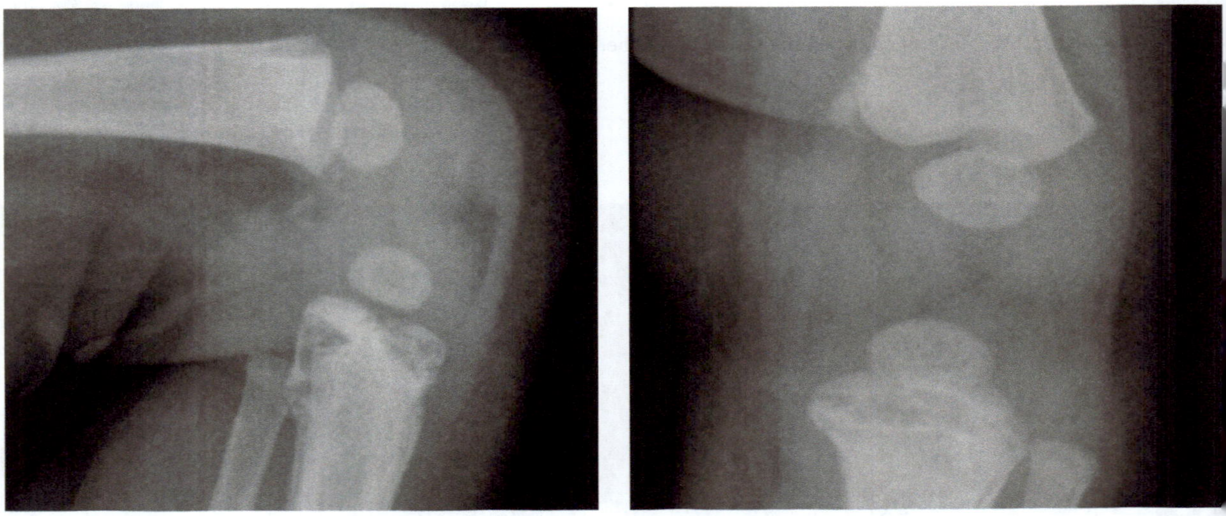

Fig. 10.10. a AP radiograph of the left knee showing metaphyseal fracture of both the distal femur and proximal tibia. **b** Lateral radiograph of the same patient shows periosteal reaction around the proximal tibia due to healing

can also occur, but this is more commonly seen post infection (particularly meningococcal septicaemia), thermal injury and irradiation.

Growth arrest due to partial or complete physeal closure occurs in between 2%–15% of physeal fractures. Bony bridging is most commonly seen to involve the distal tibia and femur (Ecklund and Jaramillo 2002). In one series injuries in the distal femur, proximal tibia and distal tibia resulted in bone bridges that required resection in 35%, 16% and 30%, respectively (Peterson et al. 1994). Fortunately these sites are relatively rare locations of physeal fractures.

Treatment depends on the size and site of the injury. The physeal bars can be resected. Optimum surgical resection results when 2 years of expected growth remain and the physeal bridge involves less than 50% of the growth plate (Langenskiold 1981).

CT or MR imaging can be used to demonstrate the size and site of bony bars. Three dimensional (3D) fat suppressed spoiled gradient recalled echo images followed by manual image reconstruction can be used to create a 3D model of the growth plate (Fig. 10.11). On these images bone bridges are visualised as low signal areas (in contrast to the high signal growth plate). This was first described by Craig et al. (1999). Sailham et al. (2004) examined 33 bony bridges in 28 children. Images were acquired in a coronal plane with the following parameters: TR/TE = 47/9 ms, flip angle 40, matrix size 256/224, slice thickness 2 mm, no gap, excitation number 2, mean field of view 140 mm. The bony bar and the growth plate were manually outlined on each coronal image. This allowed calculation of the percentage of the growth plate involved by bony bridging. Using multiplanar reformatting reconstruction (MPR) 3D models of the physis and of the bridge can be obtained (Sailhan et al. 2004).

3D MR imaging of the growth plate does have limitations. Central bony bridges are easy to identify, but lateralized ones are more difficult because the bridge often blends with the normal cortex. When processing the coronal images, (Sailhan et al. 2004) found the anterior and posterior margins of the bridges difficult to identify: in contrast to the lateral margins which were clear. This could be solved by performing both sagittal and coronal images of each growth plate. Small tongues of unossified cartilage extend from the growth plate into the metaphysis. These areas are of high signal, and it is important to recognize that these are normal days or weeks after injury, and do not result in growth arrest. In the first few months after injury, tiny defects in the physeal signal can occur, which resolve. Surgery is only indicated if a bone bridge is observed to be causing growth arrest or deformity.

10.5.2
Avascular Necrosis

The blood supply to the epiphysis is fragile. There are few vessels that cross the growth plate. The

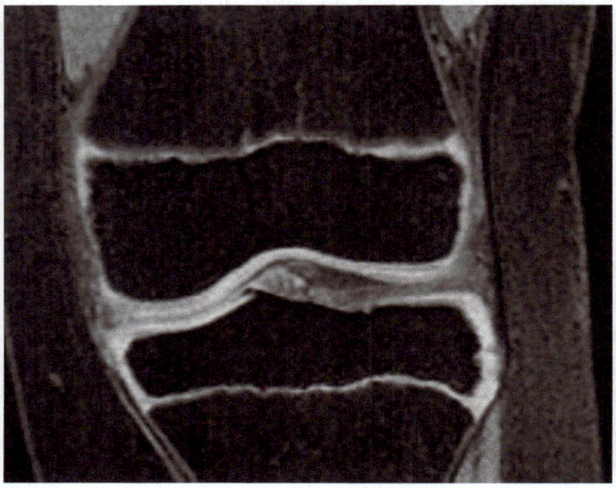

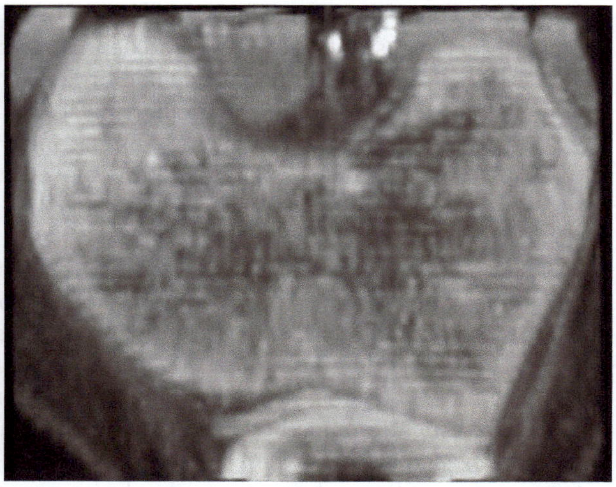

Fig. 10.11. a Three dimensional fat suppressed spoiled gradient recalled echo image showing the normal appearances of the growth plate in a 13-year-old boy. **b** 3D reconstruction of the distal tibial growth plate of the same child

radial head and proximal femoral epiphysis are particularly at risk as they are intracapsular and the supplying blood vessels run between the bone and the capsule. These are easily damaged during trauma and this can result in avascular necrosis (AVN).

Radiographs may be normal in early or mild avascular necrosis. Later findings are of sclerosis and flattening of the epiphysis. Advanced disease causes subchondral collapse and joint space narrowing. CT can show changes, but the most sensitive tool is MRI, which also has the advantage of not using ionizing radiation. MR imaging typically shows geographical lesions which have a "double line sign", i.e. on T2 images there is a hyperintense inner border parallel to a hypointense periphery. This hypointense band is the region of repair and usually enhances post contrast. Post-contrast imaging can be helpful as areas of bone marrow that do not enhance represent non-viable tissue. Decreased contrast enhancement can be seen in the early stages of AVN. Bone scans can be used; they are more sensitive at detecting early avascular necrosis compared to plain films (shown as areas of decreased uptake), but are less sensitive than MR imaging.

The International Classification grades avascular necrosis of the hip from 0 to IV.

- Stage 0: Normal imaging, but bone biopsy shows osteonecrosis.
- Stage I: Positive bone scan and/or MRI.
- Stage II: Mottled femoral head with sclerosis and/or cyst formation and/or osteopenia on the plain films, with a positive bone scan and/or MRI.
- Stage III: Crescent sign lesions and depression of the femoral head articular surface.
- Stage IV: Flattening of the articular surface with joint space narrowing and secondary acetabular changes (Stoller et al. 2004).

Treatment can be conservative, with protected weight bearing. Surgical core decompression can be helpful for patients with stage 1 or II disease. Best results are seen when less than 25% of the femoral head is involved (Beltran et al. 1990). Other methods of treatment include bone grafting, which may either be vascularised or non-vascularised (fibula). Once severe collapse has occurred salvage procedures include proximal femoral osteotomy, arthroplasty or arthrodesis.

10.6 Conclusions

The paediatric skeleton is very different to the adult skeleton and therefore reacts differently to trauma. The transitional zone between the physeal cartilage and bone, "the zone of provisional calcification", is the weakest point in the growing skeleton, and is therefore a common fracture site. Most fractures heal without long term complications. In a minority, growth arrest and avascular necrosis may occur.

References

Beltran J, Knight CT, Zuelzer WA et al (1990) Core decompression for avascular necrosis of the femoral head: correlation between long term results and preoperative MR staging. Radiology 175:533–536

Caffey J (1957) Some traumatic lesions in growing bones other than fractures and dislocations; clinical and radiological features. Br J Radiology 30:225–238

Craig JG, Cramer KE, Cody DD et al (1999) Premature partial closure and other deformities of the growth plate: MR imaging and three dimensional modeling. Radiology 210:835–843

Ecklund K, Jaramillo D (2002) Patterns of premature physeal arrest. MR imaging of 111 patients. AJR Am J Roentgenol 178:967–972

Jaramillo D, Shapiro F (1998a) Growth cartilage: normal appearance, variants and abnormalities. Magn Reson Imaging Clin N Am 6:455–471

Jaramillo D, Shapiro F (1998b) Musculoskeletal trauma in children. Magn Reson Imaging Clin N Am 6:521–536

Jaramillo D, Connolly SA, Mulkern RW et al (1998) Developing epiphysis: MR imaging characteristics and histological correlation in the Newborn Lamb. Radiology 207:637–645

Jaramillo D, Villegas-Medina OL, Doty DK et al (2004) Age related changes in the epiphysis, physis and metaphysis. Normal findings on gadolinium enhanced MRI of piglets. AJR Am J Roentgenol 182:353–360

Kleinman PK (1990) Diagnostic imaging in infant abuse. AJR Am J Roentgenol 155:703–712

Langenskiold A (1981) Surgical treatment of partial closure of the growth plate. J Pediatr Orthop 1:3–11

Ogden JA (1981) Injury to the growth mechanisms of the immature skeleton. Skeletal Radiol 6:237–253

Ogden JA, McCarthy SM (1983) Radiology of postnatal skeletal development. VIII. Distal tibia and fibula. Skeletal Radiol 10:209–220

Peterson HA, Madhok R, Benson JT et al (1994) Physeal fractures: part 1, 1979–1988. J Pediatr Orthop 14:423–430

Peterson HA (1994) Physeal fractures: part 2. Two previously unclassified types. J Pediatr Orthop 14:431–438

Rang M (1983) Children's fractures. Toronto, Lippincott

Rogers LF (1970) The radiography of epiphyseal injuries. Radiology 96:289–299

Salter RB, Harris WR (1963) Injuries involving the epiphyseal plate. J Bone Joint Surg (Am) 45:587

Sailhan F, Chotel F, Guibal AL et al (2004) Three dimensional MR imaging in the assessment of physeal growth arrest. Eur Radiol 14:1600–1608

Sofka CM, Potter HG (2002) Imaging of elbow injuries in the child and adult athlete. Radiol Clin N Am 40:251–265

Stoller DW et al (2004) Diagnostic imaging. Orthopedics 4:2–5, Amirsys Inc.

Weir J, Peter H A et al (1998) Imaging atlas of human anatomy, 2nd ed. Mosby

Non-accidental Injury

11

Stephen Chapman

Contents

S. Chapman, MD
Department of Radiology, Consultant Paediatric Radiologist, Birmingham Children's Hospital, Steelhouse Lane, Birmingham, B4 6NH, UK

11.1 Introduction

The recognition of child abuse as an evil, as opposed to a parental right, is relatively modern. The first clear medical description of the abuse of children was in 1860 when Ambroise Tardieu described the soft tissue, skeletal and intracranial injuries suffered by 32 Parisian children (Tardieu 1860; Labbe 2005). In 1946, Caffey described the association between subdural haematoma and long bone fractures and stated that the injuries "were either not observed or were denied when observed" (Caffey 1946). Further recognition of the condition followed and in 1961 when Kempe et al. (1962) coined the powerful term 'the battered child' for a multidisciplinary meeting of the American Academy of Pediatrics. Within 5 years, every US state had passed a child abuse reporting law.

Greater public and medical awareness of the condition, the increasingly broader definition of abuse to include sexual abuse and emotional maltreatment, greater emphasis on thorough investigation and, in the USA, a mandated reporter system, have combined to increase the number of reported cases of child abuse and neglect (Richman 2000). Data for the United States records that in 1974 there were 60,000 abused or neglected children (Krugman 1997); in 1997 the figure was nearly 3.2 million (Wang 1997). State child protective service agencies in the United States received reports alleging the maltreatment of approximately 4.5 million children in 2002 (US Department of Health and Human Services 2006), of whom 896,000 (12.3 per 1,000 children under 18 years of age) were determined to have been victims of abuse (19% physical abuse, 10% sexual abuse) or neglect. The large number of unsubstantiated cases serves to remind us of our huge responsibility when dealing with cases of trauma when the causation is not absolutely clear from the outset. In the 2002 United States data, 1400 children died of abuse or neglect, children under

1 year of age accounting for 41% of fatalities and children under 7 years accounted for 88%. Of the childhood fatalities that occurred in 2002, 79% involved a parent as perpetrator.

Radiologists have a critical role in identifying children who have been injured, particularly intentionally injured, and who may be injured further if the correct diagnosis of non-accidental injury is not made and the child returned to the care of the perpetrator. The radiologist's roles are listed in Table 11.1.

Table 11.1. Roles of the radiologist

- To identify the radiological findings
- To differentiate abnormalities from normal variation in the growing skeleton
- To differentiate traumatic from non-traumatic abnormalities
- To suggest a mechanism of causation for traumatic lesions
- To date the injury
- To identify or suggest an underlying skeletal abnormality that would predispose the child to fractures, either (a) when there are obvious radiographic abnormalities or (b) when the mechanism seems to be appropriate but the degree of force is less than would have been expected to cause the injury

11.2 Anatomy and Physiology of the Developing Skeleton

At birth the diaphyses or shafts of the tubular bones are composed of fetal or woven bone that lacks haversian systems. However, as periosteal-mediated appositional bone formation and remodelling enlarge the overall diameter of the shaft and the width of the cortices, mature bone becomes dominant. This early bone is very vascular and more porous than the maturing bone of older children and adults and better able to tolerate deformation. Pores retard progression of a fracture line but increase the likelihood of compression, and it is this reason that makes greenstick and torus (buckle) fractures more common in childhood (Ogden 1990). Immature periosteum also differs from that in the adult, being thicker and more loosely attached to the underlying cortex. It minimises displacement of diaphyseal fractures and is capable of faster callus and membranous bone formation (Crilly 1972). Towards the end of the bone, adjacent to the growth plate, is the metaphysis, a site characterised by decreased cortical bone and increased trabecular bone. The trabecular bone undergoes extensive remodelling as the primary spongiosa is transformed into more mature secondary spongiosa. This area of transformation is structurally weak during the period of rapid growth during infancy (Alexander 1976).

Due to the child's more flexible skeleton and increased amount of stretch allowed by the soft tissues, the majority of childhood fractures are undisplaced. Greater strength of the joint capsule and ligaments compared with the metaphyseal bone also means that fractures occur much more readily than dislocations. In the infant, hard tissues (cartilage and bone) may be considered as soft, while soft tissues (tendons and ligaments) should be considered as hard.

11.3 Patterns of Skeletal Injury

With broadening of the definition of child abuse, the percentage of children with fractures has decreased; reported frequencies vary from 11% to 55%, with age having a significant influence (Ebbin et al. 1969; Galleno and Oppenheim 1982, Herndon 1983; Kogutt et al. 1974; Lauer et al. 1974; Merten et al. 1983; Ryan et al. 1977). Ebbin et al. (1969) did not find any fractures in children over the age of 5 years. Akbarnia et al. (1974), in a series of 217 abused infants, found that 78% of fractures occurred below the age of 3 years and 50% occurred below 1 year of age. This has implications for imaging protocols (see below).

11.3.1 Subperiosteal New Bone Formation

In the infant, as opposed to the older child, the periosteum is loosely adherent to the shaft of a long bone, but is strongly attached to the physeal cartilage. Subperiosteal haemorrhage results in separation of the osteogenic periosteum from the bony cortex, but the perichondral attachment is usually preserved, resulting in maximum thickness of haemorrhage along the shaft and tapering towards the epiphysis. Subperiosteal new bone formation (SNBF) is non-specific, being seen in infectious, metabolic and neoplastic disease processes.

The importance and frequency of physiological SNBF should also be recognised (Kwon et al. 2002). Radiographically this presents as a thin well-defined density, 2 mm or less in thickness, separate from the cortex of the bone and restricted to the diaphysis (Fig. 11.1). In order of frequency the bones most commonly affected are the tibia, femur, humerus, ulna and radius. The changes are most often, but not always, bilateral and symmetrical. It is a common finding between 1 and 4 months. Outside of this age group and when ≥ 2 mm in thickness, SNBF is likely to be abnormal and should prompt further diagnostic evaluation.

When there is diagnostic uncertainty, follow-up radiographs and/or bone scintigraphy should be undertaken. SNBF may be the clue to a subtle underlying fracture and it should prompt the request for coned radiographs, other views or follow-up radiographs. SNBF without a fracture is probably the result of an applied tractional or torsional force, such as when a child is grabbed by the leg, which displaces the loosely adherent periosteum.

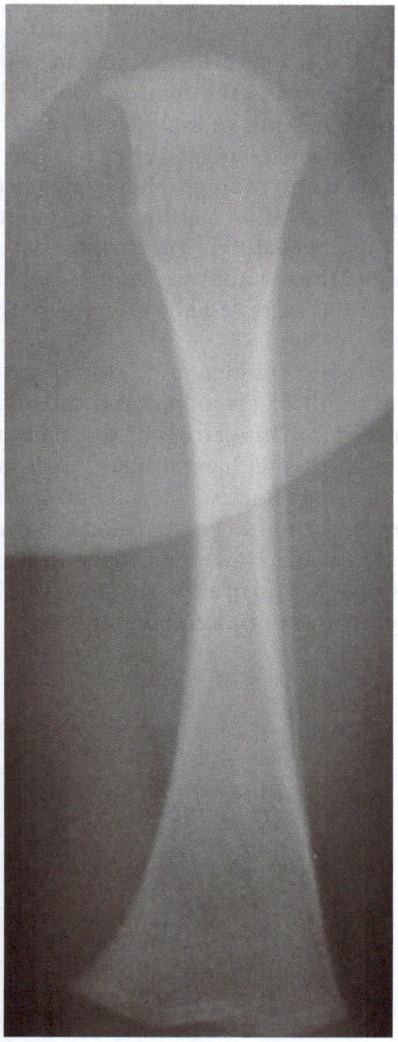

Fig. 11.1. Physiological periosteal reaction. AP view of a femur in a 2-month-old child shows a thin layer of periosteal new bone along the mid shaft that does not extend to the metaphyses

11.3.2 Metaphyseal Fractures (Classic Metaphyseal Lesion)

Metaphyseal fractures comprise approximately 20% of abuse fractures and are usually multiple. They are more common in the lower limbs and are most frequent around the knee. For many years the mechanism of injury at this site was believed to be that proposed by Caffey (1957). He stated that indirect forces transmitted through the periosteum produced avulsions of the metaphysis where it was tightly adherent. When a small fragment of bone was avulsed the radiographic finding of the 'corner' fracture resulted (Fig. 11.2). When a larger crescentic fragment of bone was avulsed and displaced or

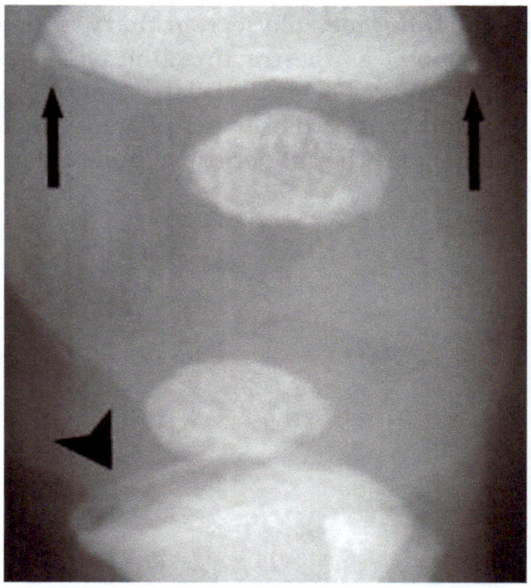

Fig. 11.2. Metaphyseal fractures. AP view of a knee shows the two typical appearances of 'corner' fractures (*arrows*) and a 'bucket handle' fracture (*arrowhead*)

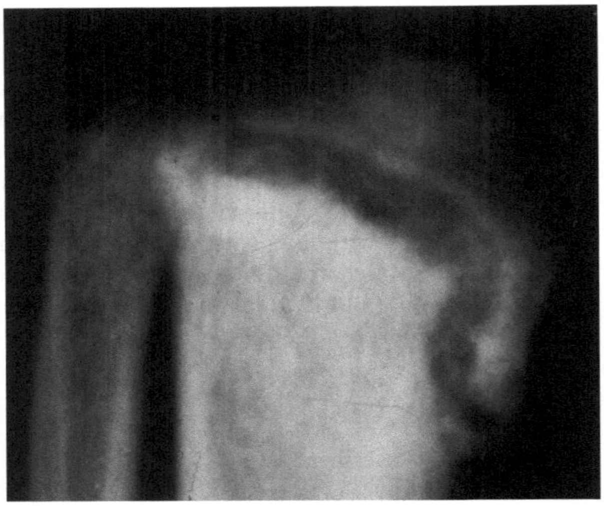

Fig. 11.3. A large bucket handle fracture. Note the thickness of the bone fragment at the periphery compared with the middle of the bone. When the thicker peripheral fragment is demonstrated without its central component, the appearances are those of a corner fracture

viewed obliquely the appearance was that of the 'bucket-handle' fracture (Figs. 11.2, 11.3).

Kleinman and co-workers have thrown new light on this classic metaphyseal lesion (CML) associated with abuse (Kleinman et al. 1986; Kleinman and Marks 1995, 1996, 1998). They have shown that the fundamental abnormality is a complete or incomplete transmetaphyseal fracture through the most immature metaphyseal primary spongiosa. Furthermore, as the fracture line passes peripherally towards the cortex it deviates away from the physis to undercut a thicker peripheral segment that encompasses the subperiosteal bone collar (Fig. 11.3). Thus, there is separation of a disk of bone, which is thin centrally and thicker peripherally. The radiographic appearance is typical, but radiographically variable. When the separated ossified disk is very thin, the radiograph is normal, although histological examination of the resected bone may demonstrate the lesion (Kleinman et al. 1986; Ruess et al. 2003). When the fracture line is wider there will be a lucent line extending across the metaphysis; the fracture line may be visible in only one plane. If the radiographic projection is such that only the thicker peripheral segment is demonstrable, then the resulting radiographic finding is the 'corner' fracture. When the entire fracture is visible and viewed obliquely, the disk appears to be further separated from the adjacent metaphysis and the 'bucket-handle' appearance results (Fig. 11.2).

Haemorrhage at the fracture line and beneath the adjacent periosteum is usually minimal or absent. SNBF is usually lacking and sclerosis along the fracture margins is inconspicuous. When healing is complete there may be no radiographic evidence of the previous injury (Fig. 11.4). Dating of these injuries is difficult. During healing, hypertrophic cartilage may extend into the metaphysis producing focal lucencies, indentations or broader scalloping of the metaphyseal margin (Fig. 11.5).

As Caffey originally pointed out, metaphyseal fractures are the result of tractional and torsional forces applied to a limb. This can occur when a limb is used as a handle or when centrifugal forces act during violent shaking. Rarely, an isolated metaphyseal fracture may be found and correlated with a plausible accidental event. However, in all other circumstances this injury in an otherwise normal child is virtually diagnostic of non-accidental injury.

a

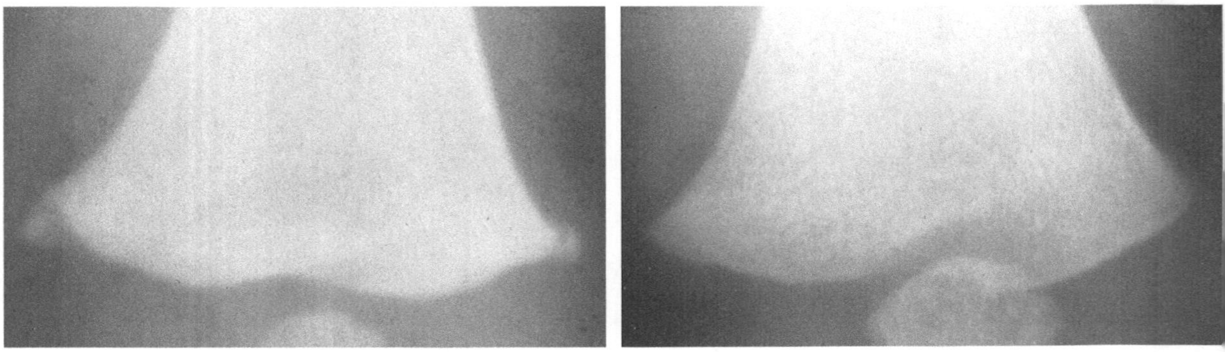

Fig. 11.4a,b. Healing of a metaphyseal fracture without the typical changes of a healing fracture. **a** Acute metaphyseal fracture. **b** Follow-up film with no evidence of callus or subperiosteal new bone formation

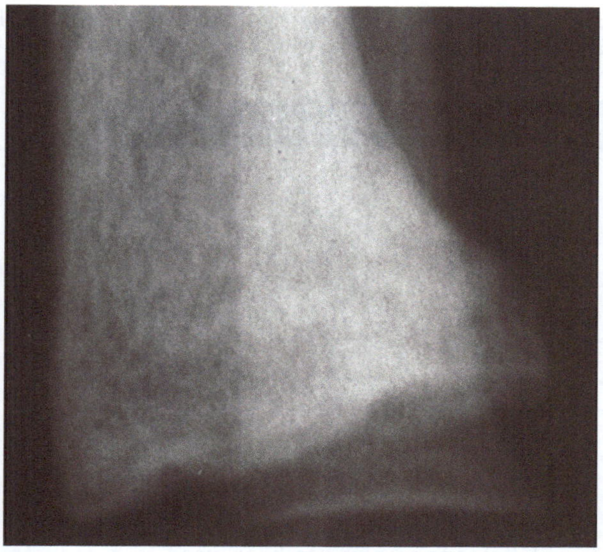

Fig. 11.5. A healed metaphyseal fracture, but with focal scalloping of its epiphyseal margin

11.3.3 Epiphyseal Separations

Fractures that involve the growth plate, with or without involvement of the adjacent epiphysis and/or metaphysis, as classified by Salter and Harris, occur most commonly as accidents. The forces which produce these physeal separations are similar to those which produce the CML, but their magnitude is greater (Kleinman and Marks 1998).

11.3.4 Shaft Fractures

In general, shaft fractures are not specific for abuse, but attain greater significance when found in a healing state, implying that the child was not brought for medical attention at the appropriate time. The most common sites are the femur and humerus followed by the tibia and forearm (King et al. 1988; Kowal-Vern et al. 1992; Thomas et al. 1991; Worlock et al. 1986). It is frequently difficult to differentiate an oblique from a spiral fracture and an individual fracture line may appear oblique in one projection and spiral in another. Although it is possible to state that each of these fracture types is the result of an indirectly applied force, determination of the exact mechanism is usually not possible. In the absence of a discrete and plausible history, solitary or multiple shaft fractures will require multidisciplinary team assessment.

Largely because of the nature of inflicted injuries in young children, it must be remembered that the published literature is not always scientifically robust. It is not always clear how a diagnosis of abuse was confirmed or refuted, or what investigations were undertaken to support the conclusions. Children are often categorised as 'abused' or 'accident' when, of course, many children should really be categorised in the grey area of 'uncertain'.

11.4 Fracture Healing

Children who present after accidental trauma virtually always have a clear history of the events associated with the injuries. When there is no history (from an infant or unhelpful parents) or when there are suspicious circumstances, one of the many pieces of the jigsaw that leads to, or excludes, a diagnosis of non-accidental injury is the dating of those injuries (Chapman 1992). Dating of fractures may highlight inconsistencies in the history. Comprehensive discussion of the dating of fractures in non-accidental injury is provided by O'Connor and Cohen (1988), although Prosser et al. (2005) stressed the lack of primary evidence on which dating is based, particularly in infants and toddlers. The changes are summarised in Table 11.2. Fracture healing is faster in younger children (Cumming 1979) and two studies have shown more rapid healing when there is a coexistent head injury, a finding of relevance in the context of non-accidental injury (Perkins and Skirving 1987; Spencer 1987). It is important to understand that radiological dating is an inexact science.

11.4.1 Radiological Changes in the Soft Tissues

Haemorrhage and inflammatory exudate begin immediately after injury. They obliterate the normal lucent fat planes and well-defined muscle boundaries, but for bones surrounded by a large muscle bulk there may be a delay of many hours before these changes are apparent radiologically. In the

Table 11.2. Timing of radiological changes in paediatric fractures. [Modified from O'Connor and Cohen (1998)]. NB The evolution of fracture healing is more rapid in the young infant compared with the older child and is influenced by lack of immobilisation and repetitive trauma

Radiological change	Earliest	Peak	Latest
Resolution of soft tissue changes (depends on severity of injury)	2–5 days	4–10 days	10–21 days
Subperiosteal new bone formation	4–10 days	10–14 days	14–21 days
Loss of fracture line definition and appearance of soft callus	10–14 days	14–21 days	
Hard callus	14–21 days	21–42 days	42–90 days
Remodelling	3 months	1 year	2 years – growth plate closure

absence of a major underlying fracture, these changes persist for a few days only, but more severe injuries may be associated with soft tissue changes that persist for longer. Interestingly, the majority of limb fractures in children are not associated with clinical bruising, either at diagnosis or in the first week after injury, and the absence of this sign should not be taken as evidence that a minimal force produced a fracture in a 'brittle' bone (Matthew et al. 1998).

11.4.2 Response of the Periosteum to Injury

Elevated periosteum is not visible radiographically until calcium accumulates in the subperiosteal haematoma and the new bone. The first appearance of periosteal new bone is dependent on the age of the child, the younger the child the earlier it appears. In the infant it can be seen, radiographically as early as 4 days after, but 7–14 days is more usual. Cumming (1979), in a study of birth-related fractures concluded that the absence of periosteal new bone 11 days after birth should suggest the possibility of abuse. Beyond the neonatal period, periosteal reaction delayed longer than 21 days may be a consequence of poor nutrition or vitamin D deficiency. The amount of subperiosteal new bone increases with repeated trauma and continuing subperiosteal haemorrhage (leading to exuberant callus formation), but chronic repetitive trauma may be of such severity as to destroy periosteal new bone as it develops, with resultant failure of the usual sequence of changes with healing.

Ultrasonography has been used to demonstrate subperiosteal haemorrhages and occult long bone fractures (Graif et al. 1988) before radiographs confirm the presence of bony injury and may be a useful supplementary investigation when attempting to date an acute injury.

11.4.3 Fracture Line Definition

Fresh fractures, including metaphyseal fractures, have sharply defined margins. With the development of an osteoclastic response to necrotic bone, the fracture ends become less well defined and the fracture widens. There are no objective criteria to estimate fracture healing using this sign but it is not apparent radiologically before 10 days and reaches a peak at 2–3 weeks.

11.4.4 Callus Formation

With the production of osteoid and its subsequent calcification and ultimate transformation into bone there is an increase in density along the fracture line. With impacted fractures and other fractures where the periosteum remains intact or little disturbed this may be the only evidence of injury and it is, therefore, a less valuable sign than subperiosteal new bone and fracture line clarity. Again, movement may inhibit or destroy endosteal callus and a fracture line may remain clearly visible after a bone has united by periosteal new bone. Endosteal soft callus is first visualised as an ill-defined increase in density and begins to form soon after the first appearance of periosteal new bone, i.e. at about 10–14 days. When lamellar bone bridges the fracture, about 1 week later, the stage of hard callus has begun. The chronology of callus formation and fracture consolidation is dependent on age. A birth-related fracture may be united at 1 month, but a similar fracture in an 8-year-old will be united at 8 weeks.

11.4.5 Remodelling

Estimation of the age of a fracture by this criterion is very difficult because initial deformity, the volume of callus produced and the age of the child are major variables. In the young infant with a stable undisplaced fracture, the remodelling process may be complete at 3 months, while the older child with an angular deformity or a markedly displaced fracture may continue to remodel for up to 2 years.

11.5 Imaging Protocols

The British Society of Paediatric Radiology and the American College of Radiology have produced guidelines for the radiological investigation of suspected abuse. It is vital that every anatomical region is imaged, including hands, feet and spine. Oblique views of the ribs are essential in order to identify these often occult fractures. High quality radiography is essential to identify subtle bony injuries, such as the CML. The continued use of the whole body radiograph (babygram) is to be deplored. The skeletal survey should be obtained during normal working hours and after the child has received appropriate analgesia. The parents/carers should be informed by the clinical staff why it is necessary.

Following a systematic literature review, KEMP et al. (2006) provided guidelines for imaging of the skeleton in suspected child abuse (Table 11.3). The yield from a skeletal survey is inversely related to age and these authors identified 2 years of age as an acceptable cut-off point. Although smaller studies have cited other indications, these authors could not find sufficient evidence to support the routine imaging of siblings of abused children or children with burns, sexual abuse, neglect or older disabled children.

Table 11.3. Recommendations for imaging of the skeleton. [After KEMP et al. (2006)]

- All children under the age of 2 years, where physical abuse is suspected, should undergo radiological investigation to exclude fractures
- Radiological investigation should be considered in children older than 2 years and disabled children on an individual clinical basis
- Either skeletal survey or bone scintigraphy alone will miss occult fractures
- Oblique views of the chest must be included in the skeletal survey
- Repeat skeletal survey at 2 weeks should be considered. As a minimum, the follow-up films should comprise a frontal chest film with both oblique views of the ribs. Follow-up radiographs increase the detection rate of fractures, assist with dating and clarify the nature of uncertain findings
- If bone scintigraphy is the first-line investigation of choice, skull radiographs and coned views of the metaphyses should be additional investigations because these are easily missed

When the first skeletal survey is equivocal, when dating is insecure or when there are continuing concerns about abuse in the presence of initially normal radiographs, a repeat skeletal survey (KLEINMAN et al. 1996; ZIMMERMAN et al. 2005), or as a minimum a repeat chest radiograph (ANILKUMAR et al. 2006) after 10–14 days may be of assistance.

Bone scintigraphy is a useful complementary investigation that may identify an additional 20% of radiographically occult injuries (MANDELSTAM et al. 2003). It is a poor tool for identifying skull and spine fractures and metaphyseal fractures (because of the high activity in the normal metaphysis), with false-negative rates range from 0.8% (STY and STARSHAK 1983) to 27% (MERTEN et al. 1983). However, it is superior to radiography for some other injuries, particularly rib fractures, especially at the costovertebral junction, undisplaced shaft fractures and subperiosteal haemorrhage (HAASE et al. 1980; JAUDES 1984; SMITH et al. 1980). A positive scan steadily becomes less so as the age of a fracture increases, but there is no definite time course and, consequently, it has no value in the dating of fractures. It should be noted that bone scintigraphy delivers a higher radiation dose to the child than a typical skeletal survey.

Ultrasonography can be a valuable tool in certain circumstances. MARKOVITZ et al. (1993) demonstrated metaphyseal fractures around the knee, while SMEETS et al. (1990) identified costo-chondral dislocation of the lower ribs. NIMKIN et al. (1995) described physeal or epiphyseal humeral injuries and advocated the role of sonography and magnetic resonance imaging (MRI), although the latter has not achieved anything like its importance for imaging of the brain and extracerebral spaces.

11.6 Upper Limb Shaft Fractures

The humerus is one of the most frequently injured long bones in abused children, probably because it is an easily accessible 'handle'. The association with abuse is inversely related to age, but as with all long bone fractures, the nature of the injury needs to be carefully considered in relation to the presenting history. There are no injuries that are specific for abuse, but excluding supracondylar fractures in toddlers, all humeral fractures are strongly suggestive (although not diagnostic) of abuse. Most fractures are spiral or oblique and are the result of twisting and/or levering forces applied to the arm against the weight of the child.

Fractures of the proximal radius and ulna are most commonly identified in association with distal humeral injuries, and are the result of hyperextension. Mid forearm fractures are typically transverse and the result of either a direct blow or levering force. Forearm fractures in a toddler, though not an infant, may occur as when an arm is raised to protect the face and head. Distal forearm fractures are indistinguishable from those seen as typical accidents in older children who fall on the outstretched arm. The history and mode of presentation are important factors in differentiating abuse from accident.

11.7 Lower Limb Shaft Fractures

There is no association between the morphological feature of a femoral fracture and the likelihood of abuse (REX and KAY 2000). Although there is some disagreement in the published literature, transverse and oblique fractures seem to be the most common type, both in abuse and accident; spiral fracture is not suggestive of abuse (KING et al. 1988, LODER and BOOKOUT 1991, SCHERL et al. 2000).

Age, however, is a significant factor in determining the likelihood that a femoral shaft fracture is due to abuse. ANDERSON (1982) reviewed 122 femoral fractures in 117 patients. In the group under 13 months of age, 15 (83%) of 18 had been abused; of 24 children under 2 years of age, 19 (79%) had been abused. BEALS and TUFTS (1983) suggested that as many as 30% of femoral fractures in children less than 4 years of age were the result of a non-accidental injury. THOMAS et al. (1991) found that 60% of femoral fractures in children less than 1 year of age were due to abuse; above the age of 2 years, 90% were accidental. In their study of 47 femoral fractures, REX and KAY (2000) noted that 13 (93%) of the 14 inflicted fractures occurred in children less than 1 year of age.

As for femoral fractures, tibial shaft fractures are not specific for abuse, although in a non-weight-bearing infant without a history of significant trauma, abuse must be given serious consideration. In the ambulant infant, a steep, vertical, undisplaced spiral or oblique fracture is likely to be a 'toddler's fracture', an accident result from a twisting fall while the foot is fixed to the ground.

11.8 Rib Fractures

Rib fractures comprise 5%–27% (AKBARNIA et al. 1974; BARRETT and KOZLOWSKI 1979; HERNDON 1983) of all fractures in abused children and are probably even more common than published figures suggest because of the difficulty in demonstrating them radiologically in the acute situation prior to the appearance of callus. Any part of the rib may be affected, and fractures are frequently bilateral and multiple, although 20% of rib fractures are solitary (CARTY and PIERCE 2002) (Fig. 11.6). Rib fractures in infancy are unusual because normal ribs are so pliable. Considerable force is required to produce them and even in children who undergo cardiopulmonary resuscitation, 99.5% do not develop rib fractures (FELDMAN and BREWER 1984; JOHN et al. 2005). Posterior rib fractures do not occur as a result of cardiopulmonary resuscitation. THOMAS (1977), in a review of over 10,000 chest X-rays of infants

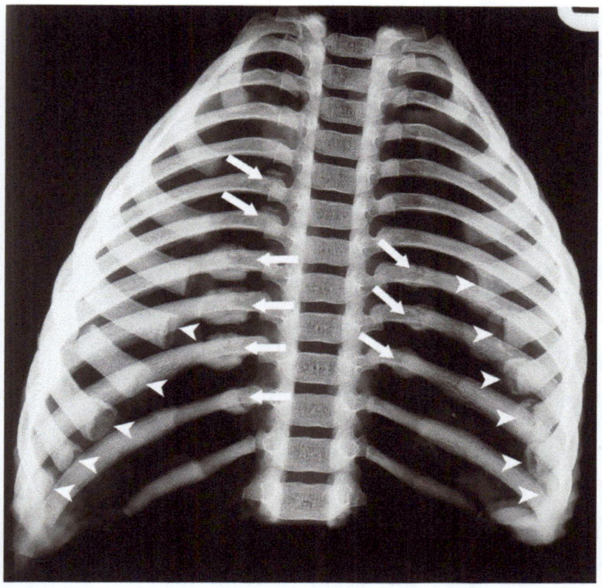

Fig. 11.6. Postmortem radiograph demonstrates multiple posterior rib (*arrows*) and costochondral fractures (*arrowheads*) of differing ages. Fractures of similar ages are aligned one with another

under 1 year of age, diagnosed fractures during life in only 25. The most commonly associated factor was prematurity. Only one infant was seen with rib fractures due to birth injury.

Metabolic bone disease is now less common in preterm infants, but may be complicated by fractures. Prolonged parenteral nutrition, prolonged jaundice, frusemide therapy and bronchopulmonary dysplasia increase the likelihood of fractures. Amir et al. (1988) found only 12 babies with fractures in 973 premature infants and the fractures were most common in the smallest infants (< 1000 g). Fractures in premature infants occur antero-laterally. Rib fractures in the absence of major trauma or underlying bone disease, even when solitary, should be considered as specific evidence of abuse (Barsness et al. 2003; Merten and Carpenter 1990; Thomas 1977; Williams and Connolly 2004) and those involving the posterior ends correlate even more strongly. Dahlenburg et al. (1989) showed that prematurity was not a major risk factor for fractures later in childhood.

In contrast to diaphyseal appendicular fractures the majority (over 81%) of rib fractures are occult (Merten et al. 1983). They most commonly result from a compressive, squeezing force applied to the chest during violent shaking. A front-to-back force results in fractures in the mid-axillary lines while lateral compression produces fractures posteriorly and at the costochondral junctions. Fractures of the posterior rib arcs carry a high specificity for abuse and result when the ribs are excessively levered on the fulcrum of the vertebral transverse process. This disrupts the ventral periosteum and cortex of the rib, usually leaving the dorsal periosteum intact. Maintenance of the posterior periosteum explains the tendency for the fracture to be undisplaced and for bleeding to be directed away from the subcutaneous tissues. The relative invisibility of the fracture line is compounded by it being frequently oriented obliquely to the X-ray beam in conventional radiographs and the superimposition of the adjacent transverse process; hence the necessity for oblique views of the ribs.

Many posterior rib fractures only become visible with the appearance of callus. In a post-mortem and radiological study, Kleinman et al. (1988) failed to identify any acute posterior rib fractures and more than 50% of healing posterior rib fractures by conventional radiography. Evidence of healing, as manifested by callus formation, was essential for reliable diagnosis of fractures near the costo-vertebral articulations. Thus failure to observe the fracture at presentation and the appearance of callus after admission to hospital is not necessarily evidence of injury after admission (Fig. 11.7).

Costochondral fractures are also subtle and will be seen during the healing phase as exaggerated cupping of the anterior end of the rib. They may be a visible sign of a major intra-abdominal injury (Ng and Hall 1998). A pleural reaction, due to haemorrhage, or lung contusion without a radiographically demonstrable rib fracture will be an indication for a radionuclide bone scan or follow-up radiographs.

11.9 Spine Fractures

Spine fractures are rare in childhood and in the absence of a history of major trauma should suggest abuse. Fractures may occur either from acute flexion/extension, as occurs during shaking, or longitudinal compression, as when buttocks are slammed down against a hard surface (Fig. 11.8).

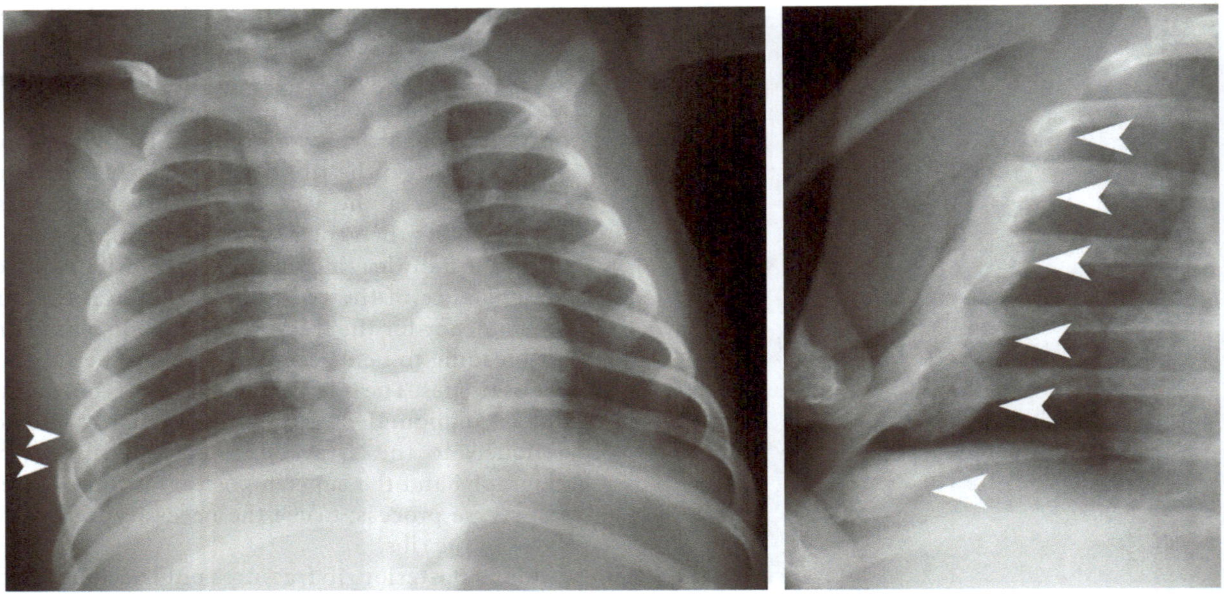

a

Fig. 11.7a,b. Multiple rib fractures that could be interpreted as appearing after admission to hospital. **a** On the admission chest radiograph the only rib fractures to be convincingly demonstrated are those involving right 6th and 7th ribs (*arrowheads*). Note also the pleural shadow immediately deep to the fractures, presumably the result of extrapleural haematoma. **b** The follow-up radiograph obtained 20 days later shows callus on the 3rd to 8th ribs (*arrowheads*). The callus has a similar appearance on each rib and the healing rib fractures lay in a line, one above the other. The fractures were, no doubt, sustained at the same time prior to admission

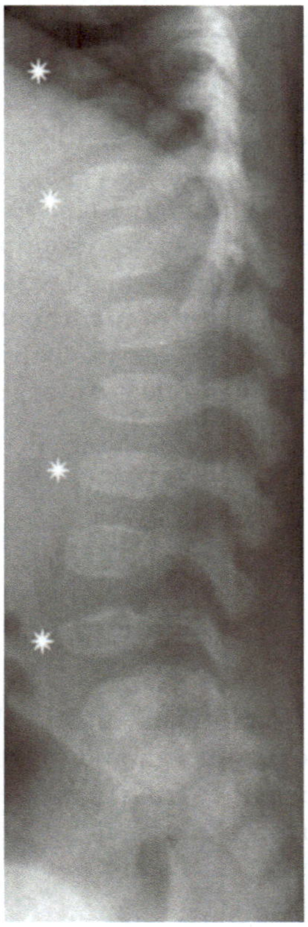

Fig. 11.8. Multiple vertebral body compression fractures (*asterisks*)

11.10 Other Unusual Fractures

With knowledge of common accidental fractures, the finding of a fracture at an unusual site will suggest an unusual mechanism of injury. In the absence of a history of an unusual mechanism, abuse should be considered. Unusual sites of fractures in infants and toddlers include phalanges (Fig. 11.9), metacarpals, metatarsals, pelvis and scapula (Fig. 11.10). Pelvic fractures have been described in association with sexual abuse (Johnson et al. 2004).

11.11 Obstetric Fractures

Clavicular fractures are by far the most frequent and may be discovered incidentally on a chest radiograph or clinically with the development of the hard lump of callus. The humerus is the commonest long bone to be fractured at birth. In Cumming's series of 23 birth related fractures the sites were clavicle, humerus and

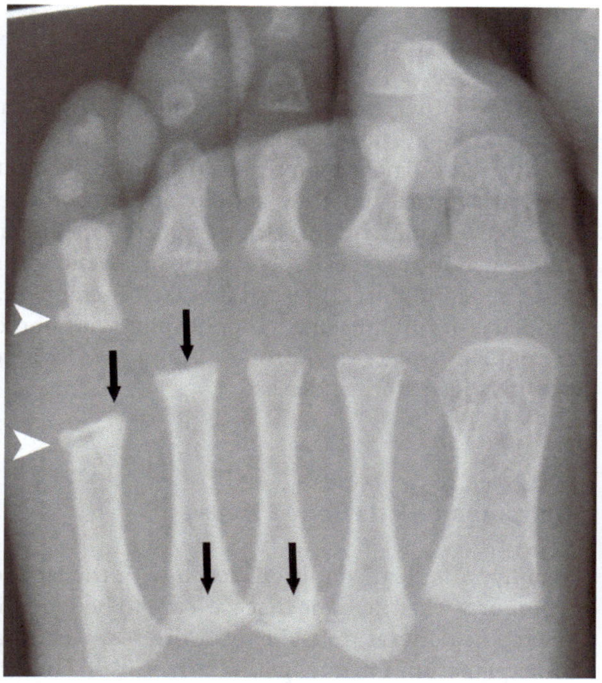

Fig. 11.9. Phalangeal and metatarsal fractures. The bases of the 3rd and 4th metatarsals show increased density because of internal callus formation

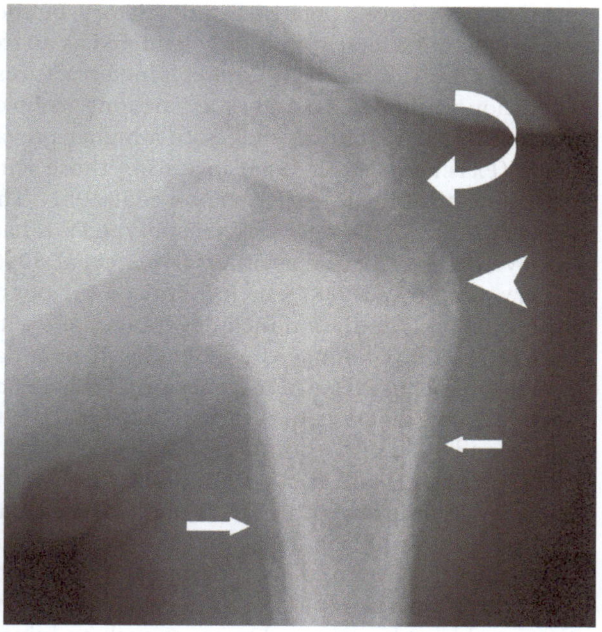

Fig. 11.10. Radiograph of the left shoulder shows a healing fracture of the tip of the acromion (*curved arrow*), the left proximal humeral metaphysis (*arrowhead*) and the associated subperiosteal new bone formation (*arrows*)

femur (Cumming 1979). He concluded that fracture at an unusual site or the absence of callus 11 days after birth should suggest the possibility of abuse. Three-quarters of all birth associated fractures of long bones occur during vaginal breech deliveries (Curran 1981). Although caesarean section has reduced the incidence of fractures, they still occur, even during easy delivery (Alexander et al. 1987). Surprisingly, rib fractures occurring at birth are very rare and are virtually confined to infants with birth weights above 4 kg who experience shoulder dystocia.

11.12 Differential Diagnosis

11.12.1 Normal Variants

There are large numbers of skeletal variations that affect the growing skeleton and those that affect the metaphysis are the most important, causing confusion with the interpretation of the CML. The most important are the 'step-off' configuration, the metaphyseal spur and metaphyseal beak. A total of 4% of infants may demonstrate focal cortical irregularity along the medial aspect of the proximal tibial diametaphysis. It is bilateral in 25% of cases (Kleinman et al. 1991).

11.12.2 Osteogenesis Imperfecta

Osteogenesis imperfecta (OI) is an inherited disorder of connective tissue resulting from abnormal quantity and/or quality of type I collagen, the major protein of bone. The phenotypic presentation is enormously varied, ranging from perinatal death to normal lifespan complicated by only a few fractures. Because fractures are a feature of the condition it must be given serious consideration in any child with unexplained fractures. There are four major types in the Sillence classification (Sillence et al. 1979), but it should be noted that there are no strict boundaries. Type IV is an uncommon type of OI (only 5% of the patients in the Sillence study) with mild to severe bone disease. Patients with this type nearly always have a positive family history, but because of white sclerae it may be considered as an explanation for the child with unexplained fractures.

Although many regard OI IV as rare, one group of authors in particular has suggested a higher prevalence (Paterson et al. 1983) including those with normal teeth, Type IV A (Paterson et al. 1987). The latter study of 78 patients with OI subtype IV A has, however, been criticised by others (Ablin et al. 1990; Carty and Shaw 1988) who have raised the possibility that the population includes individuals with NAI mistakenly diagnosed as OI. The differentiation of child abuse from osteogenesis imperfecta has been the subject of several reviews (Ablin et al. 1990; Ablin and Sane 1997; Augarten et al. 1993; Carty 1988; Chapman and Hall 1997; Smith 1995). The majority of children with OI have multiple wormian bones in the skull (Fig. 11.11) and this is an important radiological sign to be sought in any child with a fracture that is unexplained or the result of trauma that would not be expected to cause such an injury. By the time fractures begin, the majority of children with OI have osteopenia. However, this is difficult to assess radiographically because at least 30% of bone mineral must be lost before radiographs look abnormal. A further difficulty in the diagnosis of osteopenia is that there is no normal data for bone density as measured by dual energy X-ray absorptiometry (DEXA) in infants and young children. Metaphyseal fractures do occur in OI, but only in the presence of obvious bone disease with radiologically abnormal bones (Astley 1979). Skull fractures in children with OI still require a significant impact against a hard surface.

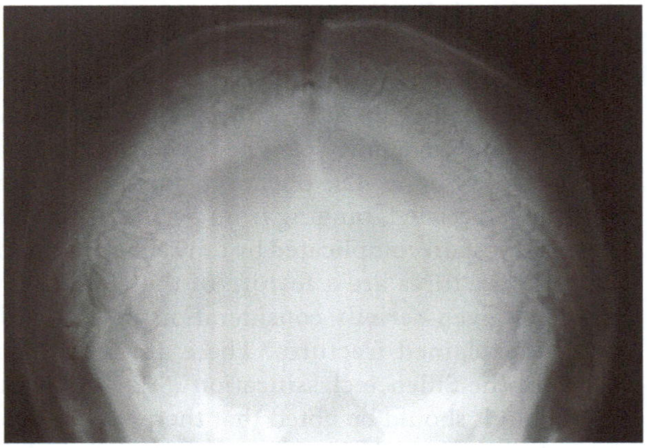

Fig. 11.11. Multiple wormian bones arranged along the lambdoid suture

11.12.3 Rarer Bone Dysplasias with Bone Fragility

There are other rare causes of bone fragility in infancy. They all have recognisable clinical, genetic and/or radiological manifestations which facilitate their diagnosis and they should not be confused with the 'normal' infant with a fracture. The list includes achondrogenesis, osteopetrosis, pycnodysostosis, mucolipidosis II (I-cell disease), metaphyseal dysplasia (type Jansen), hypophosphatasia, homocystinuria, Menke's syndrome (kinky hair disease) and glycogen storage disease.

11.12.4 Temporary Brittle Bone Disease

Two hypothetical conditions, each with the label of "temporary brittle bone disease", are to be found in the medical literature and may be offered in court as an explanation for unexplained fractures. The first described by Paterson et al. (1993) is believed by the authors to be the result of a temporary collagen synthesis defect, possibly as a result of copper deficiency or another metalloenzyme deficiency. The second, proposed by Miller and Hangartner (1999), is supposedly the result of intrauterine confinement causing a temporary defect in mineralisation. There is little scientific basis to justify the existence of either of these conditions (Chapman and Hall 1997; Mendelson 2005).

11.12.5 Other Differential Diagnoses

These are summarised in Table 11.4 and discussed by Brill et al. (1998)

11.13 Conclusions

Non-accidental injury is largely a diagnosis of exclusion. There are no fractures that are pathognomonic of abuse, but because of the mechanism of injury and degree of force required, some are highly specific for that diagnosis (Table 11.5). Correlation of the fracture, with regard to its morphology and its age, with the offered history is essential for correct interpretation

Table 11.4. Differential diagnoses of the bony lesions in non-accidental injury

Condition	Shaft fractures	SNBF	Metaphyseal abnormalities	Osteopenia	Comments
Rickets	+	+	+	+	Earliest signs are widening of growth plates and cupping and fraying of the metaphyses. Elevated alkaline phosphatase
Bone disease of prematurity	+	+	+	+	Most common in very low birth weight infants. More likely with a history of frusemide administration, prolonged ventilation and/or prolonged jaundice
Myelomeningocele	+	+	+	+/-	
Congenital insensitivity to pain	+	+	+	-	
Leukaemia	-	+	+	+	
Osteomyelitis	-	+	+	Localised	May be multifocal
Prostaglandin E1 treatment	-	+	-	-	
Congenital syphilis	-	+	+	-	
Scurvy	-	+	+	++	Not in first 6 months of life
Vitamin A intoxication	-	+	-	-	
Menke's syndrome (kinky hair disease)	-	+	+	+/-	Males with wormian bones, low serum copper and tortuous intracranial vessels
Copper deficiency	+	+	+	+	Unlikely in the absence of low birth weight, total parenteral nutrition, low-copper diet or in a term infant in the first 6 months of life
Caffey's disease	-	++	-	-	Mandible usually involved

Table 11.5. Specificity of fractures for non-accidental injury

High specificity
Classic metaphyseal lesions
Rib fractures, especially posteriorly
Unusual fractures, e.g. spine, acromion
Moderate specificity
Multiple fractures, especially bilateral
Fractures of different ages
Digital fractures, especially in a non-ambulant child
Complex skull fractures
Low specificity
Subperiosteal new bone formation
Clavicle fractures
Long bone shaft fractures
Linear skull fractures

References

Ablin DS, Greenspan A, Reinhart M, Grix A (1990) Differentiation of child abuse from osteogenesis imperfecta. AJR Am J Roentgenol 154:1035–1046

Ablin DS, Sane SM (1997) Non-accidental injury: confusion with temporary brittle bone disease and mild osteogenesis imperfecta. Pediatr Radiol 27:111–113

ACR revised standards for SS in children. http://www.acr.org/s_acr/bin.asp?TrackID=&SID=1&DID=12286&CID=543&VID=2&DOC=File.PDF. (accessed 10 September 2006)

Akbarnia B, Torg JS, Kirkpatrick J et al (1974) Manifestations of the battered-child syndrome. J Bone Joint Surg Am 56:1159–1166

Alexander CJ (1976) Effect of growth rate on the strength of the growth plate shaft junction. Skeletal Radiol 1:67–76

Alexander J, Gregg JEM, Quinn MW (1987) Femoral fractures at caesarean section. Case reports. Br J Obstet Gynaecol 94:273

Amir J, Katz K, Grunebaum M et al (1988) Fractures in premature infants. J Paediatr Orthop 8:41–44

Anderson WA (1982) The significance of femoral fractures in children. Ann Emerg Med 11:174–177
Anilkumar A, Fender LJ, Broderick NJ et al (2006) The role of the follow-up chest radiograph in suspected non-accidental injury. Pediatr Radiol 36:216–218
Astley R (1979) Metaphyseal fractures in osteogenesis imperfecta. Br J Radiol 52:441–443
Augarten A, Laufer J, Szeinberg A et al (1993) Child abuse, osteogenesis imperfecta and the grey zone between them. J Med 24:171–175
Barrett IR, Kozlowski K (1979) The battered child syndrome. Australas Radiol 23:72–82
Barsness KA, Cha ES, Bensard DD et al (2003) The positive predictive value of rib fractures as an indicator of nonaccidental trauma in children. J Trauma 54:1107–1110
Beals RK, Tufts E (1983) Fractured femur in infancy: the role of child abuse. J Pediatr Orthop 3:583–586
Brill PW, Winchester P, Kleinman PK (1998) Differential diagnosis I. Diseases simulating abuse In: Kleinman PK (ed) Diagnostic imaging of child abuse, 2nd edn. Mosby, St Louis, pp 178–196
BSPR NAI standard for skeletal surveys. http://www.bspr.org.uk/ (accessed 10 September 2006)
Caffey J (1946) Multiple fractures in the long bones of infants suffering from chronic subdural haematoma. AJR Am J Roentgenol 56:163–173
Caffey J (1957) Some traumatic lesions in growing bones other than fractures and dislocations: clinical and radiological features. Br J Radiol 30:225–238
Carty H (1988) Brittle or battered. Arch Dis Child 63:350–352
Carty H, Pierce A (2002) Non-accidental injury: a retrospective analysis of a large cohort. Eur Radiol 12:2919–2925
Carty H, Shaw D (1988) Osteogenesis imperfecta type IV A. (Letter) Acta Paediatr Scand 77:752–754
Chapman S (1992) The radiological dating of injuries. Arch Dis Child 67:1063–1065
Chapman S, Hall CM (1997) Non-accidental injury or brittle bones. Pediatr Radiol 27:106–110
Crilly R (1972) Longitudinal overgrowth of the chicken radius. J Anat 112:11–18
Cumming WA (1979) Neonatal skeletal fractures. Birth trauma or child abuse? J Can Assoc Radiol 30:30–33
Curran JS (1981) Birth associated injury. Clin Perinatol 8:111–19
Dahlenburg SL, Bishop NJ, Lucas A (1989) Are preterm infants at risk for subsequent fractures? Arch Dis Child 64:1384–1393
Ebbin AJ, Gollub MH, Stein AM et al (1969) Battered child syndrome at the Los Angeles County General Hospital. Am J Dis Child 118: 660–667
Feldman KW, Brewer DF (1984) Child abuse, cardiopulmonary resuscitation and rib fractures. Pediatrics 73:339–342
Galleno H, Oppenheim WL (1982) The battered child syndrome revisited. Clin Orthop 162:11–19
Graif M, Stahl-Kent V, Ben-Ami T et al (1988) Sonographic detection of occult bone fractures. Pediatr Radiol 18:383–385
Haase GM, Ortz VN, Stakianakis GN et al (1980) The value of radionuclide bone scanning in the early recognition of deliberate child abuse. J Trauma 20:873–875
Herndon WA (1983) Child abuse in a military population. J Pediatr Orthop 3:73–76
Jaudes PK (1984) Comparison of radiography and radionuclide bone scanning in the detection of child abuse. Pediatrics 73:166–168
John N, Maguire S, Mann MK et al (2005) Does cardiopulmonary resuscitation cause rib fractures in children? A systematic review. Arch Dis Child 90 [Suppl 11]:A41–A43
Johnson K, Chapman S, Hall CM (2004) Skeletal injuries associated with sexual abuse. Pediatr Radiol 34:620–623
Kemp AM, Butler A, Morris S et al (2006) Which radiological investigations should be performed to identify fractures in suspected child abuse? Clin Radiol 61:723–736
Kempe CH, Silverman FN, Steele BF et al (1962) The battered child syndrome. JAMA 181:17–24
King J, Diefendorf D, Apthorp J et al (1988) Analysis of 429 fractures in 189 battered children. J Pediatr Orthop 8:585–589
Kleinman PK, Marks SC Jr (1995) Relationship of the subperiosteal bone collar to the metaphyseal lesions in abused infants. J Bone Joint Surg Am 77:1471–1476
Kleinman PK, Marks SC Jr (1996) A regional approach to the classic metaphyseal lesion in abused infants: the proximal tibia. AJR Am J Roentgenol 166:421–426
Kleinman PK, Marks SC Jr (1998) A regional approach to the classic metaphyseal lesion in abused infants: the distal femur. AJR Am J Roentgenol 170:43–47
Kleinman PK, Marks SC, Adams VI, et al (1988) Factors affecting visualisation of posterior rib fractures in abused infants. AJR Am J Roentgenol 150:635–638
Kleinman PK, Marks SC, Blackbourne B (1986) The metaphyseal lesion in abused infants: a radiologic-histopathologic study. AJR Am J Roentgenol 146:895–905
Kleinman PK, Belanger PL, Karellas A et al (1991) Normal metaphyseal radiologic variants not to be confused with findings of infant abuse. AJR Am J Roentgenol 156:781–783
Kleinman PK, Nimkin K, Spevak MR et al (1996) Follow-up skeletal surveys in suspected child abuse. AJR Am J Roentgenol 167:893–896
Kogutt MS, Swischuk LE, Fagan CJ (1974) Patterns of injury and significance of uncommon fractures in the battered child syndrome. AJR Am J Roentgenol 121:143–149
Kowal-Vern A, Paxton TP, Ros SP et al (1992) Fractures in the under-3-year-old age cohort. Clin Pediatr (Phila) 31:653–659
Krugman RD (1997) Child protection policy. In: Helfer ME, Kempe RS, Krugman RD (eds) The battered child. University of Chicago Press, Chicago
Kwon DS, Spevak MR, Fletcher K et al (2002) Physiologic subperiosteal new bone formation. AJR Am J Roentgenol 179:985–988
Labbe J (2005) Ambroise Tardeau: the man and his work on child maltreatment a century before Kempe. Child Abuse Negl 29:311–324
Lauer B, Broeck ET, Grossman M (1974) Battered child syndrome: review of 130 patients with controls. Pediatrics 54:67–70
Loder RT, Bookout C (1991) Fracture patterns in battered children. J Orthop Trauma 5:428–433
Mandelstam SA, Cook D, Fitzgerald M, Ditchfield MR (2003) Complementary use of radiological skeletal survey and bone scintigraphy in detection of bony injuries in suspected child abuse. Arch Dis Child 88:387–390
Markowitz RI, Hubbard AM, Harty MP et al (1993) Sonography of the knee in normal and abused infants. Pediatr Radiol 23:264–267
Matthew MO, Ramamohan N, Bennet C (1998) Importance of bruising associated with paediatric fractures: prospective observational study. Br Med J 317:1117–1118

Mendelson KL (2005) Critical review of 'temporary brittle bone disease'. Pediatr Radiol 35:1036–1040
Merten DF, Carpenter BL (1990) Radiologic imaging of inflicted injury in the child abuse syndrome. Pediatr Clin North Am 37:815–837
Merten DF, Radkowski MA, Leonidas JC (1983) The abused child. A radiological reappraisal. Radiology 146:377–381
Miller ME, Hangartner TN (1999) Temporary brittle bone disease: association with decreased fetal movement and osteopenia. Calcif Tissue Int 54:137–143
Ng CS, Hall CM (1998) Costochondral junction fractures and intra-abdominal trauma in non-accidental injury (child abuse). Pediatr Radiol 28:671–676
Nimkin K, Kleinman PK, Teeger S et al (1995) Distal humeral physeal injuries in child abuse: MR imaging and ultrasonography findings. Pediatr Radiol 25:562–565
O'Connor JF, Cohen J (1998) Dating fractures. In: Kleinman PK (ed) Diagnostic imaging of child abuse., 2nd edn. Mosby, St Louis, pp 168–177
Ogden JA (1990) Injury to the immature skeleton. In: Touloukian RJ (ed) Pediatric trauma. Mosby Year Book, St Louis, pp 399–439
Paterson CR, McAllion S, Miller R (1983) Osteogenesis imperfecta with dominant inheritance and normal sclerae. J Bone Joint Surg Br 65:35–39
Paterson CR, McAllion S, Shaw J (1987) Clinical and radiological features of osteogenesis imperfecta type IV A. Acta Paediatr Scand 76:548–552
Paterson CR, Burns J, McAllion SJ (1993) Osteogenesis imperfecta: the distinction from child abuse and the recognition of a variant form. Am J Med Genet 45:187–192
Perkins R, Skirving A (1987) Callus formation and the rate of healing of femoral fractures in patients with head injuries. J Bone Joint Surg Br 69:521–524
Prosser I, Maguire S, Harrison SK et al (2005) How old is this fracture? Radiologic dating of fractures in children: a systematic review. AJR Am J Roentgenol 184:1282–1286
Rex C, Kay PR (2000) Features of femoral fractures in nonaccidental injury. J Ped Orthop 20:411–413
Richman HA (2000) From a radiologist's judgement to public policy on child abuse and neglect: what have we wrought? Pediatr Radiol 30:219–228
Ruess L, O'Connor SC, Quinn WJ et al (2003) An animal model for the classic metaphyseal lesion of child abuse. Pediatr Radiol 33:S112
Ryan MG, Davis AA, Oates RK (1977) One hundred and eighty-seven cases of child abuse and neglect. Med J Aust 2:623–628
Scherl SA, Miller L, Lively N et al (2000) Accidental and nonaccidental femur fractures in children. Clin Orthop 376:96–105
Sillence DO, Senn A, Danks DM (1979) Genetic heterogeneity in osteogenesis imperfecta. J Med Genet 16:101–116
Smeets AJ, Robben SG, Meradji M (1990) Sonographically detected costo-chondral dislocation in an abused child: a new sonographic sign to the radiological spectrum of child abuse. Pediatr Radiol 20:566–567
Smith FW, Gilday DL, Ash JM et al (1980) Unsuspected costovertebral fractures demonstrated by bone scanning in the child abuse syndrome. Pediatr Radiol 10:103–106
Smith R (1995) Osteogenesis imperfecta, non-accidental injury and temporary brittle bone disease. Arch Dis Child 72:169–176
Spencer R (1987) The effect of head injury on fracture healing: a quantitative assessment. J Bone Joint Surg Br 69:525–528
Sty JR, Starshak RJ (1983) The role of bone scintigraphy in the evaluation of the suspected abused child. Radiology 146:369–375
Tardieu A (1860) Étude médico-légale sur les sévice et mauvais traitments exercés sur des enfants. Ann Hyg Publ Med Leg 13:361–398
Thomas P (1977) Rib fractures in infancy. Ann Radiol (Paris) 20:115–122
Thomas SA, Rosenfield NS, Leventhal JM et al (1991) Long-bone fractures in young children: distinguishing accidental injuries from child abuse. Pediatrics 88:471–476
US Department of Health and Human Services (2006) Health Resources and Services Administration, Maternal and Child Health Bureau. Child Health USA 2004. Rockville, Maryland, http://mchb.hrsa.gov/mchirc/chusa_04/pages/0431can.htm (accessed 10 September 2006)
Wang C-T (1997) Current trends in child abuse reporting and fatalities: the results of the Annual Fifty State Survey. Center for Child Abuse Prevention Research, Prevent Child Abuse America, Chicago
Williams RL, Connolly PT (2004) In children undergoing chest radiography what is the specificity of rib fractures for non-accidental injury? Arch Dis Child 89:490–492
Worlock P, Stower M, Barbor P (1986) Patterns of fractures in accidental and non-accidental injury in children: a comparative study. Br Med J 293:100–102
Zimmerman S, Makoroff K, Care M et al (2005) Utility of follow-up skeletal surveys in suspected child physical abuse evaluations. Child Abuse Negl 29:1075–1083

Pelvic Fractures

12

Karl J. Johnson and Ed Bache

CONTENTS

K. J. Johnson, MD, MRCP, FRCR
Consultant Radiologist, Radiology Department, Birmingham Children's Hospital, Steelhouse Lane, Birmingham, B4 6NH, UK
E. Bache, MD
Consultant Paediatric Orthopaedic Surgeon, Birmingham Children's Hospital, Steelhouse Lane, Birmingham, B4 6NH, UK

12.1 Introduction

Pelvic trauma in children can result in a wide variety of different fractures and soft tissue injuries; these range from isolated, relatively benign avulsion injuries to very complex multiple pelvic fractures and joint dissociations. The type of injury will depend on the causative mechanism as well as the age and development of the child. Compared with adults, pelvic fractures are relatively uncommon in children (Schlickwei and Keck 2005) and indicate a significant high energy impact.

When assessing pelvic fractures, it is important to have an understanding of the bony anatomy and the interrelationship of the supporting ligaments within the pelvis. Additionally, with children, knowledge of the normal stages of development and the timing of the appearances of ossification of the pelvis is needed. Understanding the anatomy and development allows a more accurate evaluation of the degree of pelvic instability and the mechanism of trauma that will occur following a fracture. This is because the principle aim in the management of these injuries is to achieve stability, maintain pelvic symmetry and promote normal growth (Rieger and Brug 1997).

12.2 Incidence

Paediatric pelvic ring fractures are rare. The incidence has been estimated to between 2%–7% of all childhood fractures (Ismail et al. 1996; Junkins et al. 2001). When one compares the admissions rates of large trauma centres, pelvic fractures in adults occur in about 10% of cases as opposed to less than 5% in children. With motor vehicle and pedestrian injuries, adults are twice as likely to suffer pelvic fractures as children (Demetriades et al. 2003). Pelvic fractures in children are more likely to be associated with a pedestrian injury rather than passenger injury.

The location of fractures will depend on the age of the child and the nature and degree of force involved. If the triradiate cartilage has fused, the pelvis can be regarded as being mature whilst if it remains unfused, the pelvis is regarded as immature (Schlickwei and Keck 2005). Fractures in children with an immature skeleton have a higher propensity for anterior ring, pubic rami and iliac wing fractures, with the majority being stable injuries. When the triradiate cartilage is fused, there is increased incidence of acetabular fractures and/or pubic sacroiliac diastasis. Instability is more common in the mature skeleton.

Avulsion fractures are more common in adolescents and are associated with a better outcome and less complications.

12.3 Anatomy

The pelvis is a ring structure, composed of three bones, the sacrum and paired innominate bones. The sacrum and innominate bones articulate posteriorly at the sacro-iliac joints. The pubic bones are united anteriorly by the fibrous symphysis pubis. Each innominate bone has three primary centres of ossification, the ileum, ischium and pubis. These three centres converge at the triradiate cartilage and fuse at approximately 16–18 years of age. The pubis and ischium fuse in the region of the inferior pubic ramus at 6–7 years of age. At the time of fusion there may be an asymptomatic mass, the ischiopubic synchondrosis, which will be clearly visible on a radiograph and should not be confused with a fracture or tumour. Radiographs of the younger child will clearly demonstrate these separate ossification centres. Additional secondary ossification centres include the iliac crest, ischial apophysis, anterior inferior iliac spine, pubic tubercle, ischial spine, and lateral wing of the sacrum. These secondary ossification centres occur during adolescence and are often sites of avulsion injuries (Theumann et al. 2002). The secondary ossification centres should not be confused with fractures (Fig. 12.1a,b).

The stability of this bony ring is maintained by strong supporting ligaments which criss-cross the pelvis. Posteriorly, there is the strong posterior tension band which includes, the posterior and intraosseous sacro-iliac ligaments. These ligaments are some of the strongest in the body and run from the posterior and inferior iliac spines to the sacral ridge. There is a more superficial component, the posterior sacral iliac ligament that runs inferiorly to blend with the sacro-tuberous ligaments. These posterior ligaments resist vertical translation between the iliac bones and the sacrum (Theumann et al. 2002).

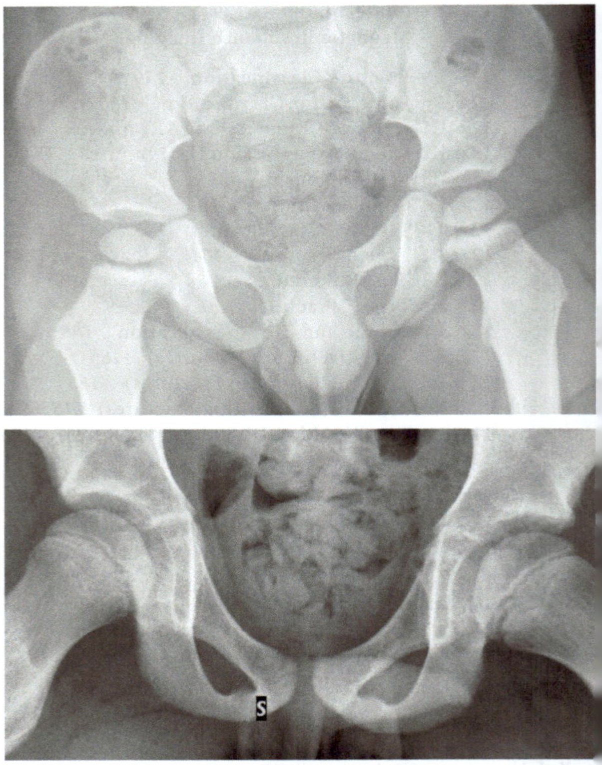

Fig. 12.1. **a** AP radiograph in a 5-year-old boy. The triradiate cartilage and the ischio-pubic synchondrosis, have yet to ossify and are seen as radiolucent areas. **b** AP radiograph in an 8-year-old boy. The ischio-pubic synchondrosis (*S*) is seen as a prominent area of ossification

Anteriorly the sacroiliac, sacro-spinous and symphyseal ligaments are transversely orientated to support the pelvic floor and resist external rotation. There are superior symphyseal ligaments which support the pubic symphysis.

The ilio-lumbar ligaments extend from the transverse process of the lower lumbar vertebrae to the superficial aspects of the anterior sacral iliac ligaments. Traction forces on these ligaments may avulse part of the transverse process and are associated with pelvic fractures (Fig. 12.2a,b).

The iliac artery and its branches run through the pelvis creating a highly vascular area. These arteries may be disrupted by shearing forces or compression injuries and can be a cause of significant blood loss resulting in hypovolaemic shock.

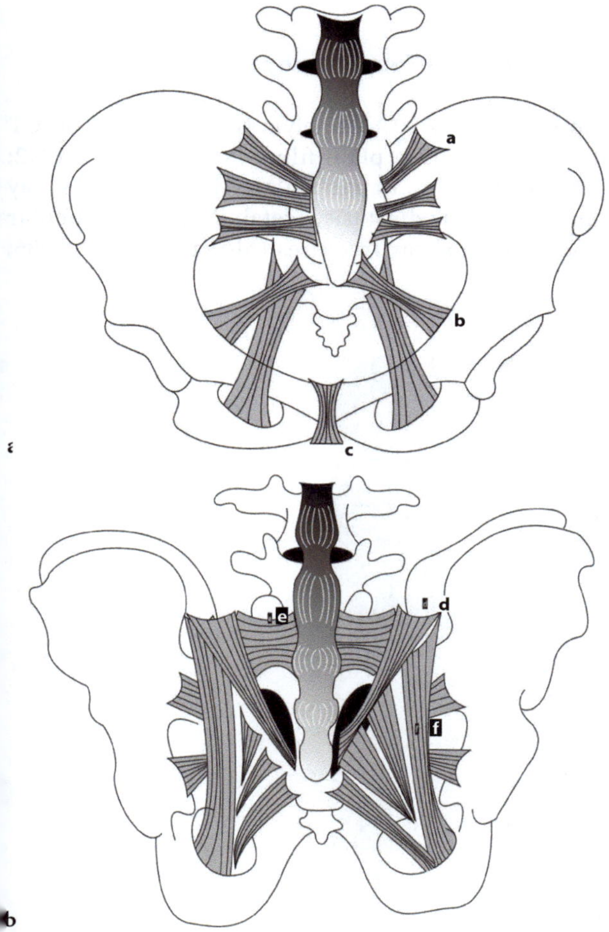

Fig. 12.2a,b. Anterior and posterior views of the pelvis **(a,b)** showing the supporting muscles around the pelvis. *a* Anterior sacro-iliac ligaments; *b* sacro spinous ligament; *c* symphysis pubis; *d* posterior sacro-iliac ligament; *e* inter-osseous sacro iliac ligament; *f* sacrotuberous ligament

12.4 Anatomical and Physiological Variations in Children

There are a number of anatomical differences between children and adults. The paediatric skeleton is more elastic than in adults, particularly around the sacroiliac joints and pubic symphysis which allows greater absorption of energy before the joint and ligaments become disrupted. A high energy impact may cause deformity of the bones rather than the fractures and joint disruption that occurs in adulthood.

At the site of many of the muscle attachments are a number of apophyses which are separated from the bone by growth cartilage. An apophysis is essentially a centre of ossification which does not lead to longitudinal growth. In children, avulsion injuries are more common at these sites, which is a reflection of the presence of the relatively weaker cartilage in these regions.

The growth plates of the ilium, ischium and pubis do not fuse completely until late in adolescence which gives the paediatric pelvis a greater opportunity for remodelling and recovery. In some cases, trauma around the growth centres can lead to premature fusion, asymmetrical development and possibly limb length discrepancy.

The triradiate cartilage and ischiopubic synchondrosis may be seen as radiolucent structures or in the older child, it may appear as an area of irregular ossification and this should not be confused with a fracture or bone tumour. Irregular areas of ossification may also be seen around the acetabulum and the iliac crest, which again are features of normal development.

12.5 Imaging

It is standard teaching on many paediatric life saving courses, that if a child is involved in a significant traumatic episode, an anterior-posterior (AP) radiograph of the pelvis along with a lateral cervical spine and chest X-ray should be obtained as part of the child's acute assessment. The rationale for this approach is that pelvic fractures can result in significant haemorrhage and be the cause for a child to be shocked. While the use of the AP radiograph is useful in initial assessment of the pelvic trauma, it is not a sensitive investigation. If there is any clinical concern about a pelvic injury then a CT examination should be performed. CT is now the investigation of choice to detect pelvic fractures, in determining the severity of an injury and in deciding the need for any surgical intervention.

12.5.1 Radiographs

The AP radiograph is useful in demonstrating pelvic fractures, but it may miss some injuries (Berg et al. 1996). While additional views such as the inlet and outlet, may detect further fractures, their use is no longer indicated if there is reasonable access to CT imaging.

The AP radiograph should be closely reviewed for signs of pelvic ring discontinuity by identifying various anatomical lines, the absence of which implies ring disruption or a fracture. These lines are the ischio-ilial line, ilio-pectineal line, and the anterior and posterior acetabular walls. The ilio-ischial line is formed by the posterior structures of the pelvis and the ilio-pectineal by the anterior acetabular structures (Ersoy et al. 1995) (Fig. 12.3).

Injuries of the posterior pelvic ring, particularly diastasis of the sacroiliac joint, may be better appreciated on pelvic inlet views which are orientated at 25° in a caudal direction. Outlet views may be useful in appreciating displacement in the vertical plane.

Avulsion fractures of the posterior inferior iliac spine and the transverse process of the 5th lumbar vertebra are rare but indicative of severe trauma. The former occurs as a result of external rotation of the hemi-pelvis which avulses the sacrospinous ligament at its insertion. The latter injury results when the ilio-lumber ligament is avulsed from the tip of the transverse process of L5 by shearing forces in the vertical plane. These injuries should arouse suspicion of pelvic instability.

12.5.2 Computerised Tomography (CT)

Approximately 30% of pelvic fractures seen on CT can be missed on plain films (Resnik et al. 1992; Berg et al. 1996). In particular, AP radiographs may miss sacroiliac diastasis, acetabular, intra-articular and vertical shear fractures (Montana et al. 1986;

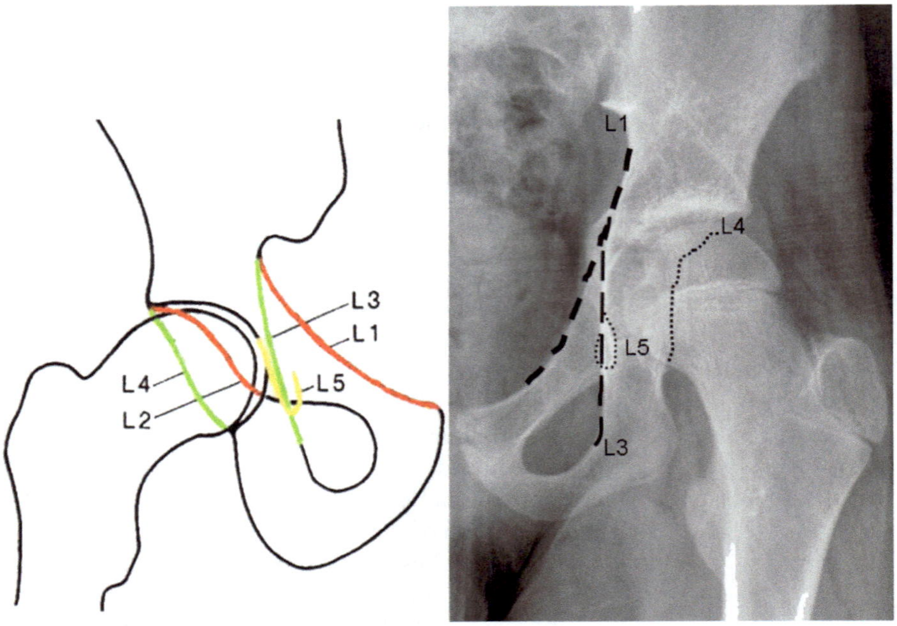

Fig. 12.3. *L1* = iliopubic or iliopectineal (arcuate) line. *L2* = anterior rim of the acetabulum. *L3* = ilioischial line, formed by the posterior portion of the quadrilateral plate (surface) of the iliac bone. *L4* = posterior rim of the acetabulum. *L5* = teardrop, formed by the medial acetabular wall, the acetabular notch, and the anterior portion of the quadrilateral plate

Resnik et al. 1992). CT will also provide additional information regarding soft tissue injury.

Some authors argue that if a child is to undergo an abdominal or pelvic CT for trauma evaluation then the AP radiograph is superfluous (Ersoy et al. 1995) and the screening pelvic radiograph should be reserved for patients in whom abdominal CT is not indicated.

12.5.2.1 CT Technique

The CT technique used in each case will depend on local machine specification and expertise. Slice thickness should be low enough to allow multiplanar (1.0–3.0 mm) reconstructions. Multiplanar reconstructions are useful in the interpretation of complex fractures and acetabular injuries. Helical CT scanning will improve this reconstruction ability. An associated abdominal examination is nearly always mandatory because of the high risk of concomitant injuries in children, so post contrast images should be standard. The timing of the contrast injection should demonstrate the vascular filling of the liver and of the major vessels within the pelvis. This timing will alter due to the age of the patient and if there is any cardiovascular compromise. Delayed images of the pelvis when there will be a contrast filled bladder are potentially useful to detect bladder rupture. Where possible, a reduction in mA from normal adult settings should always be considered as this will significantly reduce the dose to the child, who is more radiosensitive. This dose reduction can usually be achieved without adversely compromising image quality (Paterson et al. 2001).

12.5.3 Magnetic Resonance Imaging (MRI)

MR imaging has been used in particular circumstances, such as identifying intra-articular splinters, assessment of the femoral head and detecting hidden fractures, but these have been mainly performed in the elderly (Potter et al. 1994). MR imaging can be used to assess soft tissue changes around the SI joints when disruption has been identified. It has some value in assessing damage and early fusion of the triradiate cartilage (Schlickwei and Keck 2005). Its routine use in evaluating the traumatic paediatric pelvic injury has yet to be properly assessed.

12.6 Fracture Classification

The classification of pelvic fractures has been widely discussed for adult patients. In general, the classification of any paediatric injury follows adult practice, but there is less data available on paediatric injuries. The aim of any classification system is to try and determine the mechanism of injury, assess the degree of instability, aid appropriate management and if possible predict outcome. The multitude of classification systems makes comparison of incidence, mechanism of injury, morbidity and mortality between different studies difficult.

Prior to the 1980s and the routine use of CT imaging, most authors used the terms Malgaine, straddle and open book type to describe pelvic fractures. This provided limited detail regarding the type of mechanism of injury and was not particularly useful in planning the management of the patient.

Since then classification systems that related the pattern of fracture to the nature of the applied force have been introduced (Pennal et al. 1980b). This is described as the force-vector classification. There have been suggested refinements that have identified a progression in the severity of injuries and identified those fractures which are more likely to be unstable or be associated with pelvic haemorrhage and genitourinary injury (Young et al. 1986a,b; Dalal et al. 1989; Ben-Menachem et al. 1991).

Further classification systems have been described, aimed at improving the link between causation, stability and management (Dalal et al. 1989; Tile 1996a,b). The Tile AO classification identifies three types of fracture (A, B and C) based on the stability of the pelvic ring and the posterior supporting structures.

A primary paediatric classification based on a retrospective review of children's pelvic injuries that is based upon the severity of the fracture and associated prognosis has been described (Torode and Zieg 1985).

Any fracture can ultimately be classified in as many ways as there are classification systems. As with all aspects of radiology, it is important that the radiologist and treating physician use the same system and are comfortable and accepting of the classification system being used. As a consequence of the complexity of mechanisms and forces that result in acute pelvic fractures, all the injuries should be considered in the context of polytrauma management, rather than in isolation. Any classification system must therefore be seen only as a general guide to treatment. The management of each patient requires careful, individualized decision making.

12.6.1 Force Vector Classification

The forces which cause pelvic fractures are applied in three primary directions or vectors. These vectors are anterior and posterior compression (AP), lateral compression (LC) and vertical shear forces. It is possible that more than one of these vectors can be applied to the pelvis at any one time which will result in hybrid pattern and a more complex fracture (Young et al. 1986).

12.6.1.1 Anterior Compression (AP) Injuries

With anterior compression injuries, the force is applied in the AP plane, usually as a result of head-on road traffic accidents. When the compressive force is applied to the pelvis, it causes external rotation of the iliac wings, with the posterior margin of the sacroiliac joints acting as a pivot. Initially, there will be fractures of the pubic rami and disruption of the pubic symphysis. Greater degrees of external rotation of the pelvis will cause disruption of the sacral tuberous, sacral spinous and anterior sacral iliac ligaments. Finally, there is disruption of the posterior sacral iliac ligaments, causing detachment of the innominate bone from the axial skeleton. With AP compression fractures, the degree of instability will depend on the amount of force applied, so a further sub-classification is used to reflect this instability.

12.6.1.1.1 AP Type I

This is the commonest type of fracture where the majority of the impact of the trauma is confined to the anterior pubic arch and the posterior ligaments remain intact. AP radiographs of the pelvis demonstrate fractures of the pubic rami which characteristically have a vertical orientation. There may be widening and disruption of the pubic symphysis. The posterior ligaments remain intact but there may be some slight widening of the anterior sacroiliac joint from ligamental stretch rather than disruption. These injuries essentially require non-operative management (Figs. 12.4, 12.5).

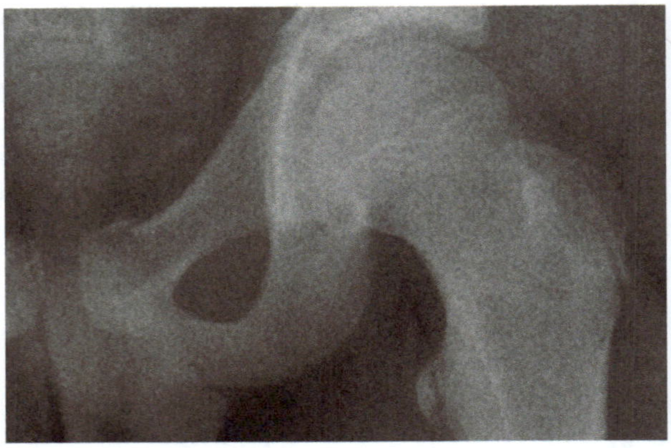

Fig. 12.4. AP Type 1 injury with a vertical fracture line in the supra-pubic ramus

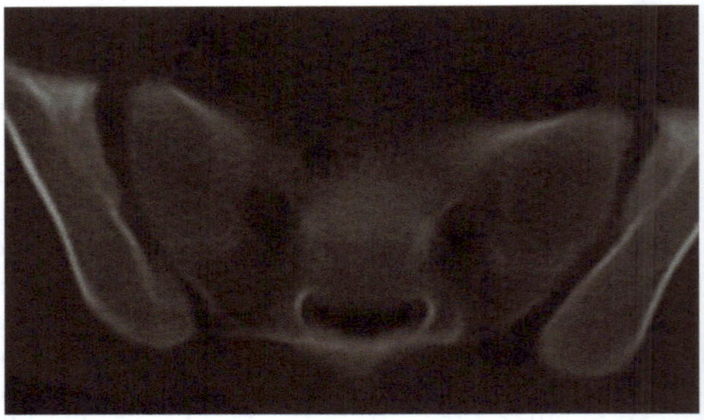

Fig. 12.5. Axial CT of the sacro-iliac joints. There is very slight widening of the right sacro-iliac joint but the posterior sacro-iliac ligaments are intact maintaining stability.

12.6.1.1.2 AP Type 2

There may be fractures of the pubic rami as in Type I. There is further diastasis of the anterior aspect of the sacroiliac joints and these are classically referred to as the open book or spun pelvis type injuries. Sacroiliac diastasis is best assessed by CT. There may be some partial instability on AP compression. In children, there may be fracturing of the adjacent bone rather than ligament rupture. This is a reflection of the relative strength of the ligaments compared with bone in the growing skeleton (Figs. 12.6, 12.7).

12.6.1.1.3
AP Type 3

This is the most severe type and results in total sacroiliac joint disruption. Features of the Type 1 and 2 pattern may be present. There is widening of the sacroiliac joint and there is diastasis both posteriorly as well as anteriorly due to the posterior sacroiliac ligament rupture. On clinical examination, the hemi-pelvis is unstable in all directions of force and typically requires operative stabilisation. It is possible for the sacroiliac joint to remain intact but there is fracture of the sacroiliac bone. Complications include bladder rupture, and vascular injury (Figs. 12.8, 12.9).

12.6.1.2
Lateral Compression (LC) Injuries

With lateral compression injuries, the forces are applied to the side of the pelvis. Lateral compression injuries are also subdivided to reflect the different degrees of severity.

12.6.1.2.1
LC Type I

This is the least severe type of injury pattern with internal rotation of the innominate bone which pivots on the anterior margin of the sacroiliac joint. There may be compression fractures of the sacrum. Pubic rami fractures are common and typically have a known oblique orientation but can be comminuted, compared with the vertical fractures of AP compression injuries (Figs. 12.10, 12.11).

12.6.1.2.2
LC Type 2

The lateral force has a more anterior orientation which will cause oblique pubic rami fractures, disruption of the posterior sacroiliac ligaments and fractures of the ileum (Figs. 12.12, 12.13).

12.6.1.2.3
LC Type 3

This is the so-called 'windswept' pelvis. There is internal rotation of the pelvis on the side of impact but external rotation of the opposite side. As a consequence, there are lateral compression injuries on one side of the pelvis with AP compression fractures on the other.

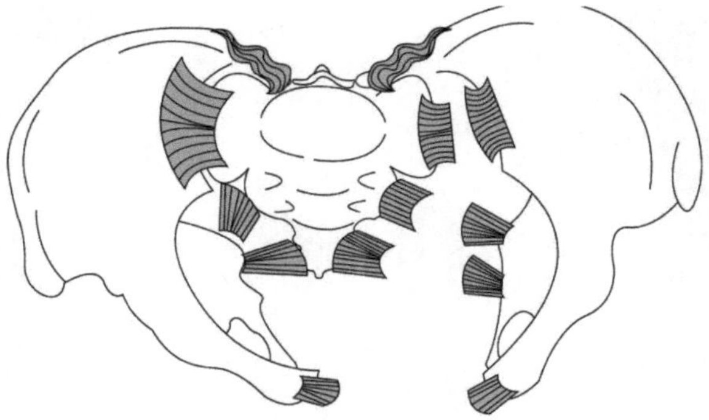

Fig. 12.6. AP Type 2 compression injury. (Images courtesy of Dr.Hughes)

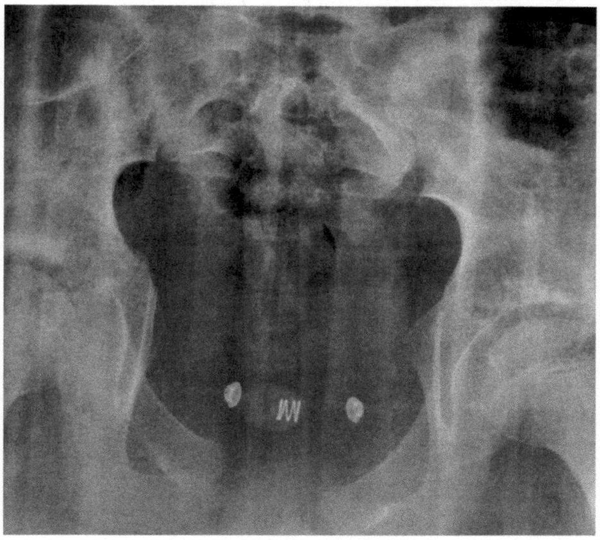

Fig. 12.7. There is diastasis of the symphysis pubis and widening of the left sacro-iliac joint. Stability was maintained as the posterior sacro-iliac ligaments remain intact. This is an AP Type 2 injury

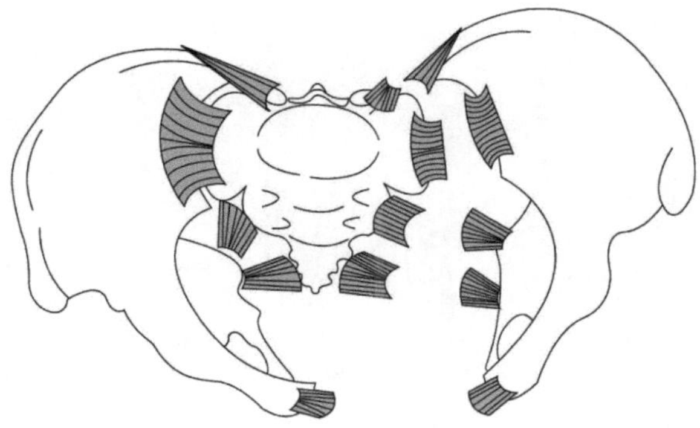

Fig. 12.8. AP Type 3 compression injury. (Images courtesy of Dr.Hughes)

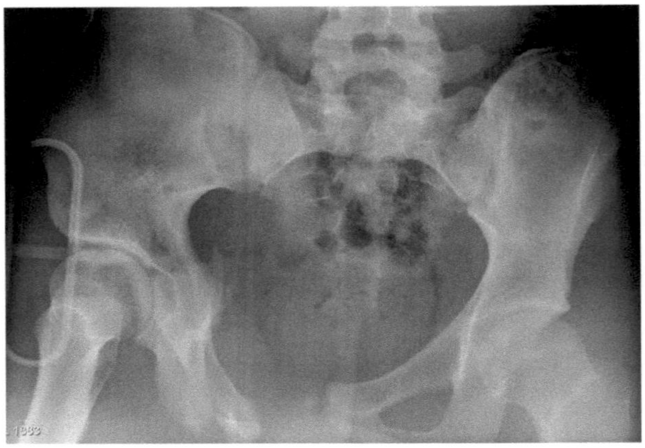

Fig. 12.9. Wide diastasis of the symphysis and of the right sacro-iliac joint. An AP Type 3 injury

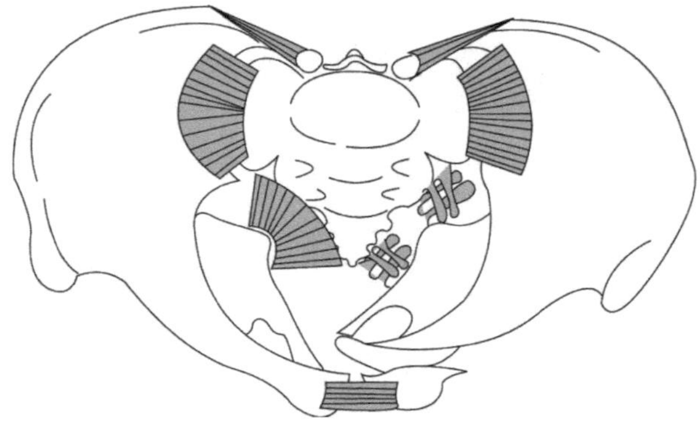

Fig. 12.10. An LC Type 1 lateral compression injury

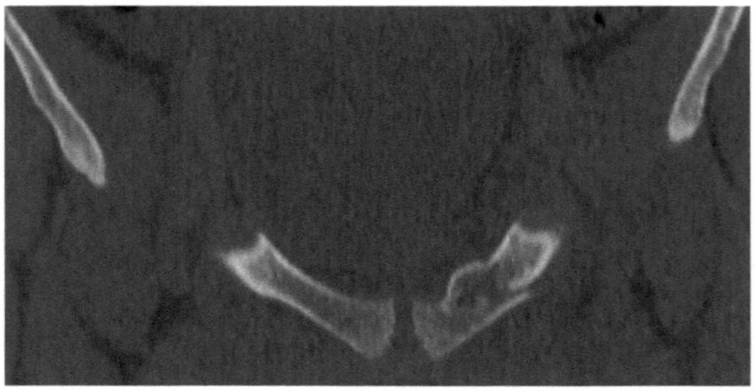

Fig. 12.11. CT coronal reconstruction showing a horizontal fracture to the left pubic ramus, indicative of lateral compression

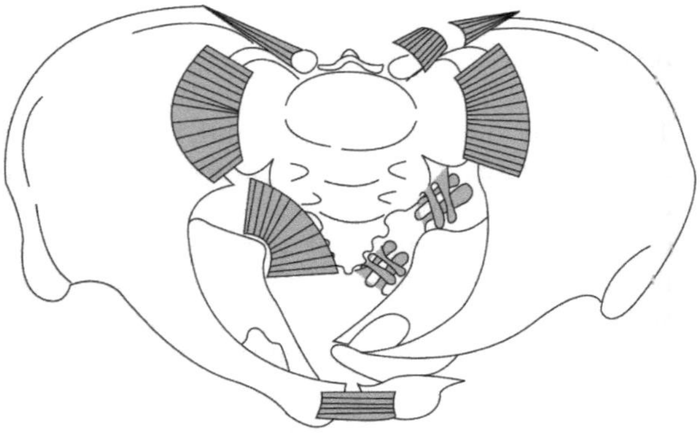

Fig. 12.12. An LC Type 2 lateral compression injury

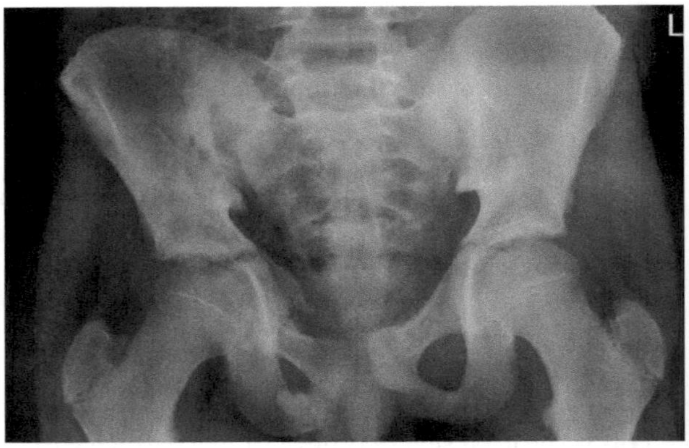

Fig. 12.13. Oblique fracture of the right supra-pubic ramus and of the right iliac blade, indicating an LC Type 2 injury

These opposing causative vectors must be recognised, as operative management could exacerbate the injury if the stabilisation forces are not applied correctly.

12.6.1.3
Vertical Shear

This is usually the result of forces transmitted through the axial skeleton from an impact into the head and shoulders through to the lower limbs. There may be symphyseal diastasis, anterior arch fractures or posterior disruption of the sacroiliac joints with cephalic displacement. Vertical injuries are often severe with disruption of all the ligaments plus associated pelvic instability. Radiographs demonstrate ipsilateral or contralateral pubic rami fractures, with disruption of the sacroiliac joint. The major differentiating feature from compression injuries is the cephalic displacement of the pelvis on the side of the impact (Fig. 12.14).

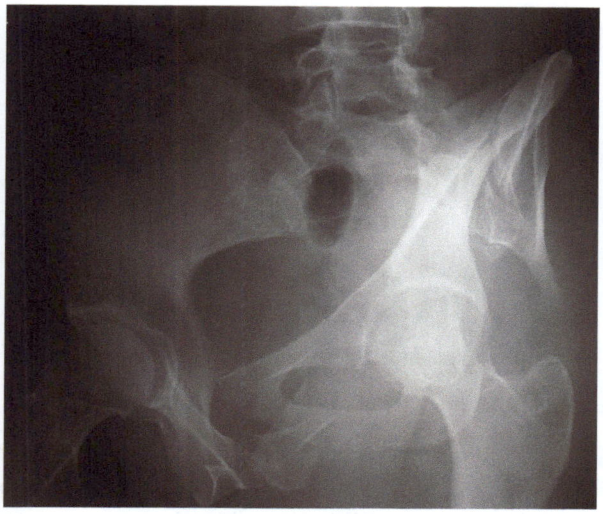

Fig. 12.14. A severe disruption of the pelvis with disruption of the symphysis and sacro-iliac joint. There is marked displacement of the left side

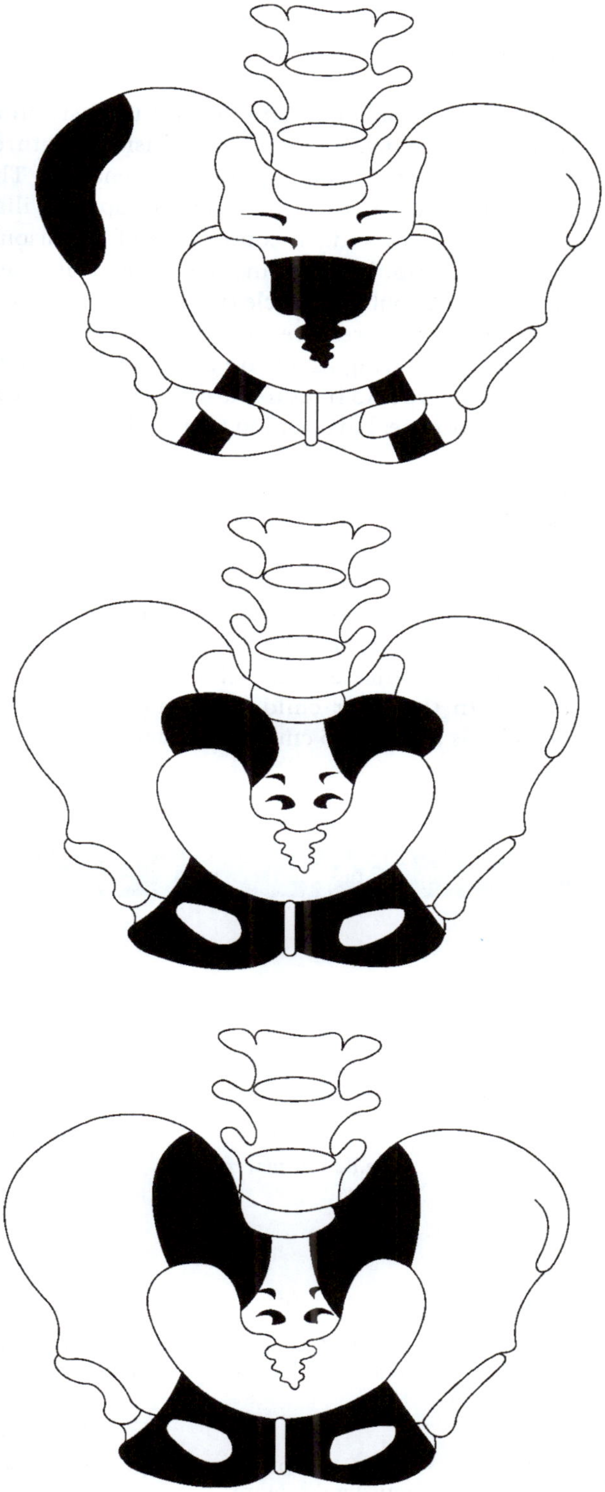

Fig. 12.15a–c. The Tile classification. The *black areas* represent fracture zones. No displacement of the posterior arch. Incomplete disruption of the posterior arch (partially stable). Complete disruption of the posterior arch (unstable)

12.6.1.4
Complex Injuries

Complex injuries are a combination of lateral compression and anterior compression injuries. It is important to recognise the complexity in view of the need to apply the appropriate external fixation.

12.6.2
TILE AO Classification

This classification system aims to link management and prognostic evaluation with the imaging findings. It is based on the work of Tile and the Association for Osteosynthesis and relates to the site of fractures within the pelvic ring (Fig. 12.15a–c). There are three classifications, A, B and C. In type A fractures, the pelvic ring is stable, type B is partially stable this includes the "open-book" and "bucket-handle" fractures which are caused by external- and internal-rotation forces, respectively. In type C injuries, there is complete disruption of the posterior sacroiliac complex. In adults, type A lesions represent 52%, type B 27% and type C 21% (Theumann et al. 2002). The classification is shown in Table 12.1.

12.6.2.1
Type A Fractures

These are incomplete fractures with no disruption of the pelvic ring. Type A1 are avulsion fractures which commonly occur in athletic teenagers. The avulsion may be from the anterior-superior iliac spine, caused by sudden contraction of Sartorious, anterior-inferior ischial spine (rectus femoris insertion), and the pubic tubercle (pectineus insertion).

Type A2 fractures are of the iliac wing, pubic rami or pelvic wing which are minimally displaced and stable. Type A3 fractures are those of the coccyx or sacrococcygeal dislocation (Fig. 12.16).

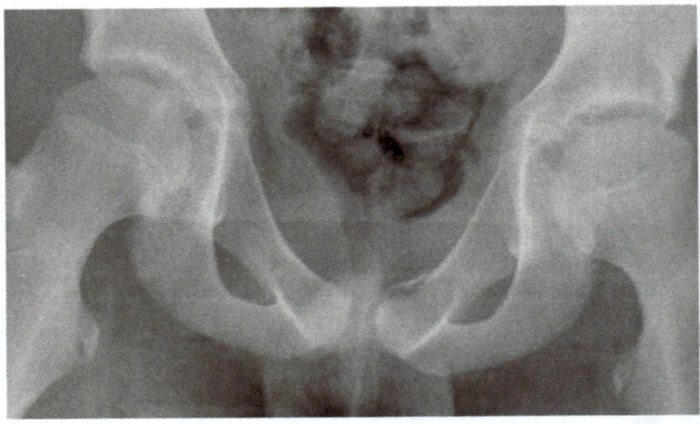

Fig. 12.16. Fracture of the left superior pubic ramus

12.6.2.2
Type B Fractures

These relate to fractures or disruption of the pubic symphysis and are associated with anterior sacro-iliac joint disruption. The posterior iliac ligament complex is unaffected and pelvic stability is maintained. In the older child, widening of the pubic symphysis beyond 2.5 cm is associated with disruption of the pelvic floor or sacrospinous ligaments. In the younger child, a considerable proportion of the pubic rami is unossified and this measurement is less reliable.

Type B1 fractures are the open book type fracture with external rotation of both iliac wings and Type B2 fractures are lateral compression injuries. Type B3 is the classical open book type fracture (Fig. 12.17).

Table 12.1. Tile/AO classification of pelvic fractures

Mechanism	Classification	Features	Stability
Type A		A1: apophyseal avulsions	Stable
		A2: stable iliac wing fractures or stable minimally displaced ring fracture	
		A3: sacro-coccygeal fractures	
Type B1	External rotation or "open-book" injuries	B1.1: unilateral antero- or sacro-iliac disruption	Partially stable (complete rupture of anterior arch, incomplete rupture of posterior arch)
		B1.2: sacral fracture	
Lateral	Type B2 Internal rotation injuries	B2.1: anterior compression fracture of the sacrum	Partially stable (complete rupture of anterior arch, Compression incomplete rupture of posterior arch)
		B2.2: partial sacroiliac joint fracture	
		B2.3: incomplete posterior iliac wing fracture	
Anterior	Type B3 Bilateral external rotation (bilateral open book)	B3.1: bilateral B1	Partially stable (complete rupture of anterior arch, incomplete rupture of posterior arch)
		B3.2: B1 and B2	
		B3.3: bilateral B2	
Vertical	Type C C1: complete unilateral rupture	C1.1: iliac fracture	Unstable (complete rupture of both anterior and posterior arches)
		C1.2: sacroiliac dislocation	
		C1.3: sacral fracture	
		C2: bilateral injury (B+C types)	
		C3: bilateral complete rupture	

12.6.2.3
Type C Fractures

These fractures are unstable injuries with disruption of the posterior sacro-iliac complex. These injuries are very rare in children. In Type C1 injuries, there is a unilateral injury of the hemi-pelvis. Type C2 are bilateral injuries of the pelvis with some partial stability on one side. Type C3 are bilateral injuries in which both hemi-pelvis are unstable.

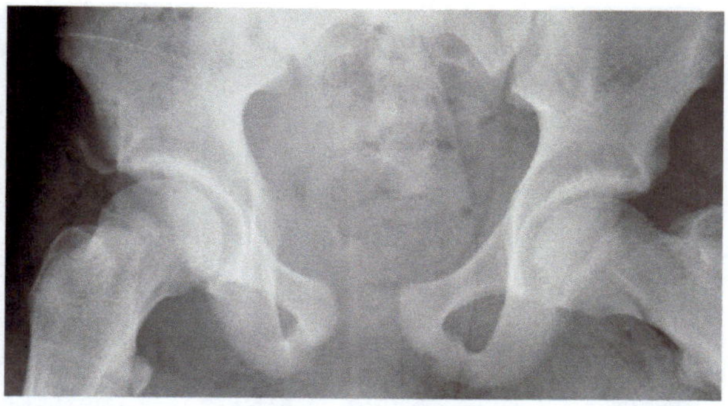

Fig. 12.17. Widening of the pubic symphysis with a fracture of the superior pubic ramus and avulsion injury from the iliac spine on the right

12.6.3
Torode and Zieg Classification

In recognition of the fact that fractures of the immature pelvis behave in a different fashion than those of adults, Torode and Zieg proposed a new classification which attempts to correlate the type of fracture with associated injuries and expected outcome (Torode and Zieg 1985) (Fig. 12.18).

12.6.3.1
Type I (Avulsion Fractures)

These are analogous to the Tile A fractures. These patients should not require admission to hospital and operative intervention is not required except if there is significant displacement in an individual who is a keen athlete (Fig. 12.19).

12.6.3.2
Type II (Iliac Wing Fractures)

These injuries are less common than similar injuries in adults and usually result from direct trauma to the pelvis.

12.6.3.3
Type III (Simple Ring Fractures)

This group includes fractures of the pubic rami or symphysis, because of the elasticity of the child's pelvis, significant displacement can occur without damage to the posterior elements of the pelvic ring (Fig. 12.20).

12.6.3.4
Type IV (Ring Disruption Fractures)

This group of fractures results in an unstable segment of the pelvic ring. It includes bilateral fractures

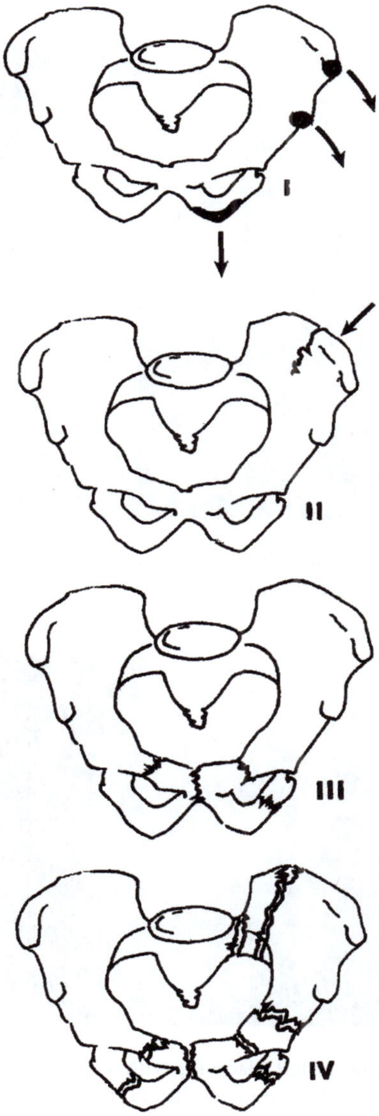

Fig. 12.18. Torode and Zeig classification of pelvic fractures. Type I avulsion injuries. Type II Iliac wing fractures (stability of the ligament complex). Type III simple ring fractures (stable). Type IV unstable fracture with ring disruption

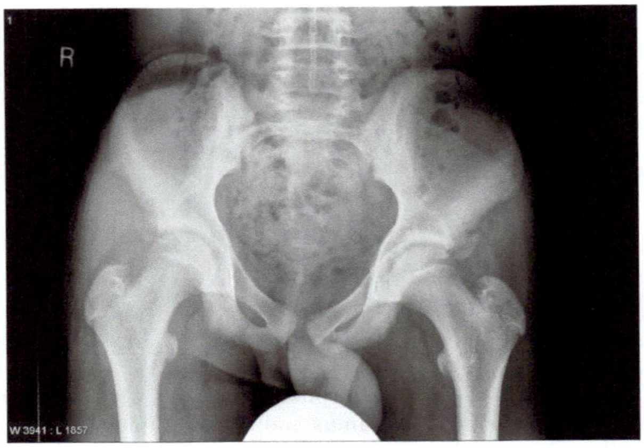

Fig. 12.19. An avulsion fracture from the anterior inferior iliac spine (Type I)

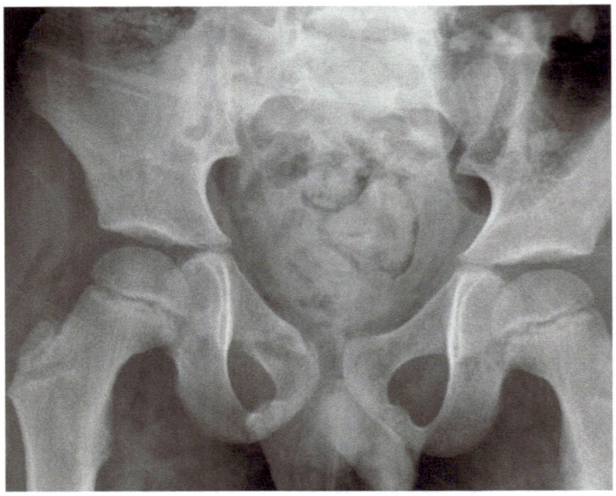

Fig. 12.20. Right superior pubic ramus fracture with minimal disruption of the pelvic ring (Type III)

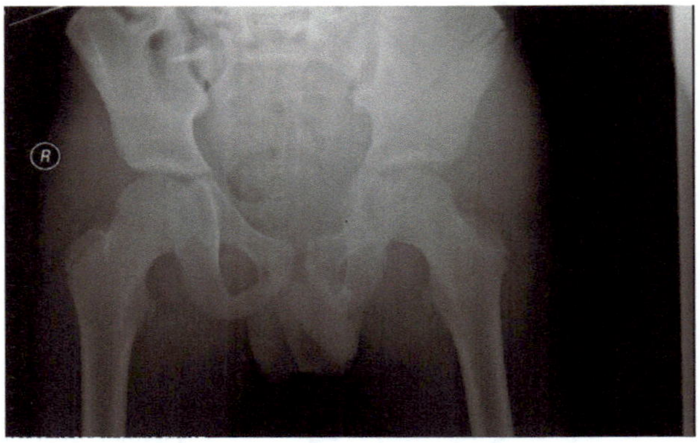

Fig. 12.21. Fracture of the left Iliac wing with widening of the left SI joint, there was clinical instability (Type IV)

of the pubic rami (straddle fractures), fractures of the anterior ring plus posterior ring and fractures of the anterior ring plus acetabulum (Fig. 12.21).

12.6.3.5
Outcome

The likelihood of associated visceral, genitourinary and neurological injuries is very low in type I and II injuries, moderate in type III and high in type IV. Type II and III injuries usually require admission to hospital for observation and analgesia and CT is often required to confirm that the fracture is not type IV. Patients are mobilised once pain allows and long term sequelae are uncommon.

Separation of the symphysis in children has a better prognosis than in adults, since it is generally an avulsion of the sleeve of the periosteum rather than a tear of the fibrocartilage. Approximately 20% of these patients may require blood transfusion because of haemorrhage.

Risks of morbidity and mortality rise significantly for type IV fractures. While the majority may still be managed non-operatively (in terms of the pelvic fracture), the patient will require several weeks of bed rest and long-term complications such as limb length inequality, closure of the triradiate cartilage and non-union are common. There has been an increasing trend over recent years to treat these fractures surgically. In particular, the advent of iliosacral screws which can be inserted percutaneously has allowed early stabilisation of the sacroiliac joint.

12.7
Acetabular Fractures

Acetabular fracture are uncommon in children, with less than 15% of children with pelvic fractures having an acetabular injury. In children, damage to the triradiate cartilage can cause long-term growth problems, with premature closure of the cartilage, dysplasia of the hip joint and subluxation of the femoral head. Injuries to the triradiate cartilage are often due to compression or crush forces. Thin slice CT imaging with multiplanar reconstruction is the most sensitive method to detect acetabular fractures (Hallel and Salvati 1977; Bucholz et al. 1982; Harley et al. 1982; Heeg et al. 1988, 1989, 1992).

12.7.1 Acetabular Anatomy

The acetabulum is comprised of a large anterior column and a smaller posterior column, together these columns create an inverted Y. The anterior column is comprised of the superior pubic ramus which continues into the iliac blade. The posterior column is shorter and more vertical and extends from the ischial tuberosity into the ileum. In addition to the two columns, there is an anterior and posterior wall which are important in maintaining hip stability (Theumann et al. 2002).

The anterior column corresponds to the iliopectineal line on an AP radiograph and the posterior column the ilioischial line. Judet views allow more detailed examination of the acetabular columns, although these have largely been superceded by CT examination. The internal (obturator) oblique view is taken with the pelvis rotated anteriorly by 45° and shows the iliopectineal line and posterior wall of the acetabulum, but again CT is more useful and allows multiplanar reconstructions.

For the external (iliac) oblique view, the pelvis is rotated in the opposite direction, allowing visualisation of the ilio-ischial line and anterior wall of the acetabulum.

12.7.2 Classification of Acetabular Fractures

In view of the relatively small numbers of acetabular injuries that occur in children, developing a classification system is difficult. A classification of injuries to the triradiate cartilage based on the Salter Harris system has been proposed (Heeg et al. 1989). Alternatively, the Judet and Letournel classification, which is widely accepted in adults, may also be used.

The Judet and Letournel classification divides fractures into ten groups, consisting of five basic elementary groups and five associated patterns. Elementary fractures run in one plane while associated patterns combine two or more of the elementary patterns (Judet et al. 1964; Pennal et al. 1980a; Heeg et al. 1988, 1989, 1992; Silber and Flynn 2002; Schlickwei and Keck 2005).

With the increased use of CT, further simplified approaches to acetabular fractures have been proposed (Harris et al. 2004a,b).

12.7.2.1 Posterior Fractures

Posterior fractures include posterior wall and column injuries. They typically occur from direct compression of the posterior wall by the femoral head from a frontal impact on a flexed knee (so-called 'dashboard injury'). This may be associated with posterior dislocation of the femoral head, but this is rare in children. It is the size and combination of a posterior wall fracture that determines the prognosis, the incidence of re-dislocation and long-term instability.

12.7.2.2 Anterior Fractures

Anterior fractures include the anterior wall and anterior column and they are often associated with other pelvic fractures. They are the result of a lateral blow to the greater trochanter when the leg is externally rotated. This is a relatively uncommon injury and typically causes minimal displacement, so surgical fixation is not usually required.

12.7.2.3 Transverse and T Type Fractures

Transverse and T type fractures are caused by high energy shearing forces. With transverse injuries, the fracture line traverses across the acetabulum in an axial or oblique orientation, dividing into upper and lower halves. The T type consists of a transverse fracture with a vertical component, the posterior column thus becomes a detached loose fragment.

12.7.2.4 Trauma to the Triradiate Cartilage

Growth in the height and width of the ileum, ischium and pubis relies on a normally functioning triradiate cartilage. Acute trauma to the growth cartilage which destroys the germinal cell layer can lead to partial or total growth arrest. A classification based around the Salter Harris type injuries has been suggested for triradiate fractures. They can be divided into three broad groups (Fig. 12.22a–j), based on Salter Harris types I, II and V. When only a portion of the growth plate is damaged, the unaffected segment will continue to grow. The outcome for type V fractures is less favourable, as fusion of the physis is more likely to occur, which can lead to progressive subluxation of the hip. Any progressive deformity will depend on the amount of the growth plate destroyed, and the age of the patient; the younger the patient, the greater the time for any deformity to progress. Severe deformity does not typically occur after early adolescence (BUCHOLZ et al. 1982). If the triradiate fuses but the cartilage continues to grow, there may be displacement of the acetabulum laterally (PONSETI 1978).

Injury to the triradiate cartilage may be missed on the initial radiograph. Those with less than 2-mm displacement have a good prognosis.

12.8 Avulsion Fractures

These are common in the adolescent age group, particularly those involved in physical activity. In acute injuries, they are the result of extreme, unbalanced and often eccentric muscle contraction. In more chronic cases, they are the result of repetitive microtrauma and overuse (TEHRANZADEH 1987; EL-KHOURY et al. 1997; STEVENS et al. 1999). The fracture occurs at the muscle attachment or tendon insertion on the bone. In adolescents, these attachments and insertions are often onto an apophysis, where the growth cartilage is an area of relative weakness. In addition, the bone in young people is relatively weaker and more elastic, so consequently it is this bone attachment that is more prone to injury than the musculo-tendinous junction. Not until early adulthood does the musculo-tendinous junction become the point of relative weakness and muscle and tendon tears the commoner injury.

In the pelvis, avulsion occurs primarily at six sites, which not surprisingly are the sites of the major muscle attachments. The three commonest sites are the anterior superior iliac spine (ASIS) (the origin of sartorius), the anterior inferior iliac spine (AIIS) (the rectus femoris origin) and the ischial tuberosity (the origin of the hamstring group). With these fractures acutely there is a clinical history of severe exertion, followed by pain and reduced function (WOOTTON et al. 1990) (Fig. 12.23).

The symphysis pubis and inferior pubic ramus are the origin of the long and short adductors and gracilis muscles. Avulsions here are typically the result of over use and discrete fractures are rarely seen. Iliac crest avulsion from abdominal musculature is rare and is associated with abrupt directional changes or repetitive microtrauma.

AP radiographs and an appropriate clinical history are all that is usually required to make the diagnosis, with an obvious avulsed fragment and soft tissue swelling seen at the point tenderness (Fig. 12.24). Comparison with the contralateral side may be helpful. In some cases, CT or MR imaging may be helpful in establishing the diagnosis (BRANDSER et al. 1995; STEVENS et al. 1999). Patients with this type of injury respond well to conservative treatment; however, if the fragment is displaced by more than 2 cm, fibrous union may occur resulting in extended disability.

In chronic cases where the presentation is less dramatic but there is a history of long-standing pain made worse with exertion, radiographs will show hypertrophic ossification at the insertion site, which may be confused with a mass lesion. The typical site and history should distinguish these changes from a tumour, but the radiographic appearances may be disturbing and if doubt remains, MR imaging can be used to exclude a mass lesion (BRANDSER et al. 1995; EL-KHOURY et al. 1997) (Fig. 12.25). Around the ischial tuberosity, these mass lesions can cause a compressive effect, leading to sciatic neuritis. Occasionally with more chronic injuries, the radiographs may be normal and MR imaging or ultrasound may be helpful in detecting inflammation at the muscle insertion.

12.9 Child Abuse

Pelvic fractures can occur as a consequence of child abuse but they are unusual. The presence of a pelvic fracture in a young premobile child without a history of significant trauma should raise the suspicion of an inflicted injury. Pelvic fractures may occur in association with other severe abdominal or pelvic injuries, they have also been described as a consequence of sexual abuse and may therefore be seen in a slightly older group of children (JOHNSON et al. 2004).

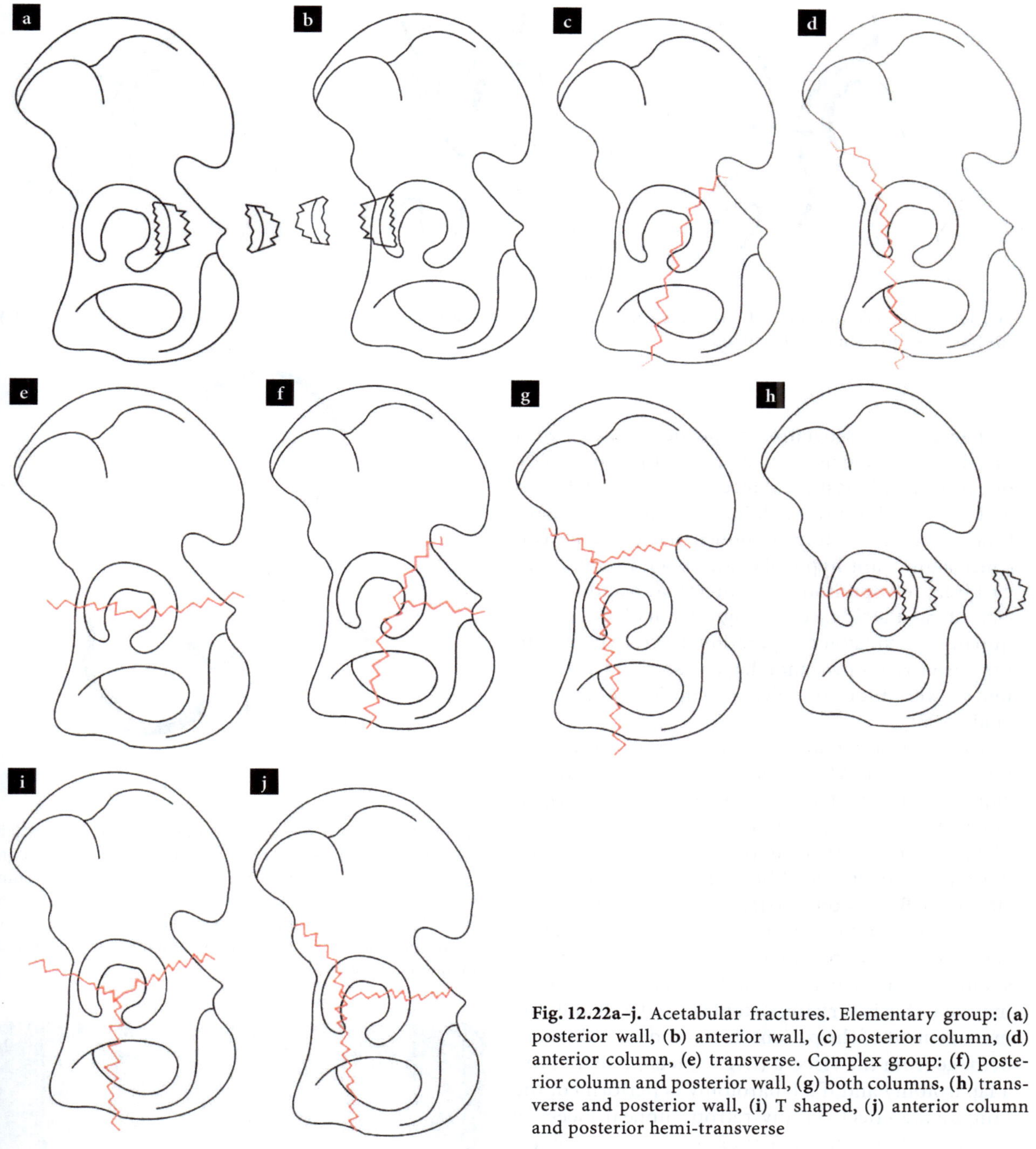

Fig. 12.22a–j. Acetabular fractures. Elementary group: (**a**) posterior wall, (**b**) anterior wall, (**c**) posterior column, (**d**) anterior column, (**e**) transverse. Complex group: (**f**) posterior column and posterior wall, (**g**) both columns, (**h**) transverse and posterior wall, (**i**) T shaped, (**j**) anterior column and posterior hemi-transverse

12.10 Complications

Pelvic fractures can be associated with significant morbidity and mortality, which reflects the high degree of impact energy associated with these injuries.

In adults, the morbidity rate in pelvic trauma ranges between 5% and 15% but may reach 50% in some cases. In 12% of cases, the death is attributable to the pelvic trauma. In children, the death rate is lower (Silber et al. 2001) and the morbidity mostly the result of associated head and neck injuries.

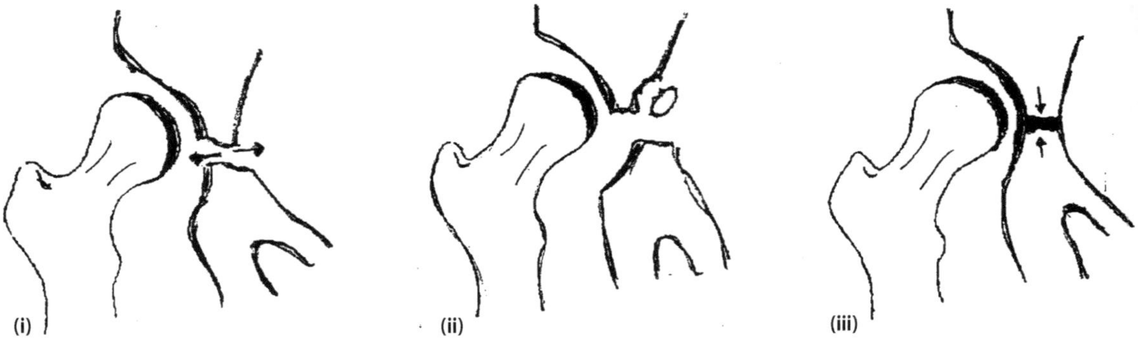

Fig. 12.23. The classification of triradiate cartridge injuries based upon the Salter-Harris classification. (**i**)Shear injury; (**ii**) fracture; (**iii**) compressive injury

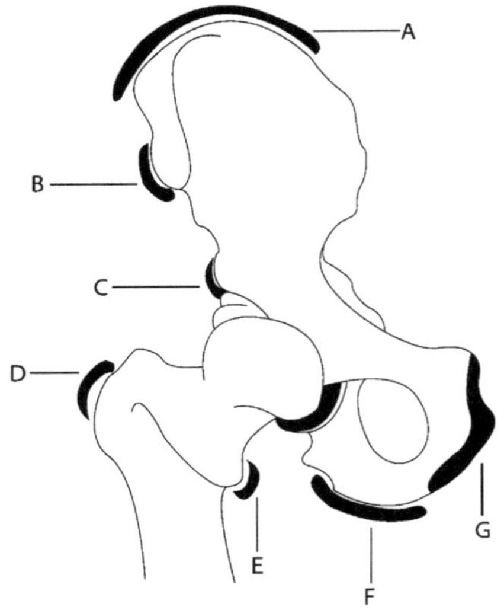

Fig. 12.24. Sites of pelvic avulsion injuries. *A*, iliac crest (abdominal muscle insertion). *B*, anterior superior iliac spine (sartorious muscle origin). C, anterior inferior iliac spine (rectus femoris origin). *D*, greater trochanter (gluteal insertions). *E*, Lesser trochanter (illiopsoas). *F*, ischial tuberosity (hamstring muscle). *G*, body of pubis and inferior pubic ramus (adductors and gracillis)

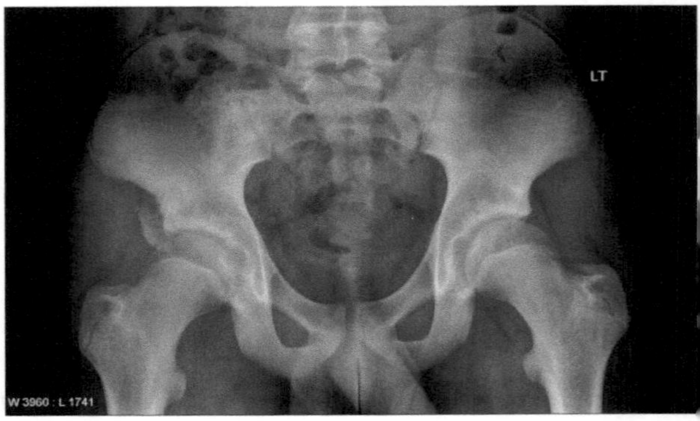

Fig. 12.25. Avulsion fracture of the right inferior iliac spine

There is an association of pelvic fractures with multi-system injuries which can occur in over 50% of cases, the highest incidence is of additional skeletal injuries, but brain, abdominal and pulmonary lesions can occur. Retroperitoneal haemorrhage can cause significant hypovolaemic shock in adults. In children, retroperitoneal haematomas occur in over 40% of paediatric cases but significant blood loss requiring transfusion or operation is rare. There is an increased risk of haemorrhage associated with the more severe types of pelvic disruption (McIntyre et al. 1993).

Haemorrhage may be either retroperitoneal or intraperitoneal. AP compression injuries with disruption of the posterior elements (Tile B1/B3, Open book, Torode IV) result in tearing of the venous plexus around the back of the pelvis and potentially massive retroperitoneal bleeding. Lateral compression (Tile B2, Torode II/III) injuries are classically associated with blunt trauma to the abdominal viscera and intraperitoneal bleeding. Ultrasound or CT should be able to distinguish the location of any haematoma, this is very important since it will alter the management of the patient. Intra-abdominal haemorrhage from the viscera (liver, spleen) may require a laparotomy and if a laparotomy is performed, the tamponade effect on any retroperitoneal bleeding may be lost and the patient exsanguinate. Exploration of the retroperitoneum is difficult and control of haemorrhage may be impossible. Any tamponade can be improved in these cases by closing the 'open book' nature of the pelvic injury. This may be achieved using a pelvic sling or an external fixator. Angiography may have a role in some cases. If bleeding is identified as being arterial (rare) it may be possible to embolise the offending vessel.

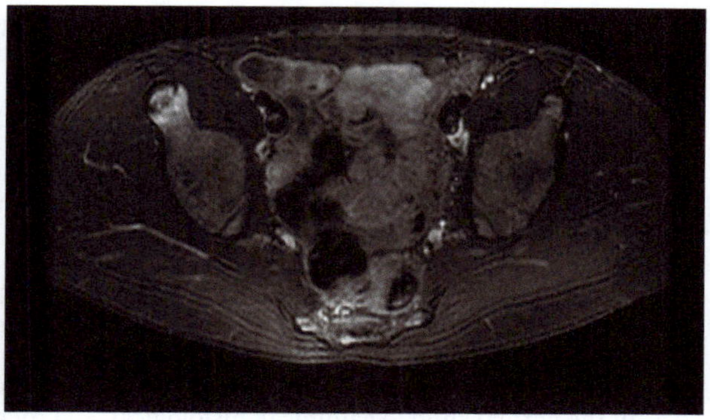

Fig. 12.26. MR image (axial STIR) of avulsion fracture of the right inferior iliac spine. There is soft tissue changes and marrow oedema around the avulsion site

Genitourinary injury is uncommon. Haematuria should prompt further investigation of the renal tract either by ultrasound or CT. Inability to pass urine in the acute setting raises the possibility of bladder rupture or urethral injury. The latter is more common in 'straddle' fractures and bruising in the perineum or blood at the urinary meatus is highly suggestive. In such instances, a urological consult is mandatory. The patient may require a cystourethrogram to assess the lower urinary tract.

Ano-rectal and gynaecological lesions are rare and often secondary to open trauma. Lower urinary tract lesions are found but it is not as common as in adults (Bond et al. 1991).

Long-term orthopaedic problems may arise from the pelvic fracture. Malunion or non-union of the pelvic ring may lead to limb length discrepancy and chronic back and hip pain. Sacroiliac injury can cause degenerative changes which can progress to fusion and disturbance of hemipelvic growth.

Late sequelae related to the bony pelvis are more likely to arise from acetabular damage. Severe damage to the triradiate may occur in up to 5% of cases (Bucholz et al. 1982; Heeg et al. 1988, 1989). Damage to the cartilage can result in separation and premature closure. Premature fusion will result in abnormal modelling of the acetabulum which may cause subluxation of the femoral head. Long-term complications include anteversion of the femoral neck, repeated subluxation, osteonecrosis and early osteoarthritis (Schlickwei and Keck 2005).

Infection can complicate these fractures either at the pin-site infection, deep within the wound or osteomyelitis.

12.11 Management

The aim with paediatric pelvic fractures is anatomic reduction and maintenance of a symmetrical pelvis. Pelvic asymmetry can be determined on the AP radiograph, from the difference in length (cm) between two diagonal lines drawn from the border of the sacroiliac joint to the contralateral triradiate cartilage. Normal anatomic variation is 4 mm of asymmetry (Keshishyan et al. 1995). An asymmetry of greater then 1.1 cm is associated with a greater degree of disability, including altered gait, sacroiliac pain and tenderness (Smith et al. 2005). In most cases, children are usually managed with bed rest, traction or pelvic slings. Most pelvic fractures in children will have a favourable outcome with this conservative approach. If the fracture is unstable or there is significant disruption of the pelvic ring, particularly vertical movement, then external fixation may be needed. This will reduce the blood loss and help alleviate any discomfort and pain. In severe cases, particularly if there is disruption of the posterior ligament complex, internal fixation may be required.

With a displaced acetabular fracture, open reduction, stable internal fixation and early motion is often indicated. Reduction of a femoral head dislocation should be paramount, as there is a relationship between the occurrence of avascular necrosis and prolonged dislocation (Heeg et al. 1989). Recurrent dislocation may occur from a capsular defect, loose fragments within the joint and remodelling of the joint.

With acetabular fractures, it is important that joint congruity is restored (Rieger and Brug 1997). If there is early bridging of the triradiate cartilage, this may be resected and replaced by fat (Langenskiold 1993). In the polytrauma patient, the other more life threatening injuries may overshadow proper fracture management.

References

Ben-Menachem Y, Coldwell DM, et al. (1991) Hemorrhage associated with pelvic fractures: causes, diagnosis, and emergent management. AJR Am J Roentgenol 157:1005–1014

Berg EE, Chebuhar C, et al. (1996) Pelvic trauma imaging: a blinded comparison of computed tomography and roentgenograms. J Trauma 41:994–998
Bond SJ, Gotschall CS, et al. (1991) Predictors of abdominal injury in children with pelvic fracture. J Trauma 31:1169–1173
Brandser EA, el-Khoury GY, et al. (1995) Tendon injuries: application of magnetic resonance imaging. Can Assoc Radiol J 46:9–18
Bucholz RW, Ezaki M, et al. (1982) Injury to the acetabular triradiate physeal cartilage. J Bone Joint Surg Am 64:600–609
Dalal SA, Burgess AR, et al. (1989) Pelvic fracture in multiple trauma: classification by mechanism is key to pattern of organ injury, resuscitative requirements, and outcome. J Trauma 29:981–1000; discussion 1000–1002
Demetriades D, Karaiskakis M, et al. (2003) Pelvic fractures in pediatric and adult trauma patients: are they different injuries? J Trauma 54:1146–1151; discussion 1151
El-Khoury GY, Daniel WW, et al. (1997) Acute and chronic avulsive injuries. Radiol Clin North Am 35:747–766
Ersoy G, Karcioglu O, et al. (1995) Should all patients with blunt trauma undergo 'routine' pelvic X-ray? Eur J Emerg Med 2:65–68
Hallel T, Salvati EA (1977) Premature closure of the triradiate cartilage. A case report and animal experiment. Clin Orthop Relat Res (124):278–281
Harley JD, Mack LA, et al. (1982) CT of acetabular fractures: comparison with conventional radiography. AJR Am J Roentgenol 138:413–417
Harris JH Jr, Coupe KJ, et al. (2004) Acetabular fractures revisited: part 2, a new CT-based classification. AJR Am J Roentgenol 182:1367–1375
Harris JH Jr, Lee JS, et al. (2004) Acetabular fractures revisited: part 1, redefinition of the Letournel anterior column. AJR Am J Roentgenol 182:1363–1366
Heeg M, Visser JD, et al. (1988) Injuries of the acetabular triradiate cartilage and sacroiliac joint. J Bone Joint Surg Br 70:34–37
Heeg M, Klasen HJ, et al. (1989) Acetabular fractures in children and adolescents. J Bone Joint Surg Br 71:418–421
Heeg M, Otter N, et al. (1992) Anterior column fractures of the acetabulum. J Bone Joint Surg Br 74:554–557
Ismail N, Bellemare JF, et al. (1996) Death from pelvic fracture: children are different. J Pediatr Surg 31:82–85
Johnson K, Chapman S, et al. (2004) Skeletal injuries associated with sexual abuse. Pediatr Radiol 34:620–623
Judet R, Judet J, et al. (1964) [Fractures of the Acetabulum.] Acta Orthop Belg 30:285–293
Junkins EP, Furnival RA, et al. (2001). The clinical presentation of pediatric pelvic fractures. Pediatr Emerg Care 17:15–18
Keshishyan, RA, Rozinov VM, et al. (1995) Pelvic polyfractures in children. Radiographic diagnosis and treatment. Clin Orthop Relat Res (320):28–33
Langenskiold A (1993) Partial closure of the epiphyseal plate. Principles of treatment. 1978. Clin Orthop Relat Res (297):4–6
McIntyre RC Jr, Bensard DD, et al. (1993) Pelvic fracture geometry predicts risk of life-threatening hemorrhage in children. J Trauma 35:423–429
Montana MA, Richardson ML, et al. (1986) CT of sacral injury. Radiology 161:499–503
Paterson A, Frush DP, et al. (2001) Helical CT of the body: are settings adjusted for pediatric patients? AJR Am J Roentgenol 176:297–301
Pennal GF, Davidson J, et al. (1980a) Results of treatment of acetabular fractures. Clin Orthop Relat Res (151):115–123
Pennal GF, Tile M, et al. (1980b) Pelvic disruption: assessment and classification. Clin Orthop Relat Res (151):12–21
Ponseti IV (1978) Growth and development of the acetabulum in the normal child. Anatomical, histological, and roentgenographic studies. J Bone Joint Surg Am 60:575–585
Potter HG, Montgomery KD, et al. (1994) MR imaging of acetabular fractures: value in detecting femoral head injury, intraarticular fragments, and sciatic nerve injury. AJR Am J Roentgenol 163:881–886
Resnik CS, Stackhouse DJ, et al. (1992) Diagnosis of pelvic fractures in patients with acute pelvic trauma: efficacy of plain radiographs. AJR Am J Roentgenol 158:109–112
Rieger H, Brug E (1997) Fractures of the pelvis in children. Clin Orthop Relat Res (336):226–239
Schlickwei W, Keck T (2005) Pelvic and acetabular fractures in childhood. Injury 36[Suppl 1]: A57–63
Silber JS, Flynn JM (2002) Changing patterns of pediatric pelvic fractures with skeletal maturation: implications for classification and management. J Pediatr Orthop 22:22–26
Silber JS, Flynn JM, et al. (2001) Analysis of the cause, classification, and associated injuries of 166 consecutive pediatric pelvic fractures. J Pediatr Orthop 21:446–450
Smith W, Shurnas P, et al. (2005) Clinical outcomes of unstable pelvic fractures in skeletally immature patients. J Bone Joint Surg Am 87:2423–2431
Stevens MA, El-Khoury GY, et al. (1999) Imaging features of avulsion injuries. Radiographics 19:655–672
Tehranzadeh J (1987) The spectrum of avulsion and avulsion-like injuries of the musculoskeletal system. Radiographics 7:945–974
Theumann NH, Verdon JP, et al. (2002) Traumatic injuries: imaging of pelvic fractures. Eur Radiol 12:1312–1330
Tile M (1996a) Acute pelvic fractures: I. Causation and classification. J Am Acad Orthop Surg 4:143–151
Tile M (1996b) Acute pelvic fractures: II. Principles of management. J Am Acad Orthop Surg 4:152–161
Torode I, Zieg D (1985) Pelvic fractures in children. J Pediatr Orthop 5:76–84
Wootton JR, Cross MJ, et al. (1990) Avulsion of the ischial apophysis. The case for open reduction and internal fixation. J Bone Joint Surg Br 72:625–627
Young JW, Burgess AR, et al. (1986a) Lateral compression fractures of the pelvis: the importance of plain radiographs in the diagnosis and surgical management. Skeletal Radiol 15:103–109
Young JW, Burgess AR, et al. (1986b) Pelvic fractures: value of plain radiography in early assessment and management. Radiology 160:445–451

The Hip Joint

13

James Metcalfe and Alan Sprigg

CONTENTS

J. Metcalfe, FRCS (orth)
Consultant Orthopaedic Surgeon, Derriford Hospital, Plymouth, PL6 8DH, UK
A. Sprigg, MD
Consultant Radiologist, Sheffield Children's Hospital, Western Bank, Sheffield S10 2TH, UK

13.1 Introduction

Interpreting images of the developing hip can be challenging due to a number of factors. The cartilaginous nature of the proximal femoral anlage means the ossified skeleton is continually changing; however, the ossification proceeds in a predictable manner and knowledge of this is important when interpreting radiographs. In addition, femoral head perfusion is precarious and can be interrupted by injuries around the hip joint. Recognising these potential pitfalls will influence the management and imaging of the hip joint following trauma.

13.2 Development

The hip and acetabulum develop from a single mass of mesenchymal cartilage. A cleavage plane forms at the 7th gestational week and by the 11th gestational week, separate cartilaginous structures for the femoral head and acetabulum have developed. The primary ossification centre of the femur develops in the middle of the diaphysis (cartilaginous model) and proceeds proximally and distally along the shaft.

At the time of birth, the proximal femur is a composite structure containing the greater and lesser trochanters and the femoral head, all as one cartilaginous mass. Ossification of the proximal femur occurs between 4–6 months post-natally. The ossific nucleus is usually visible on ultrasound 2–3 months before it appears on radiographs. The femoral head ossification centre expands, becoming hemi-spherical and the growth plate between the femoral head and the metaphysis becomes clearly identifiable on radiographs as a radiolucent area between the femoral head and metaphysis.

The greater and lesser trochanters help maintain the structure and integrity of the hip joint by providing sites for muscle and ligament attachments, but they do not add any longitudinal growth to the femur. An ossification centre appears in the greater trochanter between the ages of 5 and 8 years and by the age of 8, the geometric morphology of the femur has developed with a clearly defined femoral head and greater trochanter.

The anteversion and neck shift angle have reached their adult dimensions by early adolescence in a child who is weight bearing normally. The adolescent growth spurt is characterised by a rapid growth of the proximal femur which typically occurs between the ages of 12–14 years in girls and 13–16 years in boys. The femoral head growth plate is the first to close (Fig. 13.1).

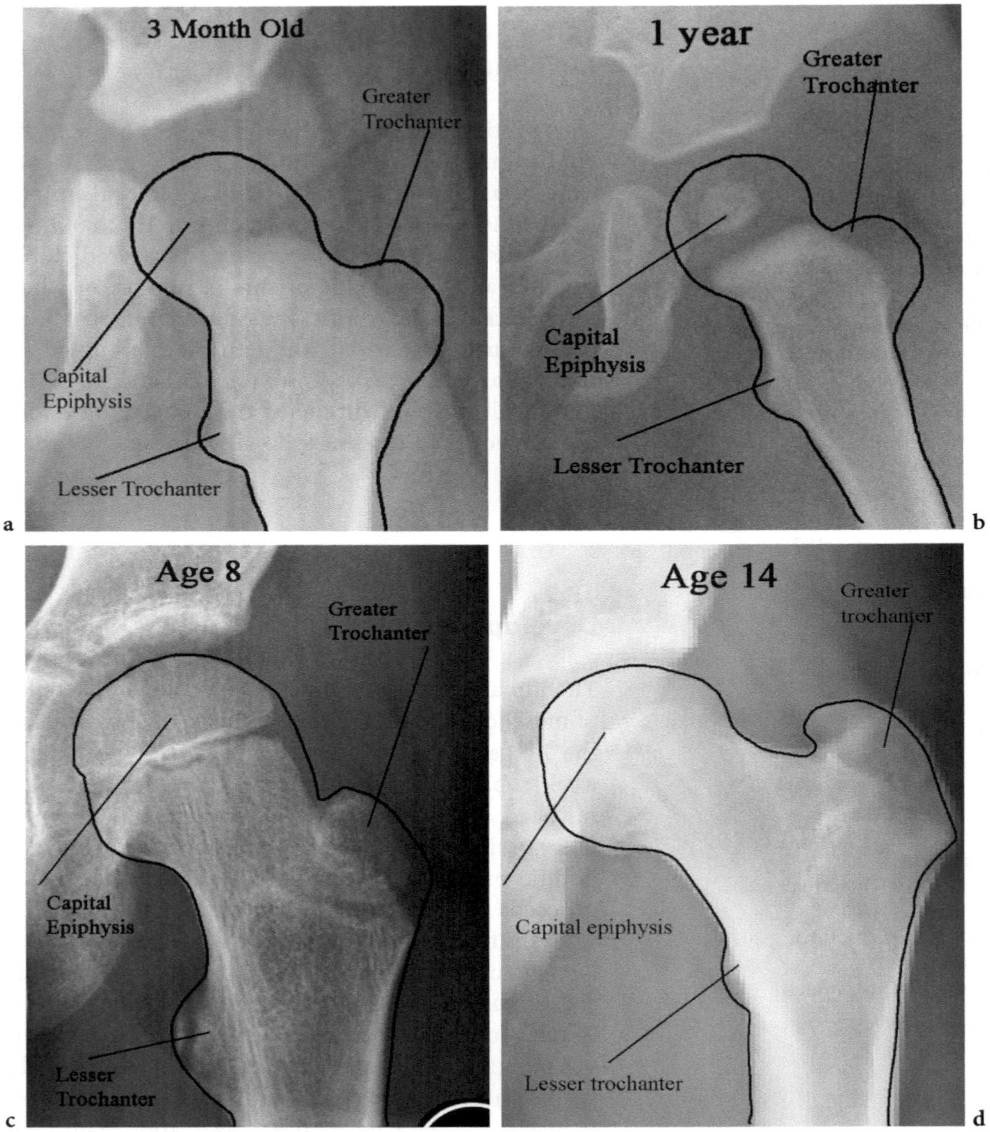

Fig. 13.1. **a** Radiographic appearance of the hip in a 3-month-old child. The ossific nucleus has not appeared. **b** Radiographic appearance of the hip by 12 months of age. The ossific nucleus is now visible. **c** Radiographic appearances in an 8-year-old. **d** Adolescent hip at the age of 14 years. The trochanters are ossified. The capital physis is closing

13.3 Vascular Supply

The femoral head is uniquely vulnerable to vascular insult. The femoral head is two-thirds of a sphere which allows a large degree of movement in three planes. This large degree of movement afforded by the hip articulation is at the cost of a precarious blood supply. Apart from the ligamentum teres, there are no soft tissue attachments to the femoral head to enable arterial supply. Consequently, the blood supply to the femoral head is provided by the ligamentum teres and from generalised perfusion around the epiphysis.

In the first year of life, metaphyseal vessels cross the physeal cartilage but after this point, the physis forms a barrier. From then onward, the blood supply is largely from branches of the circumflex vessels and to a lesser extent, the ligamentum teres.

The medial and lateral circumflex arteries form an anastomosis around the proximal femur. The lateral circumflex femoral artery predominantly supplies the greater trochanter, the anterior femoral neck and metaphysis. During the first few years of life, the artery also supplies the anterior portion of the femoral head; however, as the femoral neck grows, these vessels elongate and eventually are unable to penetrate the femoral head. The medial circumflex femoral artery supplies the lesser trochanter and provides two ascending branches (the posterior inferior and the posterior superior) for femoral head perfusion. The posterior inferior branch arises near the lesser trochanter and after penetrating the hip capsule, travels along the inferior femoral neck. The posterior superior artery penetrates the superior aspect of the hip capsule and then travels along the superior region of the femoral neck. These arteries anastamose, forming a sub-synovial ring at the articular cartilage margin. These vessels are end arteries and penetrate the femoral head.

13.4 Radiographs

The primary imaging assessment of the paediatric hip typically involves an AP radiograph of the pelvis. If it is the first presentation then lateral views are indicated. Initial trauma films should be taken without gonad protection, as this may obscure fractures. If the child is being followed up and the pathology is known, a layer of protection should be used. Obviously, the protection should be positioned so as not to obscure the pathology.

Several methods may be used to take the lateral radiograph. A frog lateral radiograph is obtained with abduction and flexion of the hips and produces both hips on one film, allowing immediate comparison. This is not always obtainable in an acute setting when the child is in pain and cannot manoeuvre the painful leg. The position of rest for the painful hip is typically in flexion and internal rotation – it is better to try and match the position of the normal hip to the abnormal, than to straighten a painful hip. Symmetrical positioning is important in hip radiography, but if this is not possible, a conventional lateral view may be the only option.

The pelvis has to withstand massive forces and the bony geometry is arranged into two columns. The anterior and posterior columns of the pelvis are recognised by tracing the iliopectineal and ilioischial lines, respectively (Campbell 2005). The iliopectineal line runs along the medial border of the iliac wing and superior aspect of the superior pubic ramus to the symphysis pubis. The ilioischial line runs along the medial iliac wing to the ischial tuberosity. Discontinuity or abnormal courses of these lines may represent a fracture.

A normal hip shows a concentric reduction of the femoral head in the acetabulum – the joint space is equidistant all around the hip. The tear-drop represents the medial wall of the acetabulum. The distance from the tear-drop to the femoral head may be compared with the contralateral side. On a perfectly positioned film, an increase in this distance is abnormal and may represent a hip effusion, infolded labrum after dislocation or intra-articular loose body entrapment after dislocation. Fibrofatty tissue within the joint (acetabulum pulvinar), septic arthritis and Perthes' disease may also give similar findings.

13.5 Ultrasound Assessment

Ultrasound is the primary assessment tool for the acutely painful hip in a young child, but not for acute trauma. Ultrasound should be performed with a linear high frequency probe. The child should be supine with the legs slightly interiorly rotated. The ultrasound probe should be placed along the line of the femoral neck and the images should include the proximal femoral diaphysis, the femoral neck and the femoral epiphysis. The iliopsoas muscles should be identified inserting into the femur. The joint capsule of the hip can be identified as a mixed echogenic area overlying the femoral epiphysis. An effusion is seen as a hypoechoic collection distending the capsule. The presence of an effusion is a non-specific finding and can occur with a variety of pathologies, including transient synovitis, juvenile idiopathic arthritis, trauma, Perthes' disease or sepsis. The presence of inflamed synovium or an echogenic effusion is again non-specific and may occur in both aseptic and septic conditions. If sepsis is considered then joint aspiration is mandatory.

13.6 Computerised Tomography (CT) Imaging

CT is a valuable imaging modality in the acute trauma setting and is available in most trauma centres. Multislice imaging produces a rapid radiological assessment, often without the need for sedation, and allows multiplanar reconstructions with three dimensional (3D) modelling. Pelvic and 3D acetabular anatomy may be difficult to assess on two dimensional radiographs. The addition of further oblique plain film views enhances the assessment but in the traumatised child, positioning for these views may not be possible and indeed may take time. Often in the setting of poly trauma, other injuries are present and CT imaging of the head, chest and abdomen are requested. Including the pelvis does not extend scanning time significantly.

3D CT scanning is a valuable adjunct to axial scanning, especially when visualising the acetabulum and quadrilateral plate. These areas are difficult to visualise on radiographs. However, fracture displacement of less than 2 mm is poorly demonstrated with the 3D scanning – emphasising the importance of reviewing source images besides the 3D model (Hayes and Balkissoon 1997). This degree of displacement in an intra-articular fracture of the acetabulum is an indication for open reduction and so careful and accurate assessment of intra-articular displacement is mandatory.

13.7 Magnetic Resonance Imaging (MRI)

The multiplanar imaging capabilities of magnetic resonance imaging (MRI) combined with its soft tissue resolution make this imaging modality very useful in the setting of trauma. In the emergency setting, MRI may not contribute to the management of the paediatric hip injury; a displaced fracture or dislocated hip are readily diagnosed on radiographs. However, when radiographs reveal little information, MR imaging reveals the occult injury. Furthermore, the integrity of the femoral capital epiphysis and the hip joint surfaces may be assessed. MR imaging is more sensitive for detecting avascular necrosis of the femoral head and may be used to assess viability before and after surgery.

13.7.1 Patient Compliance in MRI

MR imaging is a relatively hostile environment for small children. If the child is unwell, paediatric support is vital. It is important to remove all ferromagnetic material before entering the MR scan room, e.g. a ferrous Thomas splint and some external fixator devices. Adequate imaging requires a child to remain motionless for a considerable time. In the setting of hip pathology, adequate analgesia is required. In younger children, apprehension and fear may result. In this cohort of patients, sedation or general anaesthetic may be required. Careful monitoring is mandatory with the availability of MR compatible resuscitation equipment.

13.7.2 Imaging Techniques

The achievement of high resolution images is improved by the use of a phased array coil, in which the hips and pelvis are in the centre of the field of view. Enhancement with the paramagnetic contrast (Gadolinium based compound) depends on the clinical problem. A typical imaging protocol is shown in Table 13.1 (Dillon et al. 2005).

Table 13.1. MRI sequences for evaluating trauma to the hip joint

Plane	Image sequence
Coronal	T1 weighted spin echo
Coronal	Short tau inversion recovery
Axial	T2 weighted fast spin echo fat saturated
Axial	Fast spin echo proton density
Oblique sagittal	Fast spin echo proton density fat saturated

13.8 Traumatic Hip Dislocation

Traumatic hip dislocation is uncommon in children and is the result of high energy force; therefore, it is often associated with other significant injuries (Craig 1980; Salisbury and Eastwood 2000). Typically, it is the result of an axial force directed along the length of the femur, such as that which occurs when the hip is flexed and the knee impacted against the dashboard in a road traffic accident. The direction of dislocation will depend on the position of the hip at the moment of impact. If the hip is flexed and adducted, this will result in posterior dislocation. If the hip is abducted and externally rotated, this will result in anterior dislocation. Posterior dislocation is the commonest type and more frequently associated with fractures, particularly those of the posterior acetabulum.

Treatment of hip dislocation is immediate closed reduction, and should preferably be performed within 6 h of injury. This is important to lower the risk of osteonecrosis.

13.8.1 Diagnosis

Clinical presentation and history in the majority of cases are sufficient for diagnosis. AP radiographs often demonstrate abnormal continuity between the femoral head and acetabulum. Lateral films, if they can be obtained, will confirm the diagnosis.

CT is important for detecting small fractures of the acetabulum, looking for acetabular displacement and also for detecting intra-articular foreign bodies.

MR imaging can evaluate the cancellous bone, cartilage muscle ligaments and intra-articular fluid. It will also demonstrate bone contusions and muscle injury. Patients with anterior dislocation have muscle injuries in the gluteal region and anterior fascial compartment. Patients with posterior dislocation have muscle injury in the posterior fascial compartment. Nearly all patients have moderate to severe medial and anterior fascial compartment muscle injury. Gluteal injury is severe in the posterior group. MR imaging has shown that all patients with hip dislocation have significant joint effusion and haemarthrosis. In patients where it is difficult to reduce the dislocated hip, MR imaging may demonstrate imposition of the iliopsoas tendon portion of the capsule, intra-articular haematoma and ligamentum teres. Interposition of the ligamentum teres is the most likely cause of medial joint space widening following adduction (Vialle et al. 2004).

13.8.2 Complications

Complications of hip dislocation include osteonecrosis and early degenerative osteoarthritis. MR imaging is used in the identification of early osteonecrosis by visualising early fatty marrow conversion in the intratrochanteric portion of the proximal femur. Osteonecrosis develops in less than 5% of patients whose dislocation was reduced within 6 h compared with over 50% if the reduction occurred after 6 h of injury.

Osteoarthritis can occur following a traumatic dislocation, the incidence ranges from 15%–50% and this may be related to the site of the initial injury, the presence of intra-articular loose bodies and the degree of activity following the dislocation. Simple dislocations have a better prognosis than those with an associated fracture (Figs. 13.2, 13.3).

13.9 Slipped Capital Femoral Epiphysis (SCFE)

13.9.1 Clinical Presentation

Slipped capital femoral epiphysis (SCFE) or upper epiphysis (SUFE) occurs around the time of the pubertal growth spurt. It is more common in males and can be bilateral (although rarely at the same

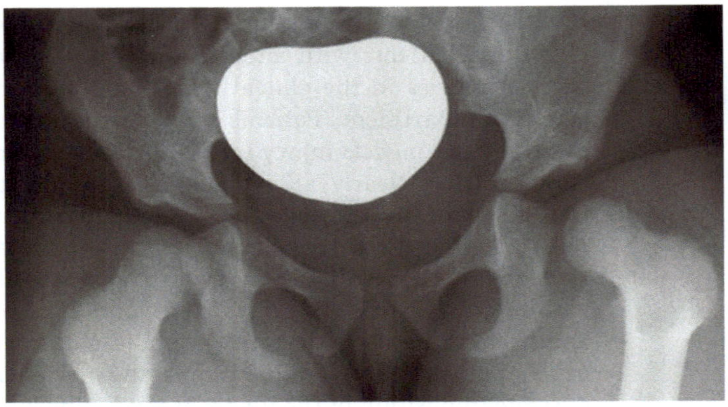

Fig. 13.2. Radiograph showing traumatic dislocation of left hip in a 3-year-old

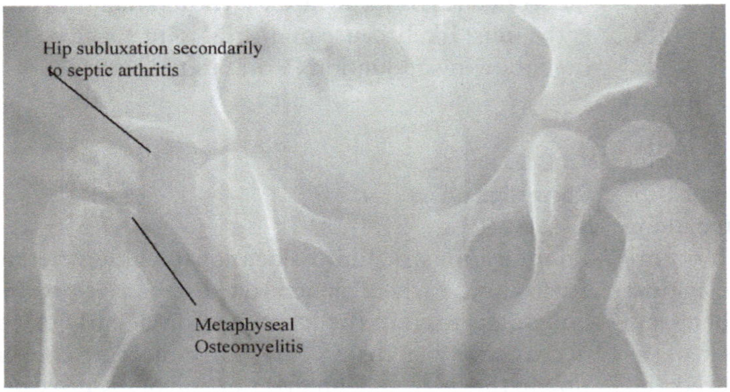

Fig. 13.3. Hip subluxation following septic arthritis. Note osteomyelitis lucency in femoral metaphysis

time) in 25% of patients. The aetiology is not entirely understood, but it would appear that the physis becomes slightly unstable, allowing the epiphysis to move with respect to the neck. The condition is more common in overweight children and patients with hormonal imbalance, particularly hypothyroidism and renal failure.

Patients present with groin and/or knee pain which may be acute or chronic. It is imperative that the condition should also be considered in patients with knee pain, since the long-term prognosis is excellent if detected early but poor if detected late.

13.9.2 Radiology

Typically, the proximal femoral epiphysis appears to slip posteriorly and medially, although it is actually the metaphysis which slips in the opposite direction. Both AP and frog lateral radiographs are indicated in any child with suspected SCFE, as the detection rate is increased. The relationship between the ossific nucleus (femoral head), femoral neck and the trochanters should be scrutinised. Early features include an ill-defined margin of the metaphysis and epiphysis adjacent to the growth plate. An actual slip may not be visible at this stage.

Normally a line extended along the superofemoral neck proximally should intersect the lateral portion of the femoral epiphysis (Klein's line) (Klein et al. 1951). In addition, a dense triangle formed by the overlapping of the inferior aspect of the metaphysis and the acetabulum is usually visible. Both these normal features are lost when the epiphysis has slipped (Bloomberg et al. 1978).

A line perpendicular to the base of the epiphysis should be parallel to the femoral neck, a deviation of > 2° is abnormal (Tins and Cassar-Pullicino 2006).

While the frog lateral view will improve the detection of subtle slips, all or none of the above radiographic signs may or may not be present and it is important that when clinical suspicion persists, further imaging should be considered (Figs. 13.4, 13.5).

SOUTHWICK (1984) described a classification based upon this angle of slippage; a slip angle of < 30° is defined as minor, 30–60° moderate and > 60° severe. The severity of slip is related to the subsequent risk of developing degenerative joint disease. SCFE may also be classified as acute, acute on chronic or chronic.

Acute slips have a history of less than 3 weeks. From a radiological perspective, a chronic slip may be identified by recognising a periosteal 'beak' of new bone posteriorly and remodelling of the femoral neck. This is most readily seen on the lateral radiograph (Fig. 13.6).

SCFE has also been described (LODER et al. 1993) as being stable or unstable. This classification is based on the ability of the patient to weight bear on the painful leg. If the patient is unable to weight bear, the slip is 'unstable' and carries a risk of avascular necrosis AVN of 50%. The risk of AVN in stable slips is 1%. If an acute or unstable SCFE is suspected, a frog lateral radiograph should not be attempted since this may precipitate further movement.

13.9.3 MRI

Whether every SCFE progresses through a phase of pre-slip is debated. Where there is no abnormality or uncertainty on radiographs, but clinical concern, then MR imaging should be considered. MR imaging will demonstrate marrow oedema around the physis with an associated joint effusion which is suggestive of an early slip or 'pre-slip'. There may also be widening of the physis in the centre or in the posterior-medial region (FUTAMI et al. 2001) (Fig. 13.7). MR imaging is also sensitive in identifying the two most feared complications of SCFE: avascular necrosis and chondrolysis.

13.9.4 Management

The standard management of SCFE is to stabilise the physis with a single screw. It should be remembered

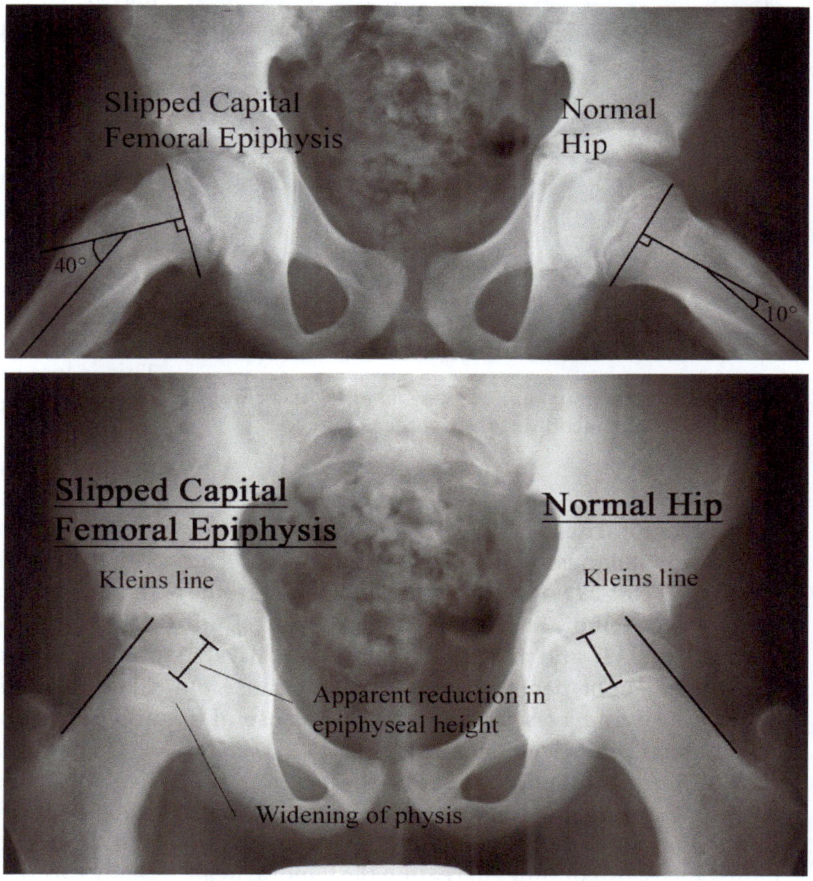

Fig. 13.4a,b. AP and frog lateral radiographs of the pelvis in a child with slipped capital femoral epiphysis

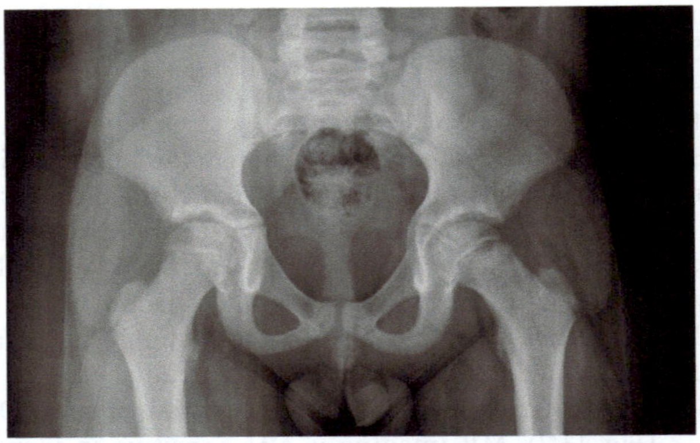
a

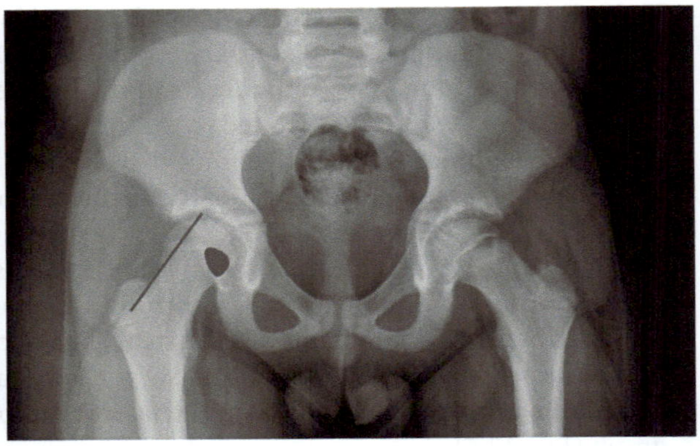

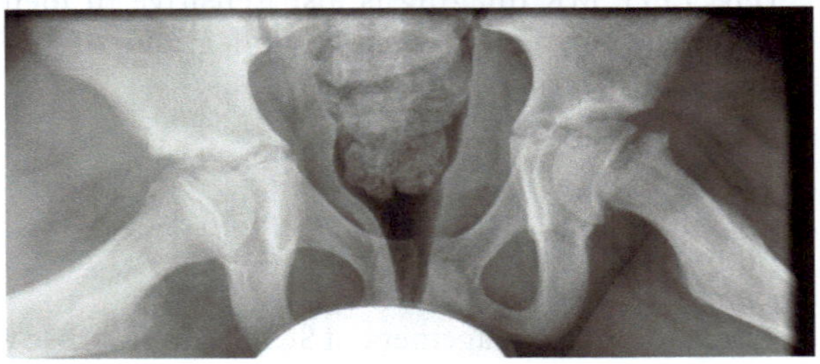
c

Fig. 13.5. a AP radiograph of the pelvis of a 14-year-old boy with left slipped capital femoral epiphysis. **b** The features of the normal right hip are emphasised on the same radiograph. A line drawn along the femoral neck intersects the epiphysis (Klein's line), and a dense triangle of bone is seen where the metaphysis of the hip overlies the acetabulum. These features are not seen on the abnormal left side. **c** The frog leg lateral radiograph of the same patient clearly shows the left slipped epiphysis

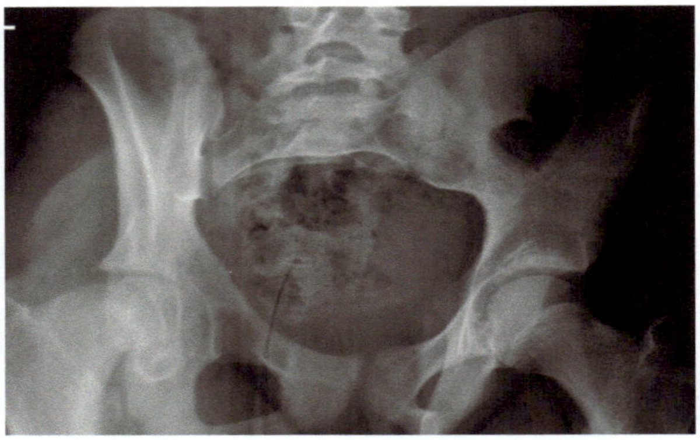

Fig. 13.6. AP radiograph of a 14-year-old girl with a chronic slip. There is remodelling of the right femoral neck

that the femoral head is spherical and penetration of the joint is a danger if the screw is misplaced. The chances of this are minimised if the screw is in the centre of the femoral head. This should be carefully checked on AP and lateral films pre-operatively. Inadvertent joint penetration is a potent cause of chondrolysis and avascular necrosis. CT is useful if doubt about pin placement exists (Fig. 13.8).

In severe slips, it may be felt that the position is so bad that pinning in situ does not present a realistic option for long-term function of the hip. In such circumstances, osteotomies to realign the femoral head may be considered. The favoured options are osteotomies through the femoral neck or osteotomies at the subtrochanteric level. These operations also carry significant risks of AVN and chondrolysis.

13.9.5 Complications

13.9.5.1 Chondrolysis

This is loss of cartilage with subsequent narrowing of the joint space and degenerative change. It may be the result of immobilisation, impingement on the metaphysis or surgical intervention (Lubicky 1996; Warner et al. 1996; Jofe et al. 2004). The incidence can be up to about 10% (Lubicky 1996; Tudisco et al. 1999). The diagnosis is suggested if there is loss of cartilage thickness of > 2 mm compared with the contralateral normal hip or cartilage thickness of < 3 mm in bilateral cases. Normal cartilage thickness is assumed to be 4–5 mm (Aronson and Carlson 1992; Hughes et al. 1999).

On radiographs, there is loss of joint space, peri-articular osteopenia and premature fusion of the growth plate. Bone marrow oedema is seen on MR imaging and increased peri-articular activity on bone scintigraphy (Mandell et al. 1992; Warner et al. 1996). In

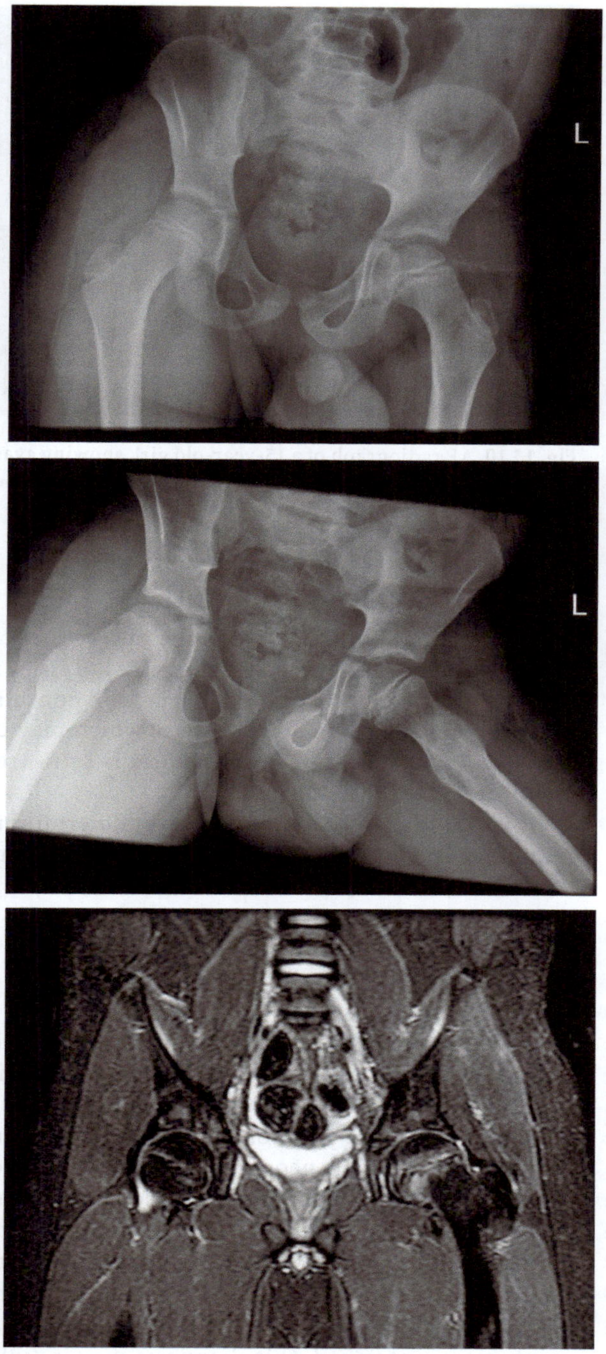

Fig. 13.7. **a** AP radiograph of a 13-year-old boy with pain in the left hip, with widening of the growth plate. **b** Frog leg lateral view of the same patient shows possible evidence of epiphyseal slip. **c** Coronal short tau inversion recovery (STIR) image of the same patient clearly shows widening of the growth plate with surrounding oedema. This patient underwent surgical pinning in view of ongoing clinical concern

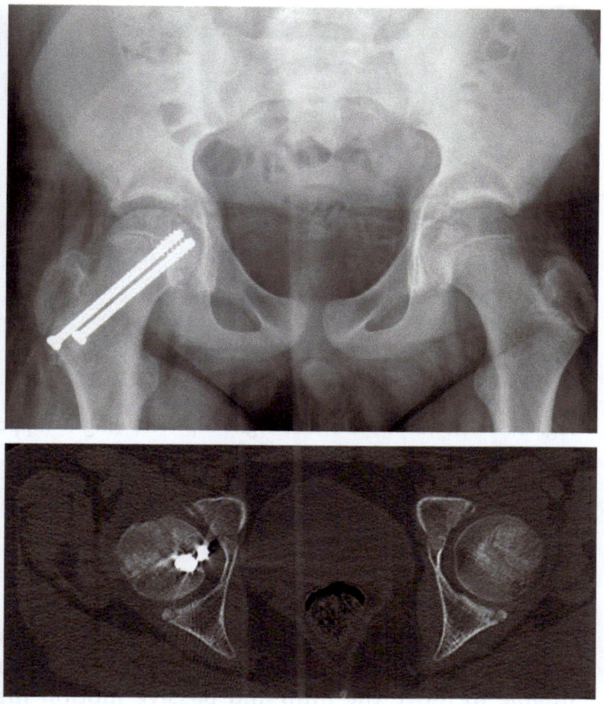

Fig. 13.8. **a** AP radiograph suggest the screws are close to the edge of the epiphysis. **b** Axial CT showing screw fixation abutting the cortical surface. Pin placement is too close to the joint surface and so were withdrawn slightly

the long term, there may be ankylosis or degenerative change within the joint. While resolution can be seen in 50% of cases (Lubicky 1996) (Fig. 13.9).

13.9.5.2
Avascular Necrosis

The risk of AVN is increased in unstable SUFE (Ballard and Cosgrove 2002; Tokmakova et al. 2003), in neck of femur or subcapital osteotomy (Arnold et al. 2002a,b) (Fig. 13.10).

13.10
Femoral Neck Fractures

13.10.1
Diagnosis

The diagnosis of hip fractures in children is relatively straightforward. Typically, there is a history

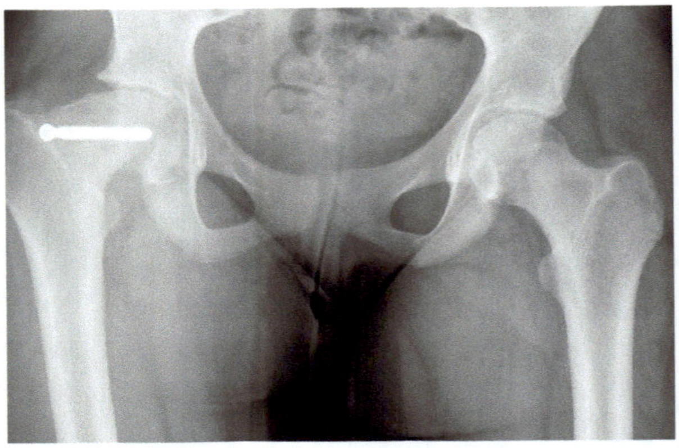

Fig. 13.9. Chondrolysis of the right hip following a slipped capital femoral epiphysis. The joint space of the right hip is reduced and there has been secondary remodelling

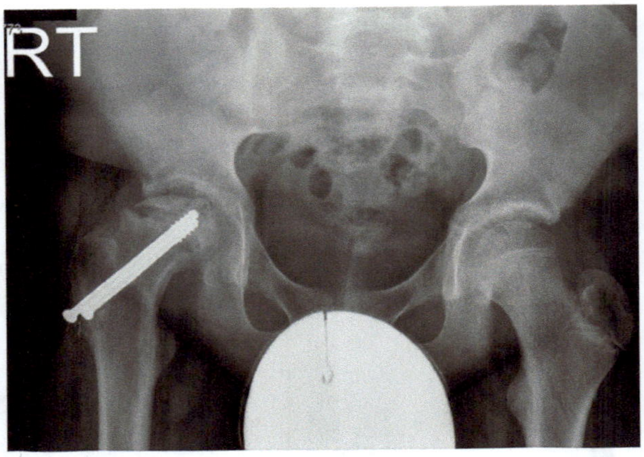

Fig. 13.10. AP radiograph of a 15-year-old girl, showing avascular necrosis of the right hip, secondary to slipped upper femoral epiphysis

of high energy trauma and the child complains of severe pain on examination (Lam 1971). They are unable to move the limb and passive motion may be limited and painful. If the fracture is displaced, the injured limb is often slightly adducted, laterally rotated and shortened. If there is associated femoral head dislocation, the leg is held in flexion, adduction and internal rotation.

Non-displaced fractures may be less symptomatic and in certain circumstances, the child may even be able to walk.

AP and lateral radiographs will typically confirm the diagnosis of a fracture and are also used in the classification. It is important to delineate the direction of the fracture line, the amount of displacement, the degree of varus deformity and the location of the femoral epiphysis.

In undisplaced fractures, the radiographs may be initially normal. MR imaging has been shown to be useful in demonstrating undisplaced fractures of the femoral epiphysis. These are seen as extensive marrow oedema which is high signal on STIR weighted images and often a low signal intensity fracture line is visible.

13.10.2 Fracture Classification

In children, the most widely used classification of hip fractures is that of Delbet (Colona 1928). Four types are described based on location. Type 1 is transepiphyseal which may or may not be associated with femoral head dislocation (IA). Type 2 is transcervical which may be displaced or non-displaced. Type 3 is cervicotrochanteric which may be displaced or non-displaced and type 4 is intra-trochanteric (Figs. 13.11–13.13).

This classification is useful both in determining treatment and prediction of complications and outcome (Canale and Bourland 1977; Lam 1971).

13.10.2.1 Type 1 Fractures

Type 1, transepiphyseal separations, are the least common type of fracture and more often seen in the younger child. There are two peaks of incidence: children less than 2 years of age and those who are 5–10 years of age. In neonates, this should be regarded as proximal femoral epiphyseolysis and can occur following difficult delivery. At this age, the femoral head, greater trochanter and lesser trochanter form one single unit and separation occurs at the chondro-osseous junction. As the proximal femoral epiphysis is unossified, this diagnosis may initially be difficult on radiographs but should be suspected in a child who holds an extremely flexed, abducted and externally rotated thigh. Similar clinical features and plain radiographic findings can occur in septic arthritis but MR imaging, ultrasound or arthrography may be helpful in confirming the diagnosis (Beaty 2006; Moon and Mehlman 2006; Shrader et al. 2007).

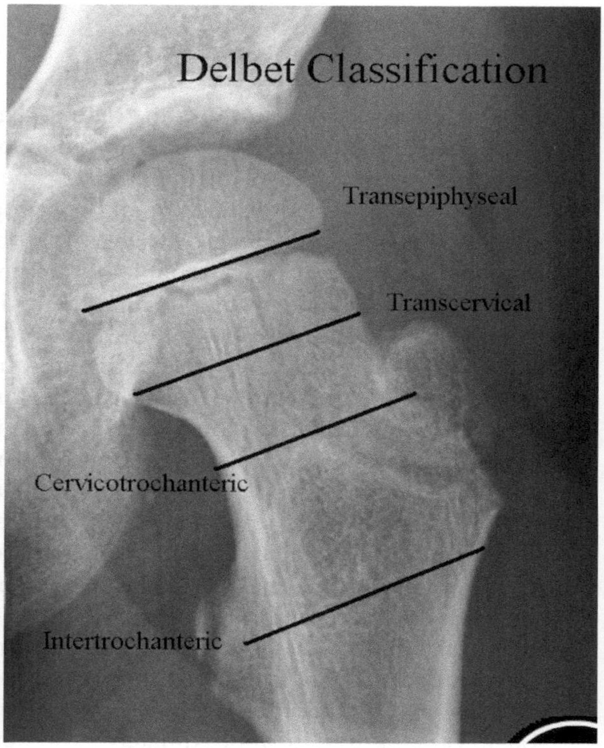

Fig. 13.11. Delbet classification of paediatric hip fractures

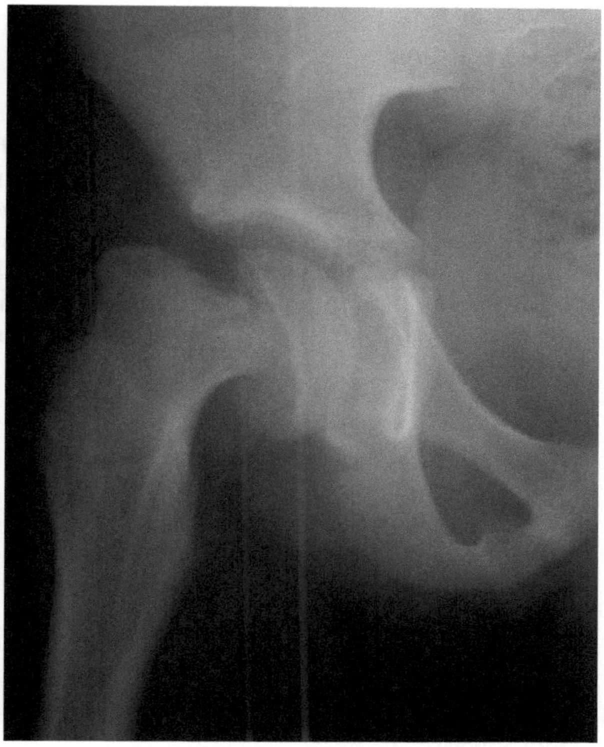

Fig. 13.12. Transphyseal fracture. There is underlying chronic epiphyseolysis

Dislocation of the femoral head can occur with proximal hip fractures and this increases the risk of osteonecrosis (100%) and premature physeal closure.

In a younger child, there is an improved prognosis than in older children because of the increased opportunity for remodelling.

13.10.2.2 Type 2 Fractures

Type 2 transcervical fractures are the most commonly seen fractures in children and adolescents. Typical aetiologies include falls and road traffic accidents. In approximately 50% of cases, the fractures are displaced. The incidence is increased at around three peak ages: 2–4 years of age, 8–9 years of age and 12–13 years of age. The incidence of osteonecrosis following a type 2 fracture is variable and reports describe between 16% and 78%. The outcome for non-displaced fractures is better than those that are displaced, although osteonecrosis can occur even in non-displaced injuries (Beaty 2006; Moon and Mehlman 2006; Shrader et al. 2007).

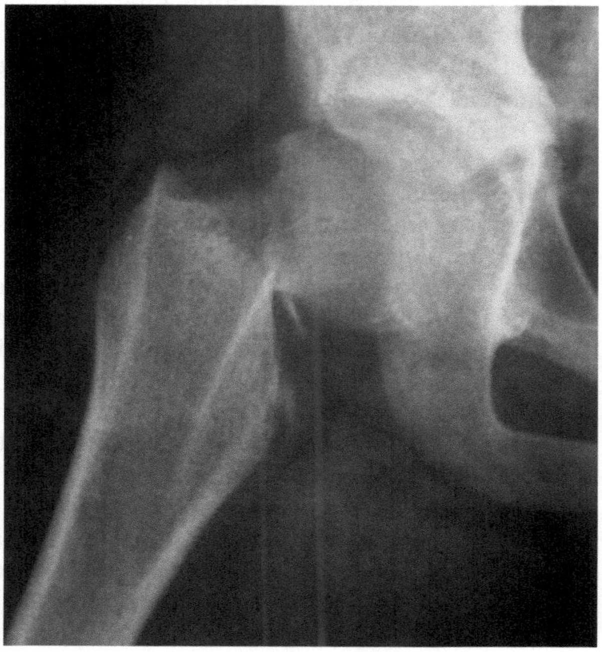

Fig. 13.13. Transcervical fracture

13.10.2.3
Type 3 Fractures

Cervico-trochanteric is the second most common type of hip fracture in a child and is the result of severe trauma. Osteonecrosis, premature physeal closure and coxa vara can occur following type 3 fractures, particularly if there is some displacement, although these complications are less common than in type 1 and 2 injuries (Beaty 2006; Moon and Mehlman 2006; Shrader et al. 2007).

13.10.2.4
Type 4 Fractures (Intertrochanteric)

Osteonecrosis is infrequent following these types of injuries and these have the best overall outcomes (Beaty 2006; Moon and Mehlman 2006; Shrader et al. 2007).

13.10.3
Complications

Osteonecrosis is the commonest complication of hip fractures in children and the occurrence is increased if there is significant fracture displacement and compromise of blood supply at the time of fracture. Immediate reduction, internal fixation and removal of intra-articular haematoma may reduce the risk of osteonecrosis but this has not been confirmed.

Osteonecrosis will usually occur within 1 year of injury. The onset may be insidious with pain and limitation of movement being the first clinical signs. Radiographs may not show any abnormality until at least 8 weeks. Typical radiological features include generalised osteopenia, widening of the joint space followed by fragmentation and sclerosis and deformity of the femoral epiphysis. MR imaging is the most sensitive test to confirm the diagnosis or define the extent of involvement. Osteonecrosis post fracture has been classified by Ratliff (1970): Type I – complete, type II – physeal, type III – metaphyseal.

Early closure of the physeal growth plate may occur following a fracture and the risk is increased if any instrumentation is passed across the growth plate. Early growth plate fusion and limb length alteration from the fracture can result in a limb length discrepancy.

13.10.4
Treatment of Hip Fractures

Complication rates are minimised if fractures are reduced early and stabilised. Closed reduction is generally possible except in the case of type 1 fractures with associated dislocation of the capital epiphysis. Hip spicas may be used to maintain the reduction in type 4 fractures, although this method of treatment is often poorly tolerated in older children and loss of position can result in non-union or coxa vara. Therefore, closed reduction and internal fixation are generally utilised. Any implant that crosses the physis risks damage and premature physeal closure. However, stability is paramount and in type 1 and many type 2 fractures, stabilisation across the physis is unavoidable. In children older than 11 or 12, premature physeal closure is of little clinical consequence, since the proximal femoral physis only accounts for 15% of limb growth. Damage may be minimised by using smooth pins but the standard implant in older children is 1 or 2 partially or fully threaded screws.

Coxa vara occurs in approximately 10%–30% of hip fractures. It may be the result of insufficient reduction in the fracture, delayed or non-union, osteonecrosis or premature closure of the physeal plate. Severe coxa vara will result in limb length shortening and can lead to early osteonecrosis. Both coxa vara and non-union can be managed by subtrochanteric valgus osteotomy.

13.10.5
Stress Fracture

Stress fractures of the femoral neck are extremely rare in children (Scheerlinck and Deboeck 1998). A history of chronicity is usually present. The fracture may occur on the superior aspect of the femoral neck (the tension side) or on the inferior side (the compression side) (Devas 1965). The radiographic features may be subtle as the fractures are mostly undisplaced. Callus at the fracture site may be visible.

Occult hip fractures have been successfully diagnosed with MR imaging despite normal radiographic findings in adults (Pandey et al. 1998). The MR imaging shows areas of intermediate signal change on the T1 weighted images traversed by a low signal (black) line. This black line has been shown to be impaction of trabecular bone (Ingar et al. 1996). Marrow oedema may be present with surrounding bleeding and this appears as signal change on T2 weighted images (Seeger and Hall 1990) (Fig. 13.14).

13.10.6 Apophyseal Avulsion Injuries

Apophyseal avulsion injuries are common around the hip and pelvis, with about 90% occurring in boys whilst playing sport. The apophysis is avulsed by strong muscle contraction. Once avulsed, the apophysis is displaced to a variable extent so the radiological signs can be very subtle. Careful comparison with the contralateral side is required on a symmetrically positioned film. The greater trochanteric apophysis may be avulsed from direct trauma.

References

Arnold P, Jani L et al. (2002a) Results of treating slipped capital femoral epiphysis by pinning in situ. Orthopade 31:880–887

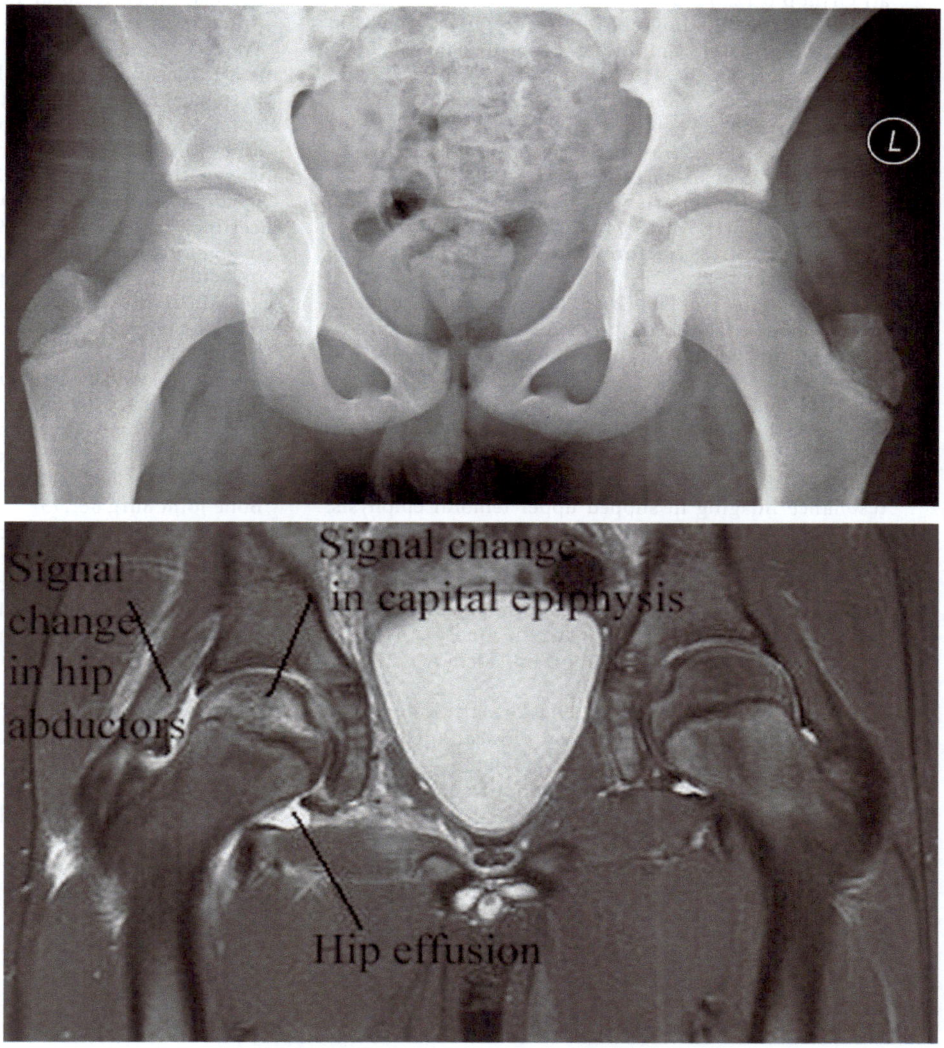

a

b

Fig. 13.14. a A normal AP radiograph of the pelvis of a 14-year-old after a fall from a height, presenting with a painful right hip. **b** T2 weighted coronal image of the pelvis. There is hip effusion and signal change in the capital epiphysis, consistent with marrow oedema. There is signal change in the abductors, consistent with traumatic oedema

Arnold P, Jani L et al. (2002b) Management and treatment results for acute slipped capital femoral epiphysis. Orthopade 31:866–870

Aronson DD, Carlson WE (1992) Slipped capital femoral epiphysis. A prospective study of fixation with a single screw. J Bone Joint Surg Am 74:810–819

Ballard J, Cosgrove AP (2002) Anterior physeal separation. A sign indicating a high risk for avascular necrosis after slipped capital femoral epiphysis. J Bone Joint Surg Br 84:1176–1179

Beaty JH (2006) Fractures of the hip in children. Orthop Clin North Am 37:223–232

Bloomberg TJ, Nuttall J, Stoker DJ (1978) Radiology in early slipped femoral capital epiphysis. Clin Radiol 29:657–667

Boero S, Brunenghi GM et al. (2003) Pinning in slipped capital femoral epiphysis: long-term follow-up study. J Pediatr Orthop B 12:372–379

Campbell SE (2005) Radiography of the hip: lines, signs and patterns of disease. Semin Roentgenol 40:290–302

Canale ST, Bourland WL (1977) Fractures of the neck and intertrochanteric region of the femur in children. J Bone Joint Surg Am 59:431–443

Colona PC (1928) Fractures in the neck of femur in childhood. A report of six cases. Ann Surg 88:902

Craig CL (1980) Hip injuries in children and adolescents. Orthop Clin North Am 11:743–754

Devas MD (1965) Stress fractures of the femoral neck. J Bone Joint Surg Am 47:728–738

Dillon JE, Connolly SA et al. (2005) MR imaging of congenital/developmental and acquired disorders of the paediatric hip and pelvis. Magn Reson Imaging Clin N Am 13:783–797

Exner GU, Schai PA et al. (2002) Treatment of acute slips and clinical results in slipped capital femoral epiphysis. Orthopade 31:857–865

Futami T, Suzuki S, Seto Y et al. (2001) Sequential magnetic resonance imaging in slipped upper femoral epiphysis: assessment of preslip in the contralateral hip. J Pediatr Orthop 10:293–303

Gekeler J (2002) Radiology and measurement in adolescent slipped capital femoral epiphysis. Orthopade 31:841–850

Hayes CW, Balkissoon RA (1997) Current concepts in imaging of the pelvis and hip. Orthop Clin North Am 28:617–624

Hughes LO, Aronson J et al. (1999) Normal radiographic values for cartilage thickness and physeal angle in the pediatric hip. J Pediatr Orthop 19:443–448

Ingari JV, Smith DK et al. (1996) Anatomic significance of magnetic resonance imaging findings in hip fracture. Clin Orth Relat Res 332:209–214

Jofe MH, Lehman W et al. (2004) Chondrolysis following slipped capital femoral epiphysis. J Pediatr Orthop B 13:29–31

Klein A, Joplin R, Reidy J et al. (1951) Roentgenographic features of slipped capital femoral epiphysis. AJR Am J Roentgenol 66:361

Lam SF (1971) Fractures of the neck of the femur in children. J Bone Joint Surg Am 53:1165–1179

Laorr A, Greenspan A, Anderson M, Moehring HD, McKinley T (1995) Traumatic hip dislocation: early MRI findings. Skeletal Radiol 24:239–245

Loder RT, Arbor A, Richards BS (1993) Acute slipped capital femoral epiphysis: the importance of physeal stability. J Bone Joint Surg Am 75:1134–1140

Lubicky JP (1996) Chondrolysis and avascular necrosis: complications of slipped capital femoral epiphysis. J Pediatr Orthop 5:162–167

Mandell GA, Keret D et al. (1992) Chondrolysis: detection by bone scintigraphy. J Pediatr Orthop 12:80–85

Moon ES, Mehlman CT (2006) Risk factors for avascular necrosis after femoral neck fractures in children: 25 Cincinnati cases and meta-analysis of 360 cases. J Orthop Trauma 20:323–329

Pandey R, McNally E, Ali A, Bulstrode C (1998) The role of MRI in the diagnosis of occult hip fracture. Injury 29:61–63

Ratliff AHC (1970) Fractures of the neck of the femur in children. J Bone Joint Surg (Br) 44:528

Salisbury RD, Eastwood DM (2000) Traumatic dislocation of the hip in children. Clin Orthop 377:106–111

Scheerlinck T, DeBoeck H (1998) Bilateral stress fractures of the femoral neck complicated by unilateral displacement in a child. J Pediatr Orthop B 7:246–248

Seeger LL, Hall TR (1990) Magnetic resonance imaging of paediatric musculoskeletal trauma. Top Mag Res Imaging 3:61–72

Shrader MW, Jacofsky DJ, Stans AA, Shaughnessy WJ, Haidukewych GJ (2007) Femoral neck fractures in pediatric patients: 30 years experience at a level 1 trauma center. Clin Orthop Relat Res 454:169–173

Southwick WO (1984) Slipped capital femoral epiphysis. J Bone Joint Surg 66:1151

Tins BJ, Cassar-Pullicino VN (2006) Slipped upper femoral epiphysis. In: Davis MA et al. (eds) Imaging of the hip and bony pelvis. Springer-Verlag , Berlin Heidelberg New York

Tokmakova KP, Stanton RP et al. (2003) Factors influencing the development of osteonecrosis in patients treated for slipped capital femoral epiphysis. J Bone Joint Surg Am 85:798–801

Tudisco C, Caterini R et al. (1999) Chondrolysis of the hip complicating slipped capital femoral epiphysis: long-term follow-up of nine patients. J Pediatr Orthop B 8:107–111

Vialle R, Pannier S, Odent T et al. (2004) Imaging of traumatic dislocation of the hip in childhood. Ped Radiol 34:970–979

Warner WC Jr, Beaty JH et al. (1996) Chondrolysis after slipped capital femoral epiphysis. J Pediatr Orthop B 5:168–172

The Paediatric Knee

14

Edward Bache, Sean Symons, and Keith Hayward

CONTENTS

E. Bache, FRCS (Orth)
Consultant Orthopaedic Surgeon, Birmingham Children Hospital, Birmingham, B4 6NH, UK
S. Symons, FRCS (Orth)
Orthopaedic Fellow, Orthopaedic Department, Royal Children's Hospital, Lemington Road, Parkville Vic. 3052, Australia
K. Hayward, FRCS
Orthopaedic Registrar, Birmingham Children Hospital, Birmingham, B4 6NH, UK

14.1 Introduction

Approximately 25% of fractures in children occur in the lower limb. The injury and fracture pattern vary with age and skeletal maturity. The peak incidence is bimodal, with high energy trauma (falls from height or motor vehicle accidents) peaking in preadolescents and sporting injuries peaking in adolescents.

It is important to understand the fracture patterns that alter with age. Initially radiographs will be obtained for skeletal trauma with MR imaging and computerised tomography (CT) being used as appropriate.

14.2 Embryology and Development

Chondrification centres of the femur, tibia and fibula appear during the 6th week of intrauterine development. The diaphyseal primary ossification centres of the femur and tibia appear at week 8. The knee joint cavity develops during week 10.

The appearance of the secondary ossification centres and the age of physeal closure are represented in Table 14.1.

14.3 Relevant Anatomy and Deforming Forces

The knee is the largest synovial joint in the body. It is a complex hinge joint which has a large range of motion, making it susceptible to instability and injury.

Table 14.1. Ossification centres around the knee

Site	Ossification		Fuses	
	Females	*Males*	*Females*	*Males*
Distal femur	Week 36 fetus	Week 36 fetus	17 years	18–19 years
Patella	3 years	4–5 years	N/A	N/A
Proximal tibia	Week 40 fetus	Week 40 fetus	16–17 years	18–19 years
Tibial tuberosity	7–15 years	7–15 years	19 years	19 years
Proximal fibula	3 years	4 years	16–18 years	18–20 years

The bones around the knee are the patella (the largest sesamoid bone in the body), the femur, the tibia and the fibula which articulate with each other to form the patellofemoral, tibiofemoral and proximal tibiofibular joints.

The largest of these joints, the tibiofemoral joint, obtains its stability from the conformity of its bony structures, the medial and lateral menisci, the medial and collateral ligaments, the anterior and posterior cruciate ligaments and the joint capsule.

Dynamic stability is provided by the muscles acting across the joint. These are principally the hamstrings which flex the knee joint and are innervated by the sciatic nerve or its branches, and the quadriceps which extend the knee and are supplied by the femoral nerve or its branches.

The quadriceps muscle attaches to the patella via the quadriceps tendon and the retinaculum medially and laterally. They are attached to the tibial tuberosity distally via the patella tendon. They are therefore integral to the stability of the patellofemoral joint.

The main movement at the knee is flexion-extension, powered by the hamstrings and quadriceps, respectively. There is also some medial (internal) and lateral (external) rotation.

The forces acting across the knee vary only slightly during the gait cycle but will dramatically increase with running and jumping.

During walking, the tibiofemoral joint has 2–4 times the body weight across it, whereas the patellofemoral joint has only 0.5 times body weight.

14.4 Indications for Radiography

Acute knee trauma is a common in children. It is important to determine from the clinical history and examination, those cases in which radiographs will alter clinical management. A number of studies, initially in adults and subsequently validated in children, have addressed this issue. The Ottawa Knee Rule was devised in 1995 (Stiell et al. 1995) which showed that a knee radiographic series was only required if there was isolated tenderness of the patella, tenderness of the head of the fibula, inability to flex the knee to 90° and an inability to weight bear. For adults, the additional parameter was age of 55 years. Studies in children (Bulloch et al. 2003; Seaberg et al. 1998; Moore et al. 2005) appear to have validated these rules. They also indicate that setting criteria reduces unnecessary radiographs.

14.5 Radiography

An AP and lateral radiograph of the knee should be standard practice in all cases of trauma. Some institutions would advocate the skyline view as part of the routine surveys. A variety of different projections have been described for a obtaining a skyline view, each one having its own eponym (Fig. 14.1) (Davies et al. 2004). Additional views may be obtained depending on the clinical suspicion, the Tunnel view (for osteochondral fractures, loose bodies and osteochondritis dissecans) and stress views.

14.5.1 Lipohaemarthrosis

An effusion in the knee joint is diagnosed when an ovoid outline is visible in the suprapatellar region

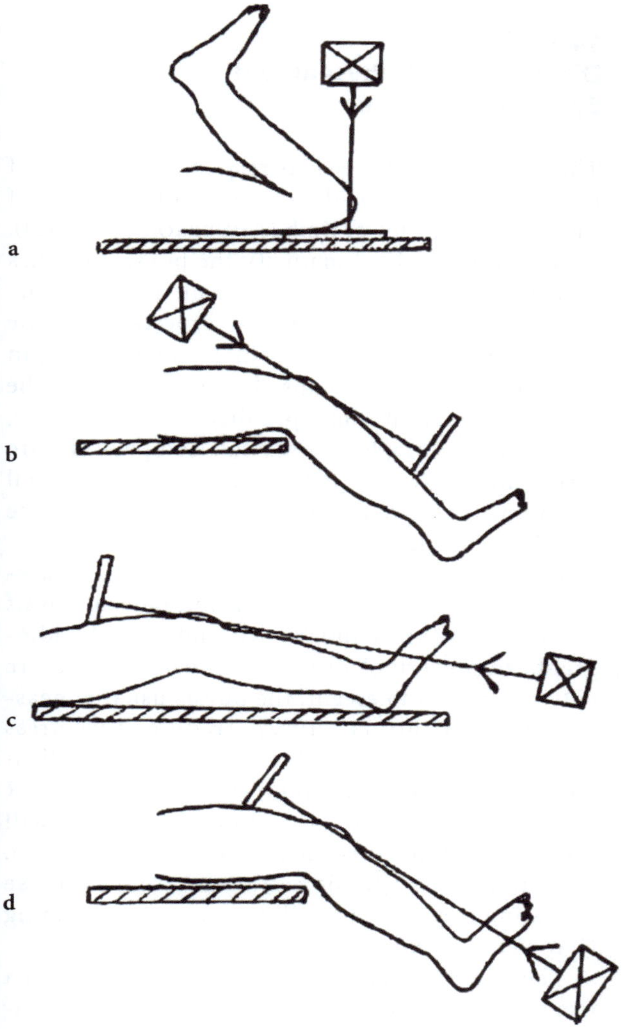

Fig. 14.1a–d. Radiographic positioning for the skyline view: **a** Settegast-prone, knee flexed 120°, vertical X-ray beam. **b** Merchant-knee flexed 45°, X-ray beam proximal to distal. **c** Laurin-knee flexed 20°, X-ray beam distal to proximal. **d** Ficat-knee flexed 30°, X-ray beam distal to proximal

due to fluid in the suprapatellar pouch on the lateral projection. This is associated with obliteration of the suprapatellar fat line (Butt et al. 1983). A lipohaemarthrosis is due to both blood and fat within the joint. If suspected, a horizontal beam lateral projection is required and this demonstrates a line separating two soft tissue densities, one of blood at the bottom and the lower density fat on top of the effusion. A lipohaemarthrosis is highly suspicious of an intra-articular fracture (Fig. 14.2).

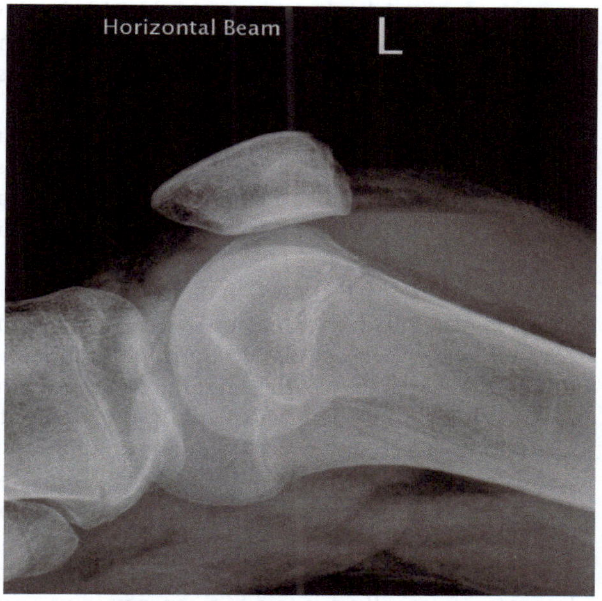

Fig. 14.2. Lateral shoot through radiograph of the knee demonstrating fat fluid interface of a lipohaemarthrosis adjacent to the patella

14.6 MR and CT Imaging

MR imaging is becoming the study of choice for pathological disorders of the knee in children, because it is painless, non-evasive and does not involve ionising radiation (Luhmann et al. 2005). In children, MR imaging is important, following trauma, in diagnosing fractures, ligamental injuries, meniscal damage and cartilage injury. Sequence choice is subjective and varies between institutions.

CT is valuable for assessing the degree of displacement of fracture fragments, in particular those involving the growth plate and articular surface. Fine slice images with multi-planar reconstruction are vital in this assessment. CT is also sensitive in detecting intra-articular bone fragments.

14.7 Distal Femoral Metaphyseal Fractures

The toddler or young child who falls from a standing height can sustain a transverse greenstick or torus fracture of the distal metaphysis. This is a low energy injury and its management depends on the degree and direction of any angulation or compression (Fig. 14.3).

Undisplaced fractures are treated non-weightbearing in a long-leg cast for 3–4 weeks. The cast should have 10° of knee flexion and some plantar flexion of the ankle, so as to relax the gastrocnemius muscles.

Fractures that have more than 10° of angulation in the sagittal (flexion-extension) plane or any in the coronal (varus-valgus) plane require manipulation under a general anaesthetic. Angulation in the plane of knee joint movement will usually remodel with growth. However, any varus or valgus angulation is poorly tolerated and will require early manipulation to a normal alignment. Any established malunion will require an early corrective osteotomy.

Fractures of the distal femoral metaphysis in adolescents are usually due to a high energy injury and can be associated with significant soft tissue trauma including damage to the major neurovascular structures around the knee. The fractures are usually unstable and require operative reduction and stabilisation.

Children with a neuromuscular disease are susceptible to insufficiency fractures of the distal femoral metaphysis due to their osteopenia. These fractures may require a manipulation and can usually be treated non-weightbearing in a long-leg cast.

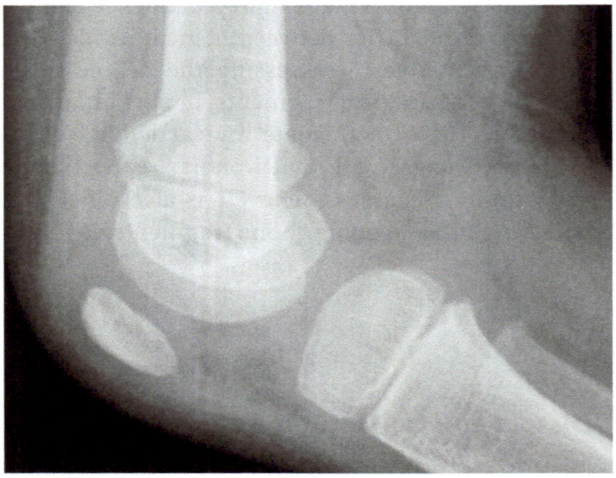

Fig. 14.3. Incomplete fracture of the distal femur

14.8 Distal Femoral Physeal and Epiphyseal Injuries

The distal femoral physis is responsible for 70% of the longitudinal growth of the femur and 37% of the length of the lower limb (Anderson et al. 1963). Approaching skeletal maturity the physis becomes increasingly undulated. As a result physeal fractures do not propagate along the hypertrophic zone but tend to damage the germinal zone resulting in growth arrest. This means that any injury to the physis increases its susceptibility to early closure, which can be complete or partial. Complete closure results in a leg-length discrepancy, whereas partial closure will also cause an angular deformity of the distal femur (Fig. 14.4).

It is important to appreciate widening, displacement and bony disruption of the radiolucent physis (Ozonoff 1979). Standard AP and lateral radiographs may overlook or underestimate the fracture pattern. In an adolescent, the physis usually measures 3–5 mm (Rogers 1992). Traditionally, stress views were used to help differentiate between ligamentous and physeal injury but increasingly, MR imaging is used to provide this information. CT will provide accurate assessment of the fracture pattern. Widening of the physis can occur from over use stress injuries and is readily seen on MR imaging (Laor et al. 1996).

The usual mechanism is a high energy trauma from a direct force to the lower thigh, most commonly a valgus/abduction force to the lateral side or hyperextension of the knee. The leg is often planted on the ground creating an axial force with some rotation. Distal femoral physeal fractures are rarer than those of the ankle or upper limb. They are associated with ligament injuries and internal derangement within the knee joint. The fractures are classified using the Salter-Harris classification; in addition, comment should be made about the degree and type of displacement. The type of displacement will provide information about the mechanism of injury.

With Salter-Harris (SH) I fractures, there is just separation through the distal femoral physis.

SH II is the commonest fracture pattern with the metaphyseal fragment often on the lateral (compression) side, due to a valgus force (Fig. 14.5). A direct anterior force will cause a hyperextension injury where the distal epiphysis is displaced anteriorly with the patella and tibia. The posterior femoral spike may cause injury to the neurovascular structures within the popliteal fossa.

SH III and IV are uncommon and they may be unicondylar or bicondylar. With SH III, the fracture line often extends through the intercondylar region and the physeal separation is of the medial condyle. It is associated with tears of the anterior cruciate ligament (ACL) (Fig. 14.6). With SH IV, the fracture usually involves the lateral metaphysis with extension into the intercondylar notch.

SH V are the result of impaction, associated with fractures of the proximal tibia and associated with consequent growth retardation.

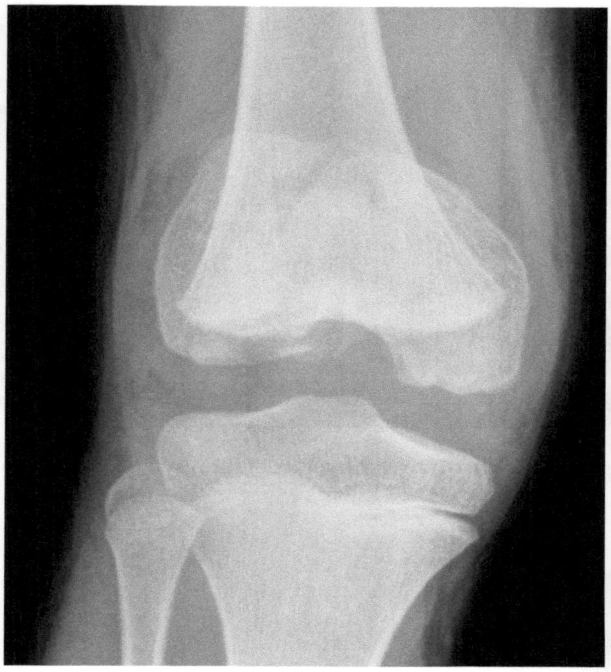
a

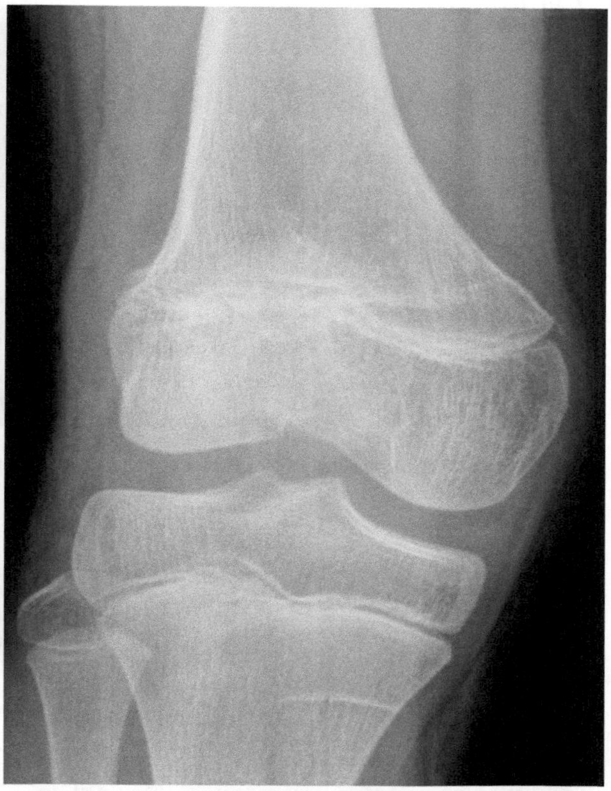
b

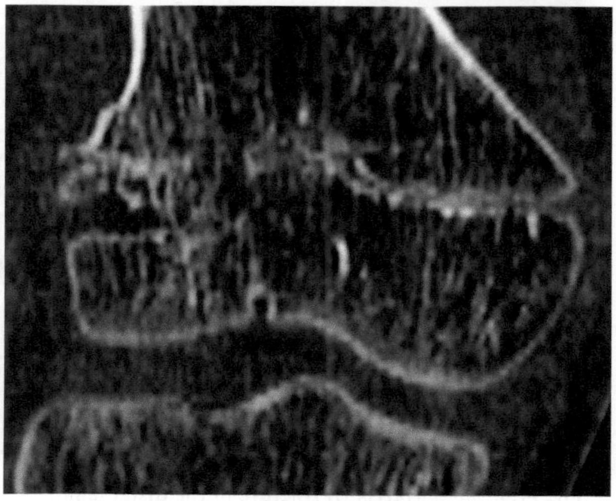
c

Fig. 14.4a–c. Fracture through the distal femoral growth plate with marked displacement of the epiphysis. Follow-up radiographs showing fusion of the central portion of the growth plate causing remodeling and deformity around the knee joint. The extent of the growth plate fusion is best demonstrated with cross-sectional imaging

a

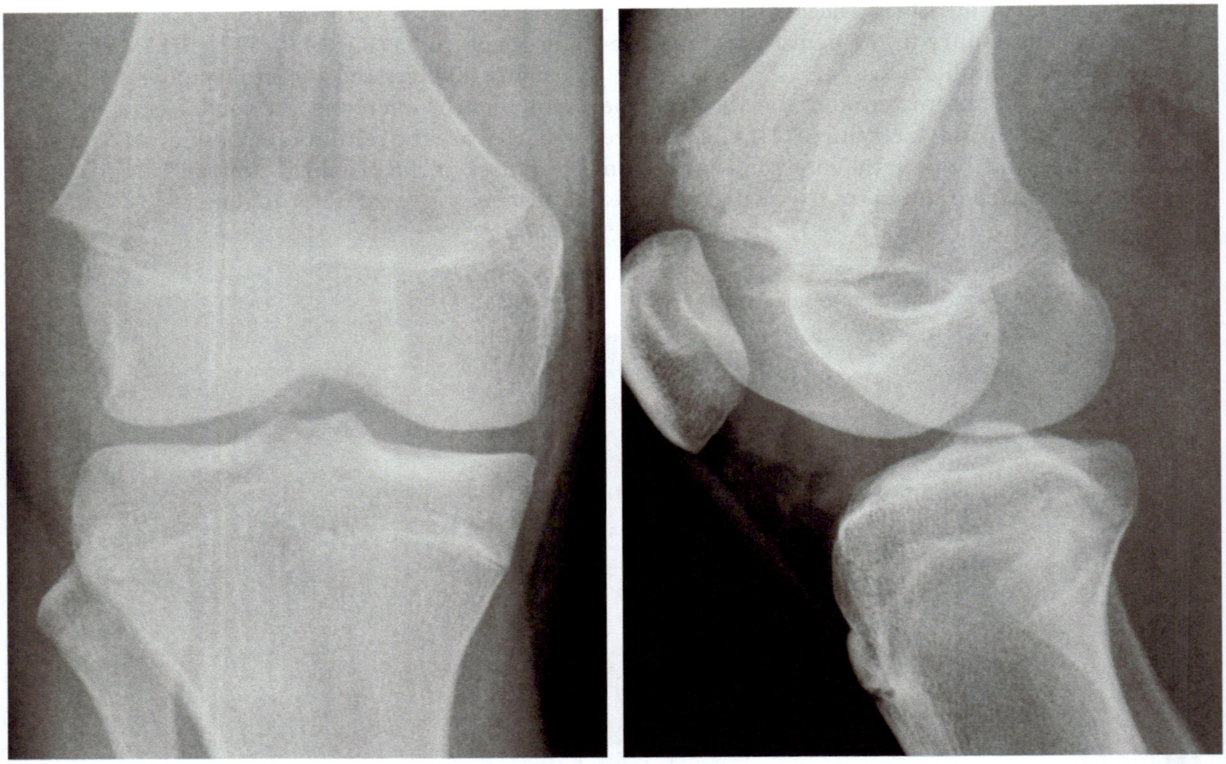

Fig. 14.5a,b. AP and lateral radiographs of the knee demonstrating a Salter-Harris II fracture of the distal femur with posterior displacement

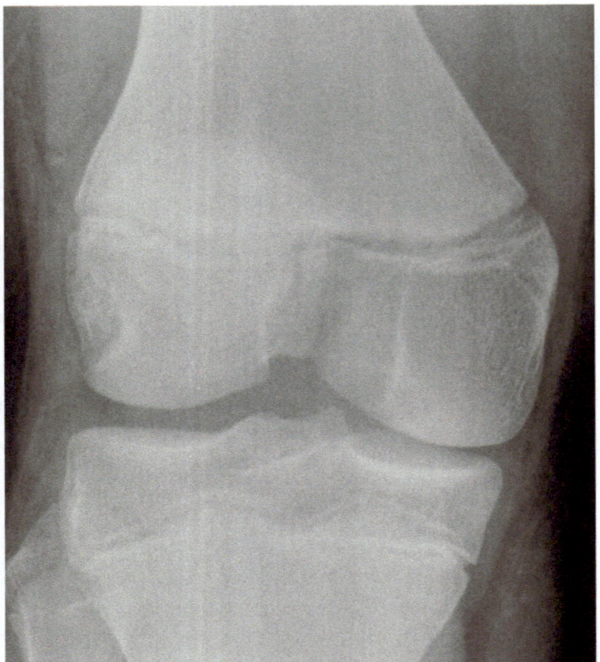

Fig. 14.6. Salter-Harris III fracture of the distal femur

14.8.1 Treatment

Radiographs will often confirm the fracture pattern and the degree of displacement, and often these injuries will reduce when the deforming force is removed, with 10° of angulation in the line of the joint being acceptable but there can be no obvious varus or valgus angulation.

Salter-Harris I and II injuries which are reducible and stable can be treated in a long-leg cast non-weight bearing for 6–8 weeks. This may fail if a sleeve of periosteum becomes interposed within the physis (Sponsellar and Beaty 1996). Unstable or irreducible fractures or SH III and IV injuries require open reduction and internal fixation, preferably using cannulated screw fixation.

SH II injuries are associated with subsequent growth disturbance usually on the contralateral side to the metaphyseal fracture, as this is the point of maximal injury of the physis.

Complications from these injuries are directly related to the severity of the deforming force. This dictates the fracture pattern, the degree of displacement and the associated soft tissue injuries. Age of the child and the rate and accuracy of the fracture reduction and stabilisation are also important factors. The radiographic signs of premature closure usually become apparent 6 months after the injury.

Accurate assessment is possible with CT scans. If less than 25% of the cross sectional area of the physis is involved it may be possible to surgically excise the bony bar and interpose a fat graft. More extensive defects cannot be excised and deformity can only then be corrected by osteotomy or staple epiphysiodesis.

14.9 Proximal Tibial Physeal Injuries and Epiphyseal Fractures

In the tibia, a proximal physeal injury with displacement of the epiphysis is rare. The mechanism is due either to a direct force to the proximal tibia or, as more commonly occurs in adolescent boys, it is due to an indirect force. This indirect force is usually anterior, causing hyperextension to the proximal tibia.

A varus or valgus angulation is caused by adduction or abduction forces, respectively. Occasionally, in boys nearing skeletal maturity, the tibia may show a flexion type injury. This occurs when taking off or landing from a jump.

One can separate these fractures using the Salter-Harris classification (Fig. 14.7):

- SH I – These are uncommon. Over 50% are displaced with the metaphysis lying medially or posteriorly.
- SH II – This is the commonest with over 50% being displaced. Usually the metaphysis lies medially due to a lateral abduction force.
- SH III – Usually the vertical fracture lies laterally with involvement of the lateral collateral ligament.
- SH IV – May involve either the medial or lateral proximal tibia. It is associated with avulsion of the ACL.
- SH V – Associated with genu recurvatum as a result of a dashboard injury.

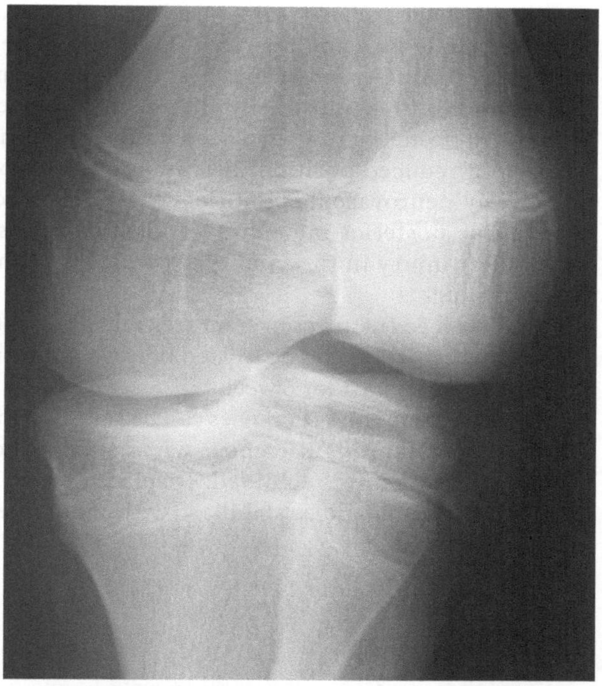
a

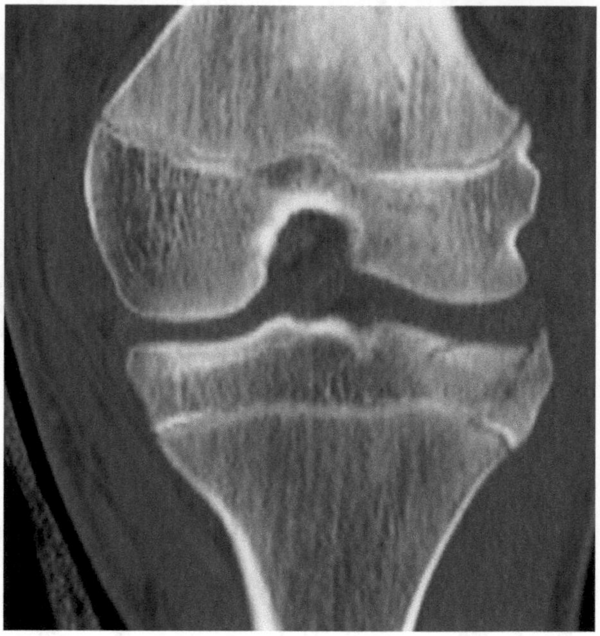
b

Fig. 14.7. a AP radiograph showing fracture of the lateral aspect of the proximal tibial epiphysis. **b** Corresponding coronal CT image demonstrating a more complex fracture pattern within the epiphysis

In older adolescents with fused growth plates fractures follow an adult pattern (Fig. 14.8). When evaluating these types of injuries, it is important to remember that minimally displaced fractures may have been severely displaced before recoiling back to a reduced position. It is important to exclude any neurovascular injuries with these fractures. The posterior metaphyseal spike can cause a vascular injury in the same way as occurs in the distal femur.

Undisplaced fractures or fractures that are stable following reduction can be treated non-weightbearing in a long-leg cast for 6 weeks.

Unstable type I and II injuries can be stabilised by crossed percutaneous Kirschner wires once reduction of the fracture is achieved. Displaced type III and IV injuries should be stabilised with cannulated screw fixation.

14.10 Tibial Tuberosity Avulsion Fractures

When assessing injuries to the tibial tuberosity, it is important to understand its normal development. At birth, there is no ossification (cartilaginous stage). The secondary ossification centre appears in the tibial tuberosity between 7 and 12 years of age (apophyseal stage). This centre is separated from the main secondary ossification centre of the proximal tibia by a cartilaginous bridge. The two centres fuse at about 16 years (epiphyseal stage) and will fuse to the metaphysis with physeal closure at about 18 (bony stage).

The ligamentum patellae (patellar tendon) is attached to the tubercle. Avulsion occurs when the traction force exceeds the combined strength of the

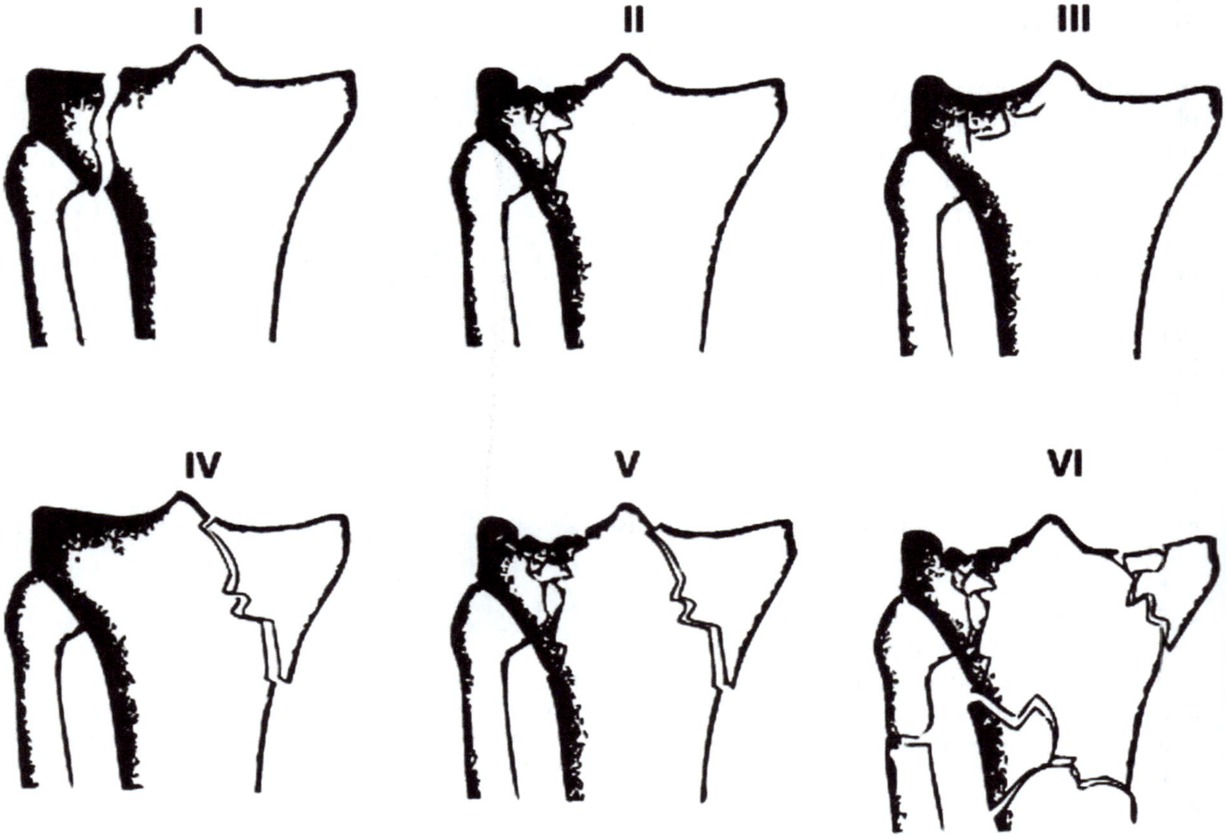

Fig. 14.8. Types of tibial plateau fractures: *I*, split fracture of the lateral tibial condyle; *II*, split fracture with associated depression; *III*, depressed fracture of the lateral tibial plateau; *IV*, fracture of the medial tibial plateau; *V*, bicondylar fracture (can be T or Y shaped); *VI*, bicondylar fracture with metaphyseal/diaphyseal association

physis underlying the tubercle, the surrounding perichondrium and periosteum.

The mechanism of injury is either a powerful active knee extension or passive knee flexion against a contracted quadriceps. It occurs in adolescents who have started the closure of their proximal tibial physis (usually boys aged 14–16 years old).

Three types of avulsion fracture have been described OGDEN et al. (1980) (Fig. 14.9).

On an AP radiograph, the tubercle lies just lateral to the midline of the tibia and its profile is best seen with slight internal rotation.

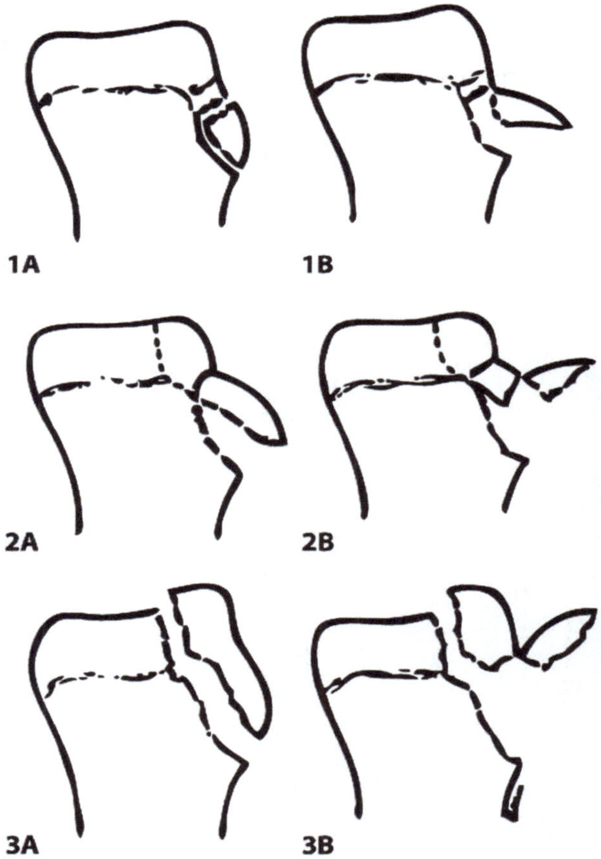

Fig. 14.9. Classification of tibial tuberosity avulsion injuries: *1A,1B*, separation of the distal portion of the physis; *2A,2B*, the separation involves the ossification centres of the tibial tubercles and tibial epiphysis; *3A,3B*, fracture/separation of the entire tubercle. In addition, there may be fracturing through the avulsed fragment (type B)

Only type 1A fractures can be treated with long-leg cast immobilisation. All other fracture types require open reduction and internal fixation. This is usually done by cannulated screws and washers. Fragmentation from previous Osgood-Schlatter's disease may make screw fixation less effective and this can be supplemented by tension band wire fixation.

Type 2 and 3 injuries may have associated intraarticular damage and the knee should be arthroscoped at the same time as fracture fixation to assess this (Fig. 14.10).

14.11 Tibial Spine Fractures

Anterior tibial spine fractures are more common in children than adults. They are caused by forced hyperextension of the knee with some rotation of the tibia on the femur. This results in a tensile force through the ACL, which has a broad attachment to the anterior tibial spine and the anterior horn of the medial meniscus.

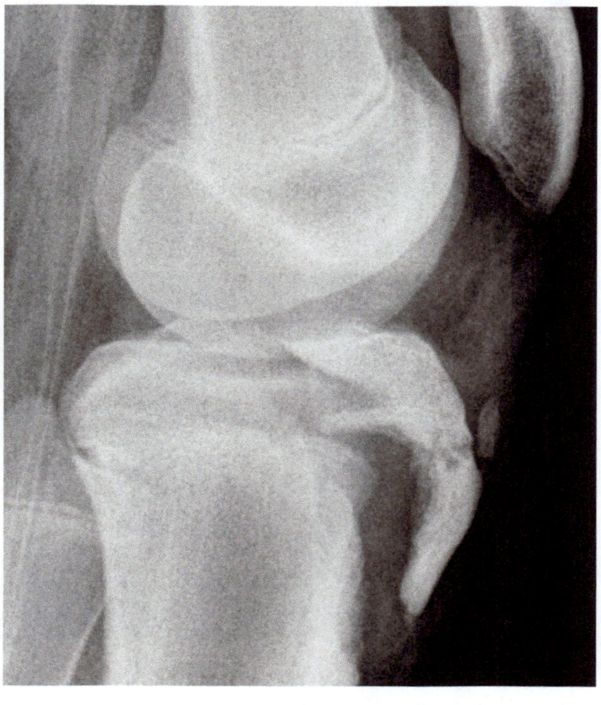

Fig. 14.10. Radiographs showing a type 3A tibial tuberosity fracture

This type of injury in an adult or older child would result in an ACL rupture. In children, the tensile strength of the ACL and the cartilaginous surface of the anterior tibial spine is greater than that of the subchondral bone. Therefore the anterior tibial spine fractures through the subchondral bone.

The patient will present with a painful swollen knee, secondary to the haemarthrosis. The knee should be assessed for an associated collateral ligament injury, with instability on varus or valgus stressing. There may be a positive anterior draw test.

AP and lateral radiographs of the knee should be obtained to assess the degree of displacement and any rotation of the fragment. In children, the avulsed fragment may be mainly unossified cartilage with only a small thin ossified fragment. CT is more sensitive in detecting tiny avulsed fragments and MR imaging will detect associated soft tissue injuries (Fig. 14.11).

Figure 14.12 illustrates the classification of the anterior tibial spine fractures by MEYERS and McKEEVER (1959). Treatment is dependent upon the degree of displacement.

Undisplaced fractures or fractures which reduce with manipulation of the knee can be treated non-weight bearing in a long-leg cast for 6–8 weeks. The aim is to prevent anteroposterior instability due to the ACL healing with increased length. There is controversy whether this is best prevented by casting the knee in hyperextension or up to 30° of flexion.

All surgeons agree that if the fragment does not reduce, especially with a grade 3 injury, the fragment requires operative reduction and stabilisation. Many procedures have been described including arthroscopic and open techniques. Fixation can be with sutures, wires or screws. Fixation should be supplemented with a long-leg cast for 6 weeks.

When the anterior tibial spine fragment displaces, it can lie on top of the anterior horn of the medial (and occasionally lateral) meniscus. This can prevent its reduction and must be looked for at the time of surgical reduction and fixation.

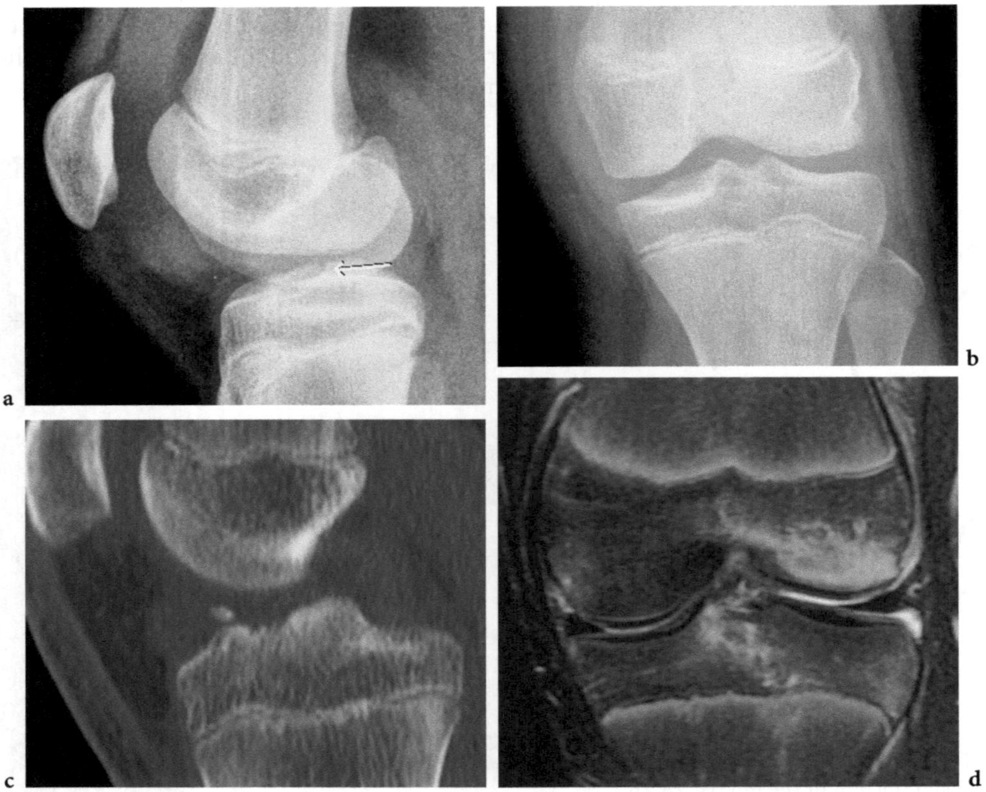

Fig. 14.11a–d. AP and lateral radiograph (**a,b**) showing an avulsed fragment from the tibial spine. The sagittal CT reconstructions (**c**) confirm the injury. The coronal T2 fat saturated MR image (**d**) shows oedema around the tibial spine as well as associated oedema in the femoral condyle

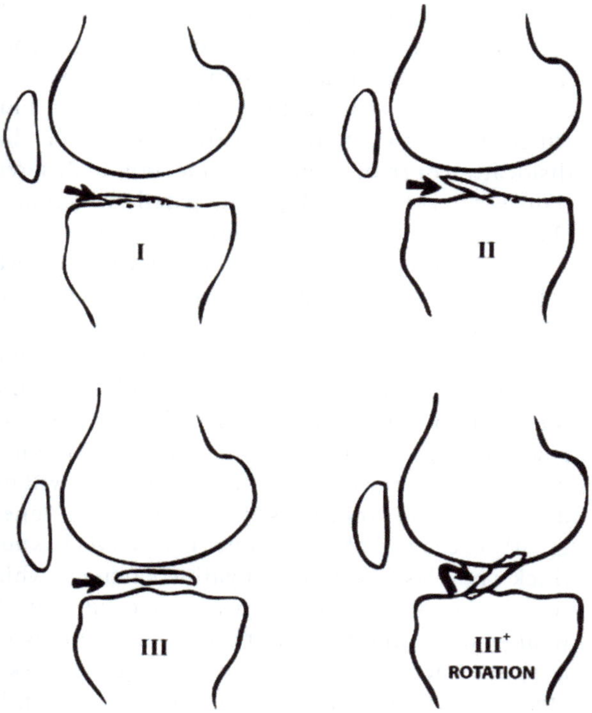

Fig. 14.12. Diagram of the different types of fracture of the intercondylar eminence of the tibia. *I*, minimal displacement; *II*, displacement of the anterior third/half of the avulsed fragment from the intercondylar eminence (beak-like deformity); *III*, the avulsed fragment is completely separated, with *III*+ the fragment is rotated so that the bony fracture margin faces into the joint (union impossible). (From Meyers and McKeever 1959)

14.12 Proximal Tibial Metaphyseal Fractures

This is a common injury which usually occurs in children of 3–8 years old. The child will have a history of a fall when running or playing and will present with a painful leg that they are reluctant to bear weight on. The leg may be swollen and the proximal tibia will be tender.

Radiographs show a torus or greenstick fracture of the proximal tibial metaphysis. The fracture line may be poorly visible or even incomplete, running from the medial (tension) side. Occasionally, there may be valgus angulation and the fibula may also be fractured.

Treatment is to place the child in a non-weight bearing long-leg cast for 4–6 weeks. Any valgus angulation must be noted and corrected. This often innocuous injury can be complicated by a valgus deformity of the tibia which may not become apparent for up to 6 months after the injury. The cause of this phenomenon is not understood but it is probably due to medial metaphyseal overgrowth. Other theories put forward are the tethering effect of the fibula, the deforming influence of the iliotibial band, the interposition of pes anserinus or periosteum medially or even an undiagnosed Type 5 Salter-Harris injury to the lateral physis. The valgus deformity usually spontaneously corrects over 2–3 years. Rarely may a corrective osteotomy of the proximal tibia is indicated.

Displaced fractures occur in adolescents and are caused by higher energy trauma. These fractures must be reduced and splinted non-weight bearing in a long-leg cast for 6 weeks.

14.13 Proximal Fibula Fractures

Fractures of the head and neck of the fibula occur rarely in isolation and are more commonly associated with proximal tibial fractures, especially compression, bicondylar and subcondylar fractures. A spiral fracture of the proximal fibula is often associated with an ankle fracture, resulting from an external rotation force. These fractures are known as Maisonneuve fractures. Fibula head fractures can occur from direct impact, valgus stress (associated with a tibial condylar fracture), and varus injuries. Varus stresses can cause avulsion of the fibular styloid at the site of the biceps tendon and fibular (lateral) collateral ligament. Peroneal nerve injury is not uncommon with these injuries. Dislocation of the proximal fibula is often missed on the initial radiograph.

14.14 Osteochondral Fractures

Most commonly these are associated with an acute traumatic lateral dislocation of the patella. The fragment is therefore usually from the lateral femoral condyle or the patella itself (Rorabeck and Bobechko 1976).

Alternatively the injury is due to an axial compressive force of the femoral condyle on the tibia. Occasionally an external shearing force against the femoral condyle will cause this injury.

The patient presents with a history of an acute injury. They will have a swollen painful knee due to the lipohaemarthrosis. This can be aspirated under aseptic conditions, which will reduce the pain and aid diagnosis – the aspirate will be bloody with fat globules in it.

The fracture is through the subchondral bone. The bony part of the fragment is usually very small and is poorly visualised on radiographs (Alleyne and Galloway 2001; Farmer et al. 2001; Matelic et al. 1995; Nietosvaara et al. 1994; Stanitski and Paletta 1998).

On the radiographs, there may be a small bony fragment within the knee joint, these can be difficult to visualise and a notch view may be helpful. CT and/or MR imaging are more sensitive in the detection of any loose fragments.

The patient may undergo a knee arthroscopy. The surgeon can take this opportunity to fully examine the knee under the anaesthetic, in particular to look for signs of a patella dislocation. The haemarthrosis is washed out. This gives better visualisation which is required to identify the area of cartilage loss and to find the dislodged fragment.

The articular cartilage lying at the edges of bare area is trimmed back to a stable cartilaginous rim. The bare bone is drilled using a fine Kirschner wire to stimulate bleeding from the subchondral bone and the formation of fibrocartilage. However, fibrocartilage is not as durable as hyaline cartilage and it is preferable to fix the osteochondral fragments if possible. This is only possible in the acute setting and really applies to large osteoarticular fragments.

14.15 Patella Fracture

These are not common injuries in children, with only 1% of patellar fractures occurring under the age of 15 (Nummi 1971; Bates et al. 1994; Crawford 1976). This is thought possibly due to the smaller extensor muscle mass, reducing the contractive forces associated with indirect injury and the cushioning effect of the surrounding cartilage.

Patellar fractures can occur from direct and indirect mechanisms, with a direct force being the commonest cause. Potential mechanisms include a powerful quadriceps contraction, a direct anterior blow which may result in an open fracture and patellar dislocation or relocation. It is important to differentiate a fracture from a bipartite patella which has a characteristic location and smooth margins.

Fractures may be classified into marginal (vertical), stellate, transverse, avulsion and comminuted (Fig. 14.13).

When a patellar fracture is suspected, radiographs of the knee are obtained, with particular reference to the lateral view. The fracture may appear incomplete with only a small bony fragment visible. However, conventional radiographs will underestimate this injury, as the cartilage component greatly exceeds that of the bone. The patella has very thick and elastic articular hyaline cartilage which remains intact and the separation occurs at the weaker subchondral layer of bone. This is known as a "sleeve fracture" and is unique to the growing skeleton. Ultrasound has been used to confirm this injury and allows assessment of fracture separation and displacement (Ditchfield et al. 2000). These most commonly occur at the inferior pole and are associated with knee extension activities, such as the high

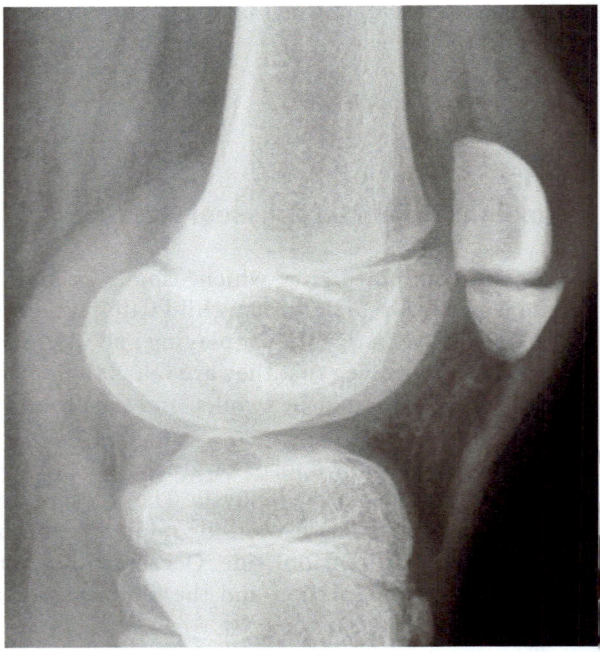

Fig. 14.13. Lateral radiograph showing a transverse fracture through the patella

jump (Fig. 14.14). Medial sleeve fractures occur with traumatic lateral dislocation of the patella. Lateral sleeve fractures are often confused with a bipartite patella. They are stress fractures caused by the pull of vastus lateralis. Superior sleeve fractures are the least common.

Medial marginal (vertical) fractures in children may traverse the entire thickness of bone or may be a medial tangential osteochondral fracture. These longitudinal orientated fractures may only be visible on an axial or oblique radiograph. Lateral vertical fractures can occur in athletes due to the pull of the vastus lateralis muscle.

Children can also sustain a transverse fracture through the mid-portion of the patella or a stellate pattern fracture. These can occur from falls with the knee in flexion or severe contraction of the quadriceps tendon. These are best seen on the lateral projection. Transverse stress fractures occur due to abnormal quadriceps pull on osteopenic bones in children with cerebral palsy.

Fractures of the patella also occur in association with femoral shaft, condylar, proximal tibia and posterior dislocation of the hip ('dashboard injury').

Undisplaced fractures can be treated with a period of splinting in a cylinder cast or brace. However, as with all intraarticular fractures, any displaced patellar fracture requires open reduction and internal fixation. Displacement of more than 3 mm is not acceptable and may disrupt the extensor mechanism (Sponseller and Beaty 1996).

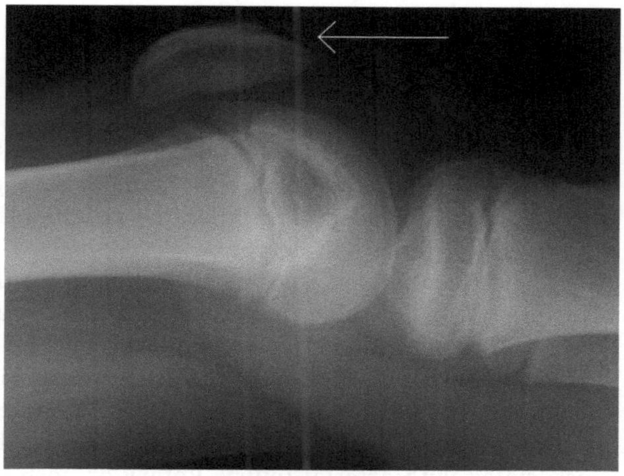

Fig. 14.14. Lateral radiograph showing a sleeve fracture of the distal pole of the patella (*arrow*)

14.16 Patellar Dislocation

Traumatic acute patellofemoral joint dislocation is uncommon in children. The patella almost always dislocates laterally. Certain anatomical variants predispose to dislocation. These include patella alta, trochlea dysplasia and genu valgum.

The mechanism is either a direct force to the medial side of the patella or a valgus force on the knee with vastus lateralis pulling the patella laterally.

A lateral dislocation causes damage to the medial patello-femoral ligament and vastus medialis obliquis. It can also cause an osteochondral fracture from either the lateral femoral condyle which may be sheared of by the patella or alternatively there may be an avulsion of the medial facet of the patella.

Usually the patella will spontaneously relocate and once reduced X-rays must be obtained. Avulsion fractures may best be seen on skyline views. However, bending the knee may be painful and the anatomy may be imaged more accurately by CT or MRI which has the added advantage of allowing assessment of the soft tissues. MR imaging will show damage to the medial retinaculum, with buckling of the lateral retinaculum, there may be an osteochondral fracture from either the lateral femoral condyle or the medial facet of the patella, bone bruising with the lateral femoral condyle and signal change within Hoffa's fat pad.

Standard treatment has been to splint the knee in a cylinder cast or extension knee brace for 3–6 weeks followed by physiotherapy and rehabilitation programme. However, recent evidence would suggest a 17% redislocation rate following the first dislocation and as high as 50% for second time dislocators (Mulford et al. 2007). This has prompted a trend towards more aggressive management and surgical reconstruction of the damaged structures. In such patients imaging is useful not only in assessing the acute injury but also predisposing anatomical variants. Much interest has been focused on the shallow trochlear groove (trochlear dysplasia) as a predisposing anatomical abnormality and this can be imaged quite clearly with both axial CT and MRI scans.

14.17 Knee Dislocation

These are rare injuries in children. They are due to high energy trauma and will result in major damage to the soft tissues around the knee, in particular the ligaments, arteries and nerves.

The dislocation is described according to the direction of tibial displacement relative to the femur. Anterior dislocation is the commonest type, and is associated with disruption of the anterior cruciate ligament, the posterior joint capsule and popliteal artery damage. Posterior dislocation can also be associated with arterial injury. Rotary or posterolateral dislocation is caused by force abduction and internal rotation. On the lateral radiograph, the femoral condyle is in profile but the tibia is rotated posterolaterally and the proximal tibiofibular joint is seen in its entirety. An early complete assessment and documentation of the neurovascular status of the leg distally is vital. Also look for signs of compartment syndrome.

The child should be taken to theatre immediately when:

- The tibiofemoral joint remains dislocated
- There is arterial damage requiring surgical repair
- There are signs of compartment syndrome

MR imaging will help define the extent of the soft tissue damage, especially to the ligaments, while arteriography will detail any arterial vessel damage, in particular an intimal tear.

Some surgeons will assess the knee under a general anaesthetic even if the joint has reduced spontaneously. The management of these injuries is controversial. Some surgeons opt for early repair and rehabilitation whilst others prefer delayed reconstruction.

When a knee dislocation is accompanied by fractures, these must be reduced and fixed early.

14.18 Proximal Tibiofibular Dislocation

Dislocation is typically classified according to the direction of displacement of the fibular head, and can occur anterolaterally, posteromedially or superiorly.

Anterolateral dislocation is the commonest and is the result of a twisting fall. On an AP radiograph, the head of the fibula is seen almost in its entirety while on the lateral view, it is completely overlaid by the tibial condyle. In posteromedial dislocation, the fibular head is overlaid by the tibial condyle on the AP radiograph but is displaced posteriorly on the lateral view. In superior dislocation, the tibia is foreshortened as a result of a shaft fracture.

Anterolateral dislocation is managed by closed reduction. The posteromedial variant often requires urgent surgery and can be associated with vascular injury.

14.19 Meniscal Injuries

Meniscal injuries in children have a similar appearance to those of adults. MR imaging is the standard investigation for meniscal injuries. The meniscus is injured when a twisting and compressive force is applied. In adolescents, the medial meniscus is most commonly injured. In children, the menisci are very vascularised and intrameniscal vessels will appear as linear areas of increased signal intensity which should not be confused with tears (Fig. 14.15). These vessels are central, horizontal, linear or possibly globular and originate from the capsular attachment of the meniscus (King et al. 1996; Luhmann et al. 2005). Meniscal tears in children are not uncommonly vertical (Busch 1990). Meniscal injury frequently accompanies ACL and PCL rupture (Ross and Chesterman 1986).

Approximately 1.5%–3 % of the population have a discoid lateral meniscus. These congenital variants are prone to tears. Discoid meniscus is diagnosed if there is continuity of the anterior and posterior horns of the meniscus on three or more consecutive sagittal images (4-mm slices), there is loss of the normal semilunar morphology and greater than 50% coverage of the lateral tibial plateau by the meniscus.

A discoid meniscus will often be asymptomatic but may cause mechanical symptoms such as pain, giving way, an effusion, and a clicking or snapping knee. Surgery to excise the central portion of a discoid meniscus can be done arthroscopically.

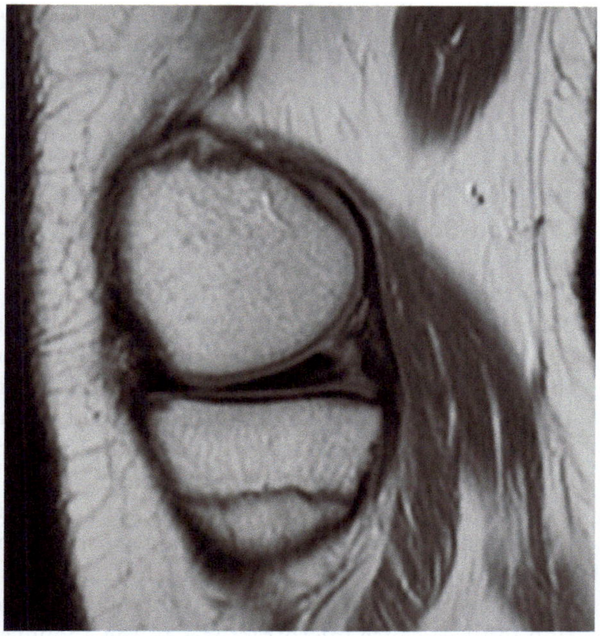

Fig. 14.15. Sagittal T1 weighted image of the knee showing high signal change within the meniscus as a consequence of normal vascular supply

14.20 Ligaments – Collaterals and Cruciates

Anterior cruciate ligament injuries (ACL) are increasingly being diagnosed in children (Shea et al. 2003), the incidence being related to skeletal maturation. Tibial avulsion fractures and partial tears are common in young children who are not skeletally mature which suggest the less rigid cartilaginous skeleton is more able to absorb the forces of trauma. In the skeletally immature, ACL injuries are more often seen in boys (Prince et al. 2005). As the child matures, complete ACL tears and associated injuries occur with frequency patterns approaching those of adults.

In children with ligamental injuries, it is important to detect associated meniscal injuries (Williams et al. 1996) and occult physeal injury as physeal arrest can occasionally occur following non-physeal injury of the lower extremity (Hresko and Kasser 1989).

Radiographs can identify associated avulsion injuries, such as Pelegrini-Stieda lesions (avulsion of the medial femoral condyle at the origin of the medial collateral ligament) and Segond lesion (avulsion fracture of the lateral tibial plateau). Segond fractures are associated with LCL, ACL and meniscal tears (Sferopoulos et al. 2006).

MR imaging is now the investigation of choice for suspected ligamental injuries. With partial tears there is increased signal intensity on T2 weighted images within the ligament but with some fibres remaining intact. With complete tears, there is total discontinuity of the ligamentous fibres with abnormal signal extending completely across the ligament.

Associated signs of ACL injury are common in children and include lipohaemarthrosis (this may indicate bony injury and a tibial avulsion injury should be excluded), contusion in the lateral femoral condyle and posterior tibial plateau, depression within the lateral condylopatellar sulcus (secondary to impaction of the lateral condyle on the tibial plateau) and Segond fractures (Prince et al. 2005).

Posterior cruciate ligament injuries (PCL), as in adults, are less common than ACL injuries. In infants and children, it must be remembered that the PCL lies in a more horizontal position than in adults and this must not be confused with injury. Secondary signs of a PCL tear include posterior subluxation of the tibia, associated tears of the ACL, meniscal tears and avulsion of the tibial insertion (Ross and Chesterman 1986).

Collateral ligament injuries are less frequent than those of the cruciates. The medial collateral ligament (MCL) is injured more commonly than the lateral ligament (LCL). Tears may be partial or complete. With a partial tear, there is increased signal intensity on T2 weighed images, the fibres are disorganised and can be thickened. There may be associated marrow oedema in the adjacent bone. With complete tears, there is lack of continuity of the ligament fibres.

Cruciate ligament surgery in skeletally immature patients is controversial. Extra-articular stabilisation procedures avoid disruption of the growth plate, but have poor long-term results. Some studies have shown that transtibial and femoral tunnels of less than 6 mm do not cause significant growth arrest. (Lo et 1997)

14.21 Osteochondritis Dissecans

There is a defect in the subchondral region of the distal femur with partial or complete separation of the bone fragment which is most often seen on the postero-lateral aspect of the medial femoral condyle (about 80% of cases), and less often seen on the posterior aspect of the lateral femoral condyle. It is more common in males aged 10–20 years old. The aetiology is unknown, but repetitive overloading is thought to contribute to fragmentation and separation of bony fragments. Initially the overlying articular cartilage remains intact. A breach in the articular surface is a precursor to possible detachment. The patient often presents with vague symptoms of knee pain, with occasional swelling. There is often a history of previous trauma. Pain is worse after activities and loose bodies may cause locking.

Prognosis depends on age of onset of symptoms; lesions occurring after growth plate closure and lesions which detach have the worst prognosis. A variety of classification symptoms based on arthroscopic or radiological findings have been described. The principle being to try and predict those lesions which are unstable and those needing surgical intervention (Kocher et al. 2001, 2007; Cepero et al. 2005; Pill et al. 2003; De Smet et al. 1997; Takahara et al. 2007).

Those predictors of instability are a large size of fragment (greater than 1 cm), fluid interface between the fragment and host bone, and cystic areas within the bone, enhancement of tissue around the fracture margins and disruption or defects within the overlying cartilage. Often fluid is seen passing through the cartilage.

On a lateral radiograph, the knee lesion may appear sclerotic, typically on the lateral aspect of the medial femoral condyle. A tunnel view may demonstrate medial condylar defects, and this may be better profiled with the knee in varying degrees of flexion. The lesion may appear sclerotic if the presentation is delayed.

Use of bone scintigraphy has been surpassed by MR imaging. With MR imaging, on T1 weighted images, the area is of low signal due to bone marrow oedema and there may be overlying thickened synovium. On T2 weighed images, there is hyperintensity due to the marrow oedema and there may be small cystic areas within the bone. Fast spin echo proton density fat saturated images are useful for assessing the overlying cartilage. MR arthrography can demonstrate contrast tracking beneath the fragment which indicates instability. It may be used to determine whether the fragment is detached. CT is useful for detecting small ossified loose fragments.

In skeletally immature patients, if the fragment remains attached, treatment is conservative with protected weight bearing. If the fragments detach, the principle is to maintain a congruous joint. Fragments smaller than 5 mm can be excised and the defects drilled to create a bleeding base. With larger fragments, especially in the weight bearing region, reduction and internal fixation should be considered.

14.22 Osgood-Schlatter Disease

The exact aetiology of Osgood-Schlatter disease is controversial. The generally excepted idea is that of a traction apophysitis of the patellar ligament on the tibial tubercle. It was described independently in 1903 by Osgood in the English literature and Schlatter in the German literature. This condition is the commonest cause of knee pain in preadolescents.

The lesion occurs when the tibial tubercle is in the apophyseal stage and the secondary ossification centre has appeared. The tibial tubercle apophysis appears between 7–9 years of age, and repeated traction injuries cause microfractures in the apophysis (Lazerte 1958).

A tendinopathy is also present (Rosenberg et al. 1992), but whether a fracture precedes the tendinopathy or vice versa is unclear.

The onset is usually gradual, with patients complaining of pain over the tibial tubercle or patellar region after activities such as running or jumping. An acute onset of pain with no preceding symptoms should alert the clinician to the possibility of a tibial tubercle avulsion.

The natural history of Osgood-Schlatter disease is self-limiting.

Although radiographs are not necessary to make a diagnosis, they are often taken. A lateral radiograph of the knee may show fragmentation of the tibial apophysis, and in chronic cases, an ossicle.

Surgery is rarely indicated, except to remove an ossicle if it is causing pain when kneeling.

Ultrasound will show the soft tissue swelling and thickening of the overlying soft issue and tendon. MR imaging will show fragmentation of the tibial tubercle, heterotopic ossification within the distal patellar tendon and non-specific oedema with a reactive bursitis.

OSD needs to be differentiated from Sinding-Larsen and Johansson syndrome which is a traction apophysitis of the distal pole of the patella.

Ultrasound is a useful adjunct to delineate involvement of bone, cartilage and the patellar tendon, as is MRI, and may be used to monitor the course of the disease.

References

Alleyne KR, Galloway MT (2001) Management of osteochondral injuries of the knee. [Review] Clin Sports Med 20:343–364

Anderson M, Green WT, Messner MB (1963) Growth and predictions of growth in the lower extremities. J Bone Joint Surg Am 45-A: 1–14

Bates DG, Hresko MT, Jaramillo D (1994) Patellar sleeve fracture: demonstration with MR imaging. Radiology 193:825–827

Bulloch B, Neto G, Plint A, Lim R, Lidman P, Reed M, Nijssen-Jordan C, Tenenbein M, Klassen TP, Bhargava R (2003) Validation of the Ottawa Knee Rule in children: a multicenter study. Ann Emerg Med 42:48–55

Busch MT (1990) Meniscal injuries in children and adolescents. Clin Sports Med 9:661–680

Butt WP, Lederman H, Chuang S (1983) Radiology of the supra-patellar region. Clin Radiol 34:511–522

Cepero S, Ullot R, Sastre S (2005) Osteochondritis of the femoral condyles in children and adolescents: our experience over the last 28 years. J Pediatr Orthop B 14:24–29

Crawford AH (1976) **Fractures about the knee in children.** Orthop Clin North Am 7:639–656

Davies AP, Bayer J, Owen-Johnson S, Shepstone L, Darrah C, Glasgow MM, Donell ST (2004) The optimum knee flexion angle for skyline radiography is thirty degrees. Clin Orthop Relat Res 423:166–171

De Smet AA, Ilahi OA, Graf BK (1997) Untreated osteochondritis dissecans of the femoral condyles: prediction of patient outcome using radiographic and MR findings. Skeletal Radiol 26:463–467

Ditchfield A, Sampson MA, Taylor GR (2000) ultrasound diagnosis of sleeve fracture of the patella. Clin Radiol 55:467–469

Farmer JM, Martin DF, Boles CA, Curl WW (2001) Chondral and osteochondral injuries. Diagnosis and management. [Review] Clin Sports Med 20:299–320

Hresko M, Kasser J (1989) Physeal arrest about the knee associated with nonphyseal fractures in the lower extremity. J Bone Joint Surg Am 71:698–703

King SJ, Carty HM, Brady O (1996) Magnetic resonance imaging of knee injuries in children. Pediatr Radiol 26:287–290

Kocher MS, Micheli LJ, Yaniv M, Zurakowski D, Ames A, Adrignolo AA (2001) Functional and radiographic outcome of juvenile osteochondritis dissecans of the knee treated with transarticular arthroscopic drilling. Am J Sports Med 29:562–566

Kocher MS, Czarnecki JJ, Andersen JS, Micheli LJ (2007) Internal fixation of juvenile osteochondritis dissecans lesions of the knee. Am J Sports Med. 35:712–718

Lazerte GD (1958) Pathogenesis of Osgood-Schlatters disease. AM J Pathol 34:803–815

Laor T, Wall EJ, Vu LP (2006) Physeal widening in the knee due to stress injury in child athletes. AJR Am J Roentgenol 186:1260–1264

Lo IK, Kirkley A, Fowler PJ, Miniaci A (1997) The outcome of operatively treated anterior cruciate ligament disruptions in the skeletally immature child. Arthroscopy 13:627–634

Lo IK, Bell DM, Fowler PJ (1998). Anterior cruciate ligament injuries in the skeletally immature patient. Instr Course Lect 47:351–359

Luhmann SJ, Schootman M, Gordon JE, Wright RW (2005) Magnetic resonance imaging of the knee in children and adolescents. Its role in clinical decision-making. J Bone Joint Surg Am 87:497–502

Meyers MH, McKeever FM (1959) Fracture of the intercondylar eminence of the tibia. J Bone Joint Surg Am 41:209–222

Matelic TM, Aronsson DD, Boyd DW Jr, LaMont RL (1995) Acute hemarthrosis of the knee in children. Am J Sports Med 23:668–671

Moore BR, Hampers LC, Clark KD (2005) Performance of a decision rule for radiographs of pediatric knee injuries. J Emerg Med 28:257–261

Mulford JS, Wakeley CJ, Eldridge JDJ (2007) Assessment and management of chronic patellofemoral instability. J Bone Joint Surg Br 89B:709–716

Nietosvaara Y, Aalto K, Kallio PE (1994) Acute patellar dislocation in children: incidence and associated osteochondral fractures. J Pediatr Orthop 14:513–515

Nummi J (1971) Fracture of the patella. A clinical study of 707 patellar fractures. Ann Chir Gynaecol Fenn Suppl 179:1–85

Ogden JA, Tross RB, Murphy MJ (1980) Fractures of the tibial tuberosity in adolescents. J Bone Joint Surg 62A:205–215

Ozonoff MB (1979) Pediatric orthopaedic radiology. Saunders, Philadelphia

Pill SG, Ganley TJ, Milam RA, Lou JE, Meyer JS, Flynn JM (2003) Role of magnetic resonance imaging and clinical criteria in predicting successful nonoperative treatment of osteochondritis dissecans in children. J Pediatr Orthop 23:102–108

Prince JS, Laor T, Bean JA (2005) MRI of anterior cruciate ligament injuries and associated findings in the pediatric knee: changes with skeletal maturation. AJR Am J Roentgenol 185:756–762

Rogers LF (1992) The knee and shafts of the tibia and fibula. In: Radiology of skeletal trauma. Churchill Livingstone, New York

Rorabeck CH, Bobechko WP (1976) Acute dislocation of the patella with osteochondral fracture: a review of 18 cases. J Bone joint Surg 58B:237–240

Rosenberg ZS, Kauelblum M, Cheung YY et al (1992) Osgood-Schlatter lesion: fracture or tendonitis? Scintigraphic, CT and MR imaging features. Radiology 185:853–858

Ross AC, Chesterman PJ (1986) Isolated avulsion of the tibial attachment of the posterior cruciate ligament in childhood. J Bone Joint Surg Br 68:747

Seaberg DC, Yealy DM, Lukens T, Auble T, Mathias S (1998) Multicenter comparison of two clinical decision rules for the use of radiography in acute, high-risk knee injuries. Ann Emerg Med 32:8–13

Shea KG, Apel PJ, Pfeiffer RP (2003) Anterior cruciate ligament injury in paediatric and adolescent patients: a review of basic science and clinical research. Sports Med 33:455–471

Sponsellar PD, Beaty JH (1996) Fractures and dislocations about the knee. In: Rockwood CA Jr, Wilkins KE, Beaty JH (eds) Fractures in children, 4th edn. Lippincott-Raven, Philadelphia

Stanitski CL, Paletta GA Jr (1998) Articular cartilage injury with acute patellar dislocation in adolescents. Arthroscopic and radiographic correlation. Am J Sports Med 26:52–55

Sferopoulos NK, Rafailidis D, Traios S, Christoforides J (2006) Avulsion fractures of the lateral tibial condyle in children. Injury 37:57–60

Stiell IG, Greenberg GH, Wells GA et al (1995) Derivation of a decision rule for the use of radiography in acute knee injuries. Ann Emerg Med 26:405–413

Takahara M, Mura N, Sasaki J, Harada M, Ogino T (2007) Classification, treatment, and outcome of osteochondritis dissecans of the humeral capitellum. J Bone Joint Surg Am 89:1205–1214

Williams JS, Abate JA, Fadale PD et al (1996) Meniscal and nonosseous ACL injuries in children and adolescents. Am J Knee Surg 9:22–26

Ankle

15

Paul Gibbons

CONTENTS

15.1 Introduction

Ankle fractures account for approximately 5.5% (Landin 1983) of paediatric fractures and the distal tibial and fibular physes are common sites of physeal injury (Peterson and Peterson 1972). The potential consequences of ankle and distal tibial physeal injury are leg length inequality, angular and torsional malalignment and post-traumatic arthritis.

P. Gibbons MBBS, FRCS (Orth), FRACS
Senior Staff Specialist, Clinical Senior Lecturer, Faculty of Medicine, University of Sydney, Department of Orthopaedic Surgery, The Children's Hospital at Westmead, Locked Bag 4001, Westmead, NSW 2145, Sydney, Australia

15.2 Relevant Anatomy

The ankle is a modified hinge joint with joint movement in essentially one plane only – plantarflexion to dorsiflexion. The lateral malleolus allows some rotation to accommodate the changing width of the talar dome, which is broader anteriorly than posteriorly.

15.3 Ossification

The distal tibial epiphysis ossifies between 6 and 24 months of age. The medial malleolus appears at 7–8 years and is complete at 10 years. It usually ossifies as a downward extension of the distal tibial ossific nucleus but may develop as a separate centre of ossification and thus be mistaken for a fracture line. The distal tibial physis closes first centrally, then medially and finally anterolaterally (Fig. 15.1), with the entire process lasting about 18 months. This sequence of closure of the distal tibial physis is important in the pattern of transitional fractures (triplane and juvenile Tillaux). Completion of distal tibial physeal closure is at around 14 years in girls and 16 years in boys.

The distal fibular epiphysis begins to ossify between 18 and 20 months of age with the physis closing 12–24 months later than the distal tibial physis.

15.4 Mechanisms of Injury

Ankle fractures are usually caused by indirect trauma with the foot fixed and forced into either

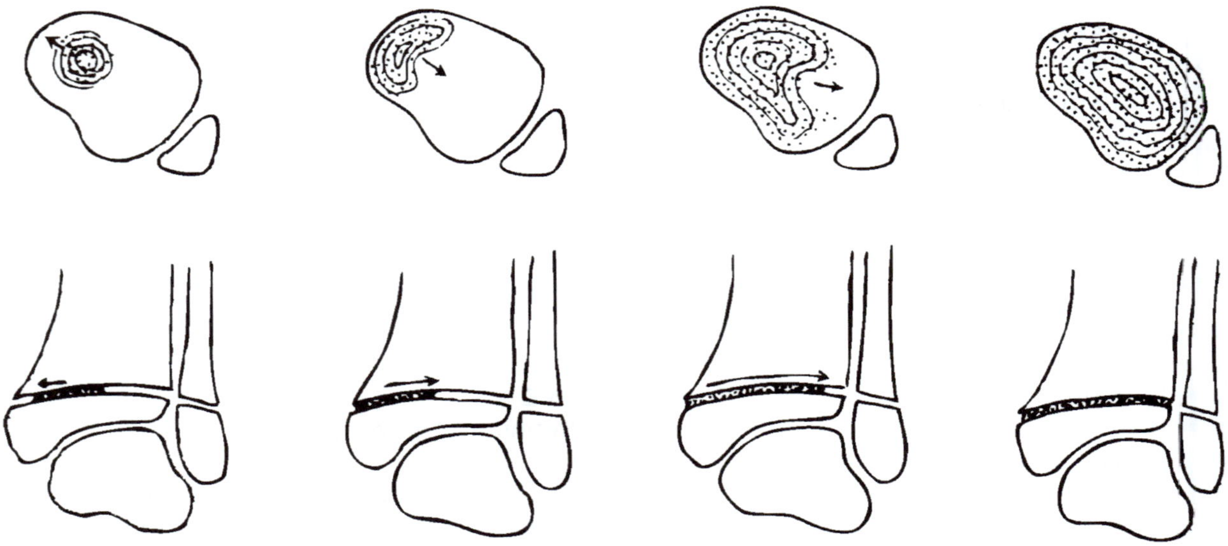

Fig. 15.1. Sequence of closure of distal tibial physis (adapted from FELDMAN et al. 1987)

dorsiflexion, plantarflexion, eversion, inversion, or external or internal rotation. Direct injuries do occur, such as in motor vehicle accidents and falls from a height. As elsewhere in children, ligamentous injuries of the ankle are uncommon because the ligaments are stronger than physeal cartilage.

15.5 Classification

In adults ankle fractures are traditionally classified according to the forces involved in producing the injury (LAUGE-HANSEN 1950). In children, the presence of the physis allows the same forces to produce different injury patterns. The Salter-Harris classification of physeal fractures is well recognised. Therefore, DIAS and TACHDJIAN (1978) modified the Lauge-Hansen classification to include the Salter-Harris classification and describe physeal injuries of the ankle in children. In the original classification there were four types of injury, each with a two-part name:

- Supination-Inversion
- Supination-Plantar flexion
- Supination-External rotation
- Pronation-Eversion external rotation

The first part of the name refers to the position of the foot at the moment of the injury. The second part indicates the direction of the abnormal force applied to the ankle. A further four types of fracture – juvenile Tillaux, triplane, axial compression and miscellaneous physeal injuries – were added later to complete the classification. Whilst this classification is useful in understanding the deforming forces of the fracture, and hence the type of manoeuvre needed to achieve a satisfactory closed reduction, the Salter-Harris classification is easier to commit to memory and provides a better predictor of outcome in terms of complications (SPIEGEL et al. 1978).

15.6 Clinical Assessment

The cardinal clinical sign of fracture is bony tenderness and careful palpation of the injured ankle will often differentiate between a fracture and a soft tissue injury. Clinical prediction rules have been shown to be useful in determining which children with ankle injuries require X-ray investigation (DAYAN et al. 2004; MYERS et al. 2005). Adherence to such rules may miss the diagnosis of a small proportion of fractures but these will generally be those of little clinical significance.

15.7 Radiological Assessment

Most ankle fractures can be adequately assessed using the standard ankle trauma series of antero-posterior, lateral and mortise views. Confusion in interpretation of radiographs can be caused by accessory centres of ossification and normal anatomical variants. In children aged 6–12 years medial (os subtibiale) and lateral (os subfibulare) accessory ossification centres are present in 20% and 1%, respectively (Powell 1961).

For paediatric ankle injuries with normal radiographs, high resolution ultrasound has been shown to be useful in diagnosing occult fractures (Simanovsky et al. 2005) and ligamentous injuries (Farley et al. 2001). The majority of these occult fractures are Salter-Harris I or II fractures of the distal fibular physis. If left undiagnosed and untreated the majority of such injuries would have a satisfactory outcome.

If there is suspected ankle instability stress views may be indicated, though they are rarely required in children.

Similarly, isotope bone scanning is rarely required in children's ankle injuries. However, it may be indicated in talar neck fractures which can be associated with avascular necrosis (Letts and Gibeault 1980).

Computerised tomography (CT) is particularly valuable in the assessment of transitional (triplane, juvenile Tillaux) and intraarticular fractures where the magnitude of displacement – both fracture gap and intraarticular or physeal step – is critical in determining whether or not operative intervention is required. CT is also extremely useful in helping the surgeon to plan the surgical approach in these situations.

Magnetic resonance (MR) imaging for acute paediatric ankle injuries conveys no real advantage over radiography (Lohman et al. 2001). It is probably as useful as CT in the assessment of transitional fractures and is also helpful in the evaluation of the articular cartilage in traumatic osteochondral lesions of the talus. Where it is perhaps most useful is in the later stages, following physeal injury, to identify and characterise physeal arrest (Futami et al. 2000; Sailhan et al. 2004).

15.8 Salter-Harris Type I and II Fractures

Respectively, these account for 15% and 40% of physeal fractures of the distal tibia (Spiegel et al. 1978). Other than standard radiographs no special studies are required as the diagnosis is generally straightforward. If there is significant displacement these fractures can, in most cases, be treated by closed reduction and cast immobilisation. Occasionally periosteal soft-tissue interposition prevents accurate reduction. In such cases the soft-tissue interposition can be removed operatively and the fracture reduced. Fixation can be achieved with a screw or smooth k-wires if desired (Fig. 15.2).

15.9 Salter-Harris Type III and IV Fractures

Since these fractures are intra-articular and disrupt the physis they more frequently require surgery than Type I or II fractures. They account for 20% and 1% of distal tibial physeal fractures, respectively (Spiegel et al. 1978). Apart from the juvenile Tillaux fracture (see below) these are supination-inversion injuries leading to a medial malleolar fracture as the medial corner of the talar dome is forced into the junction of the distal tibial joint surface and medial malleolus. This shears the medial malleolus from the rest of the epiphysis in a Type III or IV pattern. There may be an associated avulsion Type I or II fracture of the distal fibula. The degree of displacement is usually evident on plain radiographs but if required can be readily evaluated with CT. Undisplaced Type III fractures may be treated non-operatively by cast immobilisation. Undisplaced Type IV fractures are inherently unstable and because of this they, and displaced (greater than 2 mm) Type III and IV fractures, should be managed by open reduction and internal fixation. A single cannulated interfragmentary screw is usually adequate for fixation. This should remain wholly epiphyseal and not cross the growth plate.

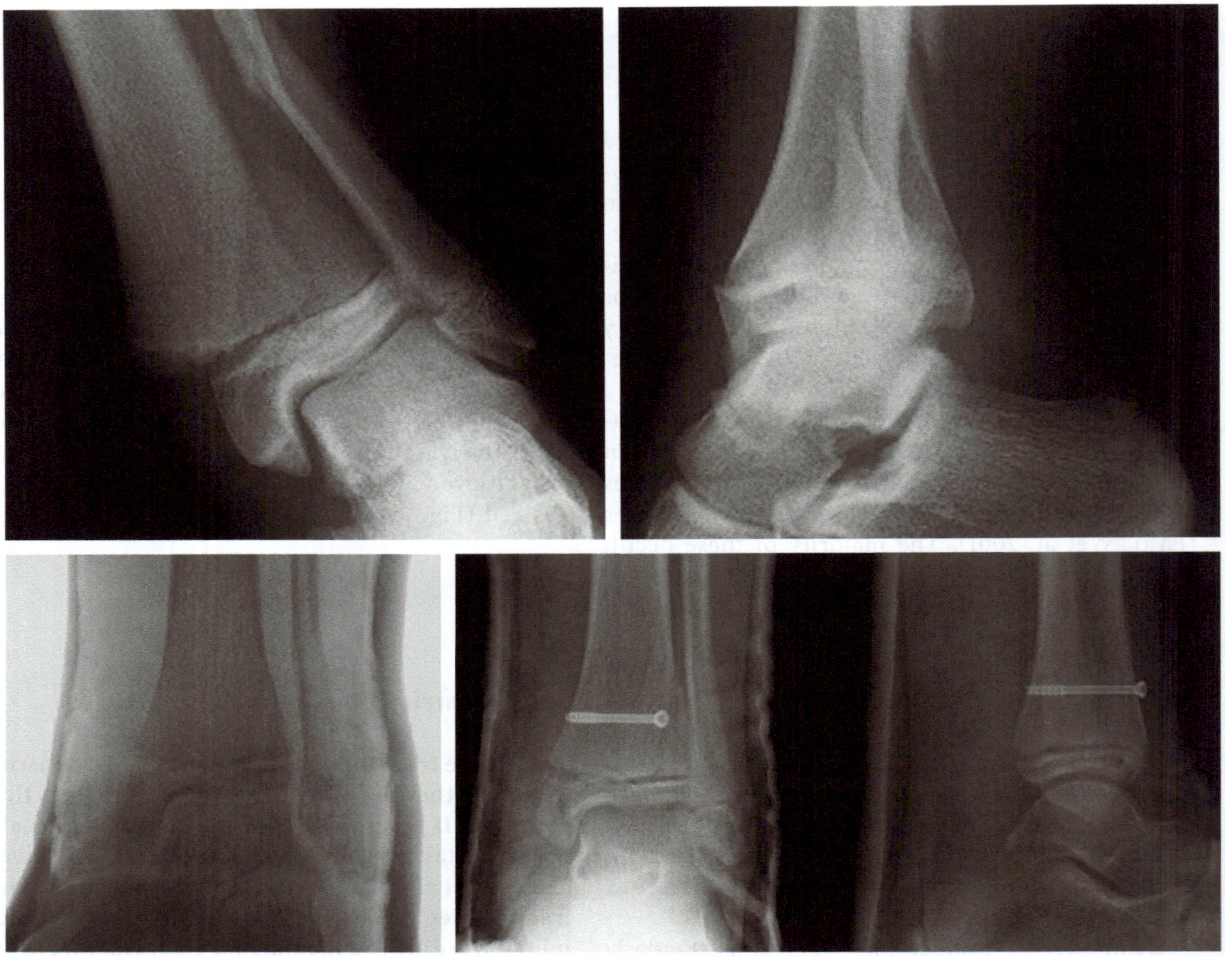

a

c

Fig. 15.2a–d. Salter-Harris Type II fracture of distal tibia. **a,b** Initial films. **c** After closed reduction the gap on the medial side of the physis was deemed to be too great (> 3 mm). **d** At open reduction interposed periosteal soft-tissue was removed from the medial side and fixation was achieved with a single cannulated screw

The potential for future asymmetric growth arrest following these fractures is well recognised. Consequently, diligent follow-up is advisable so that, should growth arrest occur, it may be identified early.

15.10 Transitional Fractures

These fractures are so-called because they occur during the adolescent transition to skeletal maturity. The distal tibial physis closes first centrally, then medially and finally anterolaterally (Fig. 15.1). This allows an area of relative weakness between the closed and open physis. Because these fractures occur around the time of physeal closure later growth disturbance is an unusual complication and consequently is not normally a consideration in management decision-making. However, they are intra-articular fractures which may predispose to post-traumatic arthritis – a factor which has a strong influence on treatment.

15.10.1 Triplane Fracture

This fracture is caused by an external rotation injury, usually whilst playing sports. It is so named because of the three planes – axial, sagittal and coronal – in which the fracture occurs. It accounts for 6% of distal tibial physeal fractures (SPIEGEL et al. 1978). The most usual pattern is the two-part triplane fracture though three- and four-part and extra-articular (Fig. 15.3) triplane fractures have been described. In about a third of cases the fibula is also fractured which may indicate a more severe external rotation force and an increased likelihood of unsuccessful closed reduction. Studies have shown (ERTL et al. 1988) that "residual displacement of two millimeters or more after reduction was associated with a less than optimum result unless the epiphyseal fracture was outside the primary weight-bearing area of the ankle". Therefore, assessment of the amount of fracture displacement at the ankle joint is critical in determining the requirement for reduction and internal fixation. On the plain films this is best seen on the mortise view (Fig. 15.4c). CT with multiplanar reconstruction (Fig. 15.4d–f) allows a more accurate assessment of displacement (BROWN et al. 2004) and also enables pre-operative planning of screw placement (Fig. 15.4g,h). Initial or, following closed reduction, residual intra-articular displacement of greater than 2 mm in any direction is an indication for open reduction and internal fixation.

15.10.2 Juvenile Tillaux Fracture

This is an avulsion injury caused by an external rotation force. It accounts for 2% of distal tibial physeal fractures (SPIEGEL et al. 1978). It tends to occur at a slightly older age than the triplane fracture because the distal tibial growth plate remains open only in its anterolateral portion. The externally rotating talus pushes the lateral malleolus posterolaterally and the anterolateral portion of the distal tibial epiphysis is avulsed, through the junction of the middle and lateral open physis, by the attachment of the anterior-inferior tibiofibular ligament. This is a Salter-Harris Type III physeal injury, the displacement of which may not be recognised on plain radiographs. CT provides accurate information on the degree of displacement and if this is greater than 2 mm reduction and internal fixation should be performed (Fig. 15.5).

15.11 Distal Fibular Fractures

These are usually Salter-Harris Type I or II fractures caused by a supination-inversion injury. They may not be evident on plain X-ray and are often incorrectly diagnosed as an ankle sprain. Ultrasound is very accurate in detecting the cortical discontinuity, periosteal elevation and subperiosteal fluid which accompanies these fractures (SIMANOVSKY et al. 2005). Where these injuries occur in isolation they should be managed in a below-knee walking cast for 3 to 4 weeks. Significantly displaced distal fibular fractures associated with Salter-Harris Type III or IV injuries usually reduce with re-

a

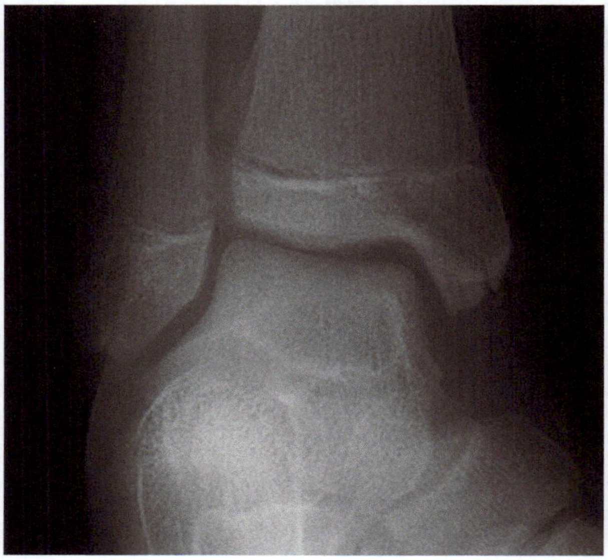

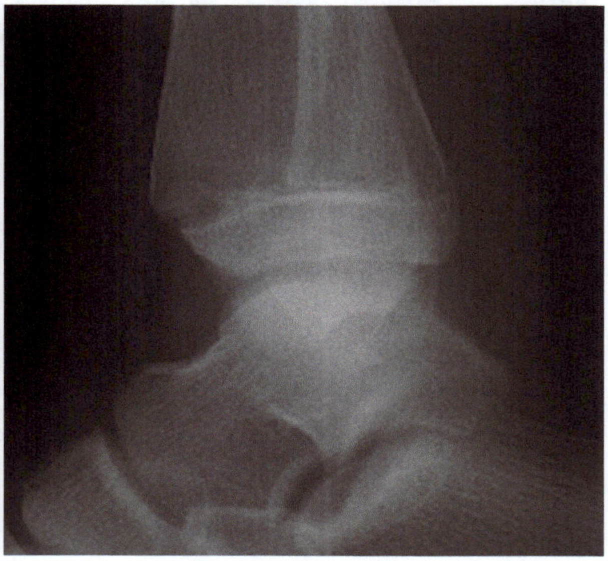

d

Fig. 15.3a,b. Extra-articular triplane fracture. The sagittal plane component exits through the medial malleolus

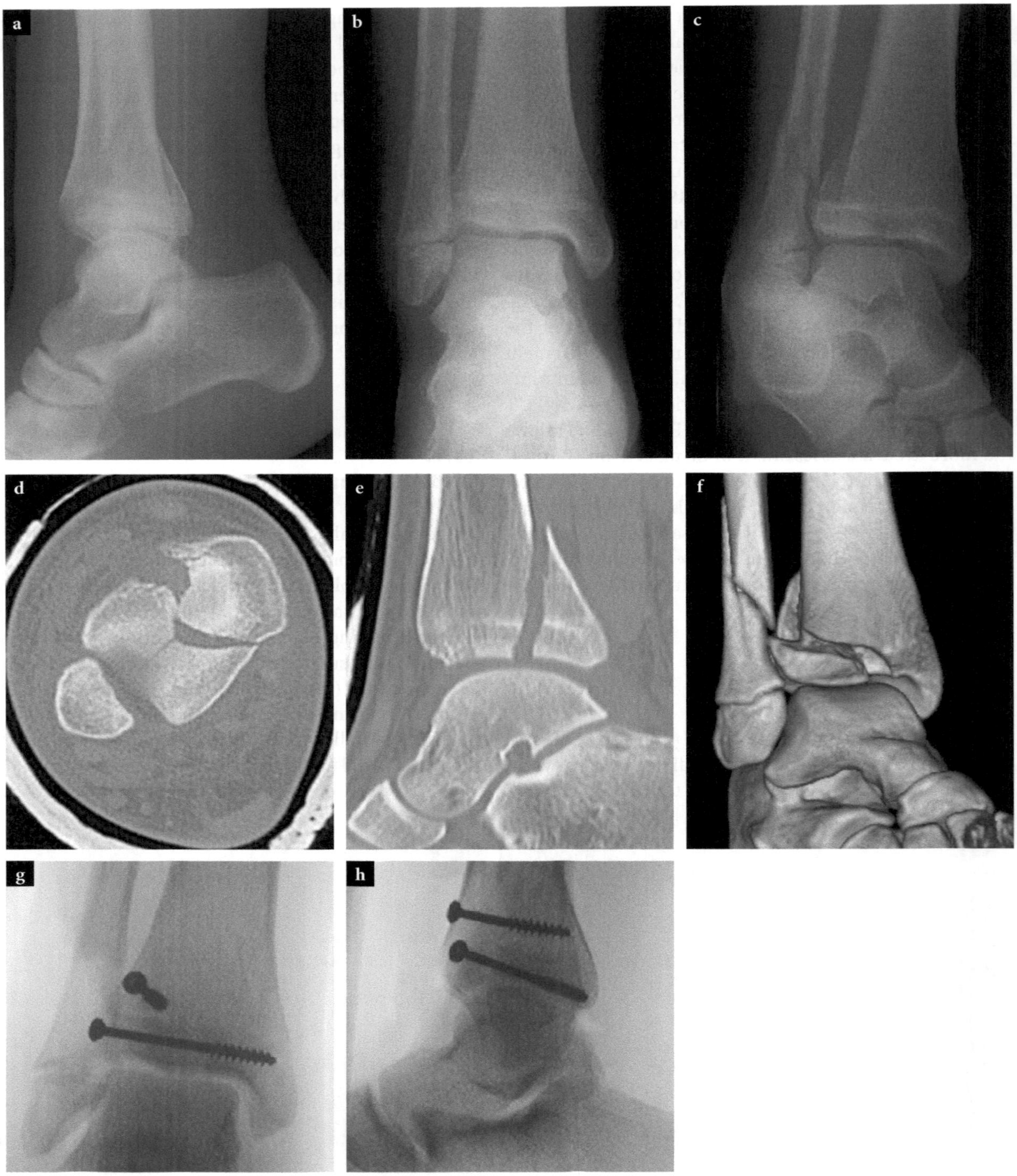

Fig. 15.4a–h. Three-part triplane fracture. **a-c** AP, lateral and mortise views; **d,e** axial and sagittal CT; **f** CT3D reconstruction; **g,h** post internal fixation

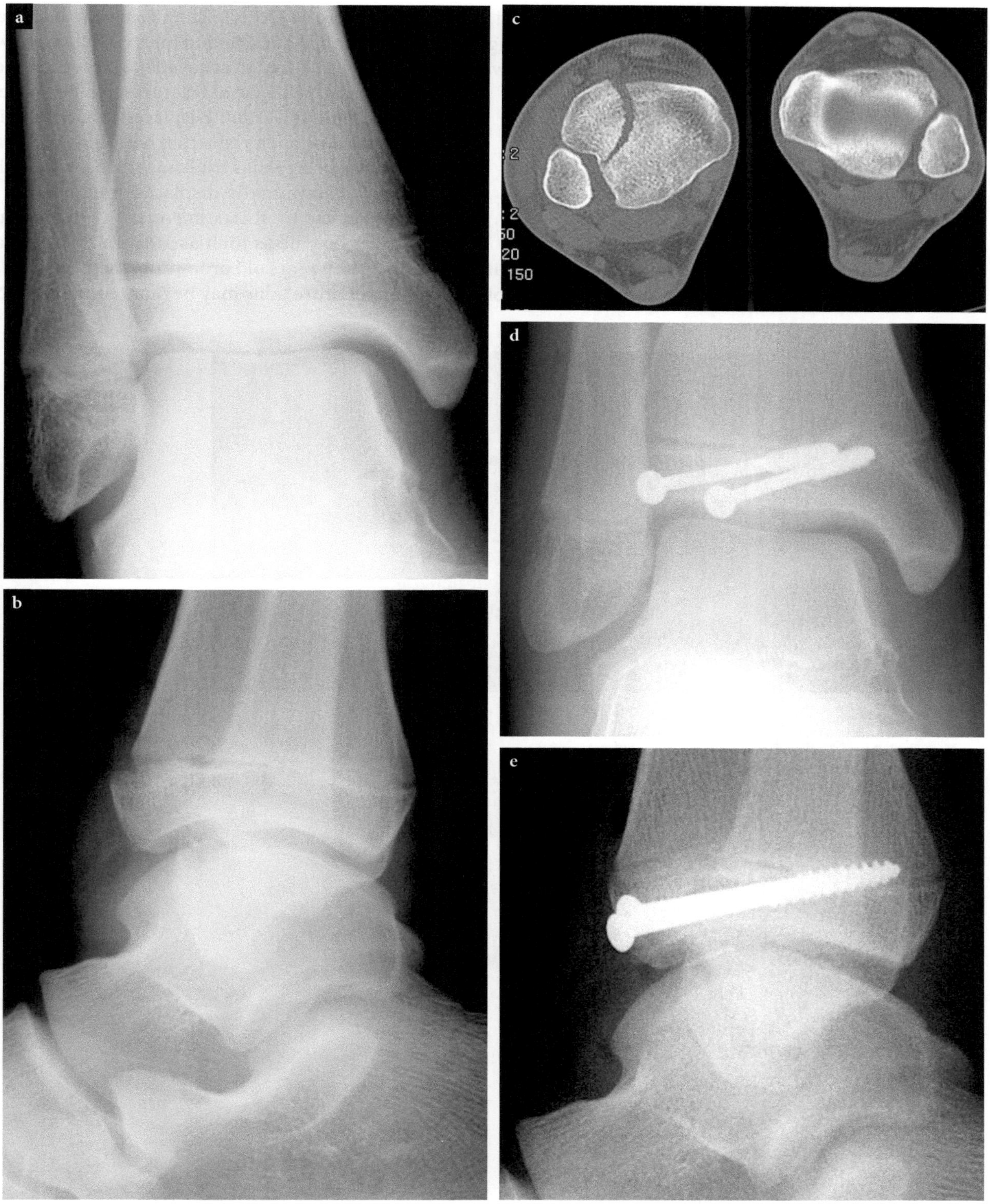

Fig. 15.5a–e. Juvenile Tillaux fracture: **a** AP and (**b**) lateral views. **c** CT axial view. **d,e** After reduction and internal fixation

duction of the tibial fracture but may require stabilisation with a smooth k-wire or, in children nearing skeletal maturity, an intramedullary cancellous screw.

15.12 Fractures of the Talus

Talar neck fractures are uncommon in children but are of importance because the associated risk of avascular necrosis (AVN). They generally occur as a result of a forced dorsiflexion injury. Oblique views or CT may be required to accurately assess displacement. Minimally displaced fractures can be treated with cast immobilisation. Displaced fractures will require closed or open reduction with internal fixation. The risk of AVN has traditionally been thought to be small in minimally displaced fractures but a literature review by Rammelt et al. (2000) calculated that it may be as high as 16%. In no case was the child over 9 years old prompting them to suggest that the immature talus may be more prone to AVN.

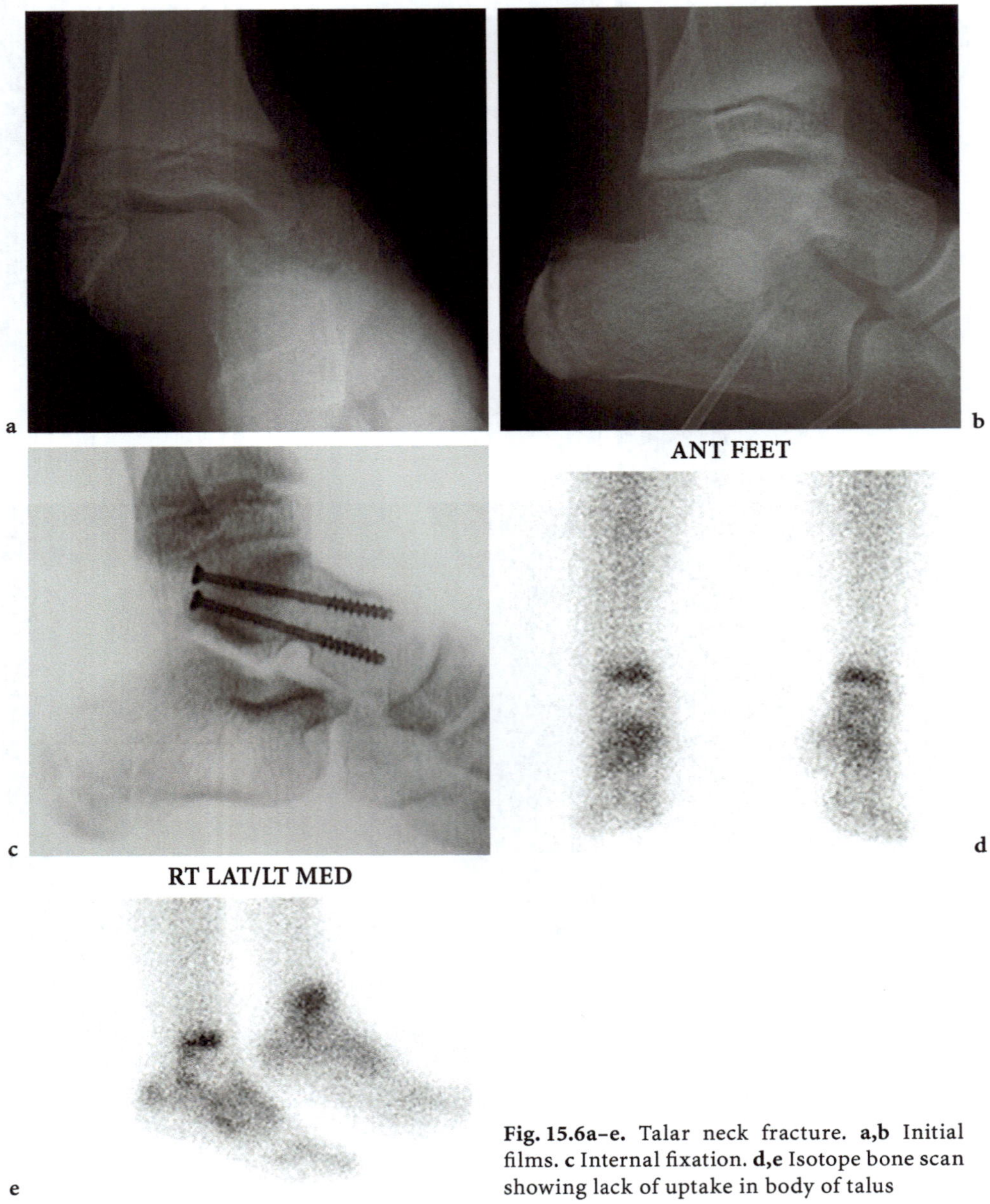

Fig. 15.6a–e. Talar neck fracture. **a,b** Initial films. **c** Internal fixation. **d,e** Isotope bone scan showing lack of uptake in body of talus

Because of this risk it is reasonable, after primary management of the injury, to check the vascularity of the talus with either isotope bone scan or MR imaging (Fig. 15.6).

15.13 Osteochondral Fracture

In the talus the terms osteochondral fracture, transchondral fracture and osteochondritis dissecans are used interchangeably. The condition is usually seen in adolescence. An associated history of trauma is identified in 64%–92% of patients (Berndt and Harty 1959; Ogilvie-Harris and Sarrosa 1999; Stone 1996) and tends to be an inversion type injury. Lateral lesions are said to be more commonly associated with trauma than medial lesions. The initial complaint is of ankle pain, swelling and a limp. Symptoms of instability and locking or clicking within the joint may also be described.

Radiographic assessment is by AP, lateral and mortise (Fig. 15.7a) views of the ankle in the first instance. Sensitivity is increased if the mortise view is performed in both plantarflexion and dorsiflexion. The radiographic classification of Berndt and Harty is most frequently used. They described four stages: Stage I is a small area of subchondral compression; Stage II is a partially detached osteochondral fragment; Stage III is a completely detached fragment which remains within its crater; and Stage IV is a fragment both detached and displaced into the joint. MR imaging is increasingly used in the assessment of these lesions and this has led to several modifications of the Berndt and Harty classification (Diapaola et al. 1991; Hepple et al. 1999). MR imaging is useful in identifying Stage I lesions where radiographs may be normal and to evaluate the overlying articular cartilage and presence of a loose fragment. A high signal rim between the osteochondral fragment and the talar bed on the T2-weighted image has attracted attention as a marker of instability of the fragment. If MR imaging is not available CT arthrography is an alternative. Both are better than plain radiographs

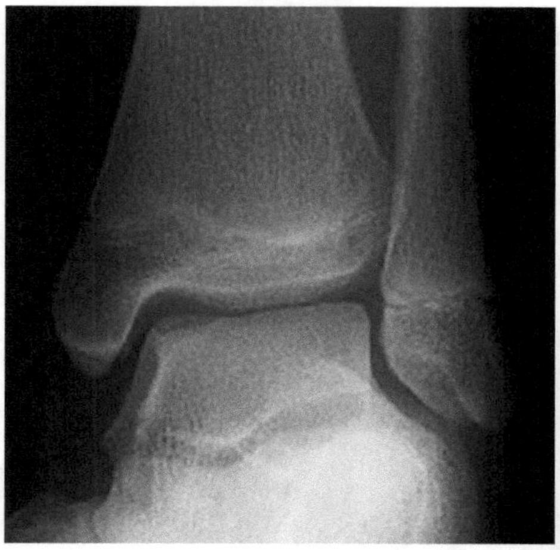
a

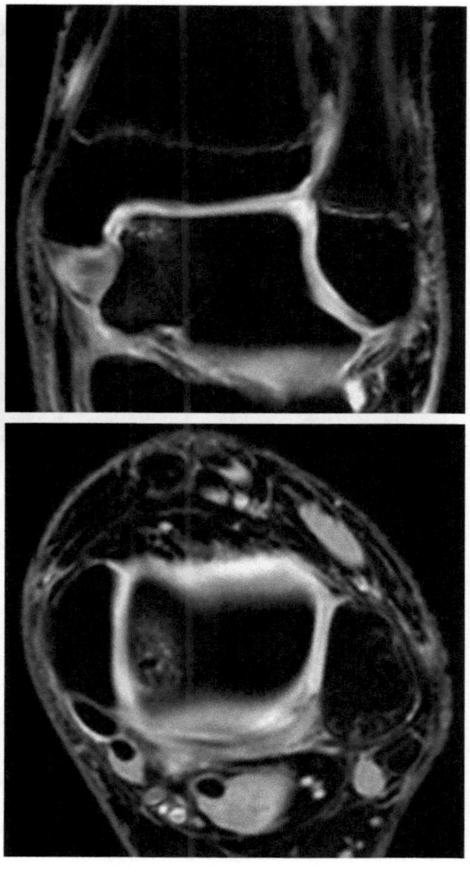
b

c

Fig. 15.7. a Mortise view showing lateral talar dome osteochondral lesion. **b,c** Coronal and axial MRI indicating precise location and extent of the lesion in revealing the extent and precise location of the lesion (Fig. 15.7b,c). Follow -up MR imaging can be used to assess healing of the lesion.

The initial treatment of Stage I and II talar OCD is non-operative with immobilization and restricted weight bearing. This achieves a good to excellent outcome in 83% (LETTS et al. 2003). Stage III and IV lesions (and Stage I and II lesions which do not respond to non-operative treatment) are treated surgically, either arthroscopically or via an arthrotomy. A variety of surgical treatments are available. These include drilling of the base of the lesion to encourage vascularisation and healing, internal fixation of larger lesions (Fig. 15.8), excision of the lesion with or without drilling of the crater, and autologous osteochondral grafting. Good to excellent results can be expected in 77% of those treated by drilling of the lesion (LETTS et al. 2003).

15.14 Open Injuries

Severe open ankle injuries tend to be caused by high-velocity motor vehicle accidents or lawn mower injuries. The pattern of injury to the underlying growth plate is variable and may not always be appreciated at the time. A degloving injury that removes the perichondrial ring of the physis occurs when the ankle is dragged across the road or pavement surface (Fig. 15.9). This is a Salter-Harris Type VI injury and later growth disturbance is not uncommon.

All open injuries should be treated with early antibiotics, debridement of devitalised tissues, fracture stabilisation (usually by external fixation spanning the ankle joint) and appropriate soft tissue coverage.

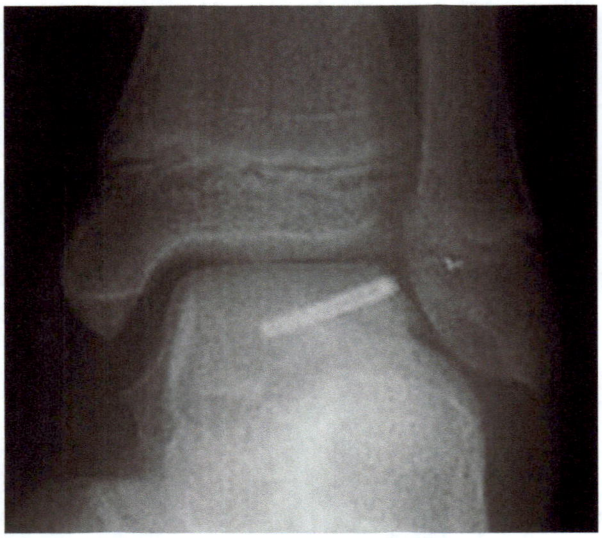

Fig. 15.8. Medial talar dome lesion after internal fixation

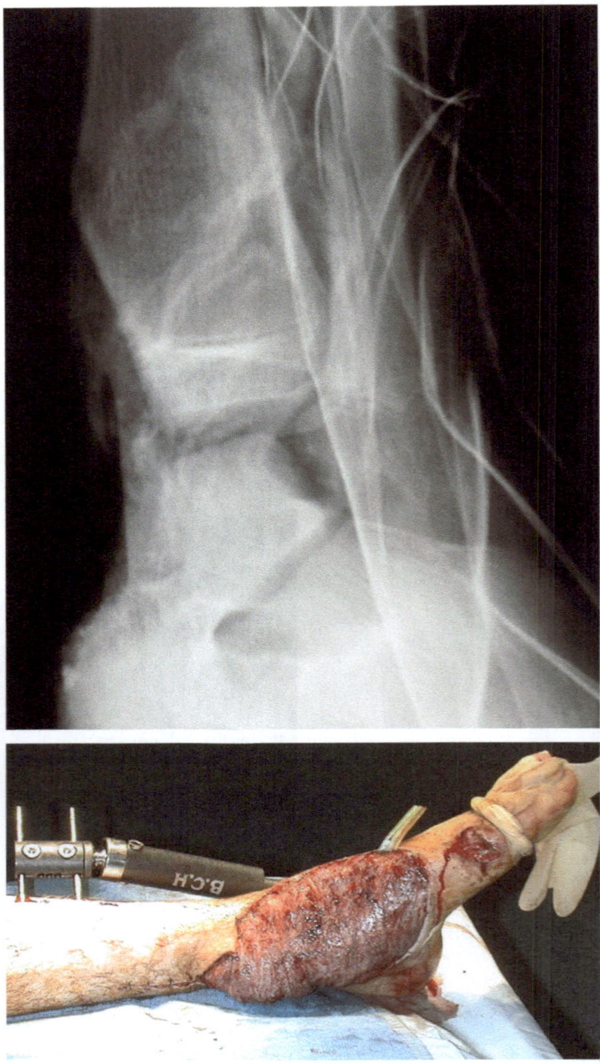

Fig. 15.9. a Degloving injury of the ankle with loss of the medial malleolus and medial part of the talus. **b** After stabilisation with external fixation and application of vascularised graft

15.15 Summary of Indications for Surgical Treatment

- Inability to obtain or maintain satisfactory closed reduction
- Displaced articular fractures
- Displaced physeal fractures (where later growth arrest likely)
- Open fractures
- Significant soft tissue injury

15.16 Outcome

The two main risks of distal tibial physeal injuries are premature physeal closure (PPC) and post-traumatic arthritis. Premature physeal closure may lead to angular deformity and/or leg-length discrepancy. Which of these occurs depends on the position and magnitude of the physeal arrest. The distal tibial physis accounts for about 3 mm per year of tibial growth which equates to 35%–40% of overall tibial length or 15%–20% of overall leg length. Obviously, the nearer the child is to skeletal maturity at the time of injury the less effect a PPC will have on growth.

Using the Salter-Harris classification in a review of 237 fractures of the distal tibia and fibula three groups of fractures were identified based on the risk of developing limb shortening, angular deformity or joint incongruity (Spiegel et al. 1978). There was a low-risk group of 89 patients, 6.7% of whom had complications, a high-risk group of 28 patients, 32% of whom had complications and an intermediate, unpredictable group of 66 patients, 16.7% of whom had complications (Table 15.1).

From this and other series, Salter-Harris Type I and II fractures of the distal tibia have traditionally been considered low risk, innocuous injuries. Recent studies have suggested that this may not be the case. Barmada et al. (2003) reviewed 92 patients with distal tibial physeal fractures and found an overall rate of PPC of 27.2%. Of the 51 Salter-Harris I or II fractures, 36% resulted in PPC. They also found in these fractures that the presence on X-ray of postreduction residual displacement and/or physeal gap (> 3 mm) was associated with a greater than three-fold increase (from 17% to 60%) in the incidence of PPC. Rohmiller et al. (2006) included patients from the above series in their evaluation of 91 Salter-Harris Type I or II fractures of the distal tibia. They reported an overall PPC rate of 39.6% with it being recognised, on average, 7.2 months after the injury. Although not statistically significant, they felt that the mechanism of injury had an effect on outcome with supination-external rotation type injuries having a PPC rate of 35% and pronation-abduction type injuries a PPC rate of 54%.

Clearly, it is important to use appropriate radiological investigations to not only identify the type of fracture in terms of Salter-Harris classification but also its severity in terms of magnitude of displacement, both before and after reduction. For this CT scans are invaluable. During follow-up close observance of growth arrest lines may provide an early indication of PPC.

Many of the studies reporting good outcome following intra-articular fractures of the distal tibial physis are of short follow-up. In triplane fractures there does appear to be a symptomatic deterioration

Table 15.1. Risk of complications in 237 fractures of the distal tibia and fibula (Spiegel et al. 1978)

Low risk complication rate 6.7%	Unpredictable complication rate 16.7%	High risk complication rate 32%
Type I and II fibular fractures	Type II tibial fractures	Type III and IV tibial fractures with > 2 mm displacement
Type I tibial fractures		Juvenile Tillaux fractures
Type III and IV tibial fractures with < 2mm displacement		Triplane fractures
Epiphyseal avulsion injuries		Comminuted tibial epiphyseal (Type V) fractures

between early and late follow-up mainly due to activity-related pain (Ertl et al. 1988), suggesting that outcome measurements should only be made some years after skeletal maturity. Caterini et al. (1991) showed radiographic evidence of ankle osteoarthritis in 29% of those who had sustained a Salter-Harris III or IV fracture at an average of 27 years previously. Again, the quality of the reduction appeared to be important.

The long-term prognosis of paediatric ankle injury is dependent upon fracture type and severity, skeletal maturity and adequacy of reduction. Of these, the orthopaedic surgeon has an influence on only the latter.

References

Barmada A, Gaynor T, Mubarak SJ (2003) Premature physeal closure following distal tibia physeal fractures: a new radiographic predictor. J Pediatr Orthop 23:733–739

Berndt AL, Harty M (1959) Transchondral fractures (osteochondritis dissecans). J Bone Joint Surg 41A:988–1020

Brown SD, Kasser JR, Zurakowski D et al (2004) Analysis of 51 tibial triplane fractures using CT with multiplanar reconstruction. AJR Am J Roentgenol 183:1489–1495

Caterini R, Farsetti P, Ippolito E (1991) Long-term follow-up of physeal injury to the ankle. Foot Ankle 11:372–83

Dayan PS, Vitale M, Langsam DJ et al (2004) Derivation of clinical prediction rules to identify children with fractures after twisting injuries of the ankle. Acad Emerg Med 11:736–43

Diapaola JD, Nelson DW, Colville MR (1991) Characterising osteochondral lesions by magnetic resonance imaging. Arthroscopy 7:101–104

Dias LS, Tachdjian MO (1978) Physeal injuries of the ankle in children: classification. Clin Orthop 136:230–233

Ertl JP, Barrack RL, Alexander AH et al (1988) Triplane fracture of the distal tibial epiphysis: long term follow-up. J Bone Joint Surg 70A:967–976

Farley FA, Kuhns L, Jacobson JA et al (2001) Ultrasound examination of ankle injuries in children. J Pediatr Orthop 21:604–607

Feldman F, Singson RD, Rosenberg ZS et al (1987) Distal tibial triplane fractures: diagnosis with CT. Radiol 164:429–435

Futami T, Foster BK, Morris LL et al (2000) Magnetic resonance imaging of growth plate injuries: the efficacy and indications for surgical procedures. Arch Orthop Trauma Surg 120:390–396

Hepple S, Winson IG, Glew D (1999) Osteochondral lesions of the talus: a revised classification. Foot Ankle Int 20:789–793

Landin LA (1983) Fracture patterns in children. Analysis of 8682 fractures with special reference to incidence, etiology and secular changes in a Swedish urban population 1950–1979. Acta Orthop Scand Suppl 202:1–109

Lauge-Hansen N (1950) Fractures of the ankle. Combined experimental-surgical and experimental-roentgenological investigations. Arch Surg 60:957–985

Letts RM, Gibeault D (1980) Fractures of the neck of the talus in children. Foot Ankle 1:74–77

Letts M, Davidson D, Ahmer A (2003) Osteochondritis dissecans of the talus in children. J Pediatr Orthop 23:617–625

Lohman M, Kivisaari A, Kallio P et al (2001) Acute paediatric ankle trauma: MRI versus plain radiography. Skeletal Radiol 30:504–511

Myers A, Canty K, Nelson T (2005) Are the Ottowa ankle rules helpful in ruling out the need for x ray examination in children? Arch Dis Child 90:1309–1311

Ogilvie-Harris DJ, Sarrosa EA (1999) Arthroscopic treatment of osteochondritis dissecans of the talus. Arthroscopy 15:805–808

Peterson CA, Peterson HA (1972) Analysis of the incidence of injuries to the epiphyseal growth plate. J Trauma 12:275–281

Powell H (1961) Extra centre of ossification for the medial malleolus in children. J Bone Joint Surg 43B:107–113

Rammelt S, Zwipp H, Gavlik JM (2000) Avascular necrosis after minimally displaced talus fracture in a child. Foot Ankle Int 21:1030–1036

Rohmiller MT, Gaynor TP, Pawelek J et al (2006) Salter-Harris I and II fractures of the distal tibia: does mechanism of injury relate to premature physeal closure? J Pediatr Orthop 26:322–328

Sailhan F, Chotel F, Guibal AL et al (2004) Three dimensional MR imaging in the assessment of physeal growth arrest. Eur Radiol 14:1600–1608

Simanovsky N, Hiller N, Leibner E et al (2005) Sonographic detection of radiologically occult fractures in paediatric ankle injuries. Pediatr Radiol 35:1062–1065

Spiegel PG, Cooperman DR, Laros GS (1978) Epiphyseal fractures of the distal ends of the tibia and fibula. A retrospective study of 237 cases in children. J Bone Joint Surg 60A:1046–1050

Stone JW (1996) Osteochondral lesions of the talar dome. J Am Acad Orthop Surg 4:63–73

Foot Fractures

16

Ed Bache, Caroline Lever, and Raj Kanwar

CONTENTS

E. Bache, FRCS
Consultant orthopaedic surgeon, Birmingham Children's Hospital, Steelhouse Lane, Birmingham, B4 6NH, UK
C. Lever, MD
Orthopaedic Specialist Registrar, Birmingham Children's Hospital, Steelhouse Lane, Birmingham, B4 6NH, UK
R. Kanwar, MD
Orthopaedic Clinical Fellow, Birmingham Children's Hospital, Steelhouse Lane Birmingham, B4 6NH, UK

16.1 Introduction

Foot fractures account for 5%–8% of paediatric fractures (Kay and Tang 2001). The metatarsals and phalanges are the most common site for injury (Green and Swiantkowsk 1998). Tarsal bones are largely cartilaginous in the young and it is thought that this accounts for the lower incidence of fractures compared with adults.

The majority of paediatric foot fractures heal well with conservative treatment. However, the change in trends of recreational activities, with some children now participating in motor sports, has meant increasing numbers of more severe foot injuries being seen in younger patients. Injuries in adolescence commonly take on similar patterns to those seen in adults.

16.2 Overview of Anatomy

A clear understanding of normal foot anatomy and anatomical variants in children must be appreciated before trying to interpret radiographs for trauma, otherwise features such as apophyses and accessory bones can be mistaken for fractures.

The foot contains 26 bones divided into three regions: the hind foot, midfoot and forefoot. The talus and calcaneum form the hindfoot. The calcaneum has three facets (anterior, middle and posterior) on its dorsal surface which articulate with the talus above forming the subtalar joint. Weight bearing is predominantly through the larger posterior facet. The irregular transverse plane formed by the talonavicular and calcaneocuboid joints constitute the Chopart joint separating the hind foot from midfoot (navicular, cuboid and three cuneiforms). Dividing the midfoot from the forefoot is the Lisfranc joint consisting of articulations of the cuboid and three cuneiforms with the metatarsal bases. The keystone for the stability of this joint is the bony architecture of the second tarsometatarsal joint. The second metatarsal is usually the longest of the metatarsal bones and its articulation with the intermediate cuneiform is recessed between the medial and lateral cuneiforms. Stability is also contributed by a strong ligamentous attachment from its base to the medial cuneiform (the Lisfranc ligament) and the intermetatarsal ligaments between metatarsals.

16.3 Ossification

All the tarsal bones ossify from single primary centres: the calcaneus ossifies at the third fetal month, cuboid just before or after birth, cuneiforms from 1 year and the navicular at 3 years. In addition the calcaneus has a secondary ossification centre on its posterior surface appearing at about 7 years of age.

The metatarsals and phalanges begin ossifying from 2 to 3 months gestation. Each has one secondary ossification centre occurring around 3 years of age and fusing at 18 years. The secondary ossification centres of the phalanges and the first metatarsal are based proximally, yet are distally based on the remaining metatarsals.

16.4 Accessory Bones

Accessory centres are commonly seen in the foot; 50 have been described (Hoerr et al. 1962) but only 20 are common. An accessory navicular, os tibiale externum, is seen on the medial or internal aspect of the navicular in 10% of children, usually after the age of 5 and more often in girls (Drennan 1992). Another variant, the os intermetatarsale, commonly situated between the bases of the first and second metatarsals can be misdiagnosed as a foreign body. Accessory ossicles can be readily distinguished from fractures by their consistent anatomical location and smooth well corticated margins.

16.5 Clinical Assessment

The Ottawa Ankle rules were developed to avoid unnecessary radiography of ankle and midfoot injuries. Radiographs are rationalised to those with a positive assessment, which for the midfoot involves any inability to walk or localised tenderness either of the navicular or the base of the fifth metatarsal. The rules have shown a high sensitivity in detecting 99% of fractures in children. If a negative result is generated the probability of a child having a fracture was 1.22% (Bachmann et al. 2003). The detection of hindfoot and forefoot injuries are not included, but radiographs are warranted if there is inability to weight bear with bony tenderness following trauma. Often the exact mechanism of injury is difficult to ascertain in a small child, especially in an unwitnessed accident and thorough examination is a must.

Full assessment of foot injuries should include careful examination of the soft tissues. Compartment syndrome of the foot can occur following foot trauma, even in the absence of a fracture, crush injuries are particularly high risk. Any significant swelling demands observation, elevation and when appropriate pressure recording or surgical decompression. Open fractures have been well documented following lawn mower injuries in the US (Vollman and Smith 2006). They should be treated following standard open fracture protocols with antibiotics and surgical debridement.

16.6 Imaging

Routine radiographs for foot trauma are the anteroposterior (AP), oblique and true lateral views. Fractures are more readily identified on the AP or oblique but a true lateral allows full assessment of displacement. Both computerised tomography (CT) and magnetic resonance (MR) imaging have roles to play in foot trauma. CT is useful in comminuted calcaneal fractures to assess joint involvement and to help plan surgical reconstruction, while MR can help diagnose ligament injuries.

Foot fractures can be missed on initial radiographs in children. With technetium bone scans it is possible to identify a fracture within 7 h of injury and to exclude one after 72 h with a normal scan (Rosenthal et al. 1976; Beaty and Kasser 2006). However, since foot fractures tend to heal well in children without sequelae, it seems reasonable to avoid the cost and radiation burden. Those in discomfort with normal initial radiographs can be immobilised in a cast with repeat clinical examination and further radiographs in 2 weeks if symptoms remain. With increased accessibility to MR imaging the use of bone scanning in children should be severely restricted.

16.7 Calcaneal Fractures

These fractures are uncommon in children accounting for less than 0.05% of all paediatric fractures (Van Frank et al. 1998). The usual mechanism is a fall from a height but unlike adults these fractures can occur following low energy trauma and stress fractures have been reported (Schmidt and Weiner 1982; Wiley 1981). Extra-articular fractures are more common than intra-articular in the skeletally immature (Inokuchi et al. 1998). Up to one third of children have associated injuries – most commonly another lower extremity fracture, with vertebral fractures being much less frequent than in adults (Schmidt and Weiner 1982).

Standard radiographs for the calcaneum are dorsoplantar, lateral and axial views. Oblique views may identify anterior process fractures (Rasmussen and Schantz 1986), but CT is the imaging modality of choice to fully assess the injury.

Bohler's angle is measured from the lateral radiograph. It is the angle formed by two lines: one drawn between the highest part of the anterior process and the highest part of the posterior articular surface, and one drawn between the same point on the posterior articular surface and the most superior point on the tuberosity (Davies et al. 2003) (Fig. 16.1). Usually it measures 25°–40° in adults and teenagers with a reduction indicating that the weight-bearing surface of the calcaneum may have collapsed. Actual measurements of Bohler's angle can be unreliable in those under 10 years of age (Ogden 2000) and a normal Bohler's angle does not exclude a calcaneal fracture. If a fracture is suspected comparison with the uninjured side values should be similar.

Böhler's angle

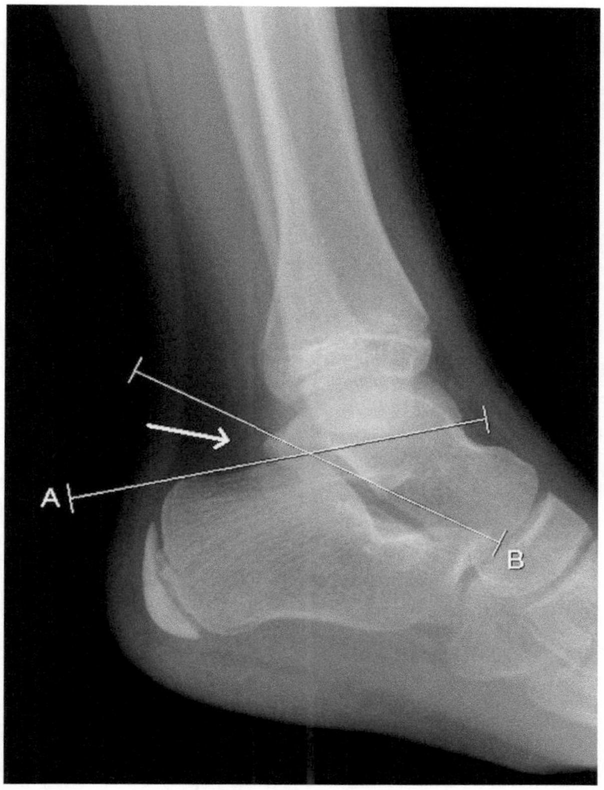

Fig. 16.1. Showing measurement of Bohler's Angle. On a lateral radiograph a line is drawn from the posterior aspect of the calcaneum to the highest midpoint (*Line A*). A second line is drawn from the highest anterior point to the highest midpoint (*Line B*). The angle of intersection at the highest midpoint is measured (*arrow*)

There are various classifications for calcaneal fractures in the literature. Schmidt and Weiner adapted the Essex Lopresti classification to include the open calcaneal fracture with bone loss seen in children following lawn mower injuries (Schmidt and Weiner 1982), thus essentially separating paediatric calcaneal fractures into extra-articular, intra-articular or complex with bone loss. Displaced fractures through the subtalar joint are further divided into tongue type or split depression type. Full assessment may require CT which provides accurate imaging of the subtalar joint. Sanders' classification of intra-articular calcaneal fractures is based on CT images. It is widely used for operative planning and can predict outcomes from surgery (Sanders et al. 1993) (Fig. 16.2, Table 16.1).

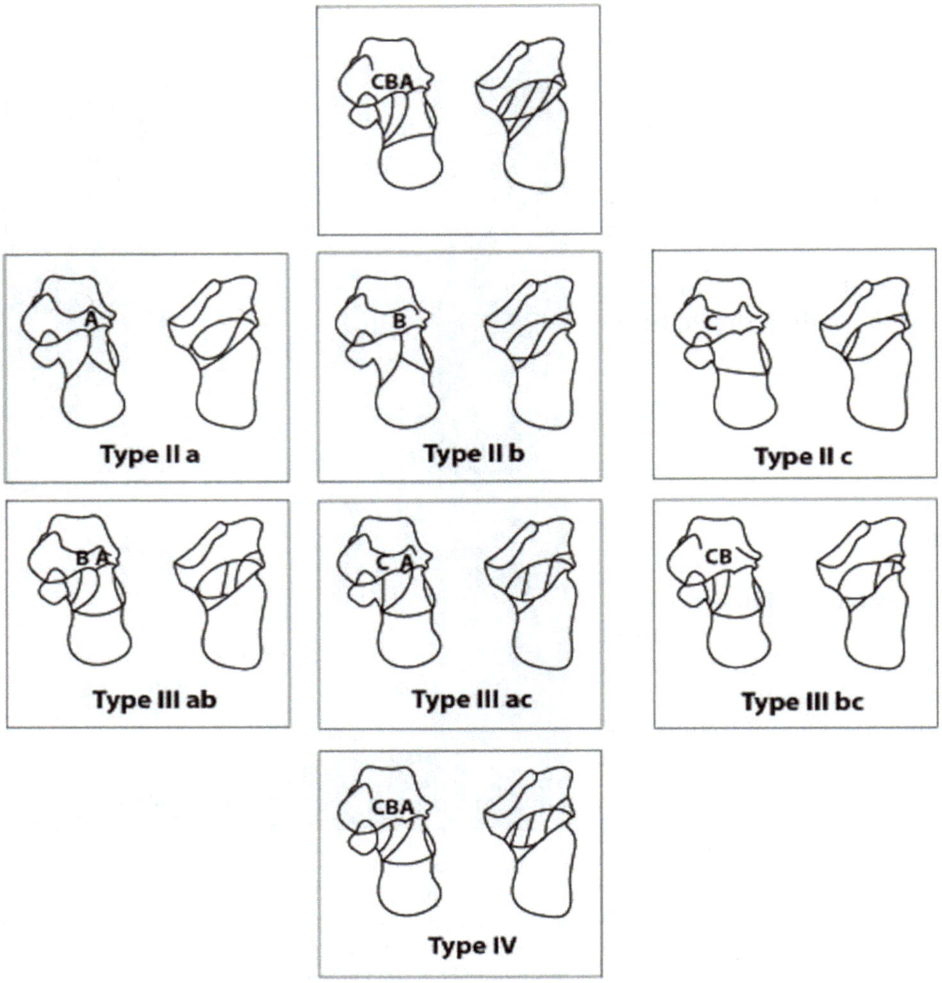

Fig. 16.2. Sanders classification based on CT images. The two images represent coronal and axial views. Type I fractures are nondisplaced and are not shown. Fracture lines *A*, *B*, and *C* describe the position of the primary fracture line in relation to the posterior facet and the subtalar joint. Line *A* divides the lateral from the central third of the calcaneum, line *B* divides the middle third from the medial third of the calcaneum and lines *C* the medial third from the sustentaculum. Types II and III fractures have two or three fragments, respectively, which are then subdivided, depending on the medial or lateral position of the primary fracture line Type IV fractures are severely comminuted. (Adapted from Sanders et al. 1993)

Table 16.1. Table of Sanders classification and suggested management

Type	Fracture pattern	Treatment
I	Undisplaced intra-articular fracture	Conservative
II	Two part displaced fracture	ORIF
III	Three part fracture with depressed central segment	ORIF
IV	Comminuted fractures	Consider fusion

Intra-articular fractures with less than 4 mm disruption of the facet joint and extra-articular fractures can be treated adequately with cast immobilisation for 4–6 weeks (Beaty and Kasser 2006) (Figs. 16.3, 16.4). As predicted by Sanders' classification, displaced intra-articular fractures are likely to require operative intervention. However, bone remodelling in children under 10 years of age can lead to a congruent subtalar joint and even significantly comminuted intra-articular fractures in this age group have satisfactory outcomes with non-operative treatment (Mora et al. 2001; Wiley 1981). Adolescents have less potential to remodel and displaced intra-articular fractures can lead to future morbidity. Their treatment should be in line with that of an equivalent fracture in an adult with open reduction and internal fixation (ORIF).

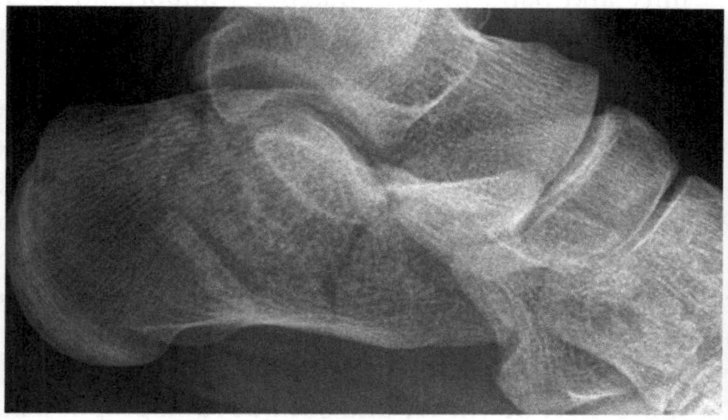

a

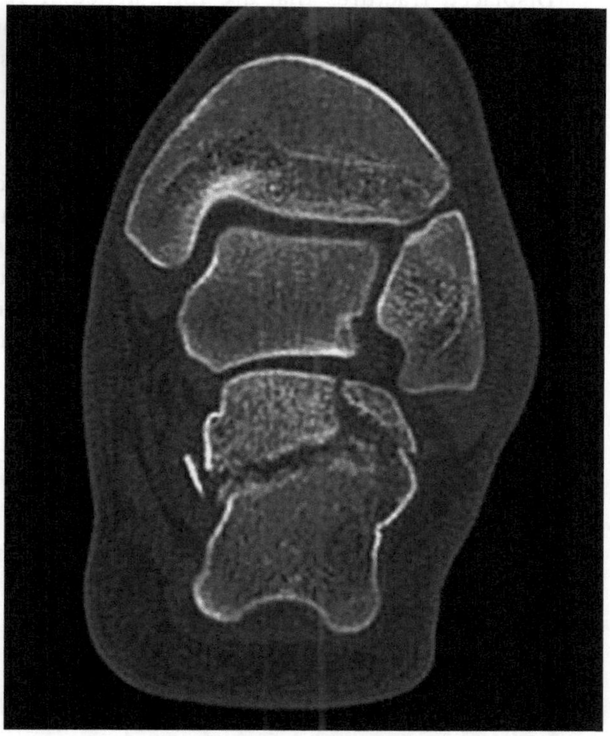

b

Fig. 16.3a,b. Calcaneal fracture in a 15-year-old boy. The radiograph does not fully detail the fracture. The coronal CT shows the fracture is predominantly on the lateral aspect of the calcaneum (type IIA)

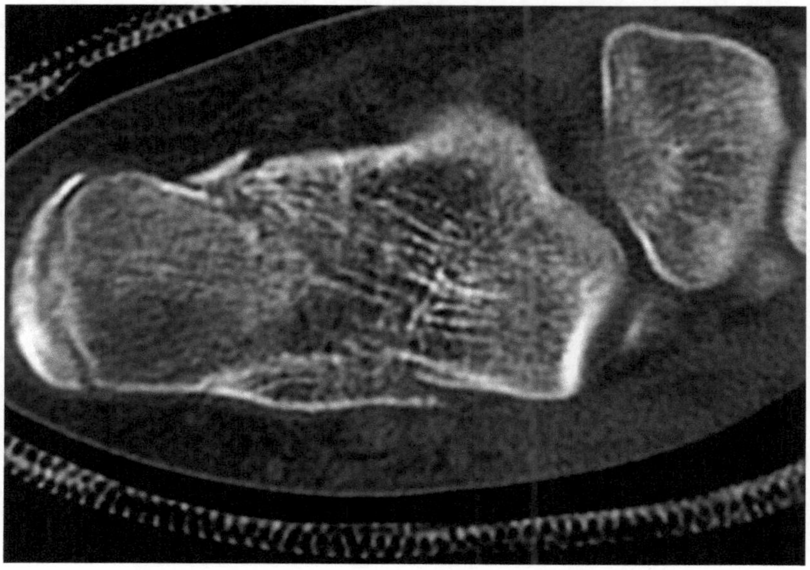

Fig. 16.4. Axial CT shows fracture on both the lateral and medial aspects of the calcaneum

16.8 Midfoot Fractures

Isolated fractures of the navicular, cuboid or cuneiforms are very rare. When they do occur they tend to be simple avulsions which can be treated symptomatically with a below knee weight bearing cast for about 3 weeks.

Displaced fractures that are intra-articular require reduction and internal fixation to restore joint congruency and prevent early degenerative changes. As with all high energy injuries these must be observed to exclude compartment syndrome.

When reviewing radiographs of the foot it is important to assess the alignment of the metatarsals to the tarsal bones. On the AP radiograph the medial margin of the second metatarsal should be in line with the medial margin of the middle cuneiform. On the oblique view the medial margin of the base of the third metatarsal should be inline with the medial margin of the lateral cuneiform (Fig. 16.5).

16.8.1 Lisfranc Injuries

The most common mechanism for injury is forced plantar flexion of the forefoot usually combined with a rotational force (Wiley 1981). Fracture dislocations of the tarsometatarsal joint are rare injuries in children but can often be overlooked. Missed Lisfranc injuries predispose to midfoot instability with chronic deformity and pain, making diagnosis important. Bruising in the sole at the level of the tarsometatarsal joint should raise specific concern for a Lisfranc injury.

AP, true lateral and oblique radiographs are required. Occasionally these injuries reduce spontaneously leaving little radiographic evidence. Fractures near the base of metatarsals should raise suspicion and prompt closer examination. The base of second metatarsal is fractured in 75% of Lisfranc injuries (Vouri and Aro 1993; Wiley 1981). A fracture of the second metatarsal with a cuboid fracture is strongly indicative. On the AP and oblique radiographs a Lisfranc fracture dislocation can be diagnosed by loss

a

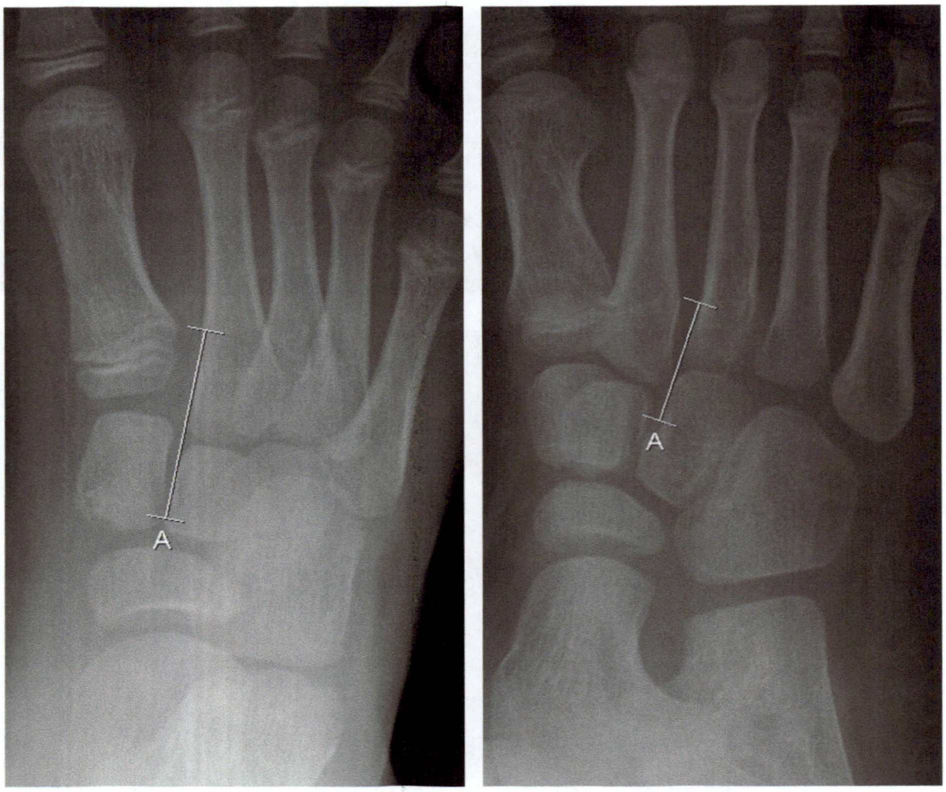

b

Fig. 16.5. **a** AP view showing the alignment of the second metatarsal with the medial margin of the medial cuneiform. **b** An oblique view showing the alignment of the medial margin of the third metatarsal with the medial margin of the lateral cuneiform of alignment between the lateral border of the first metatarsal on the medial cuneiform or the medial aspect of the second metatarsal with the medial border of the middle cuneiform, respectively.

There are two basic types of Lisfranc injuries; homolateral (or convergent) and divergent. In the homolateral type the rays displace in the same direction. In divergent type the first metatarsal displaces medially while the lesser metatarsals displace laterally (Fig. 16.6).

Again if significant swelling is present elevation and monitoring for compartment syndrome must be carried out. If there is minimal displacement cast immobilisation can begin when swelling subsides. More than 2 mm displacement requires reduction under general anaesthesia. Adequate reduction is dependent on realignment of the second tarsometatarsal joint, the keystone of the Lisfranc joint. Percutaneous K-wire fixation of the metatarsals to the cuneiforms stabilises the reduction. Open reduction is rarely needed. The prognosis for these injuries is better than in adults although complications of malunion, avascular necrosis, skin necrosis and early joint degeneration have been reported (Wiley 1981). Incomplete reduction can lead to persisting foot pain (Wiley 1981).

16.9 Metatarsal Fractures

Overall, the fifth metatarsal is the most frequently injured but patterns are age dependent. Children under 5 years age have a higher proportion of first metatarsal fractures (Owen et al. 1995). A buckle fracture of the first metatarsal in young children is commonly known as the 'bunk bed fracture' because of its frequent occurrence in children who have sustained a fall from an upper bunk (Oesterich and Crawford 1985).

Non-operative treatment for shaft fractures usually suffices (Fig. 16.7), comprising a weight bearing cast for 3–6 weeks until asymptomatic. Displacement in the coronal plane is normally acceptable but significant displacement in the sagittal plane may require reduction and K-wire fixation in the older child.

Freiberg's disease is avascular necrosis of a metatarsal head, usually the second. This should not be confused with an acute fracture. Flattening of the head and altered density help to differentiate the two (Fig. 16.8).

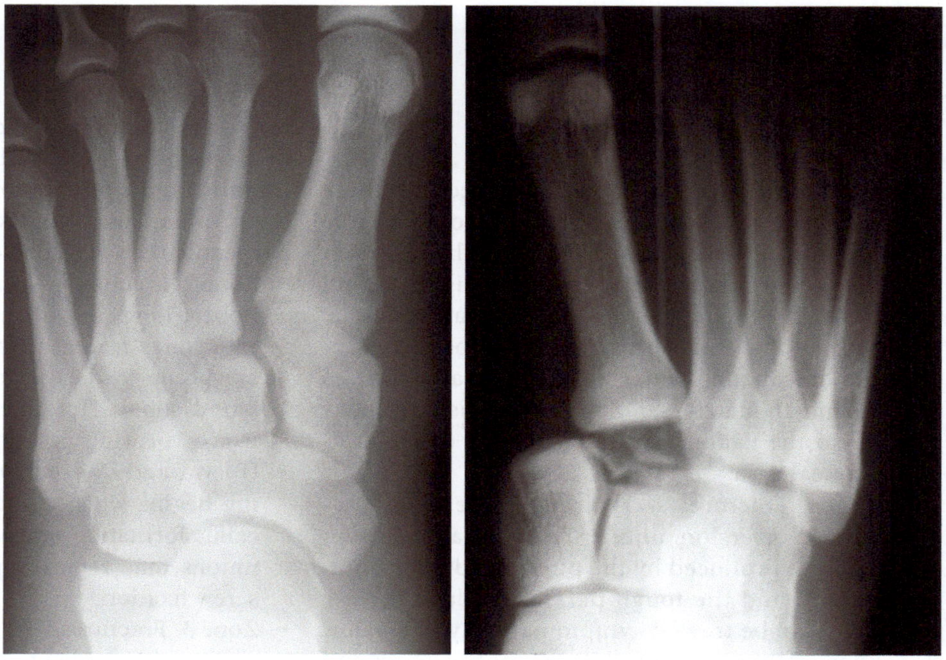

a b

Fig. 16.6. a Divergent Lisfranc injury with loss of alignment of medial border of second metatarsal and medial border of medial cuneiform. **b** Convergent Lisfranc. Note fracture fragments from second metatarsal base. (Images provided by Dr. Davies and Dr. Teh)

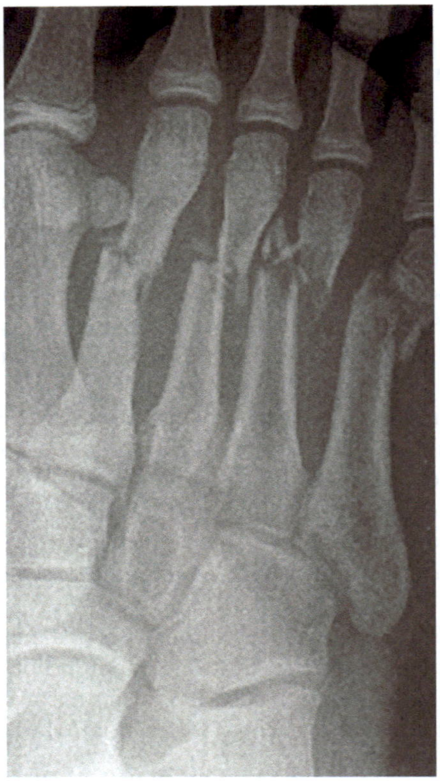

Fig. 16.7. Multiple metatarsal fractures in a 13-year-old girl

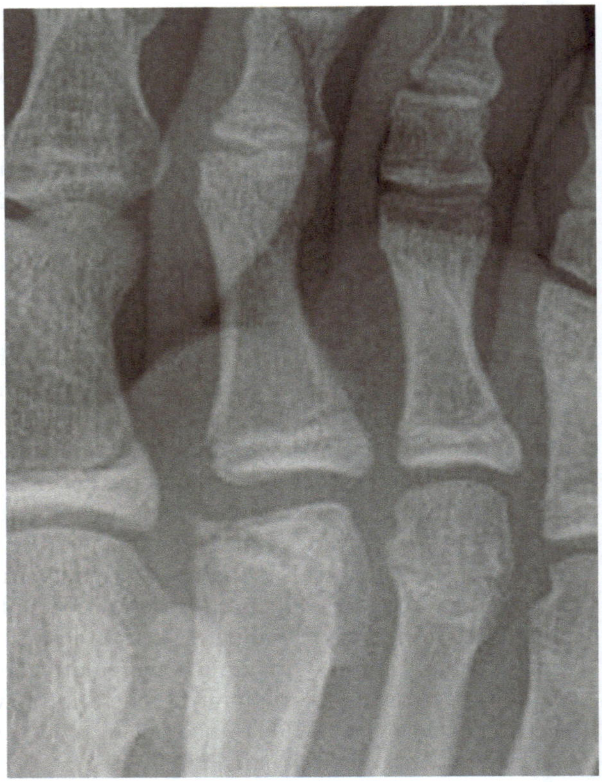

Fig. 16.8. Avascular necrosis of the second metatarsal head

16.9.1 Base of 5th Metatarsal Fractures

These fractures are typically subdivided into three types depending on their location. Zone 1 is the cancellous tuberosity, which includes the insertion of the peroneus brevis and abductor digiti minimi tendons and the lateral cord of the plantar fascia. Zone 2 is the distal aspect of the tuberosity and includes dorsal and plantar ligamentous attachments to the fourth metatarsal. Zone 3 comprises the zone distal to the ligamentous attachments to the mid-diaphyseal area.

- Zone 1 Fractures – Typically these occur following inversion injury. There is an avulsion fracture produced by the pull of abductor digiti minimi and the tough part of the lateral cord. They can be treated symptomatically in a below knee walking cast until pain resolves (Kay and Tang 2001). Surgery may be considered if significant displaced or in the rare painful non-union.

The apophyses may be mistaken for a Zone 1 fracture by the unwary. The ossification centre appears between the ages of 6 and 15 years. It can simulate a fracture but its orientation is parallel to the shaft of the fifth metatarsal unlike fracture lines which are perpendicular (Fig. 16.9).

- Zone 2 Fractures – Originally described by Sir Robert Jones in 1902 and hence often referred to as a Jones fracture (Jones 1902). These injuries are prone to delayed or non union due to their blood supply. Treatment should consist of non-weight bearing cast immobilisation for 6 weeks (Beaty and Kasser 2006). Protected weight bearing begins when clinical tenderness resides and callus formation on radiographs is evident. Non-unions may require operative intervention with screw fixation.
- Zone 3 Fractures – These injuries are seen in young athletes due to repeated stress. Acute injuries can be treated in a below knee walking cast for 6 weeks. When chronic symptoms are present intramedullary screw fixation is often needed.

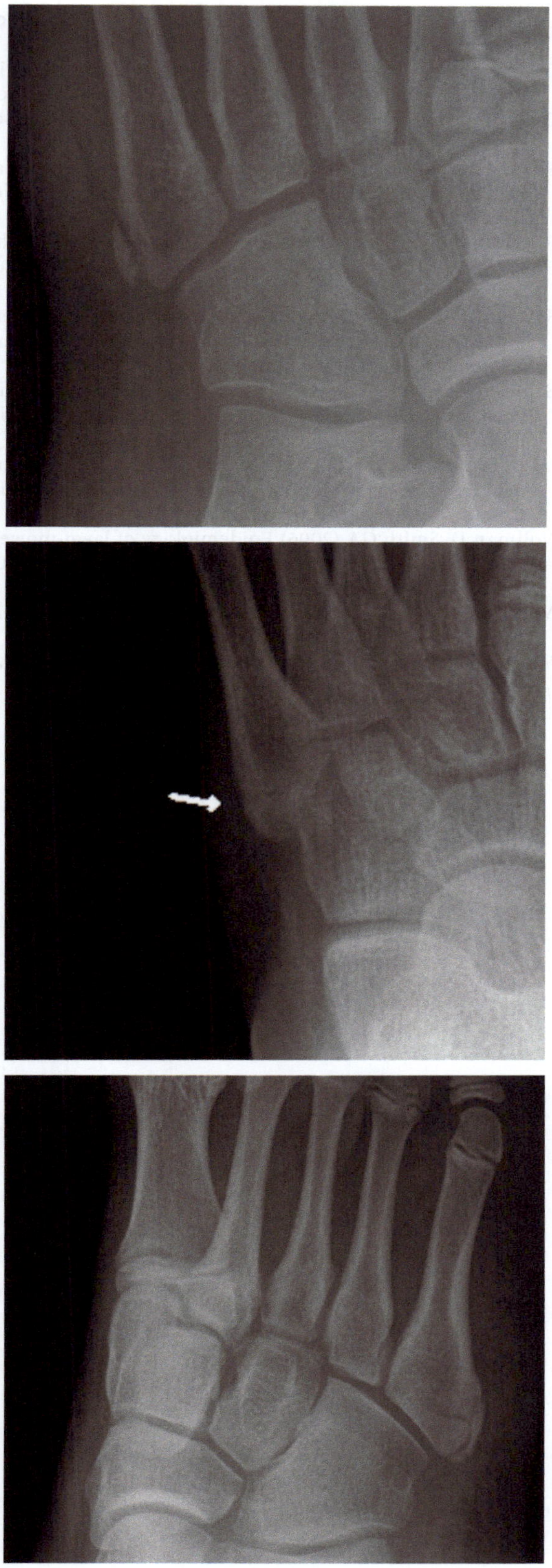
a
b
c

16.9.2 Stress Fractures

Typically these affect the metatarsals but are less common than in the adult population. Following a sudden increase in physical activity there is a history of pain with tenderness over the fracture. Initial X-rays are commonly normal but repeat films 2 weeks from the onset of symptoms show callous, allowing the diagnosis to be made. Restriction of precipitating activities for 2–3 months is all that is generally required. If there is significant discomfort immobilisation in a weight bearing cast for several weeks may help.

16.10 Sesamoids

There are typically two sesamoids located on the plantar aspect of the head of the first metatarsal. The medial sesamoid is usually larger than the lateral. On occasion it can be bipartite and should not be mistaken for fracture.

16.11 Phalangeal Fractures

The mechanism of injury is stubbing of the toe or dropping an object onto the foot. Toe injuries are not routinely imaged as management is unaltered by the images. The fractures heal well in 3–4 weeks by simple neighbour strapping. Proximal phalanx fractures of the hallux do need imaging to assess for any intra-articular displacement. Displacement of more than 3 mm with more than one third of the joint surface involved requires anatomic reduction and fixation (Beaty and Kasser 2006). Percutaneous K-wire fixation provides adequate stability in most cases.

Fig. 16.9. **a** A normal secondary ossification centre at the base of fifth metatarsal; the apophyses runs parallel to the shaft of the bone. **b** Fracture at the base of fifth metatarsal. **c** A fracture and secondary ossification centre

References

Bachmann LM, Kolb E, Koller MT, Steurer J, Riet G (2003) Accuracy of Ottawa ankle rules to exclude fractures of the ankle and midfoot: systematic review. BMJ 326:417

Beaty JH, Kasser JR (eds) (2006) Rockwood & Wilkins' Fractures in Children, 6th edn. Lippincott Williams and Wilkins, Philadelphia

Davies AM, Whitehouse RW, Jenkins JPR (2003) Imaging of the foot and ankle. Techniques and applications. Springer-Verlag, Berlin Heidelberg New York, pp 151–166

Drennan JC (1992) The child's foot and ankle. Raven Press, New York

Green E, Swiantkowski MF (eds) (1998) Skeletal trauma in children, 2nd edn. WB Saunders,Philadelphia

Hoerr NL, Pyle SI, Francis CC (1962) Radiographic atlas of the skeletal development of the foot and ankle. Charles Thomas, Springfield, 1962

Inokuchi S, Usami N, Hiraishi E, Hashimoto T (1998) Calcaneal fractures in children. J Pediatr Orthop 18:469–474

Jones R (1902) Fracture of the base of the fifth metatarsal by indirect violence. Ann Surg 35:697–700

Kay RM, Tang CW (2001) Pediatric foot fractures: evaluation and treatment. J Am Acad Orthop Surg. 9:308–319

Logan B, Singh D, Hutchings R (2004) McMinn's colour atlas of foot and ankle anatomy, 3rd edn. Mosby, Elsevier

Mora S, Thordarson DB, Zionts CE, Reynolds RA (2001) Pediatric calcaneal fractures. Foot Ankle Int 22:471–477

Oesterich AE, Crawford AH (1985) Atlas of paediatric orthopaedic radiology. George Thieme Verlag, Stuttgart

Ogden J (2000) The foot. In: Ogden J (ed) Skeletal injury in the child. Springer-Verlag, Berlin Heidelberg New York

Owen RJT, Hickey FG, Finlay DB (1995) A study of metatarsal fractures in children. Injury 26:537–538

Rasmussen F, Schantz K (1986) Radiological aspects of calcaneal fractures in childhood and adolescence. Acta Radiol Diag 27:575–580

Rosenthall L, Hill RO, Chuang S (1976) Observation on the use of 99mTc-phosphate imaging in peripheral bone trauma. Radiology 119:637

Sanders R, Fortin P, DiPasquale T et al. (1993) Operative treatment of 120 Calcaneal fractures. Results using a prognostic computed tomography scan classification. Clinic Orthop 290:87–95

Schmidt TL, Weiner DS (1982) Calcaneal fractures in children. An evaluation of the nature of the injury in 56 children. Clin Orthop Relat Res 171:150–155

Van Frank E, Ward JC, Engelhardt P (1998) Bilateral calcaneal fracture in childhood: case report and review of the literature. Arch Orthop Trauma Surg 118:111–112

Vollman D, Smith GA (2006) Epidemiology of lawn-mower-related injuries to children in the United States, 1990–2004. Pediatrics 118:e273–278

Vuori J, Aro H (1993) Lisfranc joint injuries: trauma mechanism and associated injury. J Trauma 35:40–45

Wiley JJ (1981) Tarsometatarsal joint injuries in children. J Pediatr Orthop 1:255–260

Shoulder

17

Phil Glithero

CONTENTS

17.1 Introduction

Injuries to the shoulder are reported to account for about for 8%–16% of fractures in children. Falls onto the shoulder are the usual cause of fractures of the clavicle, whilst falls onto the outstretched hand cause proximal humeral fractures. Whilst the mechanisms of injury to the shoulder in children are similar to those in adults, the fracture patterns seen differ as a consequence of the presence of the physes, with physeal separation occurring in preference to dislocation.

P. Glithero, FRCSEd (Orth)
Consultant Paediatric Orthopaedic Surgeon, Birmingham Children's Hospital, Steelhouse Lane, Birmingham, B4 6NH, UK

17.2 Clavicle

Both the clavicle and scapula initially form by membranous ossification. The clavicle secondarily develops growth cartilages at both ends. Primary ossification of the clavicle starts from two separate, lateral and medial, centres which appear by the sixth week of gestation. The medial epiphysis appears at 11–19 in girls and 14–19 in boys and fuses between the ages of 22 and 26 (Ogden and Conlogue 1979). The capsular ligaments of the sternoclavicular joint attach to the epiphysis and are stronger anteriorly. The lateral epiphysis appears after the medial and fuses rapidly. The primary stabiliser of the acromioclavicular joint is the coracoclavicular ligament acting through the inferior portion of the thickened periosteal tube around the distal clavicle.

Fractures of the clavicle result from falls onto the shoulder or lateral compression of the shoulder girdle. There is rarely any associated injury to the subclavian vessels, brachial plexus or pleura, unless the injury is due to a direct blow. Clavicular fractures have been (Allman 1967) classified into three types: type 1, middle third; type 2 distal to the coracoclavicular ligaments and type 3 medial to the sternocleidomastoid and costoclavicular ligament.

17.2.1 Middle Third Clavicle Fractures

The majority of fractures of the clavicle involve the middle third. The fracture pattern may be buckle, greenstick or displaced. Callus formation can be exuberant and, because it is subcutaneous, the prominence can be a cause of concern (Fig. 17.1). Treatment is usually symptomatic with a broad arm sling for comfort. A figure eight harness can provide additional support, especially for displaced

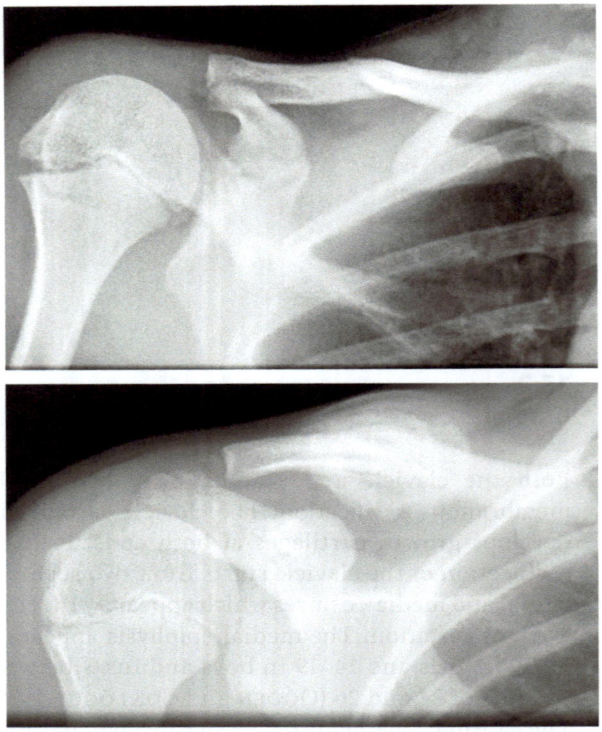

Fig. 17.1. **a** This child presented with an undisplaced fracture of the clavicle. **b** He was re-referred 12 weeks later because of concerns over the prominent callus that developed

fractures. Shoulder movements can be resumed as comfort allows and full activities resumed within 6–8 weeks. Only occasionally is operative treatment indicated, for open fractures or if skin tenting is associated with an irreducible fracture. Non-union can occur in adolescents and is treated by grafting and plating (Manske and Szabo 1985).

17.2.2 Medial Clavicle Fractures

Injuries of the medial end of the clavicle account for under 1% of clavicle fractures in children. They can occur if there is compression to the shoulder during contact sports such as ruby. Rather than the sternoclavicular dislocation seen in adults, which they mimic, these are Salter-Harris type I or II fractures (Denham and Dingley 1967). They are poorly seen on radiographs and CT or MR imaging are indicated, especially if (with posterior displacement) there is evidence of dysphagia or respiratory or vascular compromise (Fig. 17.2). If there is evidence of impingement, emergency closed reduction under anaesthesia is indicated. Once reduced posteriorly displaced fractures are usually stable and can be maintained with a figure eight harness. If there is no respiratory compromise a figure eight harness alone is sufficient and can lead to reduction. Anteriorly displaced fractures are less stable; however, as extensive remodelling occurs operative treatment is not indicated.

17.2.3 Lateral Clavicle Fractures

Injuries to the lateral end of the clavicle are more frequent than injuries to the medial end, but represent under 10% of fractures of the clavicle. Falls onto the point of the shoulder result in Salter-Harris type I or II physeal separations (Black et al. 1991) or fractures through the distal metaphysis. The distal clavicular metaphysis herniates through the thick periosteal sleeve and the acromioclavicular and coracoclavicular ligaments remain intact (Ogden 1984). Even with fractures medial to the ligaments stability is preserved. Extensive remodelling occurs and treatment is by broad arm sling.

17.2.3.1 Acromioclavicular Joint

True separation of the acromioclavicular joint occurs rarely. Distinction from physeal separations requires MR imaging, but this is not normally indicated as treatment is the same as for lateral clavicular fractures. Stress films are not routinely indicated. Full functional recovery can be expected (Taft et al 1987; Tibone et al 1992). Acromioclavicular injury in association with avulsion of the coracoid has been described (Combalia et al. 1995).

17.3 Scapula

The scapula develops multiple ossification centres which can be confused for fractures. Only the body's ossification centre is present at birth. In the first year a centre appears in the distal coracoid. A second centre appears at the base of the coracoid (the subcoracoid centre) around 10 years and forms a third of the

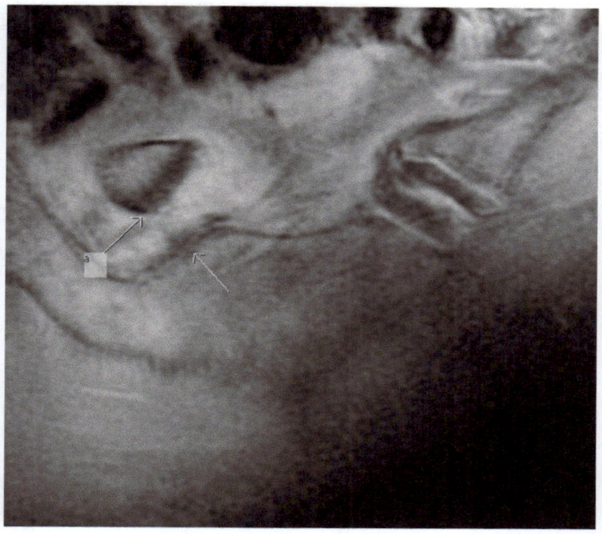

a

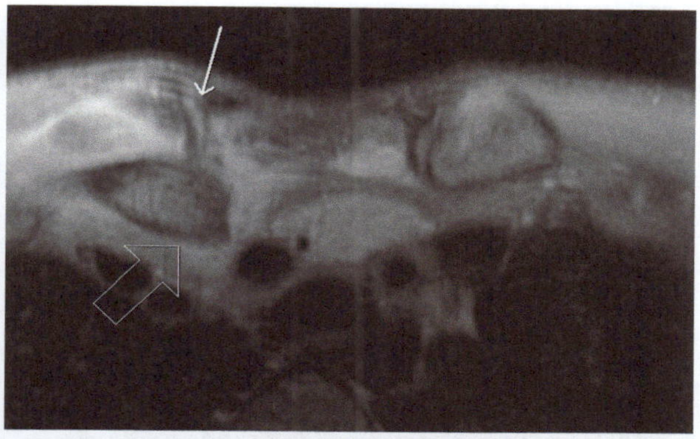

b

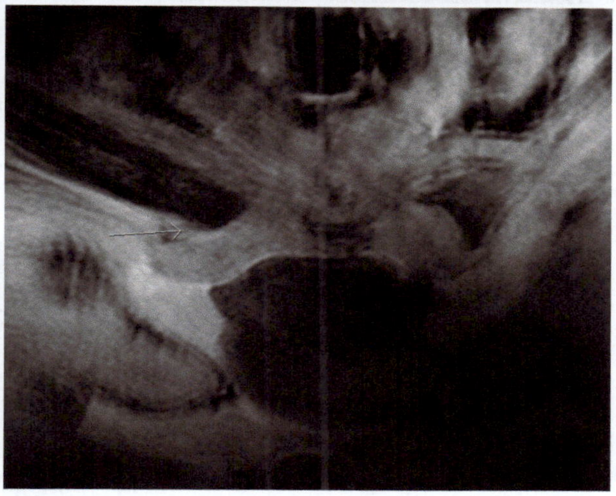

c

Fig. 17.2a-c. A teenage boy with a fracture through the most medial part of the right clavicle resulting in posterior dislocation of the clavicle. Normal appearance of the left sternoclavicular joint and clavicle. **a** Oblique axial proton density fat saturated images shows fracture on the right (*box arrow*) and normal left sternoclavicular joint (*line arrow*). **b** Axial proton density fat saturated images. On the right there is posterior dislocation of the clavicle (*box arrow*) the fracture through the medial aspect of the clavicle is seen (*line arrow*). **c** Oblique axial fast spoilt gradient echo The unossified portion of the clavicle (*bold arrow*) is seen articulating with the sternum, the clavicle (*two thin arrows*) is seen displaced posteriorly

glenoid. It fuses to the body of the scapula at around 14 in girls and 17 in boys (Fig. 17.3). At the same time a horseshoe shaped epiphysis appears forming the lower rim of the glenoid. The acromion develops multiple ossification centres at puberty which fuse at about 22 (Fig. 17.4) (Ogden and Phillips 1983; Samilson 1980). Their persistence is readily confused with fractures and failure to fuse leads to a bipartite or tripartite acromion. Additional centres appear at puberty for the vertebral border and inferior scapular angle.

Fractures of the scapula are rare and are typically the result of high energy trauma. Immediate concern is therefore with regard to associated rib fractures, pulmonary or cardiac contusion and mediastinal injury. The presence of tenderness and swelling around the shoulder indicates the possibility of a scapular fracture, which can be evaluated by CT. Indirect trauma leads to avulsion injuries (Goss 1996).

Treatment is usually by immobilisation with a sling and early mobilisation as comfort allows. Fractures of the body of the scapula are rarely displaced, but if there is significant displacement of fractures of the acromion or coracoid surgery may be indicated. Glenoid fractures may require reduction and stabilisation to maintain shoulder stability (Curtis 1990; Hardegger et al. 1984).

17.4 Shoulder Dislocation

Dislocation of the glenohumeral joint is uncommon under the age of 10, while approximately 20% of all traumatic dislocations occur between the ages of 10 and 20 (Rowe 1956). The presence of the humeral physis appears to be protective. Displacement is typically anteriorly with only 2%–4% of dislocations being posterior.

With an anterior dislocation the humeral head lies under the coracoid process on the AP radiograph (Fig. 17.5). The Y view shows the head to be displaced

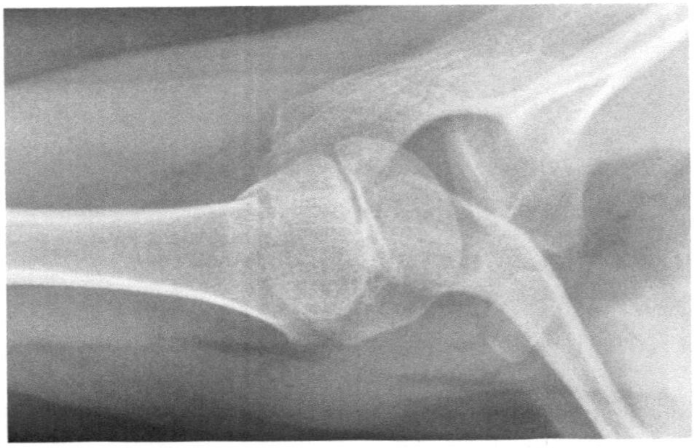

a

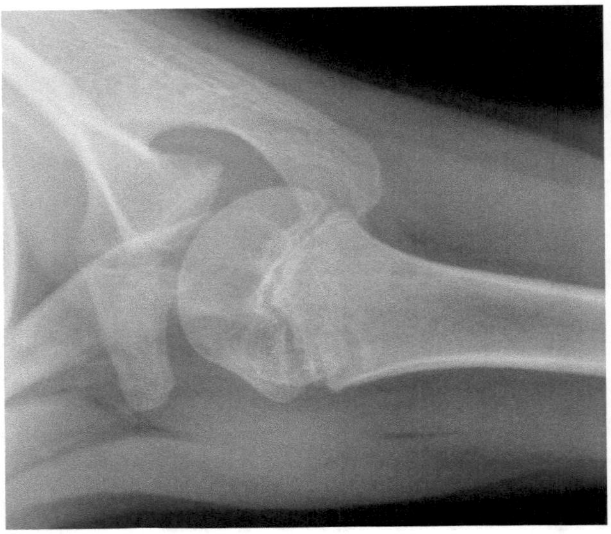

Fig. 17.3. **a** In this 10-year-old boy the distal coracoid is clearly visible, but the subcoracoid centre has yet to develop. **b** It is already present in this 9-year-old girl

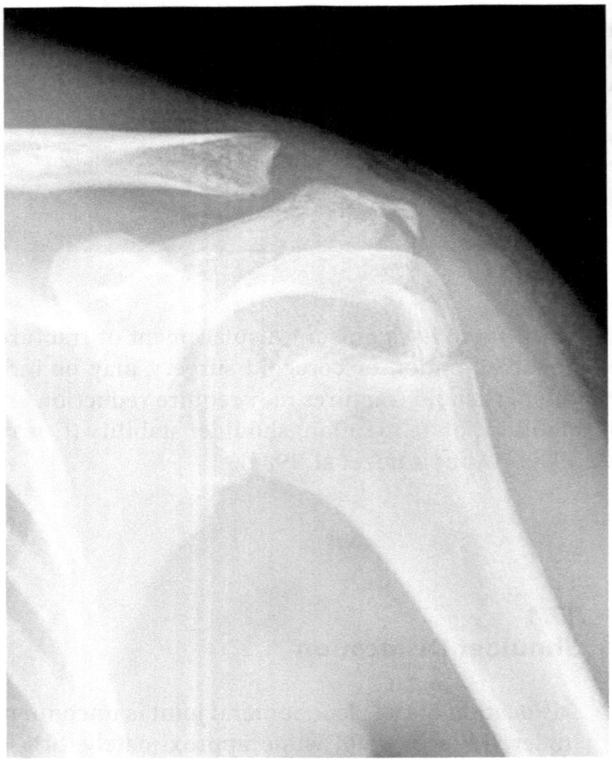

a

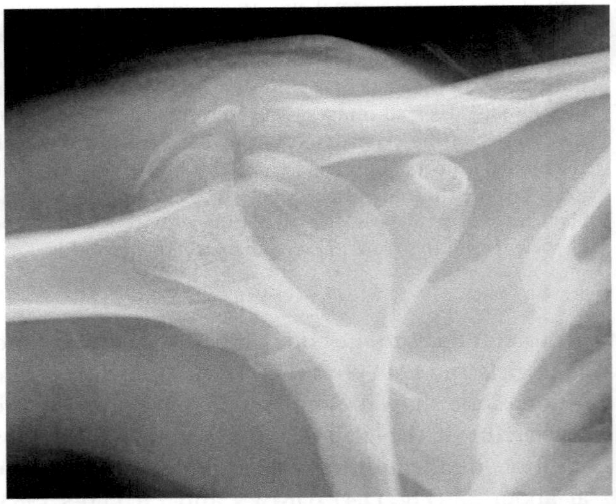

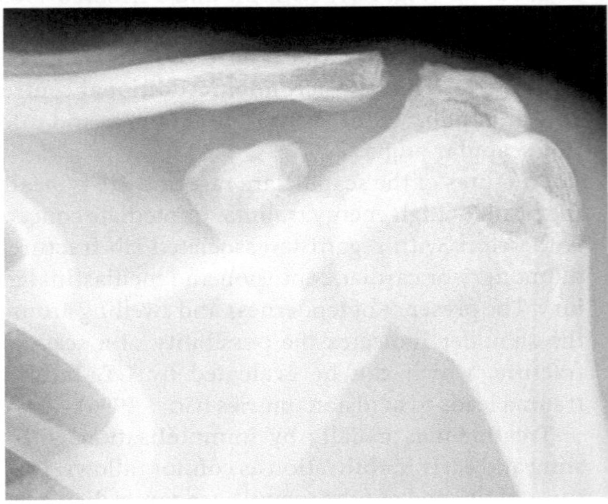

Fig. 17.4. **a** The AP view for this 12-year-old girl could suggest an avulsion from the acromion. The axillary view (**b**), however, clearly shows that this is an ossification centre. **c** In this 15-year-old the ossification of the acromion is more advanced

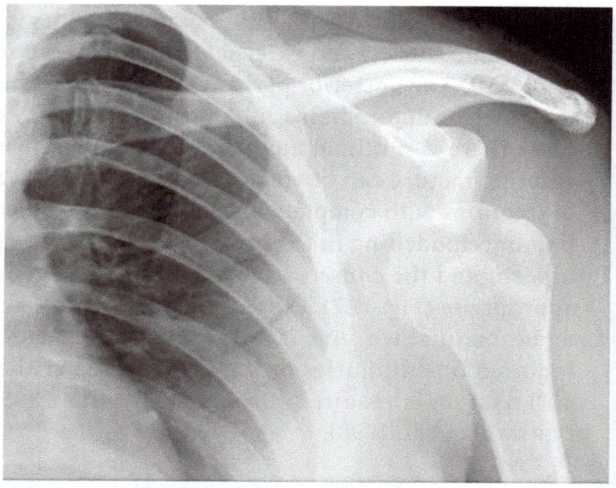

a

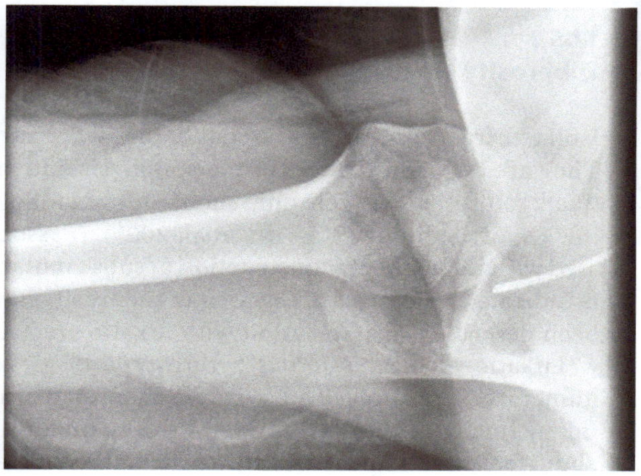

b

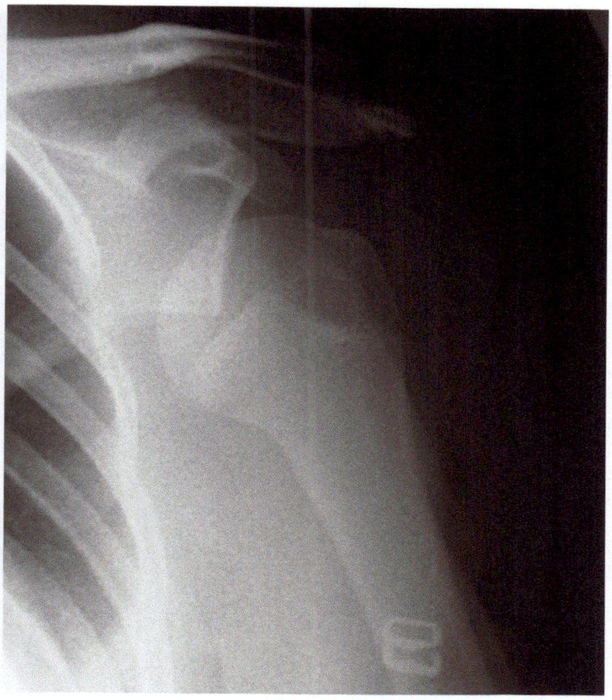

c

Fig. 17.5a-c. AP radiograph showing anterior dislocation with sub-coracoid location of the humeral head. Axial view showing anterior dislocation. Oblique view of a different child (to **a** and **b**) showing anterior dislocation

anteriorly and no longer covering the glenoid. On the oblique axial view the head of the humerus lies anterior to the glenoid. With posterior dislocations the humeral head may maintain a normal shape on the AP radiograph, in other instances the contour may be altered to resemble a 'light bulb'. On the axial view the humeral head lies posterior to the glenoid (Fig. 17.6).

Radiologically the Hill-Sachs compression lesion may be evident. The Hill-Sachs lesion is a compressive fracture of the humeral head and is an important bony sign of previous anterior shoulder dislocation and instability and is significant more common in adult patients. There may also be an avulsion injury to the glenoid rim indicative of an associated Bankart lesion (detachment of the anteroinferior capsule from the glenoid neck).

Treatment is by closed reduction followed by immobilisation for 4 weeks followed by strengthening exercises for the rotator cuff. The incidence of recurrent dislocation is unclear but probably occurs in between 60% and 85% (Hoelen et al. 1990; Kawam et al. 1997). Recurrent dislocation is an indication for surgical stabilisation.

17.4.1
Atraumatic Shoulder Instability

In the absence of a clear history of significant trauma, children presenting with dislocation of the shoulder should be considered to have atraumatic instability. This may be involuntary following a minimal event such as overarm throwing, or voluntary and is associated with inherent joint laxity (Carter and Sweetman 1960). Pain is minimal and multidirectional laxity may also be identifiable in the other shoulder. It may also be associated with congenital anomalies of the glenoid, proximal humeral deformities and emotional or psychiatric disturbance. The results of surgery in these patients are generally poor.

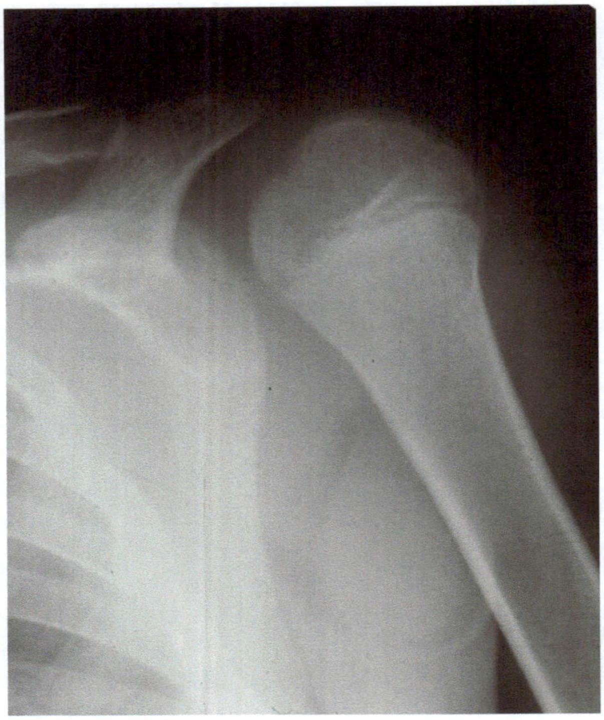

Fig. 17.6. AP radiograph of a posterior dislocation. The humeral head has a 'light bulb' type appearance

17.5 Proximal Humerus

The ossification centre of the humeral head appears at 6 months. Additional centres develop for the greater tuberosity between 1 and 2 and the lesser tuberosity by 5. The tubersosities fuse together at 5 and fuse with the head between 7 and 14. The proximal physis closes by 19 (Ogden et al. 1978). The contour of the physis can lead to misinterpretation as a fracture.

Fractures of the proximal humerus are uncommon – those involving the physis represent about 3% of physeal injuries (Schwendenwein et al. 2004). In children under 10 the fracture is typically metaphyseal, whilst in adolescence it is a Salter-Harris type II fracture. Salter-Harris type III fractures have been described in association with dislocation of the shoulder (Wang et al. 1997).

The mechanism of injury is the same as that causing a dislocation in adults. The distal fragment displaces anteriorly while the proximal fragment is pulled into flexion and external rotation by the rotator cuff. The posterior periosteum is thicker than the anterior and remains intact. In the majority of cases there is minimal angulation or displacement and the fracture can be treated conservatively. Even in fractures with complete displacement, the potential for remodelling in the proximal humerus is significant and the conservative management remains appropriate (Fig. 17.7). Closed reduction is unlikely to be maintained and if surgical management is required (open injuries or angulation greater than 60°) fixation is required (Baxter and Wiley 1986; Beringer et al. 1998).

17.5.1 Tuberosity Fractures

Isolated fractures of the lesser tuberosity are rare. They are avulsion injuries of the apophysis and are likely to present with chronic shoulder pain following a sporting injury (Levine et al. 2005). If associated with instability reconstruction of subscapularis is indicated. Fractures of the greater tuberosity have been described in association with luxatio erecta.

Luxatio erecta humeri is a rare type of glenohumeral dislocation. The pathomechanics of this injury involve either direct axial loading on a fully abducted extremity or leverage of the humeral head across the acromion by a hyperabduction force. The humeral head is dislocated inferiorly and stuck in a position of abduction. Injury to the axillary vessels and brachial plexus is not uncommon.

17.5.2 Little Leaguer's Shoulder

Repetitive over arm activities such as baseball pitching can lead to epiphysiolysis of the proximal humeral physis. It presents with shoulder pain, initially only during throwing and radiographs demonstrate widening and irregularity of the physis. There may be small subperiosteal cysts. Bone scintigraphy is normal, while MR imaging may show widening of the proximal physis, with surrounding muscle bone oedema. The condition is self limiting, but modification of activity aids resolution (Barnett 1985; Fleming et al. 2004; Song et al. 2006).

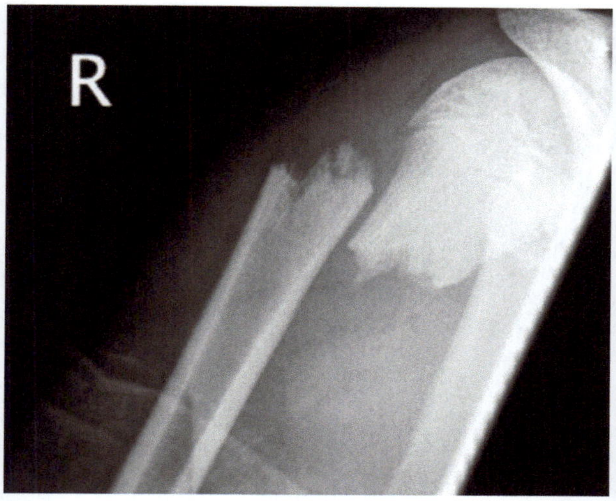

a

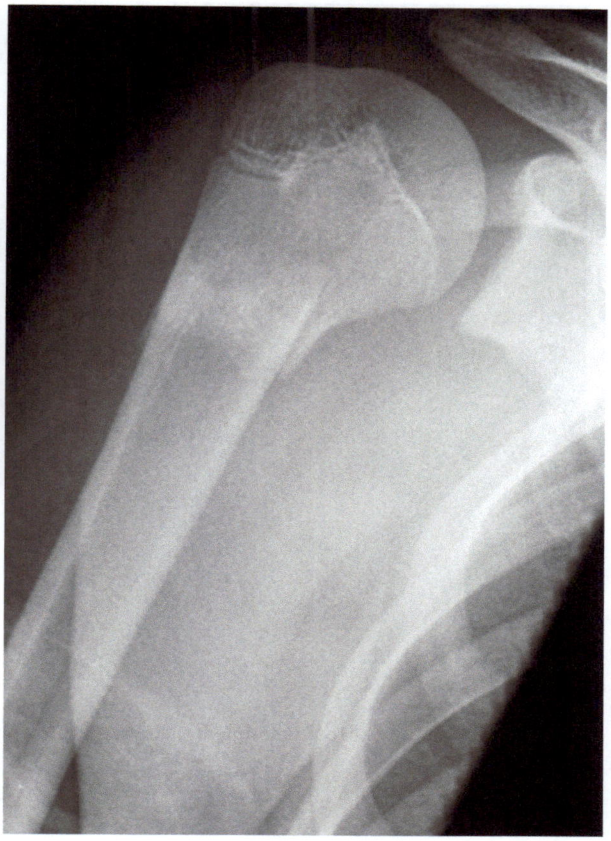

b

Fig. 17.7a,b. This 12-year-old presented with a completely displaced proximal humeral fracture (**a**). It was treated conservatively. By 4 months extensive remodelling is present and shoulder function was normal (**b**)

17.5.3 Pathological Fractures

The proximal humerus metaphysis is a common location for simple bone cysts which present following injury to the shoulder (Fig. 17.8). Radiologically the cyst is well defined and unless it has fractured there will be no periosteal reaction. The classic radiological sign, following a fracture, is the 'fallen fragment' sign in which a bone fragment sinks to a more dependent part of the cyst (Killeen 1998). Treatment may be expectant, or by aspiration and steroid or bone marrow injection, or by bone grafting.

17.6 Neonatal Shoulder Injuries

Fractures of the clavicle occur in around 1.5% of deliveries and are the commonest birth injury (Lam et al. 2002) and may be associated with brachial plexus palsy. The injury may be asymptomatic and not present until swelling has subsided and the callus mass is evident. However, the infant may present with a lack of arm movement during the neonatal period, associated with pain, swelling and crepitus. Less commonly occurring are fractures of the proximal humerus and rarely shoulder dislocation. The differential diagnosis includes brachial plexus palsy, septic arthritis of the shoulder, osteomyelitis and non-accidental injury.

Injury to the proximal humerus can be either a metaphyseal fracture or more typically a Salter-Harris type 1 physeal separation. This will not be evident on the plain film as the proximal humeral physis does not start to ossify until 3–6 months of age. The radiological finding of widening of the joint space occurs in physeal separation, dislocation, brachial plexus palsy and septic arthritis. Ultrasound may be indicated to clarify the diagnosis (Zieger et al. 1987). However, since healing is rapid at this age periosteal new bone will often be apparent within 10–14 days.

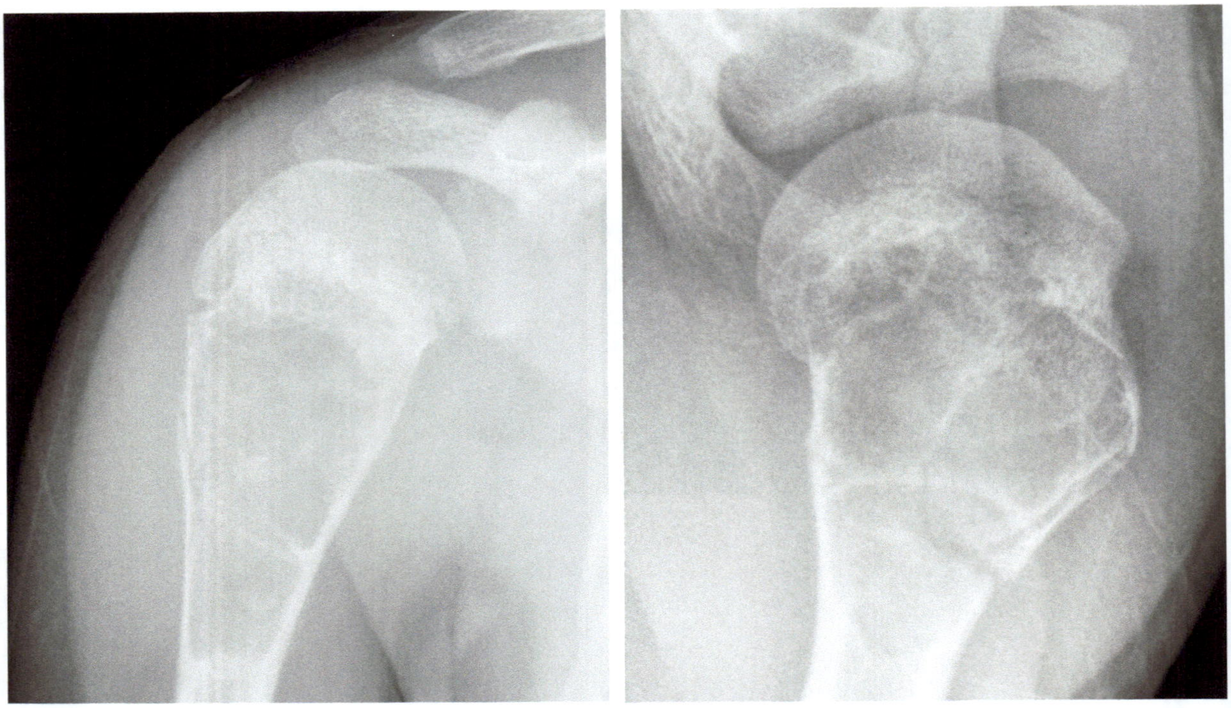

a

Fig. 17.8a,b. Fracture through simple bone cyst. Although fractures into cysts can lead to the cyst resolving, this failed to occur in this case

As healing is rapid and significant remodelling occurs, treatment is by parental reassurance and gentle handling.

17.7 Congenital Pseudoarthrosis of the Clavicle

Congenital pseudoarthrosis of the clavicle usually presents in the neonate with a lump in the line of the clavicle. Usually it is right sided and rarely bilateral. When left sided, it has been said to be associated with dextrocardia, but this is not invariable (SAKKERS et al. 1999). Unlike congenital pseudarthrosis of the tibia there is no association with neurofibromatosis. It may be confused with a birth fracture; however, repeat radiographs will not show the periosteal reaction, callus formation and remodelling that will occur following the fracture. Radiologically the proximal part is elevated and enlarged, while the lateral part is thinned, depressed and displaced behind the proximal (ALLDRED 1963). The pseudoarthrosis occurs in the middle third of the clavicle, between the primary ossification centres. The bone ends are capped by cartilage, which has the appearance of a developing physis, and are often encapsulated, forming a synovial joint (HIRATA et al. 1995).

When indicated surgical treatment requires excision of the pseudoarthrosis, grafting and plate fixation.

References

Alldred AJ (1963) Congenital pseudarthrosis of the clavicle. J Bone Joint Surg (Br) 45:312–319

Allman FL (1967) Fractures and ligamentous injuries of the clavicle and its articulation. J Bone Joint Surg (Am) 49:774–784

Barnett LS (1985) Little league shoulder syndrome: proximal humeral epiphyseolysis in adolescent baseball pitchers. J Bone Joint Surg (Am) 67:495–496

Baxter MP, Wiley JJ (1986) Fractures of the proximal humeral epiphysis: their influence on humeral growth. J Bone Joint Surg (Br) 68:570–573

Beringer DC, Weiner DS, Noble JS et al (1998) Severely displaced proximal humeral epiphyseal fractures: a follow-up study. J Pediatr Orthop 18:31–37

Black GB, McPherson JA, Reed MH (1991) Traumatic pseudodislocation of the acromioclavicular joint in children. Am J Sports Med 19:644–646

Carter C, Sweetman R (1960) Recurrent dislocation of the patella and of the shoulder: their association with familial joint laxity. J Bone Joint Surg (Br) 42:721–727

Combalia A, Arandes JM, Alemany X, Ramon R (1995) Acromioclavicular dislocation with epiphyseal separation of the coracoid process: report of a case and review of the literature. J Trauma 38:812–815

Curtis RJ (1990) Operative management of children's fractures of the shoulder region. Orthop Clin North Am 21:315–324

Denham R, Dingley A (1967) Epiphyseal separation of the medial end of the clavicle. J Bone Joint Surg (Am) 49:1179–1183

Fisher NA, Newman B, Lloyd J, Mimouni F (1995) Ultrasonographic evaluation of birth injury to the shoulder. J Perinatol 15:398–400

Fleming JL, Hollingsworth CL, Squire DL, Bisset GS (2004) Little Leaguer's shoulder. Skeletal Radiol 33:352–354

Gibson DA, Carroll N (1970) Congenital pseudarthrosis of the clavicle. J Bone Joint Surg (Br) 52:629–643

Goss TP (1996) The scapula: coracoid, acromial, and avulsion fractures. Am J Orthop 25:106–115

Hardegger FH, Simpson LA, Weber BG (1984) The operative treatment of scapular fractures. J Bone Joint Surg (Br) 66:725–731

Hirata S, Miya H, Mizuno K (1995) Congenital pseudarthrosis of the clavicle. Histologic examination for the etiology of the disease. Clin Orthop Relat Res 315:242–245

Hoelen MA, Burgers AM, Rozing PM (1990) Prognosis of primary anterior shoulder dislocation in young adults. Arch Orthop Trauma Surg 110:51–54

Kawam M, Sinclair J, Letts M (1997) Recurrent posterior dislocation of the shoulder in children: the results of surgical management. J Pediatr Orthop 17:533–538

Killeen KL (1998) The fallen fragment sign. Radiology 207:261–262

Lam MH, Wong GY, Lao TT (2002) Reappraisal of neonatal clavicular fracture: relationship between infant size and neonatal morbidity. Obstet Gynecol 100:115–119

Levine B, Pereira D, Rosen J (2005) Avulsion fractures of the lesser tuberosity of the humerus in adolescents: review of the literature and case report. J Orthop Trauma 19:349–352

Manske DJ, Szabo RM (1985) The operative treatment of mid-shaft clavicular non-unions. J Bone Joint Surg (Am) 67:1367–1371

Ogden JA, Conlogue GJ, Jensen P (1978) Radiology of postnatal skeletal development. The proximal humerus. Skeletal Radiol 2:153–160

Ogden JA, Conlogue GJ, Bronson ML (1979) Radiology of postnatal skeletal development. III. The clavicle. Skeletal Radiol 4:196–203

Ogden JA, Phillips SB (1983) Radiology of postnatal skeletal development. VII. The scapula. Skeletal Radiol 9:157–169

Ogden JA (1984) Distal clavicular physeal injury. Clin Orthop 188:68–73

Sakkers RJ, Tjin A, Ton E, Bos CF (1999) Left-sided congenital pseudarthrosis of the clavicula. J Pediatr Orthop B 8:45–47

Song JC, Lazarus ML, Song AP (2006) MRI findings in Little Leaguer's shoulder. Skeletal Radiol 35:107–109

Rowe C (1956) Prognosis in dislocation of the shoulder. J Bone Joint Surg (Am) 38:957–977

Samilson RL (1980) Congenital and developmental anomalies of the shoulder girdle. Orthop Clin North Am 11:219–231

Schwendenwein E, Hajdu S, Gaebler C, Stengg K, Vecsei V (2004) Displaced fractures of the proximal humerus in children require open/closed reduction and internal fixation. Eur J Pediatr Surg 14:51–55

Taft TN, Wilson FC, Oglesby JW (1987) Dislocation of the acromioclavicular joint: an end result study. J Bone Joint Surg (Am) 69:1045–1051

Tibone J, Sellers R, Tonino P (1992) Strength testing after third-degree acromioclavicular dislocations. Am J Sports Med 20:328–331

Wang P Jr, Koval KJ, Lehman W, Strongwater A, Grant A, Zuckerman JD (1997) Salter-Harris type III fracture-dislocation of the proximal humerus. J Pediatr Orthop B 6:219–222

Zieger M, Dorr U, Schulz RD (1987) Sonography of slipped humeral epiphysis due to birth injury. Pediatr Radiol 17:425–426

Elbow Injuries

18

Edward Bache

CONTENTS

18.1 Incidence

Approximately 65%–75% of fractures in children occur in the upper limb, principally due to their tendency to fall on an outstretched hand. Most fractures occur at the distal radius with less than 10% of them occurring at the elbow. Of the elbow injuries, the vast majority are at the distal end of the humerus with the supracondylar fracture being the commonest, followed by lateral condyle fractures.

E. Bache, FRCS (ortho)
Consultant Paediatric Orthopaedic Surgeon, Birmingham Children's Hospital, Steelhouse Lane, Birmingham, B4 6NH, UK

An estimation of the distribution of fracture patterns about the elbow is supracondylar (70%), lateral condyle (15%), medial epicondyle (10%), olecranon (5%), radial neck (1%), medial condyle (1%), capitellum (1%), T condylar (<1 %).

The peak age of elbow fractures in children is between 5–10 years. While some authors have noted a higher incidence in girls, others have noted a higher incidence in boys.

18.2 Embryology and Development

Chondrification centres of the humerus are evident at around 6 weeks of intrauterine age (12 mm embryo). The elbow joint cavity appears at about 9 weeks (27 mm embryo), with the radio-humeral and the ulno-humeral cavities developing separately. The two cavities fuse after about 1 week. Muscles and tendons get demarcated by the 9th week. At the end of 30 weeks, the bony architecture of the elbow is well defined. At birth, ossification centres are only present in the metadiaphyses of the humerus, radius and ulna.

Six separate centres of ossification appear at certain ages and fuse in a specific pattern (Table 18.1; Fig. 18.1) and vascular changes occur at the same time.

Knowledge of the timings of these events is important in determining the type of injury and the possibility of avascular necrosis following trauma. The pattern of appearance of these ossification centres around the elbow is very consistent and has been used to determine bone age by various authors. The order of appearance of the various ossification centres can be remembered by the acronym CRITOE [capitellum, radial head, internal (medial) epicondyle, trochlea, olecranon, external (lateral) epicondyle].

18.3 Blood Supply

Damage to the blood supply about the elbow, either as result of injury or following surgery may affect its subsequent growth and function. It is supplied proximally by branches of the brachial artery and distally by branches from the radial and ulnar arteries. The distal humerus is supplied by vessels running posteriorly. There is no anastomosis between the blood supply to the metaphyseal region and the ossific nuclei.

The blood supply to the trochlea is via two terminal interosseous branches of the recurrent ulnar artery, the lateral trochlea and medial trochlea arteries. The medial artery may be damaged in fractures of the medial condyle, leading to avascular necrosis.

The blood supply to the capitellum is via end arterioles from the inferior ulnar collateral artery crossing the olecranon fossa posteriorly into the lateral condyle to the ossific nucleus of the capitellum. This predisposes to avascular necrosis following displaced capitellar fractures.

Table 18.1. Centres of ossification, ages and fusion patterns

Site	Ossification		Fuses	
	Females	*males*	*Females*	*males*
Capitellum	1–11 Months	1–26 Months	14–16 Years	14–16 Years
Medial epicondyle	5–8 Years	7–9 Years	20 Years	20 Years
Medial trochlea	7–11 Years	8–13 Years	14–16 Years	14–16 Years
Lateral epicondyle (extracapsular)	8–11 Years	9–13 Years	Puberty	Puberty
Proximal radius (intracapsular)	4 Years	5–6 Years	14–17 Years	14–17 Years
Olecranon	8–9 Years	10–11 Years	Puberty	Puberty

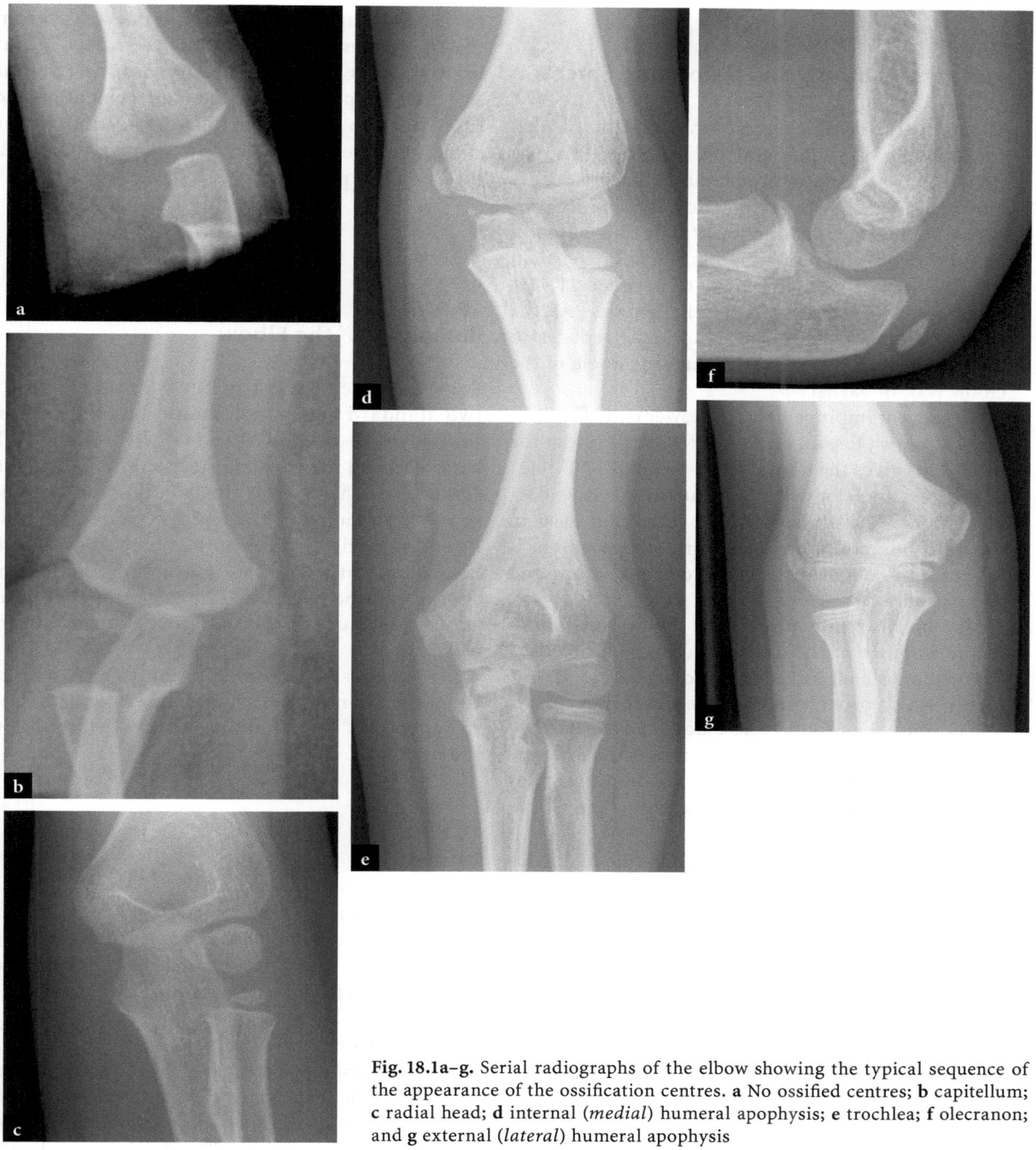

Fig. 18.1a–g. Serial radiographs of the elbow showing the typical sequence of the appearance of the ossification centres. **a** No ossified centres; **b** capitellum; **c** radial head; **d** internal (*medial*) humeral apophysis; **e** trochlea; **f** olecranon; and **g** external (*lateral*) humeral apophysis

18.4 Relevant Anatomy and Deforming Forces

The elbow is a complex hinged synovial joint which consists of the ulno-humeral, radio-humeral and the radio-ulnar articulations. Flexion-extension occurs mostly at the ulno-humeral articulation while pronation supination is a function of the radio-humeral and the radio-ulnar articulation. In full extension, the elbow has a carrying angle of between 11°–16° of valgus with a greater angle in females. As the elbow flexes to 60°, the carrying angle reduces to zero, while in full flexion, the carrying angle of the elbow is 6° of varus.

To prevent impingement, the lower end of the humerus has two fossae, one at the front and one at the back. This gives the human elbow a range of 0°–142° of flexion extension with 5° of further passive flexion. About 9° of abduction and adduction exist in the ulno-humeral joint. This range of movement is essential to complete the full arc of pronation and supination.

The bony architecture of the elbow contributes to the stability of the joint, which is reinforced by the medial (ulnar) and lateral (radial) collateral ligaments, which provide most of the stability.

The muscles around the elbow can be divided into groups for convenience. These groups define the internervous planes, which are important for various different surgical approaches to the elbow. The groups are as follows:

- Flexor group: Supplied by the musculocutaneous nerve, this group comprises of the brachialis and the biceps.
- Extensor group: Supplied by the radial nerve, this group is made up of the triceps and the anconeus.
- Flexor pronator (medial) group: Supplied by the median and ulnar nerves, this group comprises of the pronator teres, flexor carpi radialis, palmaris longus, flexor carpi ulnaris, and the flexor digitorum superficialis.
- Lateral (wrist extensor) and supinator: Supplied by the radial and the posterior interosseous nerve, this group consists of the supinator, extensor carpi radialis longus, extensor carpi radialis brevis, extensor digitorum communis, and the extensor carpi ulnaris.

The elbow joint is a lever type joint and the muscles that act around it are at a significant mechanical disadvantage, which can result in excessive joint reaction forces. The construct of the elbow, including the forces that are transmitted during various activities, help determine the management of fractures and also aid in reduction and fixation. Understanding these forces is vital to diagnose and treat these injuries properly.

18.5 Radiology of the Elbow

For all children having an injury to the elbow, the two standard views that should be obtained are the anteroposterior (AP) view with elbow fully extended and the forearm fully supinated (if possible). The other view is the lateral with the elbow at 90° of flexion and the forearm in neutral position. Comparison views of the other elbow should not be part of normal radiographic practice and should only be performed in exceptional circumstances, because of the radiation exposure to the child.

As previously discussed, it is important to assess the ossification centres around the elbow. The internal apophysis should always appear before that of the trochlea.

18.5.1 Landmarks

When reviewing an elbow radiograph, there are important landmarks and measurements that should be reviewed to confirm the adequacy of the radiograph and to assess for any pathological changes.

Anteroposterior view (Fig. 18.2):

- Metaphyseal diaphyseal angle is the angle formed between the long axis of the humerus and the line drawn between the lateral and the medial epicondyle. This ranges from 72°–95°, with considerable inter- and intra-observer error, and so is not very reliable (Keats et al. 1966).
- Humero-ulnar angle is the angle formed between the long axis of the humerus and the long axis of the ulna. This angle depicts the carrying angle of the elbow. This ranges from 154°–178° and is greater in females (Keats et al. 1966).

- Angulation of the lateral physis in respect to the long axis of the shaft of the humerus (shaft physeal angle) is also known as the Baumann angle (Baumann 1929). It is important to have the humerus parallel to the radiographic plate with a perpendicular X-ray beam for an accurate measurement of this angle. This angle is subtended by the longitudinal axis of the humerus and a line through the coronal axis of the capitellar epiphysis. This angle has a mean value of 70° (range 64°–81°) (Williamson et al. 1992).

18.5.2 Lateral View

Important landmarks and lines should be assessed on a lateral view of the elbow (Fig. 18.3):

- The teardrop or hourglass sign is formed by the anterior margin of the olecranon fossa and the posterior margin of the coronoid fossa with the capitellum forming the inferior portion. The capitellum and trochlea (if ossified) should be super-

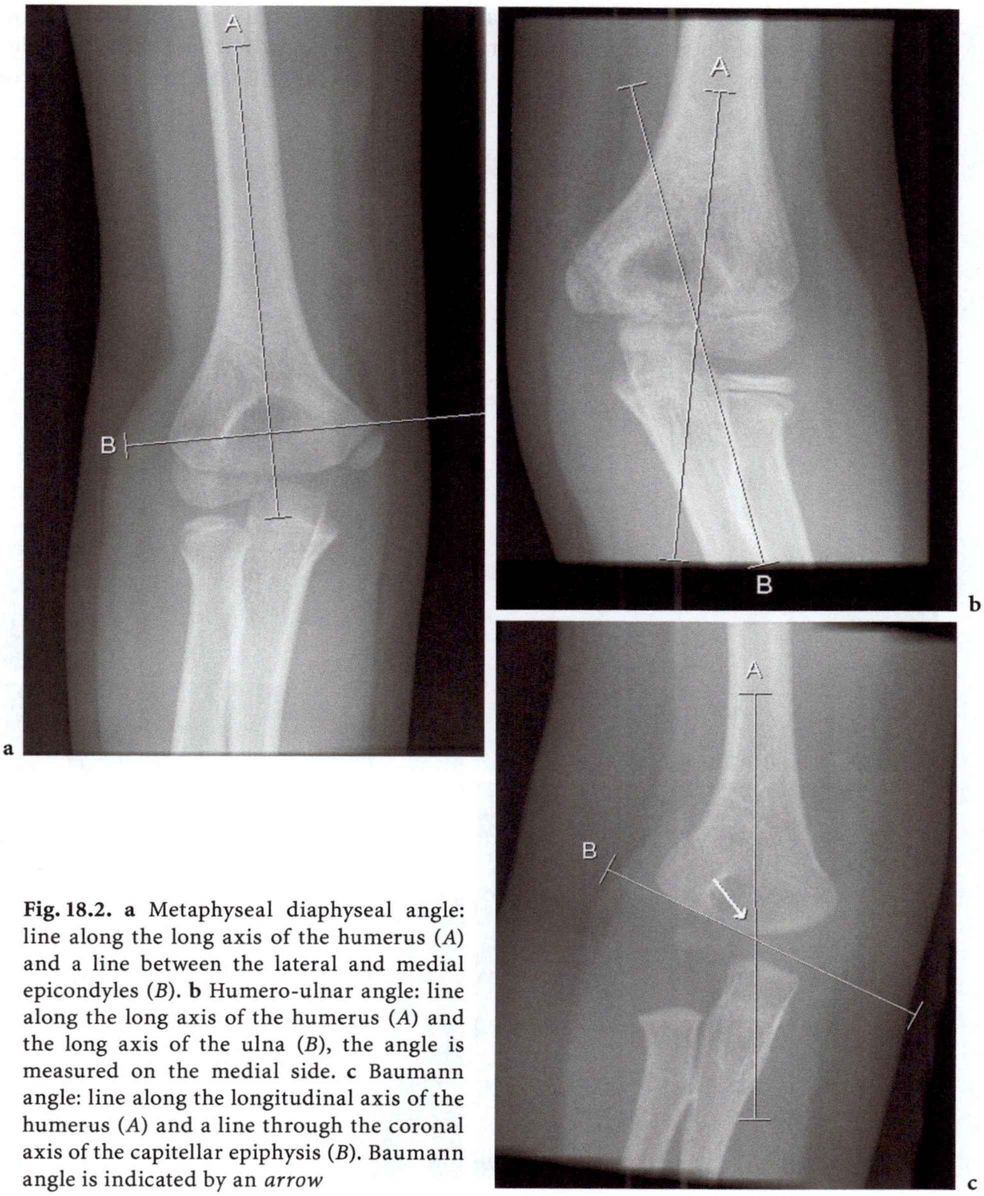

Fig. 18.2. a Metaphyseal diaphyseal angle: line along the long axis of the humerus (*A*) and a line between the lateral and medial epicondyles (*B*). **b** Humero-ulnar angle: line along the long axis of the humerus (*A*) and the long axis of the ulna (*B*), the angle is measured on the medial side. **c** Baumann angle: line along the longitudinal axis of the humerus (*A*) and a line through the coronal axis of the capitellar epiphysis (*B*). Baumann angle is indicated by an *arrow*

imposed. These lines indicate that a correctly positioned lateral radiograph has been obtained and as such, the remaining observations are valid.

- The angle formed by the long axis of the shaft and the long axis of the capitellum can be used to determine rotation and angulation.
- A longitudinal line drawn along the anterior cortex of the humerus should traverse the middle third of the capitellum (Rogers et al. 1978).
- A line drawn along the centre of the proximal radius should intersect the capitellum (the radiocapitellar line). Failure to do so suggests dislocation of the radial head. This rule is always valid on a true lateral image, in all stages of flexion (Storen 1959).
- A line extended from the anterior aspect of the coronoid should just touch the superior aspect of the capitellum.

18.5.3 Fat Pad

The articular surfaces of the elbow are contained within the joint capsule, which also encloses non-articular surfaces, including the coronoid, radial fossa and olecranon fossae. It attaches just distal to the coronoid and olecranon processes. The whole of the radial head is within the capsule.

Three fat pads lie over the capsule, the anterior over the coronoid fossa, the posterior over the olecranon fossa and a third over the supinator as it wraps over the radius. Fracture, haematoma and effusion into an intact capsule may cause capsular distension, which can distort these fat pads, improving their visibility and identifying occult fractures (Fig. 18.4). In the setting of acute trauma, a visible

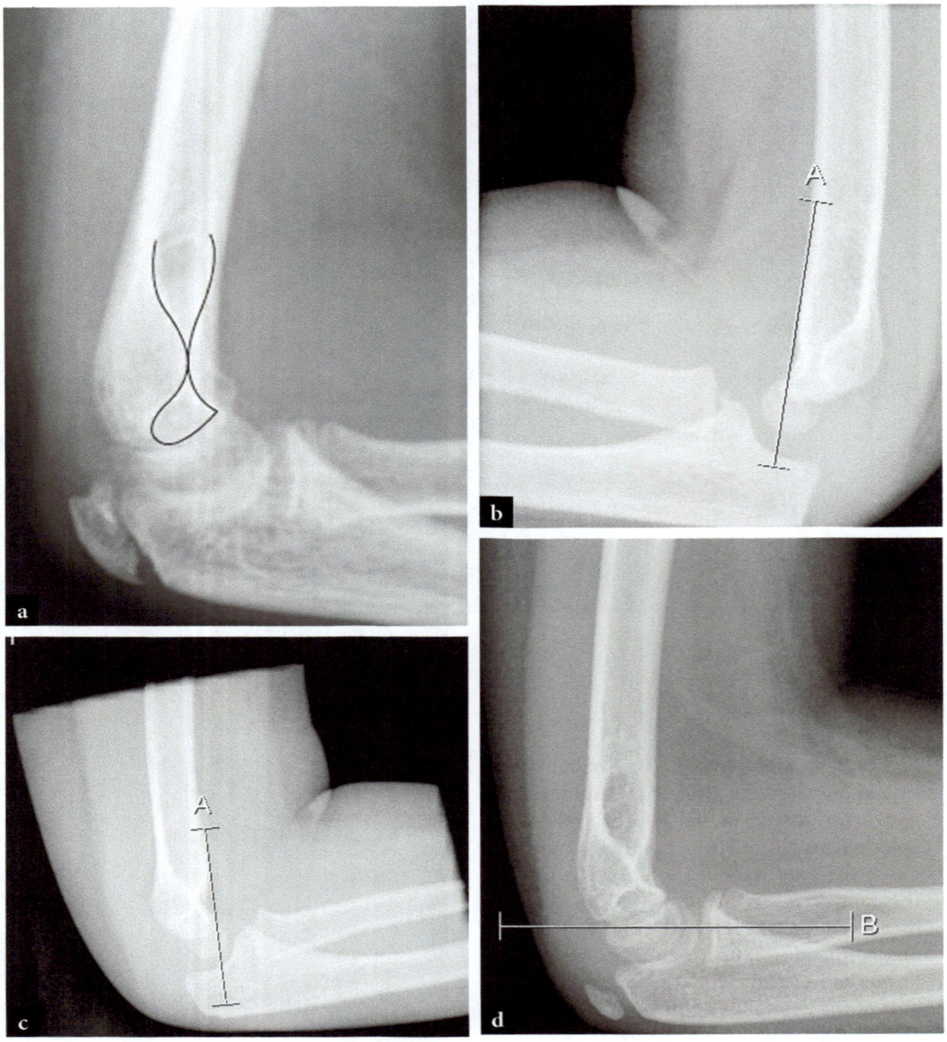

Fig. 18.3. a The teardrop or hourglass sign formed by the anterior margin of the olecranon fossa and posterior margin of the coronoid fossa with capitellum – the inferior portion. These indicate a correctly positioned lateral view. **b** A line along the anterior cortex should traverse the middle third of the capitellum – the anterior humeral line. **c** A supracondylar fracture with displacement and alteration of the normal relationship of the capitellum and humerus. **d** A line along the centre of the radius should intersect the capitellum – the radio-capitellum line

posterior fat pad should be regarded as abnormal, due to an occult injury, particularly of the radial head or an undisplaced supracondylar fracture. A visible anterior fat pad may be normal but if displaced anteriorly then it is regarded as abnormal (Skaggs and Mirzayan 1999). The absence of visible fat pads does not exclude the presence of a fracture.

The medial and lateral epicondyles are extracapsular and fractures of these structures are not associated with capsular distension or displacement of the fat pads.

18.6 Supracondylar Fractures

Supracondylar humeral fractures are the commonest fractures in children under the age of 7. Complications are common, with rates of nerve injury reported between 6% and 16% (Lyons et al. 2000), and a high incidence of malunion leading to cubitus varus/valgus. The majority of fractures are extension type, sustained from a fall on an extended upper extremity. They result in posterior displacement of the distal fracture fragment. Hyper-extensibility of the elbow has been postulated as a risk factor for this type of injury; however, a study (McLauchan et al. 1999) aimed at proving this, has found no supporting evidence.

Flexion type fractures, with anterior displacement of the distal fragment, account for less than 1% of supracondylar fractures (Blount 1977). These types of fractures are usually caused by a direct blow to the posterior aspect of the flexed elbow and are often very unstable.

It is important to distinguish between flexion and extension fractures, since flexion injuries almost always require surgical stabilisation and often open reduction (Fig. 18.5). The rest of the limb should be examined since ipsilateral forearm fractures have been reported in 3%–13% of supracondylar fractures (Roposch et al. 2002).

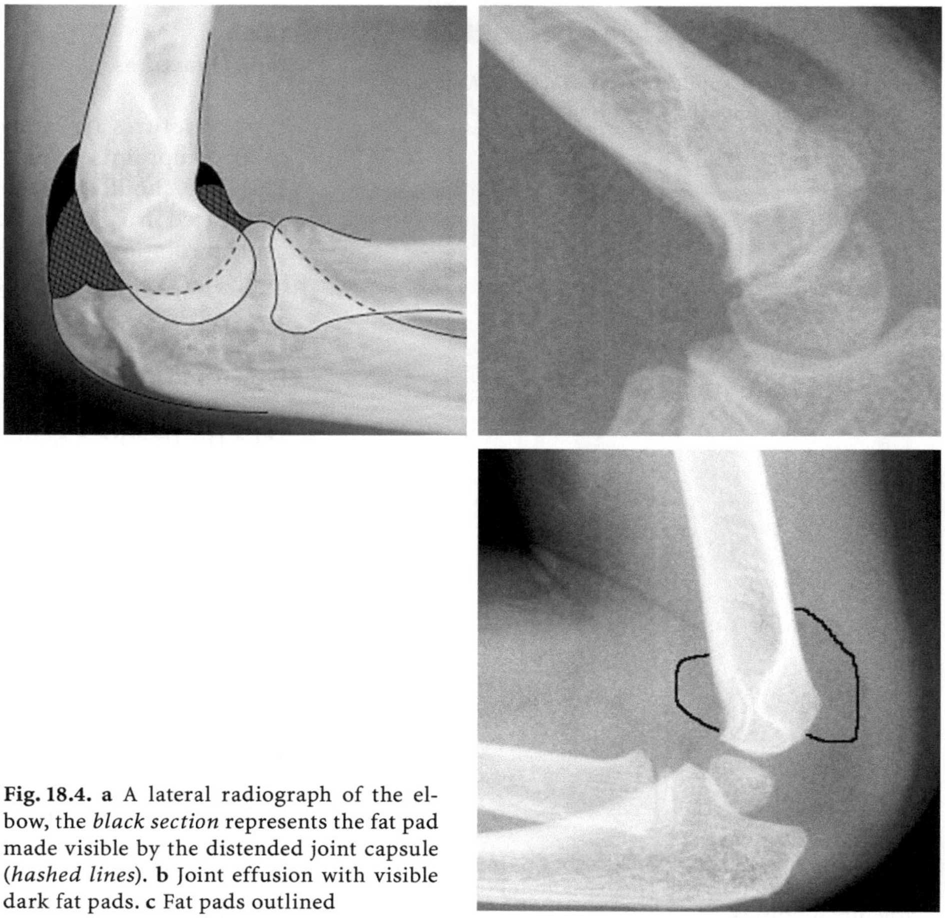
a b c

Fig. 18.4. **a** A lateral radiograph of the elbow, the *black section* represents the fat pad made visible by the distended joint capsule (*hashed lines*). **b** Joint effusion with visible dark fat pads. **c** Fat pads outlined

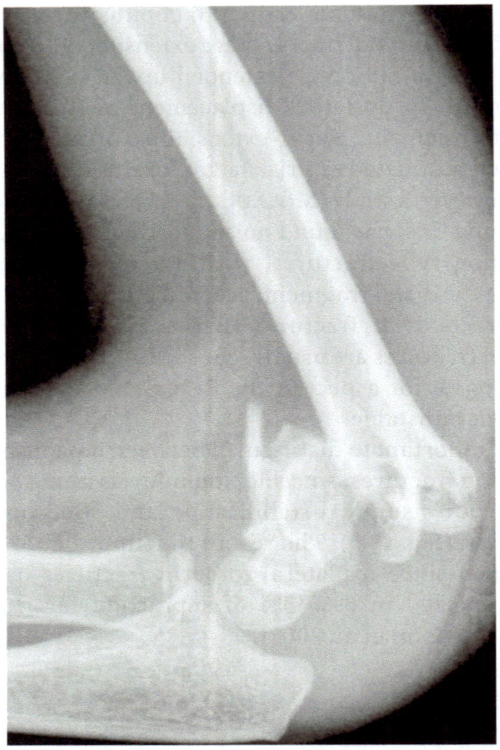

Fig. 18.5. Flexion supracondylar fracture. Anterior displacement of the distal fragment

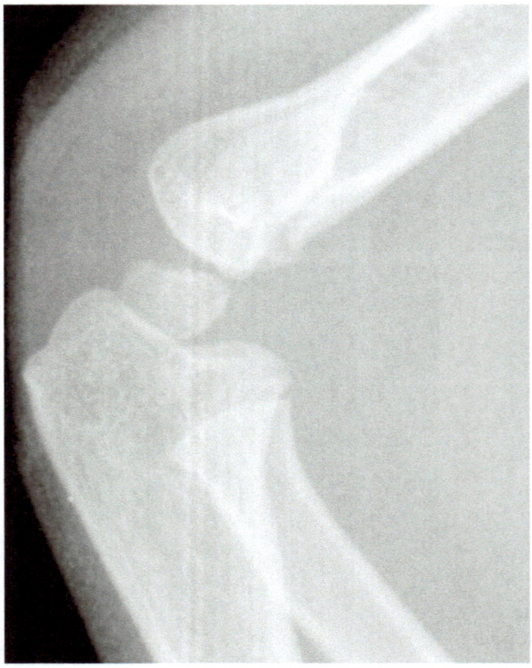

Fig. 18.6. Gartland type I extension supracondylar fracture (undisplaced)

18.6.1 Classification

The most commonly used classification system for extension type fractures is that of GARTLAND (1959), who divided these fractures into three categories. Type I fractures are minimally displaced. Type II fractures have an intact posterior cortical hinge, with some posterior angulation. This type of fracture is sometimes subclassified into types A and B, depending on whether there is simple posterior angulation or angulation plus malrotation respectively. Type III fractures have complete disruption of the cortex with displacement. They again may be subdivided into posteromedial or posterolateral, depending on the direction of displacement of the distal fragment. This may have implications on the likelihood of injury to neurovascular structures.

18.6.2 Management

18.6.2.1 Type I Fractures

Type I fractures are rarely a problem, with neurovascular compromise being extremely rare (Fig. 18.6). The limb should be assessed in the usual manner and placed in a plaster back slab in 90° of flexion and neutral rotation (O'HARA et al. 2000). Three weeks in plaster is usually sufficient.

18.6.2.2 Type II and III Fractures

Type IIA fractures reduce with flexion of the elbow (Fig. 18.7). This position can be maintained with a plaster cast or adhesive tape. The greater the flexion, the greater the stability; however, excessive flexion may cause vascular problems.

18.6.3 Surgical Management

All type III fractures require surgical stabilisation (Fig. 18.8). In addition, any type II fracture with malrotation (IIB) will be inherently unstable and may drift into varus or valgus (Fig. 18.9). Again, fixation should be strongly considered. The usual method is to use percutaneous K-wires. Common

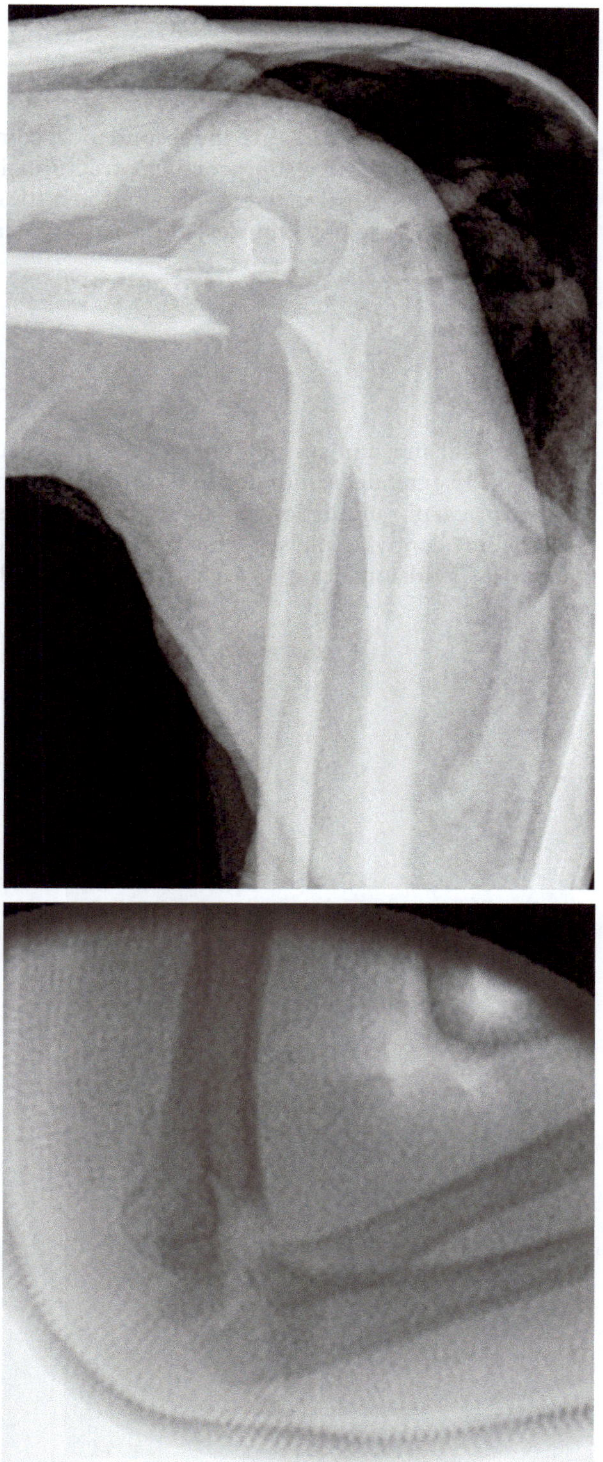

a

b

Fig. 18.7. **a** Gartland type II supracondylar fracture. Note intact posterior periosteal hinge. **b** Flexion of elbow leads to reduction of fracture

configurations are either two or more lateral wires or crossed medial and lateral wires. Maintenance of rotational stability is of paramount importance and most studies would suggest that this is best achieved with crossed wires (Lee et al. 2002; Mostafavi and Spero 2000). Divergent lateral wires may be a suitable alternative, but parallel lateral wires give the poorest stability and should be avoided. The concern with placement of the medial wire is penetration, contusion or kinking of the ulna nerve. The nerve may be difficult to palpate due to swelling, and its position is notoriously difficult to predict, indeed 16% may be subluxed anteriorly (Childress 1975). A rate of 2%–3% of ulna nerve injury is commonly reported, there are few reports, however, of permanent damage to the nerve, with most symptoms resolving over 3–6 months (Lyons et al. 1998).

18.6.4 Vascular Complications

Vascular compromise occurs in 0.5%–5% of supracondylar fractures of the distal humerus. Typically, there is absence of the radial pulse. Most surgeons initially manage these injuries by urgent closed reduction of the fracture followed by crossed K-wire stabilisation. In most instances, the radial pulse will then return. If the pulse does not return and the arm is clearly ischaemic, immediate exploration is indicated. However, the arm may be pulseless but well perfused, the so-called 'pulseless pink hand'. In this instance, opinion as to the best form of treatment is varied. Some authors advocate observation (Sabharwal et al. 1997), some investigation by arteriogram/MR angiogram and some would favour immediate exploration of the vessel (Schoenecker et al. 1996; Karlsson et al. 1986). The collateral circulation around the elbow is excellent and the limb can be adequately perfused even if the brachial artery is completely occluded. Vascular injury usually results from grade III fractures where the distal fragment is displaced posterolaterally. The proximal fracture surface pierces the brachialis and presses on the brachial vessel and often the median nerve which is in close proximity. Clinically, telltale bruising may be visible in the cubital fossa with puckering of the skin. The vessel is rarely divided but intimal tears can occur, leading to thrombosis. When closed reduction is attempted, the vessel can be dragged through the brachialis and become tented down to the fracture site. More rarely, the vessel may run through the fracture gap, even when the radiological reduction appears satisfactory. Sometimes the vessel can be in spasm and the pulse therefore not palpable. However, this should resolve over 24 h. An arteriogram would be advocated if the pulse has not returned at this stage (Fig. 18.10).

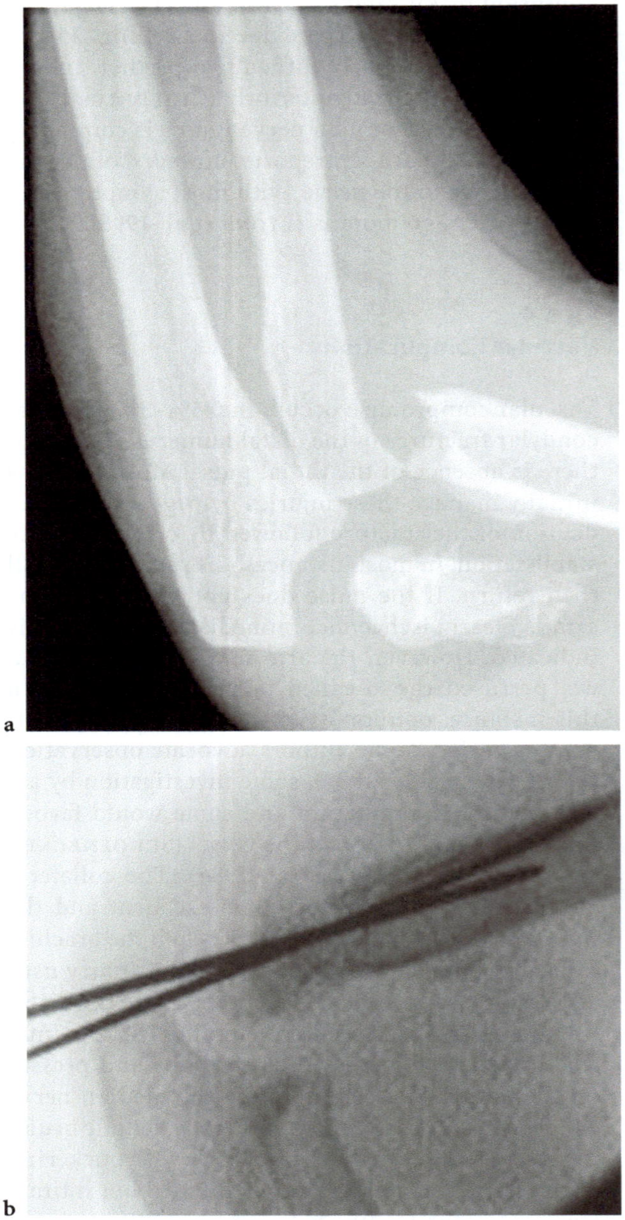

Fig. 18.8. **a** Lateral radiograph of type III extension supracondylar fracture with posterolateral displacement of the distal fragment. **b** Internal fixation with crossed K-wires

18.7 Lateral Condyle Fracture

Lateral condylar fractures are the second most common elbow injury after supracondylar fractures in children. They are estimated to form between 10%–20% of paediatric elbow injuries, and have a typical age range from 5–10 years old.

18.7.1 Mechanism

The typical mechanism of injury is a large varus force on an extended supinated forearm, causing the extensor carpi radialis longus and brevis to avulse the lateral condylar physis. This may cause either a partial avulsion, leaving a cartilaginous epiph-

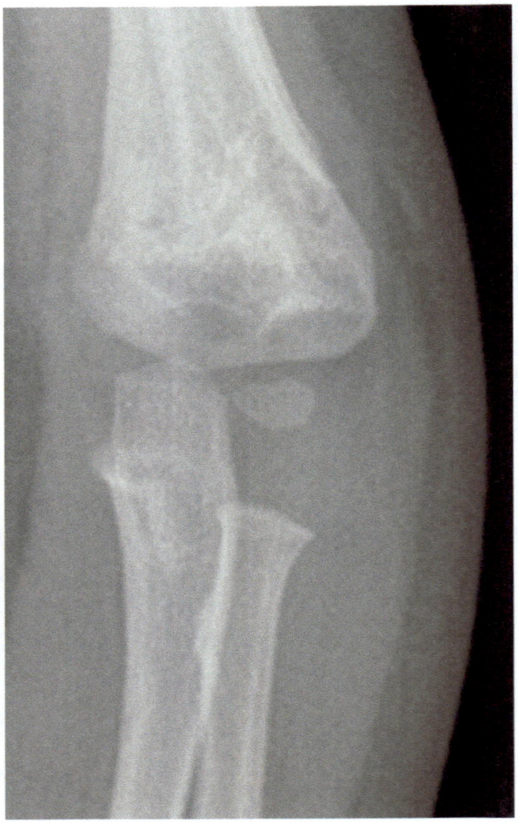

Fig. 18.9. Malunion of grade IIb supracondylar fracture, resulting in varus deformity (cubitus varus). Although of little functional significance, such 'gunstock' deformities are often cosmetically unacceptable

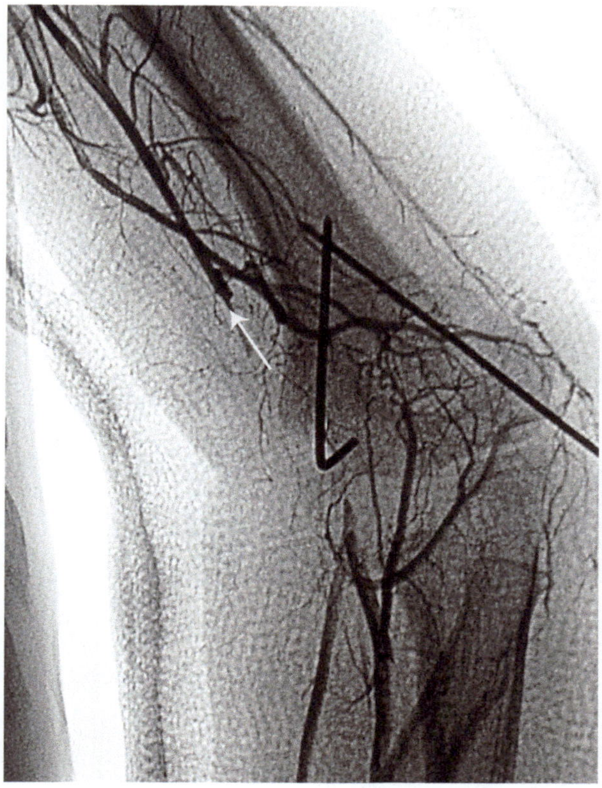

Fig. 18.10. Arteriogram demonstrating abrupt block to flow in the brachial artery. Note the excellent collateral circulation

yseal hinge, or a total separation of the condyle. The fracture line originates in the posterior-lateral metaphysis. There may be an associated soft tissue tear through the brachioradialis. With significant displacement, the anterior and posterior edges of the elbow capsule may become torn. A variant of this fracture is an articular cartilage sleeve fracture. More rarely, a valgus injury can lead to fracture of the lateral condyle by a shearing mechanism.

18.7.2 Classification

Milch (1964) classified by position of the fracture line:

- Milch Type I (Fig. 18.11): The fracture line exits lateral to the capitellar trochlear groove and the lateral crista remains intact for the ulna to articulate with. This corresponds to a Salter-Harris type IV physeal injury.
- Milch Type II: The fracture line exits medial to the capitellar trochlear groove and the lateral crista (the ridge on the side of the trochlea groove) is with the fracture fragment making the humero-ulnar joint unstable. This corresponds to a Salter-Harris type II physeal injury.

This radiological classification has been shown to correlate poorly with intra-operative findings but is often used to describe the fracture (Mirsky et al. 1997).

Jacob et al. (1975) classified the fracture according to degree of displacement and rotation:

- Jacob I Incomplete undisplaced fracture
- Jacob II Fracture displaced in the anterior-posterior plane
- Jacob III Major displacement with no soft tissue hinge

18.7.3 Diagnosis

Clinical examination reveals a laterally swollen elbow, tender at the fracture site, which is increased by active flexion of the wrist. Interpretation of the AP and lateral radiographs depend on the degree of ossification of the capitellum and the extent of the displacement. The lesser the degree of ossification, the harder it is to assess the full extent of the injury. In infants, where there is no ossification of the distal humeral epiphysis, lateral condylar injury may be confused with physeal separation or dislocation of the joint. Physeal separation is the commonest of these injuries in infants less than 1 year old. Often the only sign of injury is a small sliver of displaced metaphyseal bone.

18.7.4 Treatment

Stability of the fracture is dependent on whether the lateral condyle has an intact articular cartilage hinge. This is not evident on radiograph and whilst MR imaging has been used to demonstrate the fracture line and distinguish between complete and incomplete fractures, this is not usually indicated in normal practice (Horn et al. 2002).

Finnbogason et al. (1995) utilised plain radiographs to determine fracture stability:

- Type A Fracture through the lateral humeral condyle with a minimal lateral gap (stable)

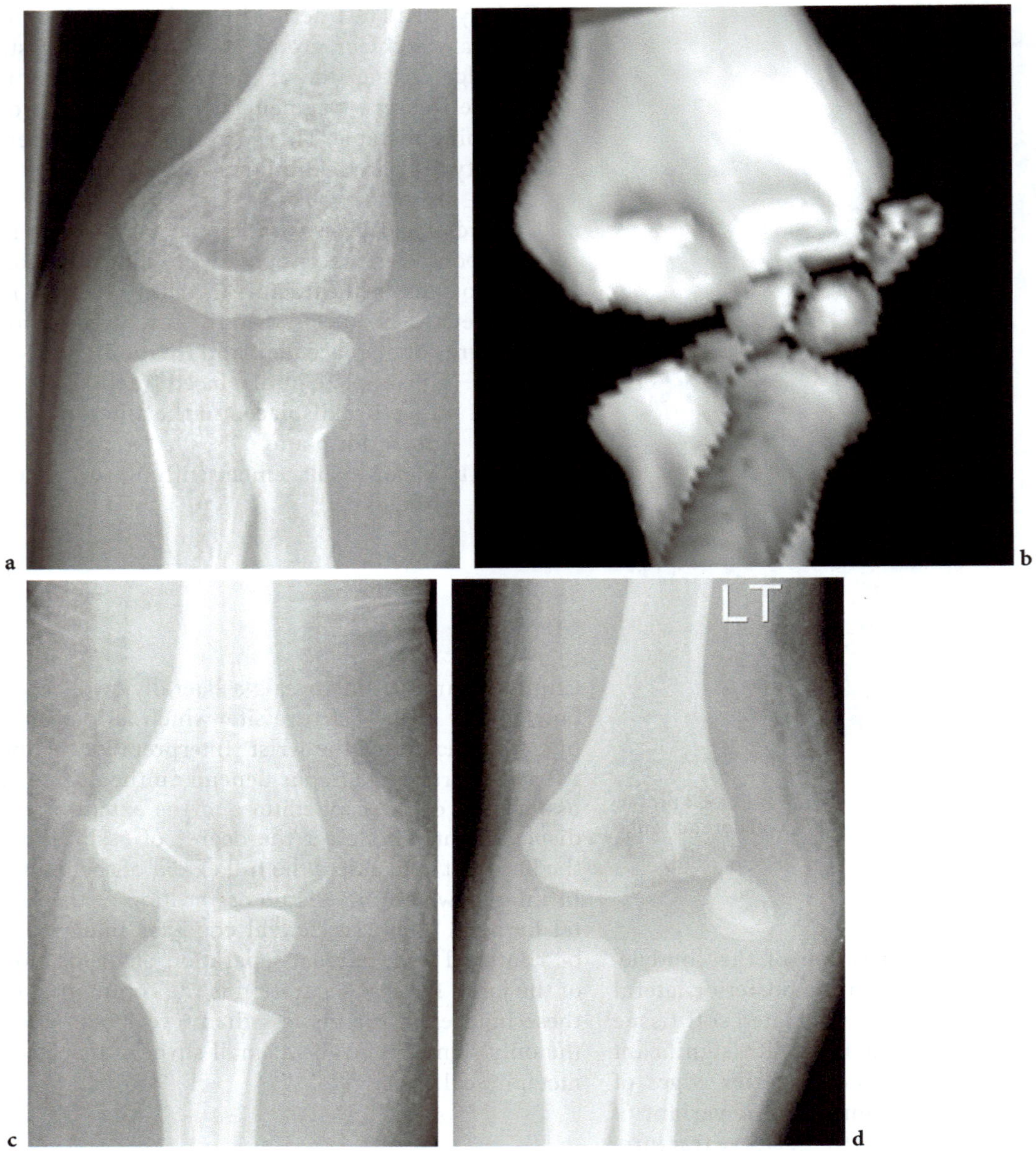

Fig. 18.11. a Milch type I fracture of the lateral condyle. **b** corresponding CT image showing the fracture through the capitellum (Milch type I or Salter Harris type IV). **c,d** Milch type II fracture in different patients

- Type B Fracture through the lateral condyle to the epiphyseal articular cartilage with a lateral gap (risk of displacement undefinable)
- Type C Fracture into the joint with a gap as wide medially as laterally (unstable)

Since the fracture fragment is located posterolaterally in most cases, the fracture line is best evaluated on internal oblique radiographs (Song et al. 2007).

18.7.4.1 Non-operative

Minimally displaced fractures of less than 2 mm are likely to have an intact cartilage hinge and may be treated non-operatively. Early follow-up is required, so that if significant displacement occurs, operative reduction can then be carried out. The elbow is placed into a back slab in 90° of flexion and supination to allow swelling to reduce. A radiograph at 7 days follow-up is required to ensure that no displacement has occurred. The elbow is then returned to a complete above elbow cast for 4–5 weeks.

18.7.4.2 Operative

A lateral condyle displaced by more than 3 mm requires reduction and internal fixation. Lateral condyle fractures are less likely to be associated with neurovascular compromise and surgical exploration is not generally indicated out of hours.

Some fractures may be reduced by closed manipulation and stabilised by percutaneous K-wires. Evaluation of fracture reduction may be aided by intraoperative arthrogram. The most stable and therefore ideal configuration of K-wires is for a common entry point on the lateral edge of the condyle, with one wire running transversely to the medial condyle, and the second at about 60° aiming at the medial cortex above the olecranon fossa.

Type III and non-reducible type II fractures require open reduction and fixation.

In a younger child, K-wires should be used to hold the reduction, whilst in an older child with a large fragment, a single cannulated screw may be used.

18.7.4.3 Follow-Up

The patient should be reviewed in clinic with a radiograph after 7 days to confirm displacement has not occurred, and the K-wires removed between 3 and 4 weeks later.

18.7.4.4 Complications

Recognised complications of lateral condylar fractures include nonunion, malunion, cubitus varus or valgus, osteonecrosis and a limitation of range of motion from the development of scar tissue (Skak et al. 2001).

Nonunion develops if the lateral condyle is displaced, or inadequately stabilised. Bone grafting and internal fixation are recommended.

Cubitus valgus occurs following nonunion when the lateral condyle fragment moves laterally and proximally. It can also lead to the development of a tardy ulnar nerve palsy as the valgus deformity stretches out the nerve. Supracondylar osteotomy with ulnar nerve transposition may improve function.

Cubitus varus deformity is thought to occur either due to in-filling of the fracture gap or following overgrowth of the capitellum. It is normally small (<5°) and does not cause functional impairment. This occurs more commonly in the younger patients (Foster et al. 1985).

Osteonecrosis of the capitellum is associated with wide dissection extending to the posterior aspect of the capitellum whilst attempting to reduce the lateral condyle which compromises the blood supply which enters posteriorly.

Radiographic changes after the healing of the fracture may show a deepening of the trochlear groove known as 'fish tailing' and is associated with malreduction, but is of no proven functional significance unless severe (Fig. 18.12) (Rutherford 1985).

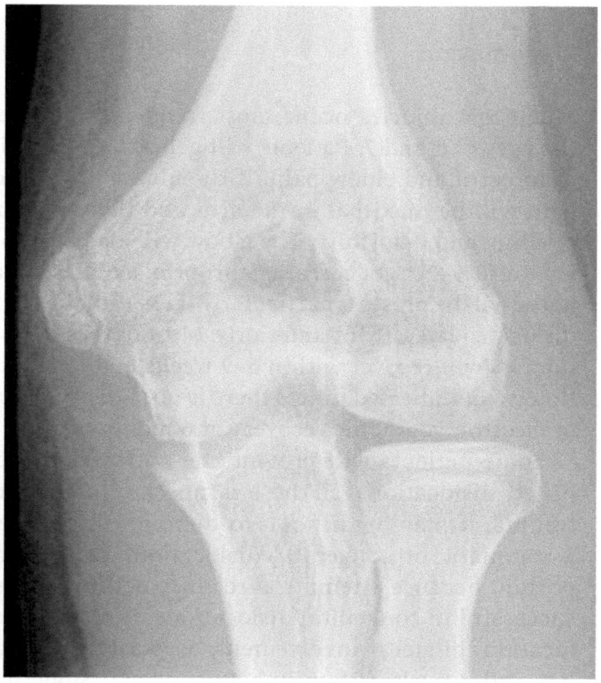

Fig. 18.12. Fish tail deformity of the distal humerus

18.8 Monteggia Lesions

The Monteggia lesion is dislocation of the radial head associated with a forearm injury. This should not be confused with the Galeazzi injury which is fracture of the radius and dislocation of the distal radioulnar joint.

The dislocated radial head is an easily missed lesion, not infrequently resulting in litigation. The forearm fracture is readily identified and attention is drawn away from the co-existing elbow injury. It is vital that for long bone fractures, the adjacent joints are both imaged and properly reviewed.

18.8.1 Mechanism

Three mechanisms have been proposed for Monteggia injuries: hyperextension of the joint, direct blows and hyperpronation. Most falls onto the outstretched limb occur with the arm pronated and in this position, the ligamentous restraints around the proximal radioulnar joint are most lax, predisposing to dislocation.

18.8.2 Presentation

Monteggia injuries occur most frequently between the ages of 5 and 7. Patients will generally complain of forearm and elbow pain. If the ulna is fractured, pain will be maximal in the arm and there may be swelling and deformity. The elbow will also be swollen. In 10%–20% of cases, a neuropraxia of the radial nerve will be present, particularly if the radial head is dislocated laterally or anteriorly. Most of these nerve injuries will recover within 6–9 weeks and intervention is not indicated unless there is no sign of clinical or electromyographic recovery at 6 months.

Some patients will present late with well established dislocations. If there is no clear history of trauma, it may be difficult to distinguish between a traumatic or congenital dislocation. This is important because attempts at reconstruction are less successful in congenital dislocations. Posterior dislocation, bilateral involvement, associated anomalies and a positive family history would suggest a congenital problem.

18.8.3 Classification

The standard classification for Monteggia lesions was described by Bado (1967):

- Type 1 Fracture of the ulnar shaft with anterior dislocation of the radial head. This accounts for 70% of children's Monteggia fractures.
- Type 2 Posterior dislocation of the radial head with associated fracture of the ulna. Rare in children.
- Type 3 Lateral dislocation of the radial head with metaphyseal fracture of the ulna. Second commonest fracture in children.
- Type 4 Anterior dislocation of the radial head with fracture of both the ulna and radius. Rare in children.

A number of 'equivalent' lesions have also been described. Commonest of these is the Type 1 variant Where the radial head is dislocated anteriorly but the ulna has plastic deformation rather than a fracture. Other variants include dislocations with associated radial neck fractures, olecranon fractures and dislocations of the ulnar-humeral joint. In some respects, the 'pulled elbow', commonly seen in infants, can also be considered a Bado I equivalent. The injury occurs when the elbow has traction applied, usually resulting in hyperextension and pronation. The radial head subluxes through the annular ligament but does not truly dislocate and radiographs are either normal or will show an effusion with elevation of the fat pads.

18.8.4 Imaging

When imaging any long bone injury, it is imperative to include both the joint above and the joint below. Whilst Galeazzi lesions are rare in children, Monteggia lesions are not uncommon. It should also be stressed that the joint must be imaged in two planes. The elbow may look normal on the AP view but dislocation of the radial head is readily appreciated on the lateral projection. A straight line drawn up the shaft of the radius should intersect the capitellum in both AP and lateral views, irrespective of the degree of flexion of the joint (Fig. 18.13).

Careful inspection of the radiographs is recommended when considering surgery in late presenting

Monteggia lesions. The articular surface of the radius is normally concave where it articulates with the capitellum. When the radial head has been dislocated for some time, the head becomes convex. This makes relocation of the joint difficult. Similar appearances may also occur in congenital dislocations of the radial head. In this instance, the dislocation is always posterior and thus confused with type II injuries.

18.8.5 Management

In acute presentations, the dislocated radial head can generally be reduced by closed means. Under general anaesthesia, the elbow is flexed to enable reduction. In younger children, the associated ulna fracture does not require internal fixation and plaster cast will suffice. This should be applied in flexion and supination. In older children, it may be difficult to maintain reduction unless the ulna is stabilised with either an intramedullary rod or plate and screws. If the radial head is irreducible, the joint should be explored. The annular ligament may be torn and blocking reduction.

Pulled elbow does not require manipulation under anaesthesia. The forearm is flexed and supinated. Often this results in a gratifying pop and the child resumes normal activity. If this manoeuvre is unsuccessful, simply resting the arm in a sling will allow swelling in the annular ligament to subside and the radial head will reduce within 2–3 days.

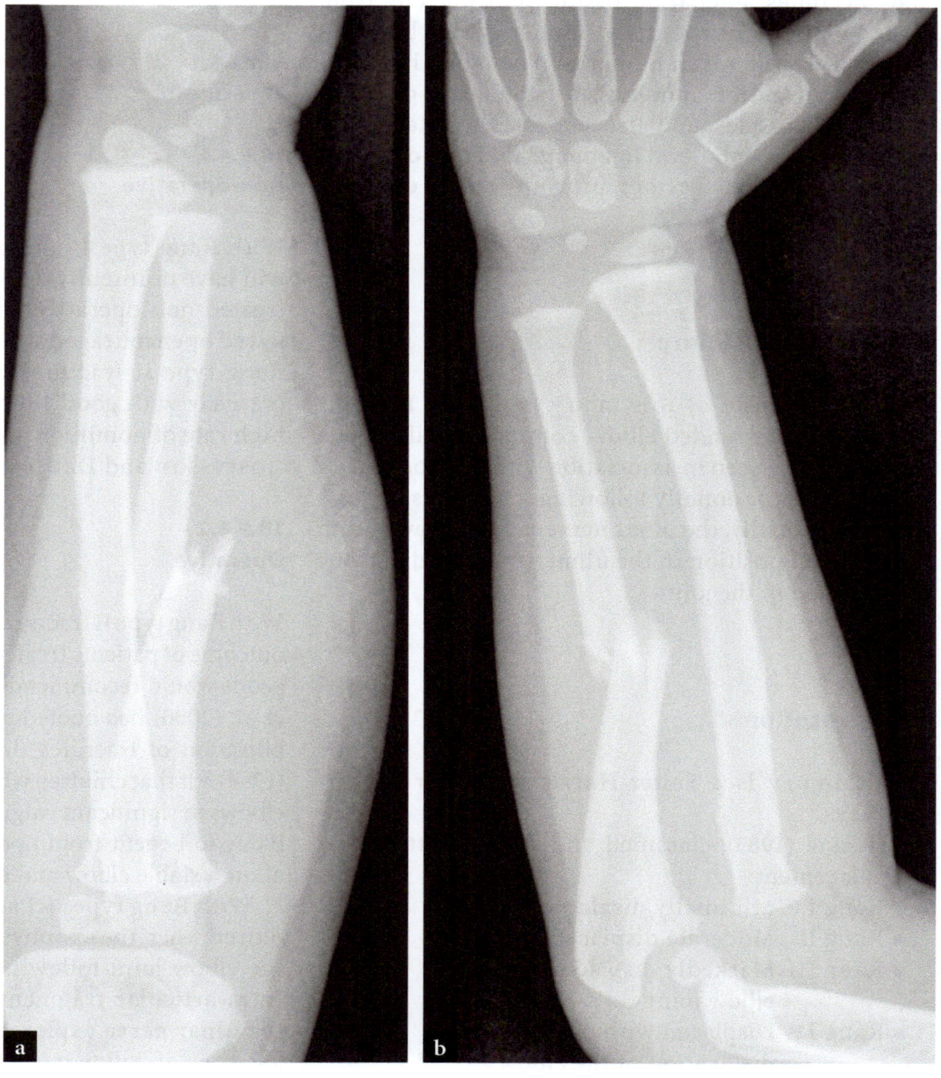

Fig. 18.13a,b. Type I Monteggia fracture with plastic deformation of the ulna. **a** AP radiograph shows minimal displacement and dislocation could easily be missed. **b** Lateral radiograph clearly demonstrates the dislocated radial head

The decision to operate on established dislocations is difficult. In the long-term, patients may well develop a restriction in elbow flexion and progressive valgus deformity leading to tardy ulnar nerve palsy. Open reduction with reconstruction of the annular ligament (Bell Tawse 1965) with ulnar osteotomy can prevent valgus instability but is less successful in regaining lost motion.

18.9 Medial Epicondyle Fracture

Avulsion fractures of the medial epicondyle are seen between the ages of 9 and 15, after the apophysis becomes a separate ossification nucleus from the epiphysis of the distal humerus and before it fuses with the distal humerus. The medial epicondyle is a traction apophysis for the flexor group of forearm muscles, and also serves as an attachment for the ulnar collateral ligaments and the joint capsule. This injury accounts for up to 10% of elbow fractures.

18.9.1 Mechanism of Injury

The mechanism of this injury is usually a valgus force on an extended elbow, commonly following a fall. It is also seen in association with a dislocated elbow, and occasionally following a vigorous throw.

Occasionally, the ulnar nerve may be drawn from its normal position in the ulnar groove and become entrapped in the joint.

18.9.2 Classification

This injury is a Salter-Harris type I or type II injury.

Rang (1983) classified the injury patterns by displacement:

- Rang I Minimally displaced <2 mm
- Rang II Moderate displacement
- Rang III Markedly displaced within the elbow joint
- Rang IV Displaced with postero-lateral dislocation of the elbow

18.9.3 Diagnosis

Based on AP and lateral radiographs, the normal curve following around the medial condyle is disrupted. In type III injuries, it can be easy to misinterpret the radiographs as normal, since the fragment may be difficult to identify, particularly on the AP view. It is important that the acronym CRITOE is used to assess the ossification centres about the elbow joint. The medial epicondyle ossifies before that of the trochlea. If the trochlea is seen then the medial epicondyle must be present (Fig. 18.14). A displaced medial epicondyle lying within the elbow joint should not be confused with the ossification centre of the trochlea. The diagnosis should always be considered if the epicondyle cannot be visualised at an age when it should be present.

18.9.4 Treatment

18.9.4.1 Non-operative

With Rang type I injuries, the majority of patients will have minimally displaced fractures and may be treated non-operatively in cast for 3–4 weeks, followed by encouraged active mobilisation (Fig. 18.15). Rang type II fractures have been treated non-operatively with good functional outcomes, despite a high rate of nonunion and some residual symptoms (Josefsson and Danielsson 1986).

18.9.4.2 Operative

With Rang type II fractures, despite the good long-term outcome of patients treated non-operatively, some surgeons would recommend operative fixation. Haxhija et al. (2006) has quoted good results for surgical stabilisation of fractures displaced >4 mm. Huurman (1994) felt that children who will routinely subject their elbows to significant valgus stress, such as athletes, are likely to benefit from open reduction and fixation to allow a stable elbow and early mobilisation.

With Rang types III and IV, open reduction is required when the apophysis has become entrapped in the elbow joint following a dislocation (Fig. 18.16). Intra-articular fragments may be washed out and the ulnar nerve explored. In the case of elbow dislocation, if following reduction, the epicondyle is found to be in a satisfactory position, surgical stabilisation is not necessary.

18.9.5 Chronic Injury

Chronic stress injury of the medial epicondyle can cause degeneration of the common flexor tendon and enlargement, sclerosis, fragmentation and physeal widening around the medial epicondyle. It is often found in children involved in throwing sports due to repeated valgus stress around the elbow. It is often called 'little leaguers elbow'.

MR imaging will show oedema within the common flexor tendon and muscle belly and around the apophysis. The physis is widened and irregular. The apophysis may be avulsed and can be displaced inferiorly.

Clinically, there may be a palpable mobile epicondyle, crepitus and tenderness.

18.10 Medial Condyle Fractures

This type of fracture is seen rarely but the complication rate is high (Leet et al. 2002).

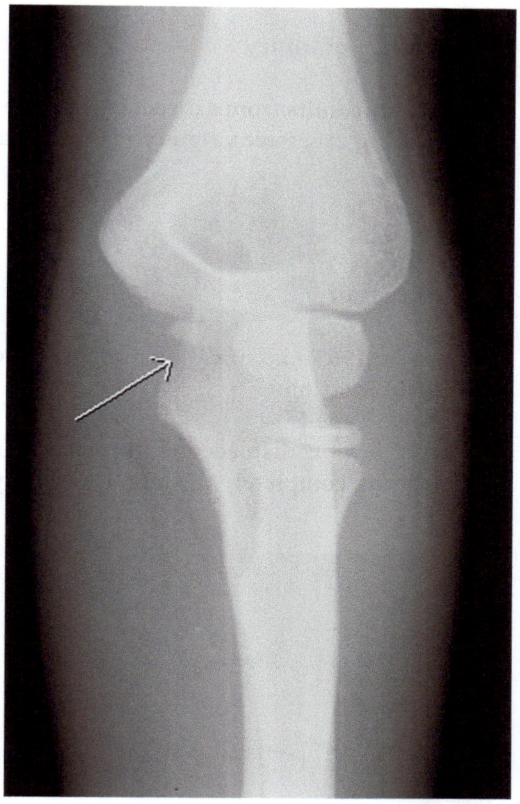

Fig. 18.14. AP radiograph showing a displaced medial epicondyle within the joint mimicking the trochlea. The epicondyle was replaced at surgery

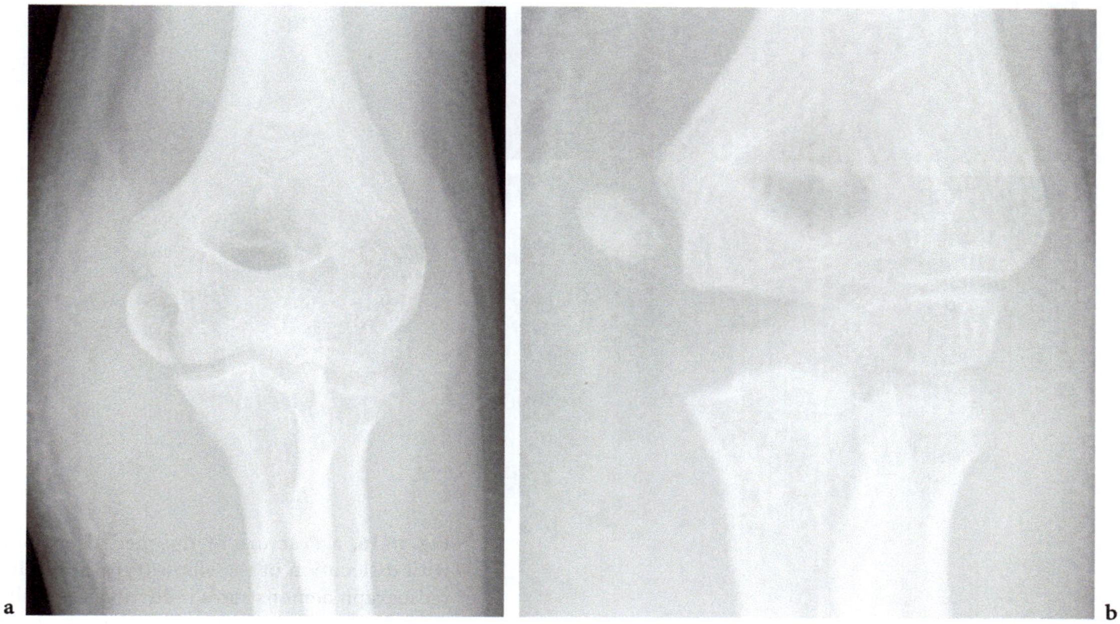

Fig. 18.15a,b. Two children with moderately **a** and minimally **b** displaced fractures of the medial epicondyle

18.10.1 Mechanism of Injury

This injury results from a direct blow to the condyle, or following excessive valgus stress in pronation on the elbow.

18.10.2 Classification

Kilfoyle (1965) classification by degree of displacement and rotation:

- Kilfoyle Type I
  Partial or non-displaced with fracture line not extending completely through the epiphysis.
- Kilfoyle Type II
  Complete fracture through the articular surface may be displaced laterally but not rotated.
- Kilfoyle Type III
  Fracture which is complete, displaced and rotated with loss of relationship of the radial head against the capitellum.

18.10.3 Diagnosis

Until the trochlea ossifies, this fracture is difficult to differentiate from an epicondylar fracture but as this is an intra-articular injury, there is normally a positive fat pad sign.

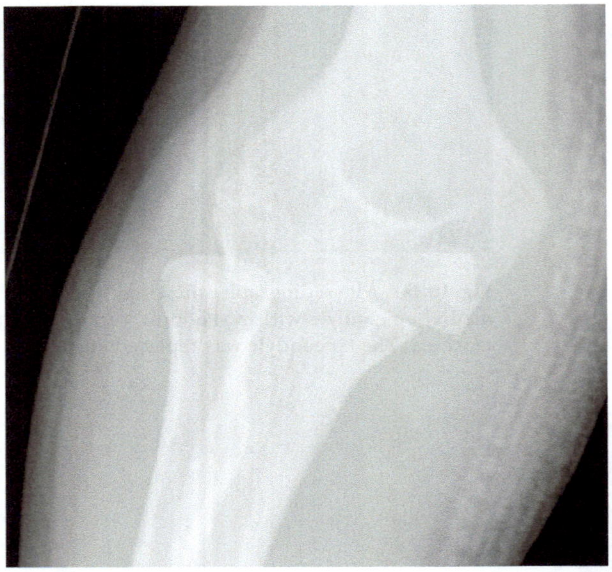

a

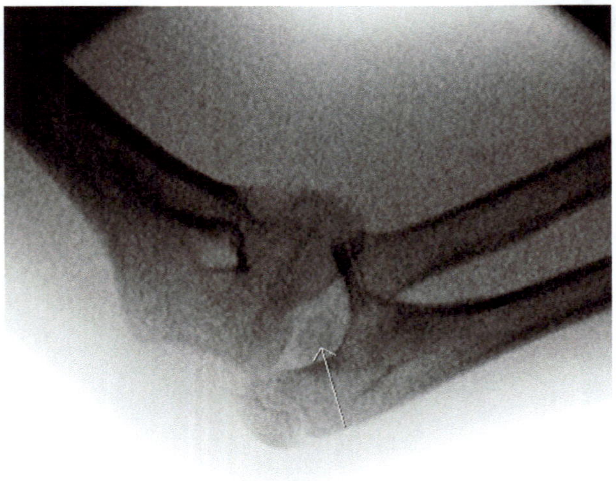

b

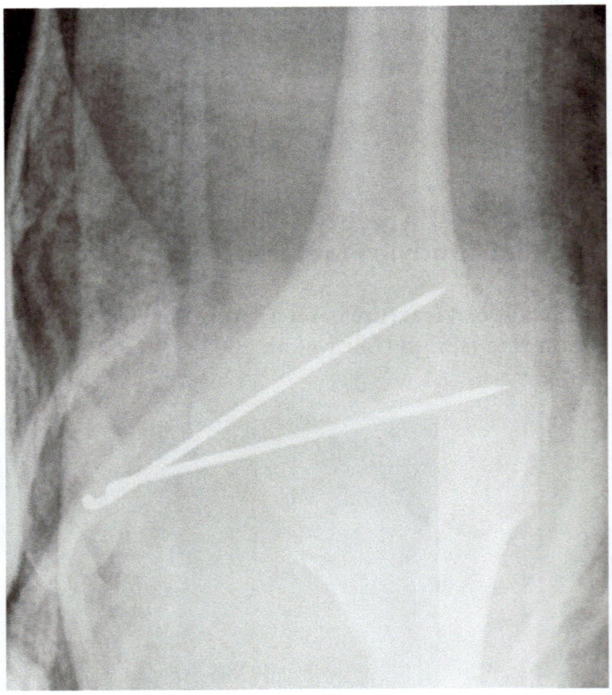

Fig. 18.16. **a** Fracture of the medial epicondyle associated with dislocation of the elbow (type IV). **b** Image intensifier radiograph demonstrates reduction of the elbow but the epicondyle is stuck in joint rather than in an anatomical position – arrowed. **c** Epicondyle fixed in correct position.

18.10.4 Treatment

Type I injuries only require immobilisation, while type II injuries will require stabilisation of the fracture, either using closed reduction and percutaneous K-wire, or if this fails, open reduction and K-wiring. Type III injuries require open reduction and K-wiring.

The surgical incision is made along the medial supracondylar ridge. The ulnar nerve is located and protected. Care is taken to limit excessive soft tissue stripping to avoid vascular injury to the trochlea ossific nucleus. The elbow is immobilised at 90° of flexion with the forearm in neutral.

18.10.5 Complications

Type II and III fractures risk avascular necrosis of the trochlea, leading to limited elbow function.

18.11 Radial Head and Neck Fractures

Fractures of the radial neck may be isolated injuries but can occur in association with medial epicondyle avulsions, fractures of the olecranon and dislocations of the elbow joint.

18.11.1 Mechanism of Injury

Radial neck fractures occur when following a significant valgus compression applied to the forearm, the lateral condyle presses against the radial head. The weak radial neck, largely composed of cancellous bone, fails which leads to angulation and displacement of the radial head. Normally, the radial neck is angulated laterally at 12.5° to the long axis of the radial shaft in the AP plane and 3.5° anteriorly. The axis of rotation is within the radial neck. An injury in which there is a significant translocation of the radial head away from the radial neck will alter the arc of rotation of the radial head, causing a cam effect and resulting in a limitation of rotation of the forearm.

The radial head may also be displaced following dislocation of the elbow, either during dislocation or following subsequent reduction.

18.11.2 Classification

Jeffery (1950) has classified the primary displacement of the radial head:

- Type A Salter-Harris type I or II
- Type B Salter-Harris type IV
- Type C Metaphyseal with or without angulation, translocation or completely displace

Judet and Judet (1974) classified the angular displacement of the radial neck (Fig. 18.17):

- Type I Undisplaced
- Type II <30° Angulation
- Type III 30°–60°
- Type IV (a) 60°–80°
  (b) >80°

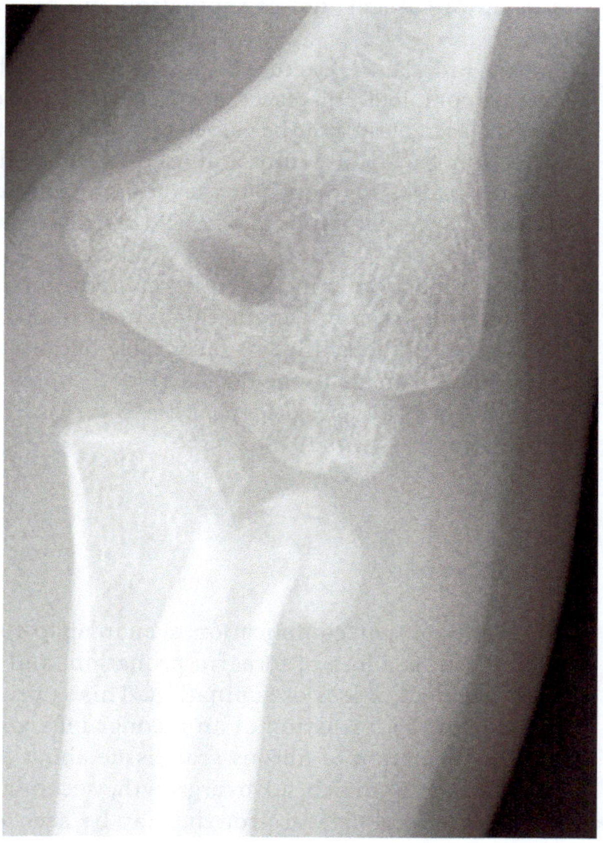

Fig. 18.17. Judet type IVa fracture of the radial neck

18.11.3 Diagnosis

In addition to AP and lateral radiographs, the child may complain of referred pain in the wrist and increased tenderness on forearm supination/pronation.

18.11.4 Treatment

With radial neck injuries where the angulation is up to 30°, a non-operative approach is usually employed as this will normally remodel and does not require intervention (Schmittenbecher et al. 2005).

Fractures with up to 45° of angulation, in children less than 10 years old, are treated expectantly by many surgeons. In older children, fractures with more than 30° angulation should have reduction in theatre under image intensifier, using closed, percutaneous or open techniques. The aim is to restore at least 60° of supination and pronation.

If the radial neck fracture is metaphyseal and the fracture completely displaced, then a flexible wire or nail, with a bent tip, may be passed up the medullary canal from the distal radius and used to reduce the proximal radial fragment onto the radius by rotation of the nail (Metaizeau et al. 1993; Prathapkumar et al. 2006).

Open reduction is indicated if percutaneous reduction fails, but only if angulation is more than 45°. The results are generally less favourable because of the risks of damage to the delicate blood supply to the radial head and because the initial injury is likely to be worse (Evans 1999b).

18.11.5 Complications

The most common complication, seen in up to 40% of children, is a loss of forearm pronation, and to a lesser extent, a loss of supination. This is probably due to the formation of an incongruous joint and the formation of fibrous scar tissue about the radial head. Radial head overgrowth, secondary to increased epiphyseal growth, may be seen on radiograph but does not seem to cause functional impairment.

Since the proximal epiphysis of the radius is entirely intracapsular, it has a precarious vascular supply and injury can result in avascular necrosis. This is more likely if the delicate soft tissue attachments are damaged further by surgical open reduction of the joint and this should be avoided for all but the most extreme cases when other methods of closed reduction have failed. Rates of avascular necrosis exceed 25% following open reduction.

Other less common complications include nonunion, radio-ulnar synostosis and myositis ossificans.

18.11.6 Reversal of the Radial Head

Rarely, the radial head is completely displaced, often lying adjacent to the capitellum. This fracture can occur during the reduction of a dislocated elbow if there is an undisplaced radial neck fracture (Fig. 18.18). The radial head may be reduced by closed manipulation aided by manipulation with percutaneous K-wire. One should be careful to make sure that the reduced radial head is not rotated 180° (Wood 1969).

18.12 Olecranon Fractures

Olecranon fractures are occasionally seen in children and account for about 5% of fractures about the elbow. Fortunately, the majority of injuries are minimally displaced, and are managed non-operatively. A significant number of fractures have associated injury either to the elbow or to the wrist.

These include fractures of the radial neck, lateral condyle, distal radius and subluxation of the radial head (Evans 1999a). Physeal fractures are rare and the majority of injuries are metaphyseal fractures. As with any other intra-articular fracture, it is important to restore the articular surface if the fracture is displaced.

18.12.1 Classification

Fractures are classified into physeal fractures and metaphyseal fractures.

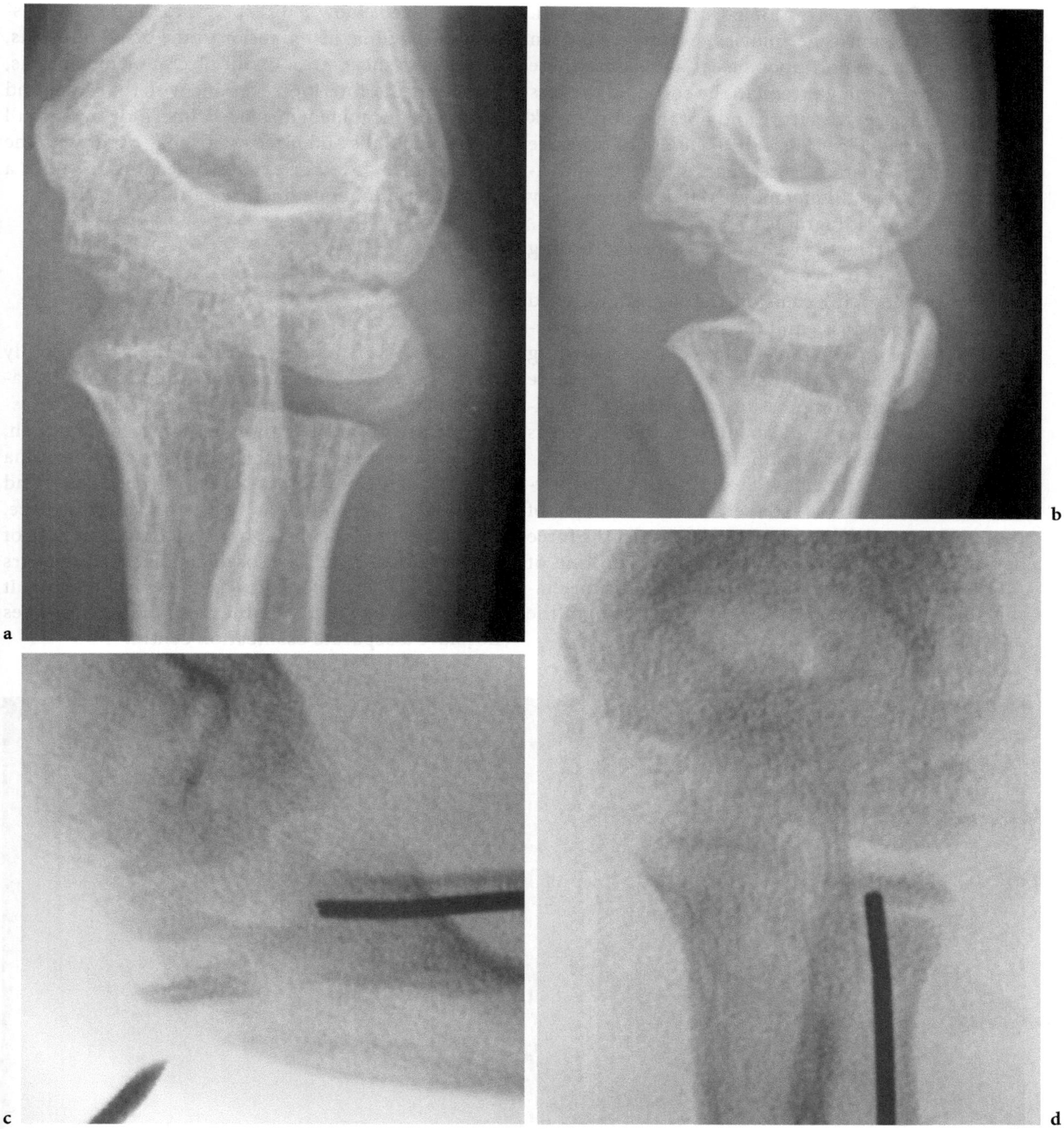

Fig. 18.18. **a,b** AP and lateral radiographs of radial neck fracture displaced by reduction of the dislocated elbow. Radial head lies adjacent to the capitellum. **c** Intraoperative radiographs showing intramedullary nancy nail and percutaneous wire used to manipulate the femoral head. **d** Post reduction film

Physeal fractures are Salter-Harris type I and II. They are avulsion type injuries. Younger children tend to sustain type I apophyseal avulsions where the fracture line may extend to the coronoid process almost like a sleeve fracture and not therefore break the articular surface (Fig. 18.19). Older children are more likely to sustain Salter-Harris type II equivalent injuries. A small metaphyseal flake of bone may be apparent on radiographs.

Metaphyseal fractures can be classified according to mechanism of injury. The majority of injuries occur with the elbow in extension, the olecranon locked in the olecranon fossa and the maximum stress developed in the proximal metaphyseal region leading to fracture. When a valgus stress is applied, there may be associated compression fractures of the radial neck and avulsion of the medial epicondyle. Varus stress is associated with radial head subluxation.

Injuries with the elbow flexed during a fall occur as the olecranon is stressed over the fulcrum of the trochlea as the triceps attempt to resist the force acting on the distal ulna (Fig. 18.20). The line of fracture is oblique and intra-articular. This mechanism may also produce an extensor avulsion of the apophysis.

In a flexed elbow, a direct blow to the posterior aspect of the ulna, just anterior to the distal humerus, can cause a shear stress on the olecranon metaphysis, breaching the anterior cortex and with the radius and distal ulnar fragment displaced anteriorly by the pull of the brachialis and biceps. This may occur with the elbow either flexed or extended, leading to either a transverse or oblique fracture pattern (Table 18.2).

18.12.2 Radiographs

Good quality AP and lateral radiographs will usually be the only necessary imaging. Apophyseal separations may occur in younger children before the ossific centre of the olecranon has appeared. At birth, the edge of the proximal metaphysis of the ulna extends to the midpoint of the semilunar notch and should be perpendicular to the articular surface. By the age of 6, the metaphysis encompasses 75% of the semilunar notch. The ossification centre appears between the ages of 8 and 9 and may be bipartite. It should also be noted that the coronoid process does not have a separate ossification centre.

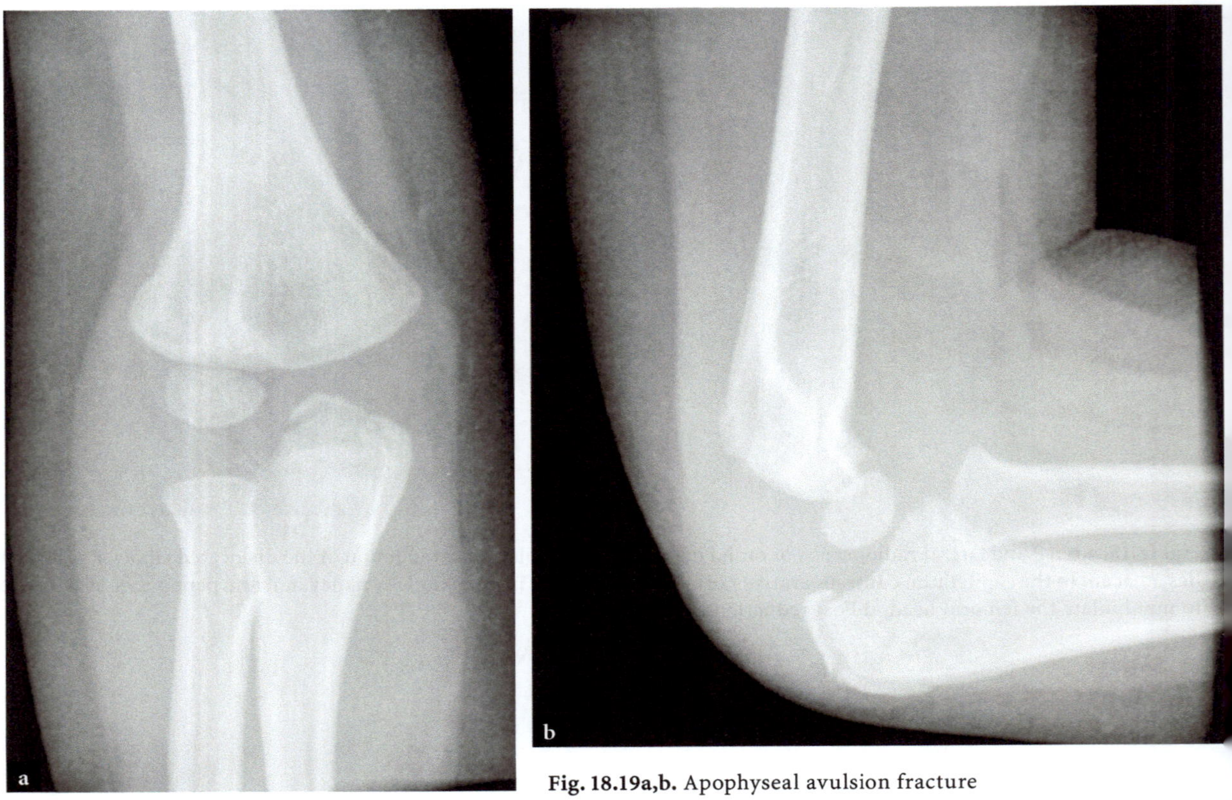

Fig. 18.19a,b. Apophyseal avulsion fracture

Table 18.2. Fracture pattern relative to flexion or extension

Wilkins	Position	Loading force	Injury
A	Flexion	Across trochlea	Posterior aspect ulnar metaphysis and extensor mechanism
B	Extension	Valgus	Ulnar metaphysis fracture +/- medial epicondyle avulsion +/-radial neck fracture
B	Extension	Varus	Ulnar metaphysis fracture +/- radial head subluxation
C	Flexion	Shear	Transverse fracture through ulnar metaphysis with intact extensor mechanism
C	Extension	Shear	Oblique fracture through ulnar metaphysis with intact extensor mechanism

18.12.3 Treatment

18.12.3.1 Non-operative

Undisplaced, less than 2 mm, flexion type injuries may be immobilised in a cast in limited flexion at only 45°, and carefully followed up to ensure displacement does not occur.

Extension injuries are reduced by placing the arm into full extension, correcting the varus or valgus, treating the associated injury such as radial head or medial condyle fracture, before immobilising in a cast for 3 weeks in slight flexion.

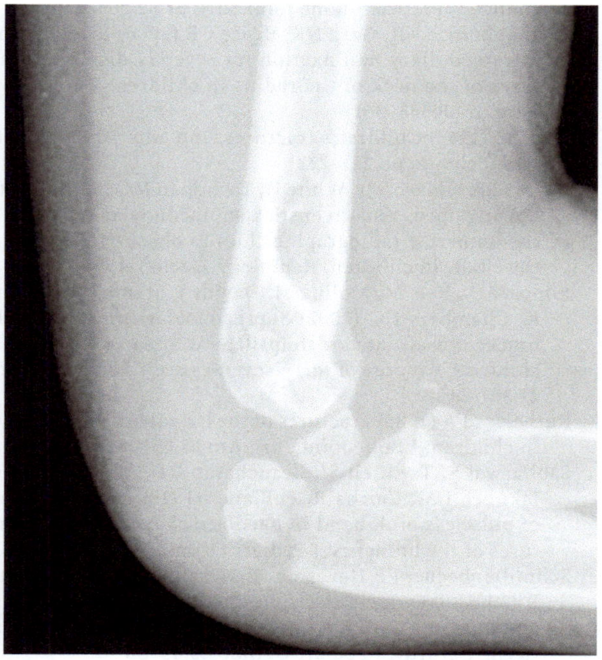

Fig. 18.20. Flexion type (Wilkins A) fracture of the olecranon through the metaphysis

Fractures which have an intact extensor side periosteal hinge, as a result of a shear type injury, can be reduced by flexing the elbow past 90°, correcting varus/valgus and casting in the reduced position.

18.12.3.2 Operative

Operative treatment is required to stabilise displaced flexion fractures of more than 3 mm and fractures with more than 2 mm step-off on the articular surface. Operative techniques available to fix the fracture include tension band wiring over twin K-wires, tension band screw, and the use of a screw and biodegradable suture. Tension band wiring and K-wires can cause irritation and may require removal. Compression screw adds to stability due to compression and is less irritating as the screw head can be counter sunk. Biodegradable sutures provide sufficient strength until healing has occurred before degrading, as healing takes place more rapidly in children (Wilkins 1991). Shear or oblique fractures without an intact extensor mechanism, should be stabilised. This is achieved either with oblique bicortical screws or, in older children, with a plate and screws.

18.12.3.3 Follow-Up

Follow-up radiography to exclude displacement of the fracture should occur at 7 days.

18.12.4 Complications

Treated isolated fractures of the olecranon have been shown to have an excellent long-term outcome (Gicquel et al. 2001). Delayed union and malunion are possible complications of early displacement of those fractures treated nonoperatively and are the reason for early review.

The most common feature overall is a small loss of extension and flexion which has been noted in a minority of patients (GRAVES and CANALE 1993).

References

Bado JL (1967) The Monteggia lesion. Clin Orthop Relat Res 50:71–86
Baumann E (1929) Beiträge zur Kenntnis der Fracturen am Ellenbogengelenk. Bruns Beitr klin Chir 146:1–50
Bell Tawse AJS (1965) The treatment of malunited anterior Monteggia fractures in children. J Bone Joint Surg (Br) 47B:718–723
Blount WP (1977) Fractures in children. Robert E Krieger, Huntingdon, p 26
Childress HM (1975) Recurrent ulna nerve dislocation at the elbow. Clin Orthop 108:168–173
Evans MC, Graham HK (1999a) Olecranon fractures in children. J Pediatr Orthop 19:559–569
Evans MC, Graham HK (1999b) Radial neck fractures in children: a management algorithm J Pediatr Orthop Part B 8:93–99
Finnbogason T, Karlsson G, Lindberg L, Mortensson W (1995) Nondisplaced and minimally displaced fractures of the lateral humeral condyle in children: a prospective radiographic investigation of fracture stability. J Pediatr Orthop 15:422–425
Foster DE, Sullivan JA, Gross RH (1985) Lateral humeral condylar fractures in children. J Pediatr Orthop 5:16–22
Gartland JJ (1959) Management of supracondylar fractures of the humerus in children. Surg Gynecol Obstet 109:145–154
Gicquel P, De Billy B, Karger CS, Clavert JM (2001) Olecranon fractures in 26 children with mean follow-up of 59 months. J Pediatr Orthop 21:141–147
Graves SC, Canale ST (1993) Fractures of the olecranon in children: long term follow up. J Pediatr Orthop 13:239–241
Haxhija EQ, Mayr JM, Grechening W, Hollworth ME (2006) Treatment of medial epicondylar apophyseal avulsion injury in children. Oper Orthop Traumatol 18:120–134
Horn BD, Herman MJ, Crisci K, Pizzutillo MacEwen GD (2002) Fractures of the Lateral humeral condyle: role of the cartilage hinge in stability. J Pediatr Orthop 22:8–11
Jakob R, Fowles JV, Rang M, Kassab MT (1975) Observations concerning fractures of the lateral humeral condyle in children. J Bone Joint Surg Br 57:430–436
Jeffery CC (1950) Fractures of the head of the radius in children. J Bone Joint Surg Br 32:314
Josefsson PO, Danielsson LG (1986) Epicondylar elbow fractures in children Acta Orthop Scand 57:313
Judet H, Judet J (1974) Fractures et orthopedie de l'enfant. Maloine, Paris, pp 31–39
Karlsson J, Thorstien T, Thorleifsson R, Arnason H (1986) Entrapment of the median nerve and brachial artery after supracondylar fractures of the humerus in children. Arch Orthop Trauma Surg 104:389-391
Keats TE, Teeslink R, Diamond AE, Williams JH (1966) Normal axial relationships of the major joints. Radiology 87:904–907
Kilfoyle RM (1965) Fractures of the medial condyle and epicondyle of the elbow in children. Clin Orthop 41:43–47
Lee SS, Mahar AT, Miesen D, Newton PO (2002) Displaced pediatric supracondylar humerus fractures: biomechanical analysis of percutaneous pinning techniques. J Pediatr Orthop 22:440–443
Leet AI, Young C, Hoffer MM (2002) Medial condyle fractures of the humerus in children. J Pediatr Orthop 22:2–7
Lyons JP, Edwin A, Hoffer MM (1998) Ulnar nerve palsies after percutaneous cross-pinning of supracondylar fractures in children's elbows. J Pediatr Orthop 18:43–45
Lyons ST, Quinn M, Stanitski CL (2000) Neurovascular injuries in type III humeral supracondylar fractures in children. Clin Orthop 376:62–67
Mclauchan GJ, Walker CRC, Cowan B, Robb JE, Prescott RJ (1999) Extension of the elbow and supracondylar fractures in children. J Bone Joint Surg Br 81:402-405
Metaizeau JP, Lascombes P, Lemelle JL, Finlayson D, Prevot J (1993) Reduction and fixation of displaced radial neck fractures by closed intramedullary pinning. J Pediatr Orthop 13:355–360
Milch H (1964) Fractures and fracture dislocations of humeral condyles. J Trauma 4:592–607
Mirsky EC, Karas EH, Weiner LS (1997) Lateral condyle fractures in children: evaluation of classification and treatment. J Orthop Trauma 11:117–120
Mostafavi HR, Spero C (2000) Crossed pin fixation of displaced supracondylar humerus fractures in children. Clin Orthop 376:56–61
O'Hara LJ, Barlow JW, Clarke NM (2000) Displaced supracondylar fractures of the humerus in children. Audit changes practice. J Bone Joint Surg Br 82:204–210
Prathapkumar KR, Garg NK, Bruce CE (2006) Elastic stable intramedullary nail fixation for severely displaced fractures of the neck of the radius in children. J Bone Joint Surg Br 88:358–361
Rang M (1983) Children's fractures, 2nd edn. JB Lippincott, Philadelphia, pp 221–232
Rogers LF, Malave S Jr, White H, Tachdjian MO (1978) Plastic bowing, torus and greenstick supracondylar fractures of the humerus: radiographic clues to obscure fractures of the elbow in children. Radiology 128:145–150
Roposch A, Reis M, Molina M, Davids J, Stanley E, Wilkins K, Chambers HG (2002) Supracondylar fractures of the humerus associated with ipsilateral forearm fractures in children: a report of forty-seven cases. J Pediatr Orthop 21:307–312
Rutherford A (1985) Fractures of the lateral humeral condyle in children. J Bone Joint Surg Am 67:851–856
Sabharwal S, Tredwell SJ, Beauchamp RD, Mackenzie WG, Jakubec DM, Cairns R, LeBlanc JG (1997) Management of pulseless pink hand in paediatric supracondylar fractures of the humerus. J Pediatr Orthop 17:303–310
Schmittenbecher PP, Havernick B, Herold A, Knorr P, Schmid E (2005) Treatment decision, method of osteosynthesis, and outcome in radial neck fractures in children: a multicentre sturdy. J Pediatr Orthop 25:45–50
Schoenecker PL, Delgado E, Rotman M, Sicard GA, Capelli AM (1996) Pulseless arm in association with totally displaced supracondylar fracture. J Orthop Trauma 10:410–415

Skaggs DL Mirzayan R (1999) The posterior fat pad sign in association with occult fracture of the elbow in children. J Bone Joint Surg Am 81:1429–1433

Skak SV, Olsen SD, Smaabrekke A (2001) Deformity after fracture of the lateral humeral condyle in children. J Pediatr Orthop Part B 10:142–152

Song KS, Kang CH, Min BW, Bae KC, Cho CH (2007) Internal oblique radiographs for diagnosis of non-displaced or minimally displaced lateral condylar fractures in children. J Bone Joint Surg Am 89:58–63

Storen G (1959) Traumatic dislocation of the radial head as an isolated lesion in children; report of one case with special regard to roentgen diagnosis. Acta Chir Scand 116:144–147

Williamson DM, Coates CJ, Miller RK, Cole WG (1992) Normal characteristics of the Baumann angle, an aid in assessment of supracondylar fractures. J Pediatr Orthop 12:636–639

Wilkins KE, Morrey BF, Jobe FW, Kvitne RS, Coonrad RW, Figgie HE, Jupiter JB, Inglis AE, Wright PE, Burns EB (1991) The elbow. Instr Course Lect 40:1–87

Wood SK (1969) Reversal of the radial head during reduction of fractures of the neck of the radius in children. J Bone Joint Surg Br 51:707–710

The Hand and Wrist

19

Greg John Irwin and Roderick Duncan

CONTENTS

G. J. Irwin, BMSc (Hons); MB ChB; FRCS (Edin); FRCR
Consultant Paediatric Radiologist, Diagnostic Imaging, Royal Hospital for Sick Children, Dalnair Street, Glasgow, Scotland G3 8SJ, UK
R. Duncan, MB ChB; FRCSEd (Orth)
Consultant Paediatric Orthopaedic Surgeon, Orthopaedic Department, Royal Hospital for Sick Children, Dalnair Street, Glasgow, Scotland G3 8SJ, UK

19.1 Introduction

The hand and wrist are the most common sites of skeletal injury in children (Hastings and Simmons 1984), with fractures of the distal end of the radius being the most common (Landin 1997). Wrist fractures are usually the result of falls, the ubiquitous 'FOOSH' (fall on out-stretched hand) on the X-ray request, or sports related injuries. Again these are common injuries of childhood, with 42% of all fractures of the radius and ulna occurring in children up to the age of 14 (Chung and Spilson 2001).

Hand fractures show a bimodal age distribution, with toddlers suffering distal phalanx fractures associated with soft tissue lacerations often caused by crushing injuries in doors. The larger second peak occurs around age 14 years with proximal phalanx and metacarpal fractures predominating. The most commonly injured ray is the little finger, followed by the thumb and ring finger (Vadivelu et al. 2006). Under the age of 6 injuries tend to occur at home, and from age 6 to 12 injuries are predominantly sports related (Valencia et al. 2005). Right and left hands are injured with equal frequency, and fractures are seen more often in boys than girls (Bhende et al. 1993). A review of hand and fingertip injuries presenting to an emergency department in Florida (Fetter-Zarzeka and Joseph 2002) showed that radiographs were performed in two thirds of all patients, but only 20% of these showed fractures, dislocations or foreign bodies.

The diagnosis of fractures in children can be difficult, and it is essential to ensure that the clinical signs correlate with the appearances seen on the radiographs. Fractures in children are different from those in adults for a variety of reasons. Whilst children's bones are weaker than those of adults, they are more plastic and able to absorb more energy before breaking (Currey and Butler 1975). Fractures may be incomplete, and are generally better supported than in adults by a thicker periosteum. Many forearm and hand fractures will do well without operative intervention, aided by the potential of children's bones to remodel. This is particularly true in younger children, and in those fractures located nearer to the physis. There are, however, several fracture types which can be problematic, and whose early recognition is essential to allow the best treatment. These will be discussed in the following regional sections.

It should be noted that different departments have their own thresholds for intervention in the treatment of various injuries. It is therefore neither practical nor desirable to attempt to be overly dogmatic regarding the exact degree of displacement or angulation that requires operative intervention in a particular fracture. Intra-articular fractures should be reduced anatomically, and they may often require open reduction and internal fixation.

Rehabilitation of the child with hand injuries is different from adults. Although stiffness is less of a problem in the paediatric population, the hand should usually be immobilised with the wrist in slight dorsiflexion, the metacarpo-phalangeal (MCP) joints in 90 degrees of flexion, and the inter-phalangeal joints in full extension (position of immobilisation). Compliance is often poor in very young children, and adequate immobilisation can be challenging. Elevation to minimise swelling is essential and the use of 'boxing glove' padded bandages with or without a volar/dorsal plaster slab is recommended.

19.2 Distal Phalanx

19.2.1 Extraphyseal Fractures

The extraphyseal (distal) portion of the distal phalanx is commonly fractured as part of a crush injury in children around the age of 2 years. This is the most frequent type of hand fracture in young children. Trapping a finger tip in a door is the archetypal aetiology (Ljungberg et al. 2003). Fractures may be comminuted (Fig. 19.1) or transverse, or more rarely a longitudinal splitting fracture occurs, which can extend to the physis or joint (Fig. 19.2). Management of the soft tissues is the main concern as fracture union is very rarely a problem. A stable soft tissue repair of the skin and the nail bed is required. A fingernail that has been avulsed can be retained as a splint. Additionally, a longitudinal K-wire can be inserted across the distal interphalangeal joint (DIPJ) to supplement the soft tissue repair in unstable fractures (Fig. 19.3) (Salazard et al. 2004).

In older children, the tendon of flexor digitorum profundus may become avulsed from the volar metaphysis of the distal phalanx. This produces an inability to flex the DIPJ. This rare fracture is sometimes called a rugby jersey injury, as it occurs when a shirt is forcefully gripped and pulled during a tackle. This results in forced extension of the flexed DIP joint. These injuries are important to diagnose, as they often require surgical treatment.

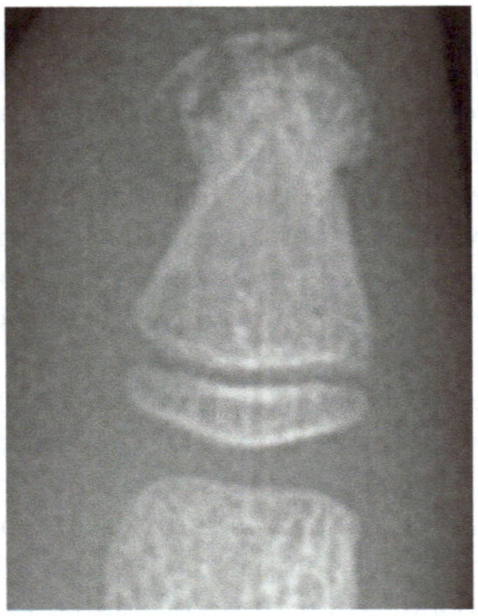

Fig. 19.1. Comminuted fracture of the thumb distal phalanx

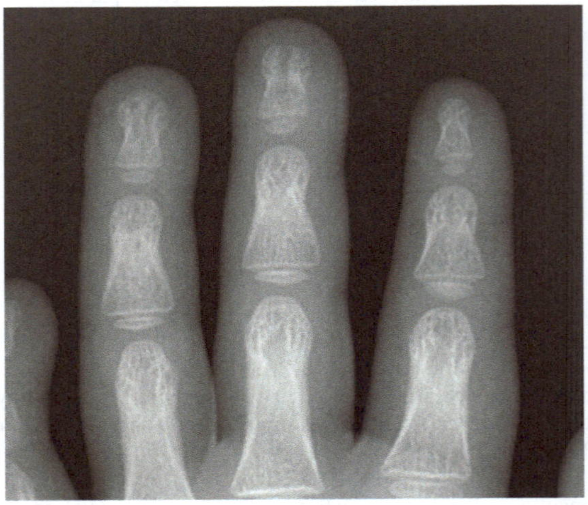

Fig. 19.2. Vertical crush fracture of the index finger distal phalanx

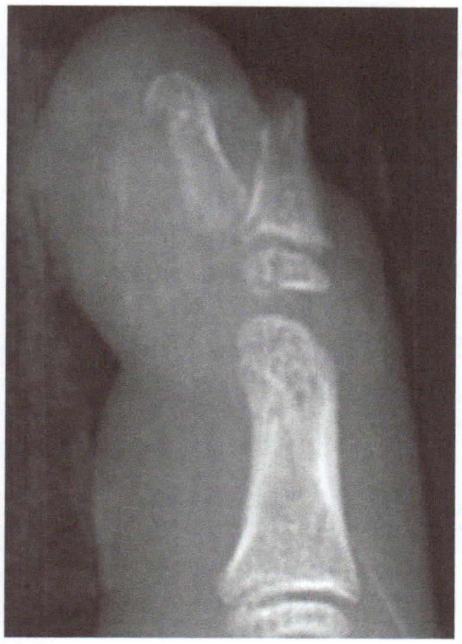

Fig. 19.3. Unstable crush fracture

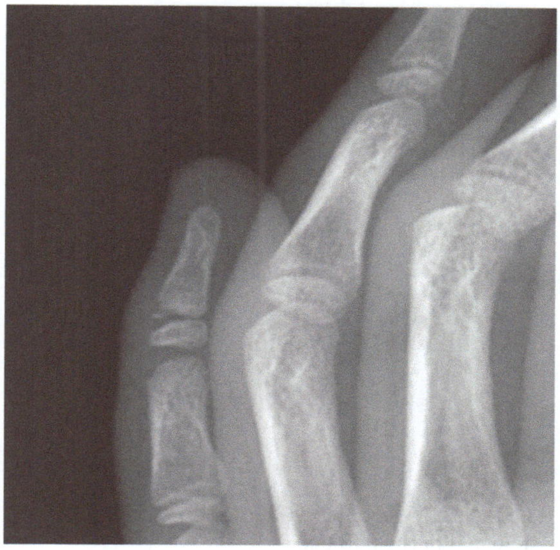

Fig. 19.4. Salter-Harris II fracture of the distal phalanx

19.2.2 Physeal Injuries

A mallet finger deformity is acquired by an axial load or forced flexion applied to an extended fingertip, and is often the result of a ball hitting the fingertip. In children, the deformity may be associated with an angulated Salter-Harris I or II fracture, which does not involve the DIP joint surface (Fig. 19.4). The angulation at the physis is maintained by the flexor tendon which inserts distal to the physis, and the extensor tendon which inserts proximally on the epiphysis, and therefore cannot extend the fingertip. More equivalent to adult mallet finger injuries are Salter-Harris III or IV fractures of the distal phalanx, which involve avulsion of the bony attachment of the extensor tendon (Cornwall and Ricchetti 2006).The great majority of closed mallet fractures are treated with closed reduction and splinting (Graham and Waters 2001).

Surgical treatment may be required in certain cases, such as where there is a Salter-Harris III or IV fracture with a large dorsal fragment of over 50% of the joint surface, or where there is an open fracture. Another specific case is the Seymour fracture (Seymour 1966) where a mallet deformity is associated with avulsion of the nail bed from the eponychial fold (Fig. 19.5). Reduction of this fracture can only be achieved after removal of interposed nail bed matrix at operation. Another problem fracture occurs where there is a Salter-Harris I or II fracture with extrusion or dislocation of the physis (Fig. 19.6). These rare injuries require operative intervention to restore the joint and the extensor mechanism.

19.3 Middle and Proximal Phalanges

19.3.1 Condyle Fractures (Intra-articular)

Various fracture patterns occur involving one or both condyles with an intra-articular element. Fractures can be associated with subluxations or dislocations of the joint (Weiss and Hastings 1993). Unicondylar fractures may be hard to identify radiographically, particularly on the frontal or dorsi-palmar (DP) view. The lateral view should be carefully examined to ensure that the condyles at the distal end of the phalanx lie at the same level. An overlap, the double density sign, indicates a unicondylar fracture (Graham and Waters 2001). However, this appearance can also be created spuriously by angulation of the finger in the coronal plane, and oblique views may be useful. It is important to recognise these intra-articular fractures, because malunion results in joint incongruity, which predisposes to degenerative changes. Surgical correction of a malunion is difficult. Delayed identification of the fracture also

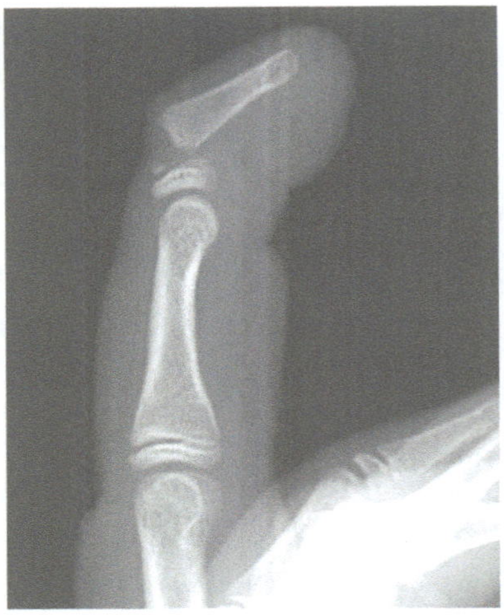

Fig. 19.5. A Seymour fracture, with avulsion of the nail bed

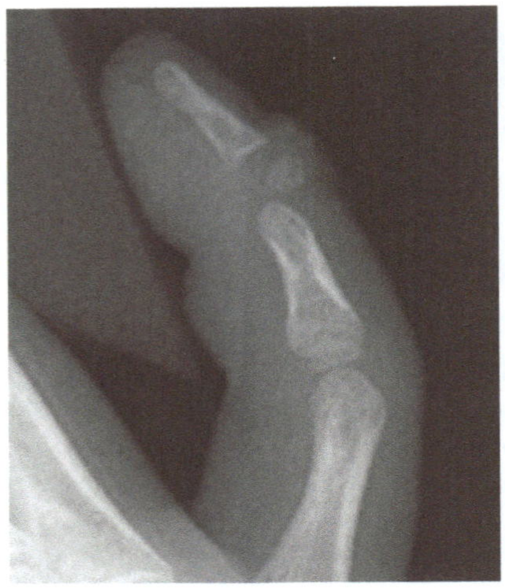

Fig. 19.6. Dislocation of the terminal phalanx epiphysis

reduces the chances of anatomical reduction. Displaced fractures are likely to need internal fixation after closed or open reduction (Fig. 19.7).

19.3.2 Phalangeal Neck Fractures

Fractures of the neck of the middle or proximal phalanx are extra-articular fractures, sometimes called subcondylar fractures. Occasionally the separated phalangeal head may be mistaken for an epiphysis, but there is no epiphysis at the distal end of the phalanx. As with all phalangeal fractures, it is important to obtain adequate radiographs, preferably true DP and lateral projections with further views as necessary, to demonstrate the full extent of the injury. Dressings and buddy strapping obscure subtle findings, and should be postponed until after the radiograph (Fig. 19.8). Fractures of the phalangeal neck tend to tilt into extension, leaving the volar side of the proximal fracture projecting as a spur into the subcondylar fossa (Figs. 19.9, 19.10). This can create a mechanical block to flexion of the joint. Closed reduction is usually successful in the acute phase (Cornwall and Ricchetti 2006), and pinning to maintain reduction reduces the risk of malunion and nonunion (Al Qattan 2001). Undisplaced fractures achieve excellent results with splinting alone, although careful clinical assessment is required as radiographs may under-represent the residual deformity.

19.3.3 Phalangeal Shaft

Fractures of the diaphysis of the middle and proximal phalanges are less common than those around the joints. Fracture types are transverse, oblique or spiral (Fig. 19.11). Dorsal tilting of the distal fragment is seen in angulated or displaced fractures (Fig. 19.12). It is essential to identify and correct any rotational deformity of phalangeal fractures, as it does not have the same remodelling potential as planar angulation.

19.3.4 Proximal Phalanx

This is the most common location for phalangeal fractures. The little finger is particularly affected, especially in the 9–12 year age group (Rajesh et al. 2001). The pattern most usually seen has been called the extra-octave fracture (Rang 1983), a Salter-Harris II fracture of the ulnar side of the base of the little finger, with ulnar deviation. The name comes from the presumed advantage gained by a pianist in having a wider span (Fig. 19.13). Closed reduction is readily accomplished by using a pencil in the webspace between the little and ring fingers and the application of an adduction force to the little finger. Some authors contend that the fracture line is actually juxta-epiphyseal, lying entirely in the metaphysis 1–2 mm distal to the physis (Barton

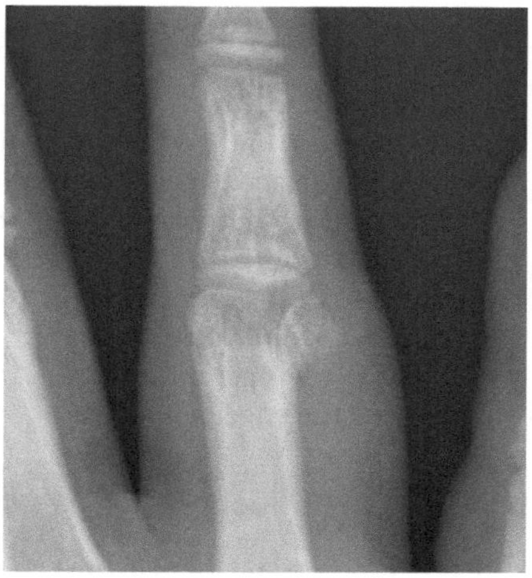

Fig. 19.7. Proximal phalanx rotated unicondylar fracture

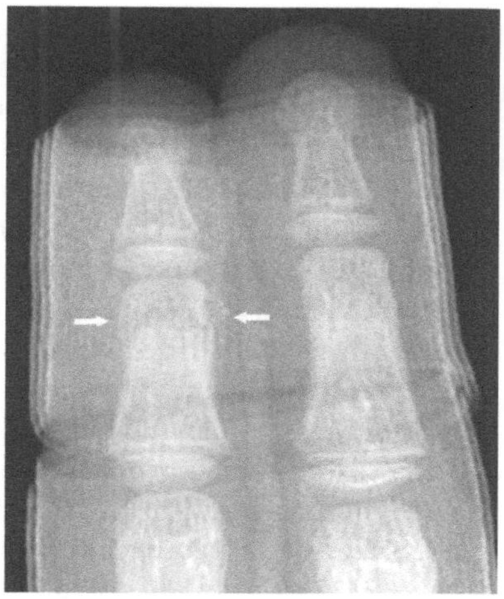

Fig. 19.8. Phalangeal neck fracture (*arrows*) largely obscured by strapping

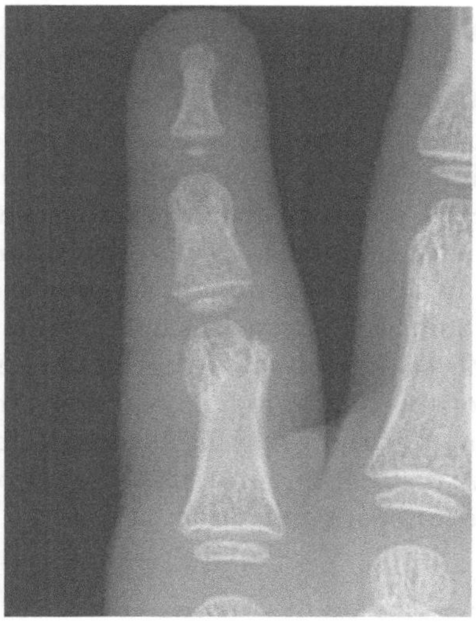

Fig. 19.9. Phalangeal neck fracture, frontal view

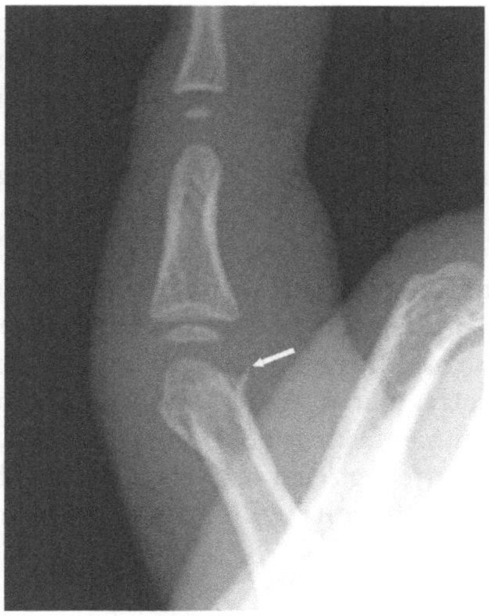

Fig. 19.10. Phalangeal neck fracture, lateral view. A bony spur projects into the subcondylar fossa (*arrow*)

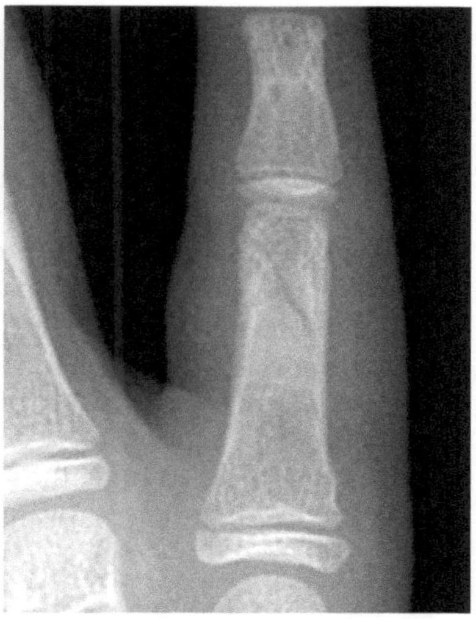

Fig. 19.11. Spiral fracture of the phalangeal shaft

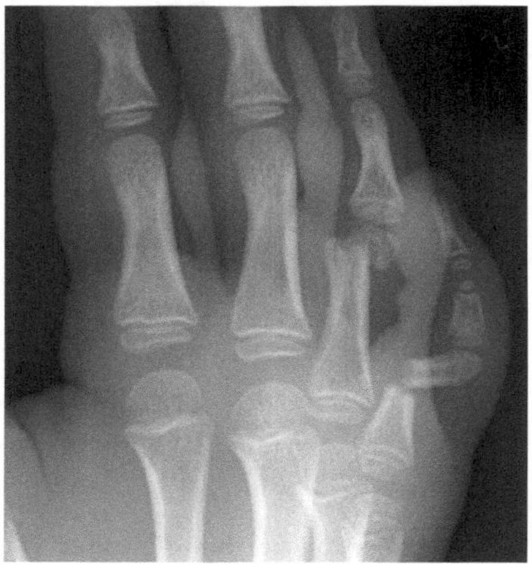

Fig. 19.12. Fractures of phalangeal neck and shaft with typical dorsal angulation

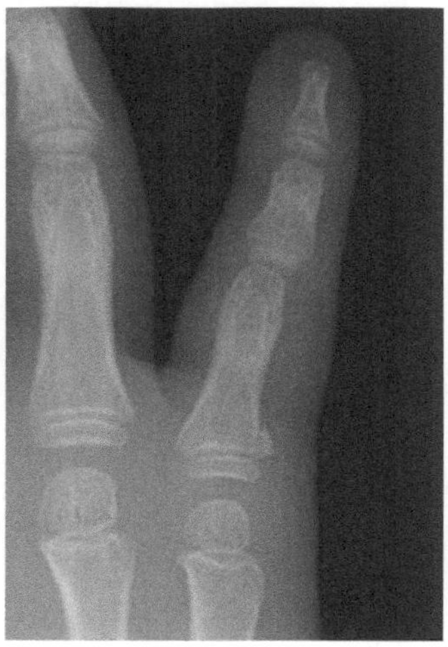

Fig. 19.13. The 'extra octave' fracture

1979; Beatty et al. 1990) (Figs. 19.14, 19.15). A series of 34 of these injuries showed mildly displaced fractures all did well with closed reduction and splinting, whilst 6 of 16 severely displaced fractures required Kirschner (K-) wire fixation, one following open reduction (Al Qattan 2002). Displacement is assessed by drawing 'Campbell's lines' (Campbell 1990) through the centre of the phalangeal neck and metaphysis. This line normally passes through the centre of the metacarpal head regardless of radiographic projection, and in mildly displaced fractures still crosses some part of the head. If the angulation is such that the line misses the metacarpal head completely, the fracture is termed severely displaced (Fig. 19.16). Campbell's straight line method is also useful for identifying metacarpophalangeal joint dislocations.

19.3.5 Volar Plate and Central Slip Avulsion Fractures

Volar plate injuries occur due to forced hyperextension of the proximal interphalangeal joint (PIPJ). There is avulsion of the insertion of the volar plate from the epiphysis at the base of the middle phalanx volarly, often only seen on the lateral or oblique radiographs (Fig. 19.17). Large fragments may require internal fixation. If they are unrecognised or progress to malunion, a swan neck deformity will develop (hyper extension at the PIPJ and flexion at the DIPJ).

Extensor hood central slip avulsion fractures are rare, and are visualised as tiny bony avulsions from the dorsal surface of the epiphysis at the base of the middle phalanx. Displaced bony fragments require internal fixation. Elson's test (Elson 1986) will demonstrate central slip integrity. If the extensor slip is ruptured, the child will be unable to extend the PIPJ of the injured finger if the MCPJs are flexed to 90 degrees over the edge of a table.

19.3.6 Interphalangeal Dislocations

In children's fingers, the physes are weaker than the supporting soft tissue structures, so fractures are more common than dislocations. The distal interphalangeal joint usually dislocates with the terminal phalanx lying dorsal to the middle phalanx. This injury can appear normal on frontal radiographs, but the lateral view is diagnostic. DIPJ dislocations are often open injuries. Dislocations at the proximal interphalangeal joint may occur in any direction, but again the dorsal direction is the most common. Avulsion of the collateral ligament from the proximal phalangeal origin may be demonstrated (Fig. 19.18). These dislocations are usually easily reduced and stable following reduction.

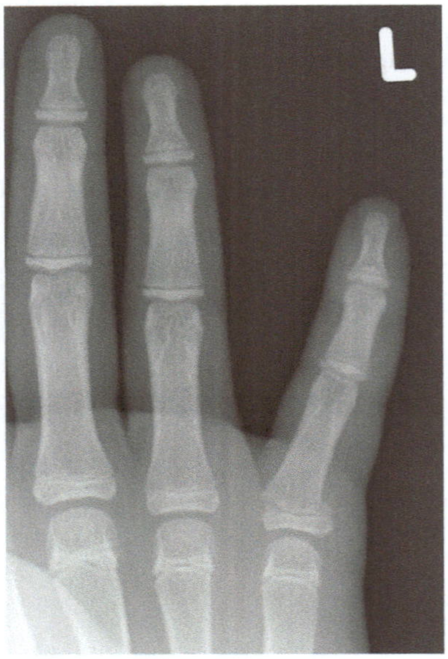

Fig. 19.14. Juxta-epiphyseal extra octave fracture

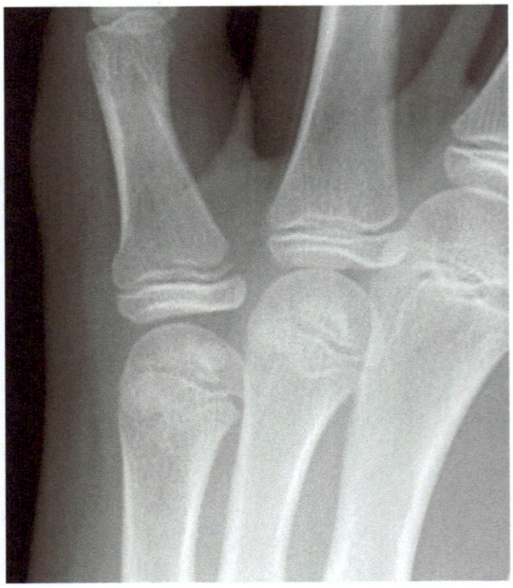

Fig. 19.15. Oblique view of another juxta-epiphyseal extra octave fracture. The fracture line parallels the physis

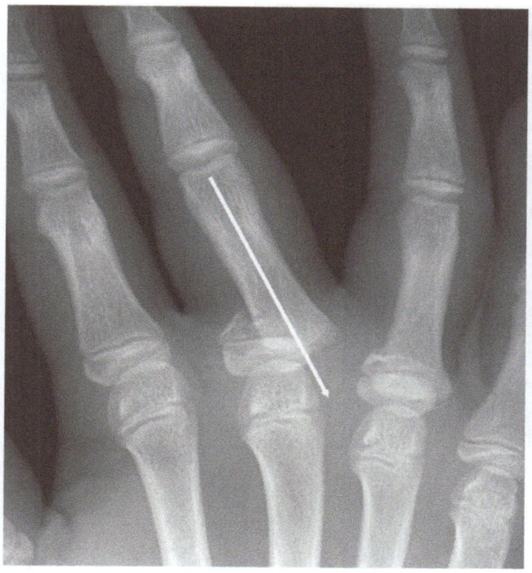

Fig. 19.16. Campbell's straight line method indicates a severely displaced phalangeal fracture

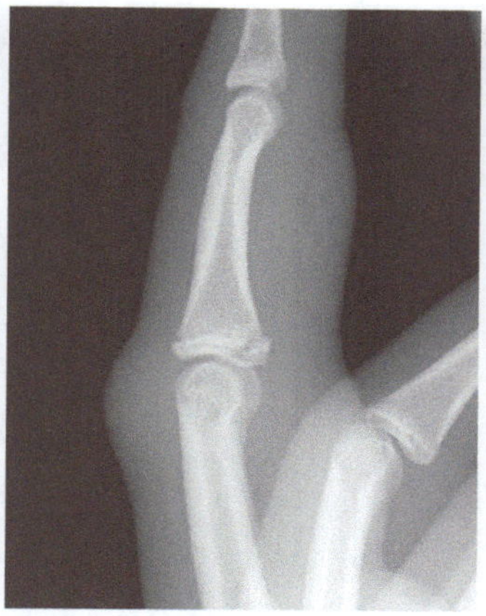

Fig. 19.17. Volar plate avulsion fracture

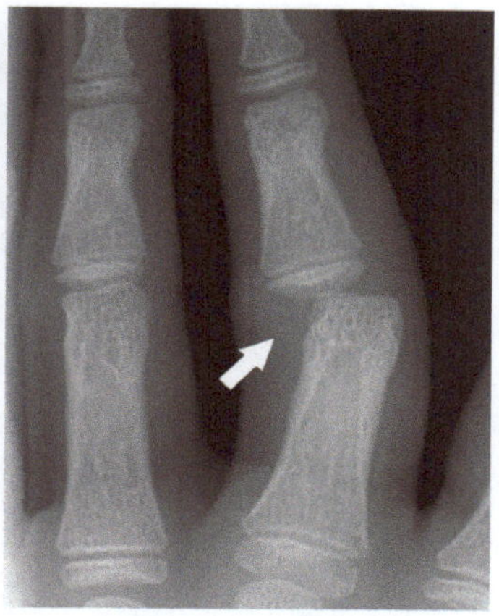

Fig. 19.18. Small avulsion fracture of the collateral ligament associated with proximal interphalangeal joint dislocation

19.4 The Metacarpals

Relative to the phalanges the metacarpals are reasonably protected, although several series of hand fractures found the fifth metacarpal to be the most frequently injured bone (Rajesh et al. 2001; Vadivelu et al. 2006). Incidence peaks in older schoolchildren, when the mechanism of injury is usually punching, or involvement in contact sports.

19.4.1 Metacarpal Epiphysis and Physis

Fractures involving the epiphysis and physis of the finger metacarpals are uncommon (Mahabir et al. 2001). Epiphyseal fractures are rare, and non displaced fractures may heal well (Fig. 19.19). Displaced split fractures of the epiphysis may need open reduction to restore articular congruity (Graham and Waters 2001). Intra-articular fractures of the epiphysis are important to identify as they are associated with joint effusions. If these effusions are under enough pressure, blood flow to the epiphysis may be sufficiently compromised to cause avascular necrosis. Preventative joint aspiration may be considered (McElfresh and Dobyns 1983).

Of the finger metacarpal fractures involving the physis, 85% are Salter-Harris type II, with a similar mechanism of injury to metacarpal neck injuries (Fischer and McElfresh 1994). Even so, there are proportionately less fractures affecting the physis in the metacarpals than in the phalanges, possibly due to a more stable arrangement of the collateral ligaments (Cornwall 2006). Salter-Harris II fractures rarely need open reduction (Fig. 19.20), and unstable fractures can be pinned percutaneously. The extent of physeal injuries may not be apparent on initial

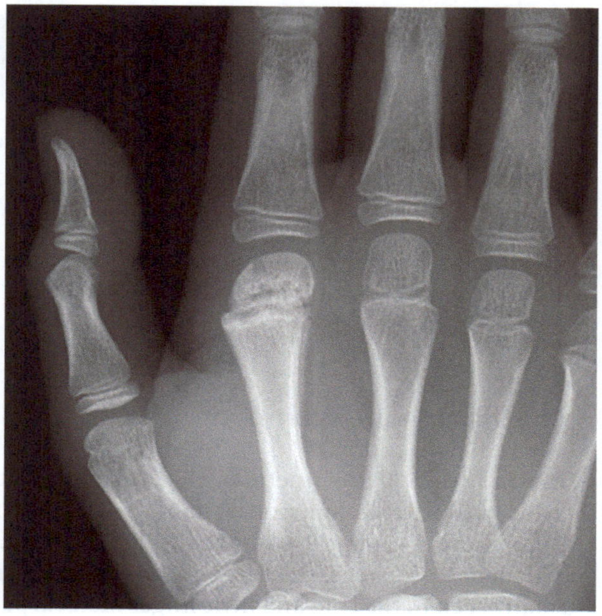

Fig. 19.19. Healing fractures of the index finger metacarpal head and neck

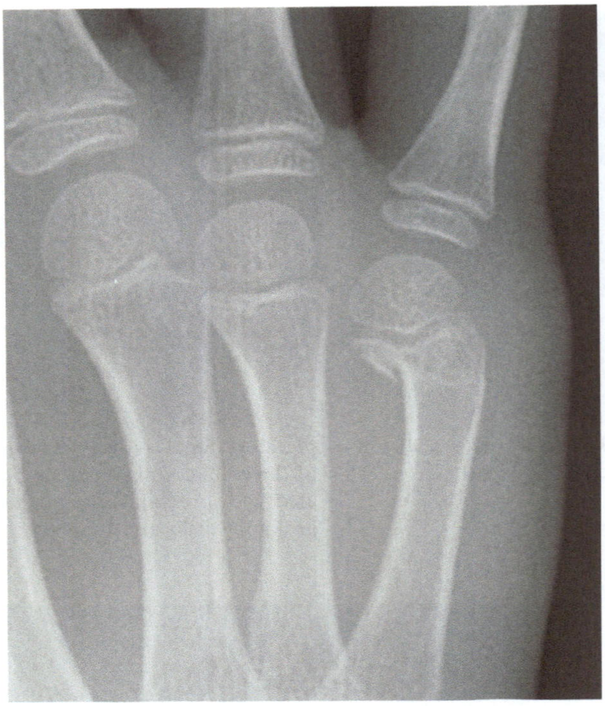

Fig. 19.20. Salter-Harris II fracture of the little finger metacarpal

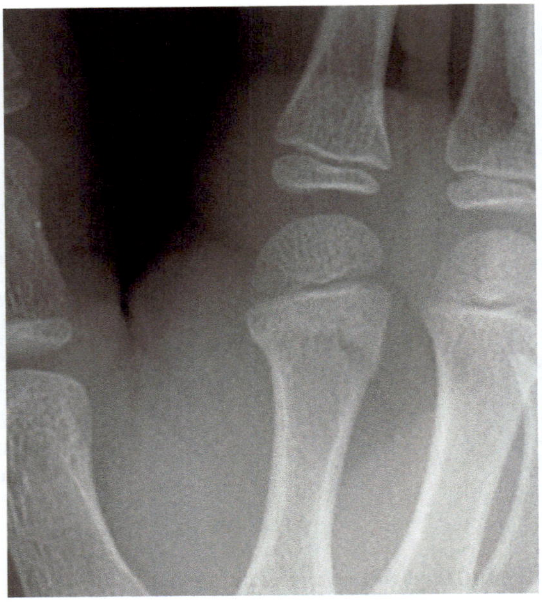

Fig. 19.21. A 7-year-old boy punched his brother, sustaining a transverse buckle fracture of the index metacarpal neck

radiographs, and physeal damage may impair longitudinal growth (LIGHT and OGDEN 1987).

19.4.2 Metacarpal Neck Fractures

In a study of 293 hand fractures, the neck of the fifth metacarpal was the commonest hand fracture in the 13–16 year age group (RAJESH et al. 2001). These are analogous to boxer's fractures in adults, and are usually seen in the ring and little finger metacarpals (Fig. 19.21). They occur when the axial loading force, commonly generated by a punch, is applied tangentially to the epiphyseal head (knuckle) from a dorsal direction. The force is transmitted to the weaker neck, causing a transverse fracture with a dorsal apex (i.e. volar angulation of the distal fragment).

Undisplaced fractures can be expected to heal without problems. The degree of acceptable angulation is not universally agreed, but more angulation is acceptable incrementally from the second to fifth metacarpals. The deformity is in the plane of the adjacent joint so remodelling is usually good, although loss of prominence of the knuckle of the little finger is the norm. A degree of extensor lag may be seen after splinting is discontinued. Although closed manipulation may be performed occasionally, open surgical treatment is not usually required.

19.4.3 Metacarpal Shaft Fractures

Most metacarpal shaft fractures are spiral, indicating a torsional injury (RAJESH et al. 2001). As in the phalanges, careful assessment is required of rotational deformity, although this is probably more easily performed clinically than radiologically. Treatment is similar to phalangeal injuries. If stabilisation of the metacarpal is required to maintain reduction, K-wires which pass from the fractured metacarpal across to the adjacent, intact metacarpal can be inserted.

19.4.4 Fractures of the Base of the Metacarpal

Injuries at this site are not common. The little finger sustains more metacarpal base fractures than the other finger metacarpals, and metaphyseal buckle fractures may be seen as a result of punching. Higher energy injuries , such as a fall from a height or a crushing injury, may cause intra-articular fractures of the base associated with carpometacarpal (CMC) joint subluxation or dislocation (Sandzen 1973). This region is difficult to assess with radiographs, and multiple oblique views may be required. If clinically relevant, CT scanning can be performed where doubt persists.

19.4.5 Metacarpophalangeal Dislocations

The MCP joint is the most frequently dislocated joint in the child's hand, usually a dorsal dislocation of the index finger. This digit also has the highest proportion of complex or irreducible dislocations. The volar plate ruptures from its insertion on the metacarpal as the proximal phalanx moves dorsally, and may become interposed between the articular surfaces, blocking reduction. The metacarpal head may also become fixed by the surrounding soft tissues (Kaplan 1957). Open reduction of these complex dislocations is usually required.

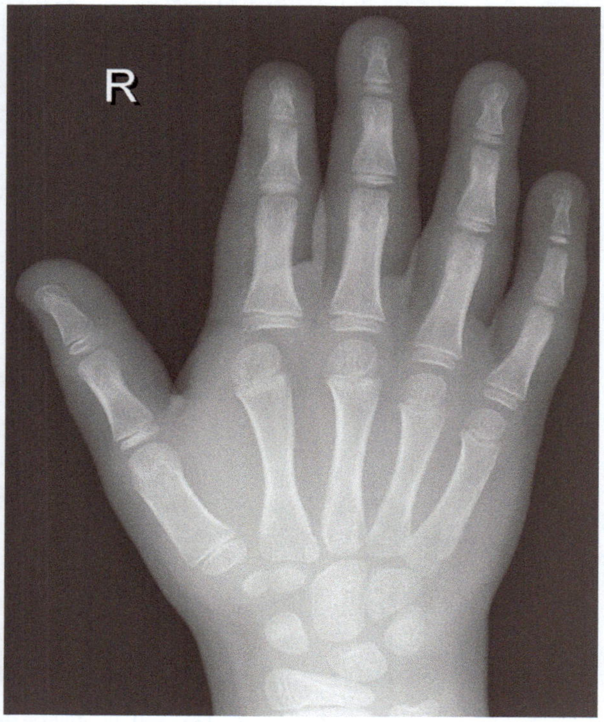

Fig. 19.22. Frontal view shows slight misalignment of the index finger metacarpophalangeal joint

The radiographs in MCP joint dislocations may be more difficult to evaluate than expected. On the DP view, the only abnormality visible may be alteration in the width of the MCP joint. Campbell's straight line method may be of use, as described previously. The oblique views, however, usually show a 'bare' metacarpal head in the palm (Figs. 19.22, 19.23).

19.4.6 Carpometacarpal Dislocations

These are rare injuries. If associated with fractures of the metacarpal base, the dislocations are analogous to Bennett's fractures of the thumb (Sandzen 1973). Post-reduction these injuries tend to redislocate, and often require stabilisation (Graham and Waters 2001).

19.5 The Thumb

The thumb has a distinct anatomy, with a bony structure similar to a finger without the metacarpal, i.e. the physis is located at the proximal end of the distal phalanx, middle phalanx and metacarpal (Kozin 2006). The collateral ligament insertions are different at the interphalangeal joint and the metacarpophalangeal

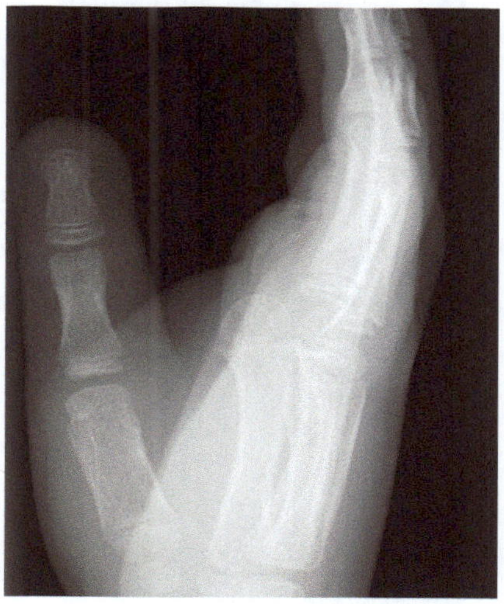

Fig. 19.23. Lateral view reveals the bare metacarpal head indicating metacarpophalangeal joint dislocation

joint, which accounts for the frequency of Salter-Harris II fractures at the former and type III fractures at the latter. Two common anatomical variants seen in the thumb metacarpal are the pseudoepiphysis and double epiphysis, situated distally (Fig. 19.24). These should not be confused with fractures.

19.5.1 Paediatric Skier's Thumb

A sprain of the ulnar collateral ligament (UCL) is the commonest skiing related injury in adolescents (Deibert et al. 1998). In adults, rupture of the ligament is known as gamekeeper's or skier's thumb, but isolated UCL rupture is very rare in children (Davies et al. 2002). Forced abduction and extension at the thumb metacarpophalangeal joint more usually causes a Salter-Harris III fracture with avulsion of the UCL (Fig. 19.25) (Wyatt and Beattie 1995). This is an important injury as it can destabilise the MCP joint, and impairs pincer grip. If there is doubt about the integrity of the UCL then fluoroscopic screening, after appropriate analgesia, is very valuable. Displaced fractures may require open reduction and internal fixation (Campbell 1990) and complete ligament injuries require repair, as they do not heal with conservative treatment. In younger children, Salter-Harris I and II fractures of the thumb base predominate, and instability at the fracture site may mimic UCL avulsion.

19.5.2 Dislocation of the Thumb MCP Joint

The thumb is vulnerable to hyperextension injury, often during sporting activity. Dislocations may be classified radiologically, with implications for the chance of successful closed reduction (Bohart et al. 1982). Incomplete dislocations allow the proximal phalanx to perch on the dorsum of the metacarpal (Fig. 19.26). The collateral ligaments are still intact, and closed reduction is usually successful. Simple complete dislocations are characterised by the dorsal displacement of the proximal phalanx, with marked angulation relative to the long axis of the metacarpal (Fig. 19.27). Here the collateral ligaments may be completely disrupted, but the volar plate is not interposed within the joint in the major-

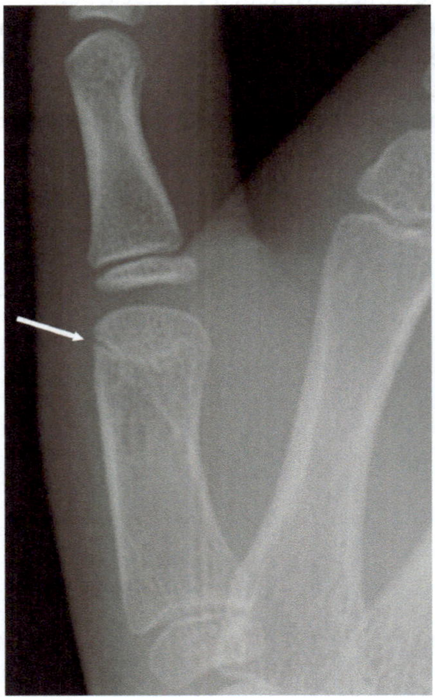

Fig. 19.24. Pseudoepiphysis at the distal thumb metacarpal (*arrow*), a common normal variant

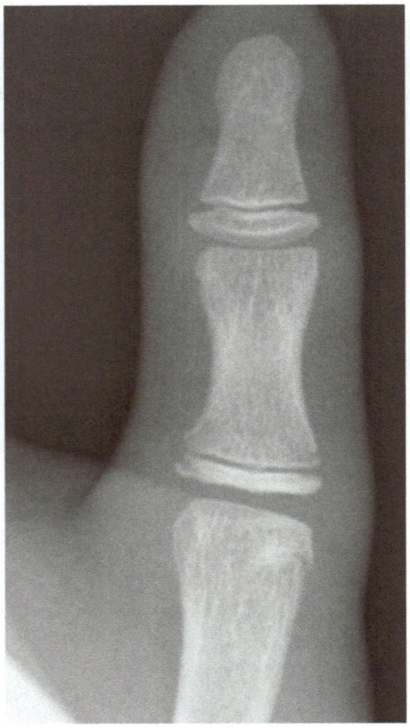

Fig. 19.25. Avulsion fracture of the ulnar collateral ligament at the thumb metacarpophalangeal joint

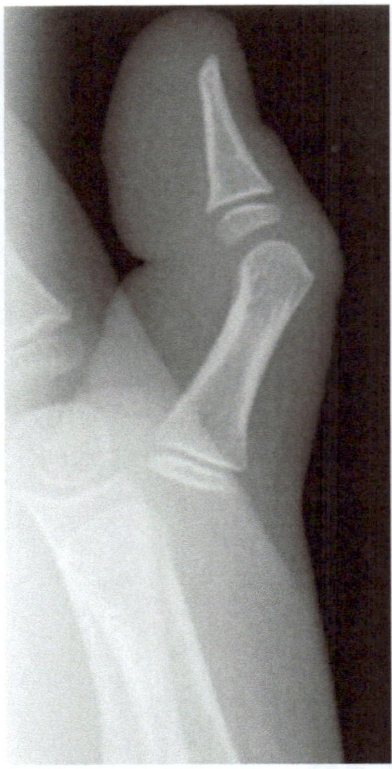

Fig. 19.26. Incomplete dislocation of the thumb metacarpophalangeal joint

ity of occasions. Closed reduction using longitudinal traction in the extended position, followed by flexion is usually possible. Complex complete dislocations are the most severe type of injury. The radiographs are misleadingly less dramatic, as the long axis of the dislocated proximal phalanx lies parallel to the thumb metacarpal. Open reduction is usually required to remove the interposed volar plate from within the joint (Bohart et al. 1982).

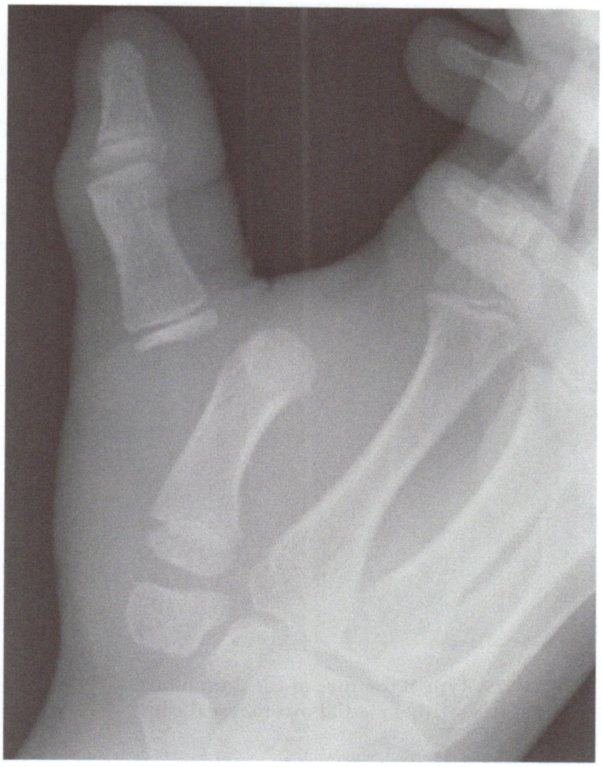

Fig. 19.27. Simple complete dislocation of the thumb metacarpophalangeal joint. (Image courtesy of Dr. John Morrison)

19.5.3 Fractures of the Thumb Metacarpal Base

Fractures of the head and shaft of the thumb metacarpal are similar to those seen in the other digits in terms of treatment. Fractures of the base of the metacarpal, however, deserve special attention due to their potential impact on thumb function (Graham and Waters 2001). Four categories are described. Type A fractures are extra-articular fractures of the shaft, usually in the proximal third of the metacarpal with a transverse or oblique orientation (Fig. 19.28). There is often apex lateral angulation, with medial impaction. Good remodelling can be expected due to the proximity to the physis.

Type B and C fractures are Salter-Harris II injuries. Type B injuries are the more common, and have the metaphyseal spur on the medial side, and apex lateral angulation due to the pull of abductor pollicis longus (Fig. 19.29). Type C fractures have the opposite pattern, i.e. the spur is lateral and the angulation is apex medial (Figs. 19.30, 19.31). Angulated Type C fractures are more difficult to treat by closed reduction than type B, but both are problematic.

Type D fractures are intra-articular Salter-Harris III or IV injuries of the proximal thumb metacarpal, resembling the adult Bennett's fracture (Fig. 19.32). These injuries are fortunately not common, as they can be very difficult to treat. Open reduction and internal fixation are often required

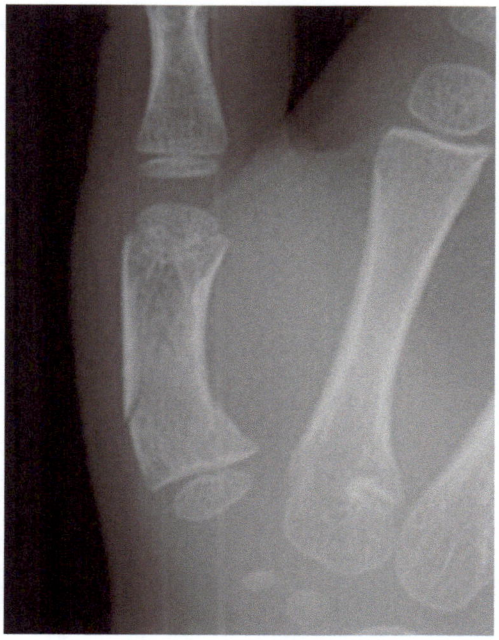

Fig. 19.28. Type A fracture of the thumb metacarpal proximal third

19.6 The Carpals

Fractures and dislocations of the carpal bones are rare, and a child with a painful wrist following trauma is much more likely to have injured the distal radius (Fig. 19.33). Carpal bone fractures are uncom-

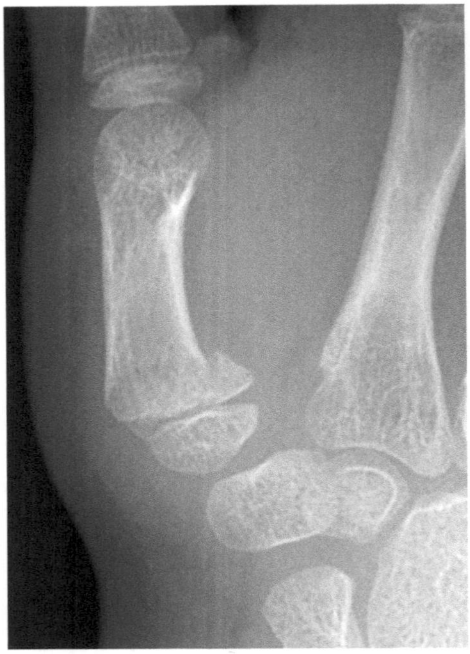

Fig. 19.29. Type B fracture of the thumb metacarpal base with a medial metaphyseal spur

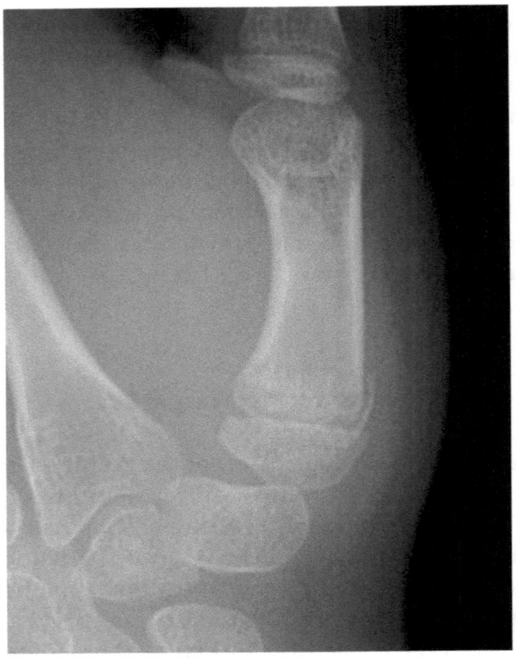

Fig. 19.30. Type C fracture of the thumb metacarpal base with a lateral metaphyseal spur

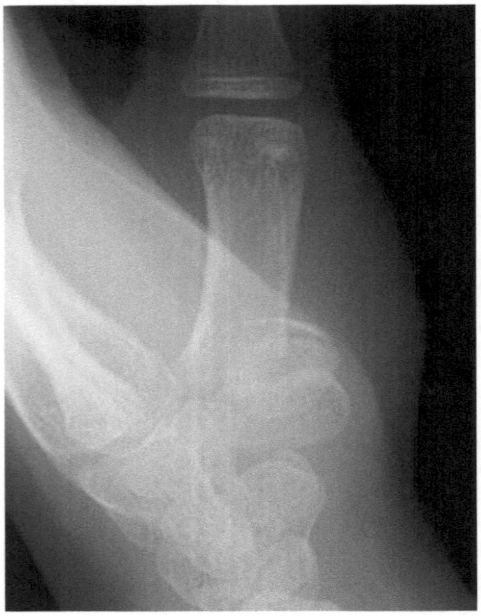

Fig. 19.31. Type C fracture of the thumb metacarpal base, lateral view reveals marked displacement

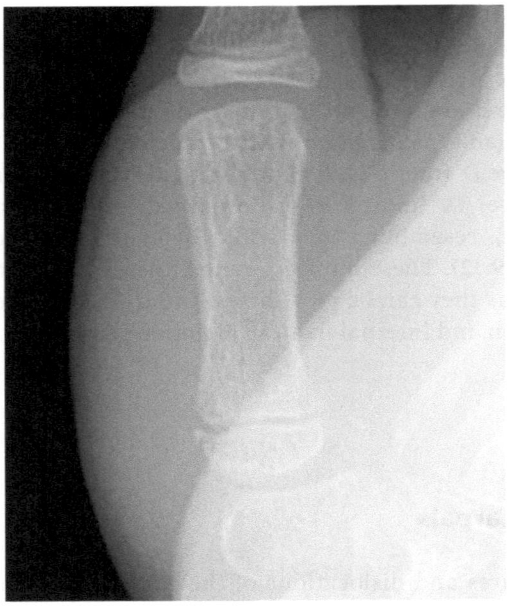

Fig. 19.32. Small Salter-Harris III fracture at the base of the thumb metacarpal, type D fracture

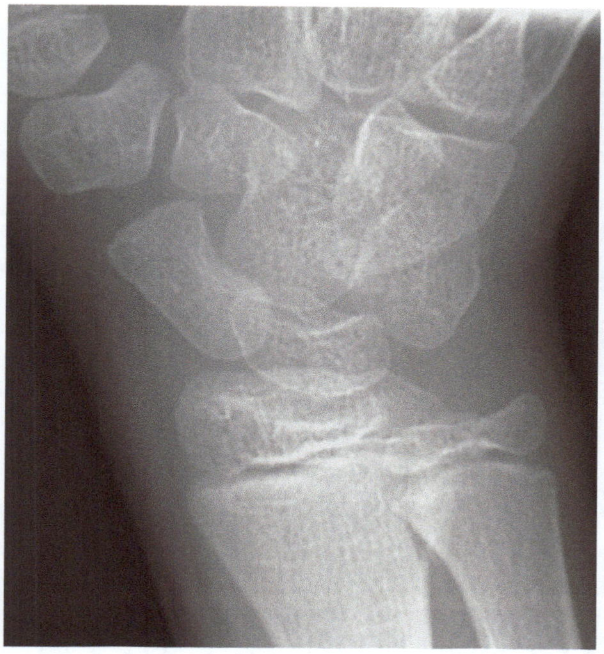

Fig. 19.33. Scaphoid views of the wrist performed in a 12-year-old boy show a dorsal buckle fracture of the radius

mon in the younger child as the carpal bones form through enchondral ossification, and the developing ossification centres are therefore protected within a cartilaginous coat of decreasing thickness until skeletal maturity.

19.6.1 The Scaphoid

The ossific nucleus of the scaphoid appears around 4–6 years of age, and ossification is complete at 13–15 years. As in adults, the scaphoid is the most frequently injured carpal bone. The incidence of fractures is extremely low in the first decade, thereafter rising to a peak in the late teens to mid twenties (Grad 1986). Unlike adults, fractures of the distal pole are more common than of the waist (Fig. 19.34). These fractures represent ligamentous avulsion injuries, with failure through the bone rather than the stronger soft tissues. Middle third fractures occur in older children and adolescents, whilst proximal pole fractures are rare. Many fractures are the result of direct trauma to the wrist rather than a fall on the outstretched hand (Vahvanen and Westerlund 1980).

If the initial radiographs are negative, but mechanism of injury and clinical examination suggest scaphoid injury, casting and repeat radiographs 2 weeks later is recommended (Graham and Waters 2001). This is because occult scaphoid fracture rates of 12% have been reported (Christodoulou and Colton 1986). Non-union is fortunately very rare in treated acute scaphoid fractures in children. Even late presenting fractures generally do well with immobilisation (Vahvanen and Westerlund 1980). With increasing availability of other imaging modalities this repeat radiograph approach is being superceded.

Bone scans have been used to investigate suspected scaphoid fractures, but involve a significant radiation dose (Beeres et al. 2005), more recently magnetic resonance imaging (MRI) has been shown to have better specificity (Breitenseher et al. 1997). A normal initial MRI scan has a negative predictive value of 100% for scaphoid fractures, and may yield other clinically important information (Cook et al. 1997). If the facility exists, then early MR imaging significantly alters the management of children with suspected scaphoid injuries (Johnson et al. 2000). Complex regional pain syndromes can be seen in teenagers with wrist injuries and it is important to exclude serious injury promptly in order that movement can be regained and stiffness prevented.

19.6.2 The Other Carpal Bones

Fractures of the other carpals are very rarely seen in children (Goddard 2005). The capitate may be injured in isolation, or more typically, in conjunction with other carpals, particularly the scaphoid (Anderson 1987). Rare cases of lunate dislocations have been reported, usually associated with other injuries (Giddins and Shaw 1994) (Fig. 19.35). Open reduction and repair of the intercarpal ligaments is advised.

19.7 Distal Radius and Ulna

19.7.1 Metaphyseal Fractures

Forearm fractures, particularly in the distal third, are common injuries in children. Standard two view

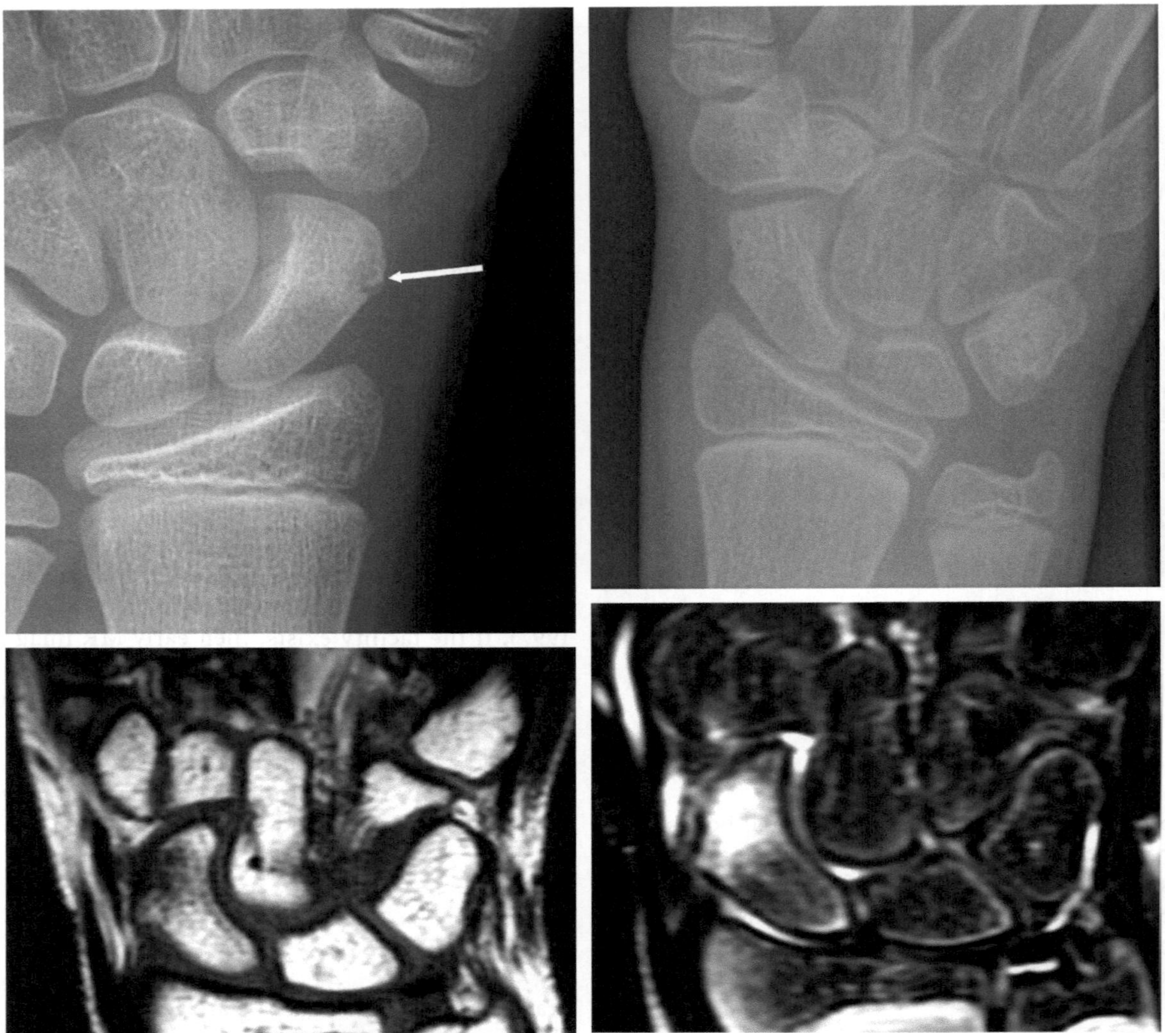

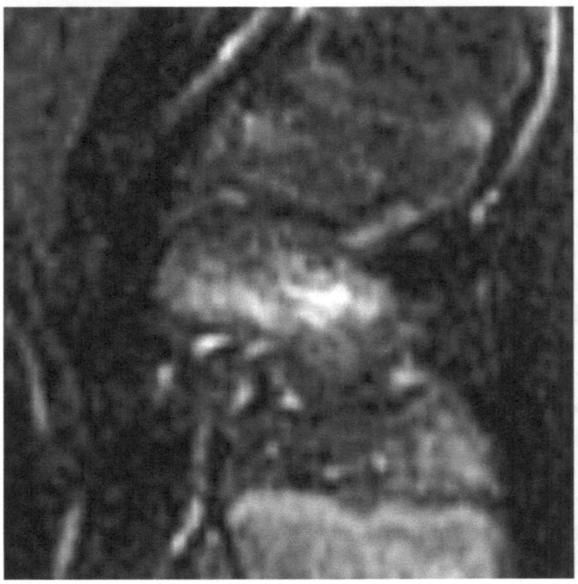

Fig. 19.34. a Small avulsion fracture from the distal pole of the scaphoid (*arrow*). **b** AP radiograph of the wrist in a different child shows possible cortical irregularity of the scaphoid (other scaphoid d views were obtained but were non-diagnostic). **c** Coronal T1 weighted image shows low signal change in the upper pole of the scaphoid. **d** Coronal T2 fat saturated image shows oedema in the upper pole of the scaphoid confirming a fracture. **e** Sagittal STIR image in another child shows a high signal band through the scaphoid confirming the presence of a fracture

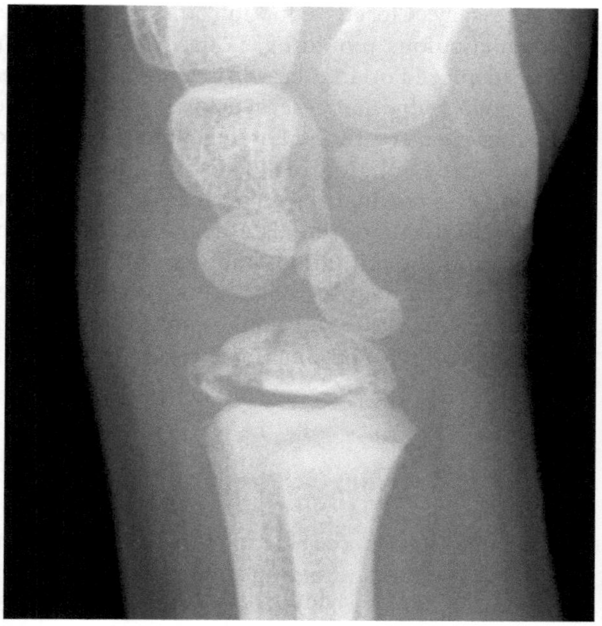

Fig. 19.35. Lunate dislocation and radial epiphyseal fracture. (Image courtesy of Dr. Andrew Downie)

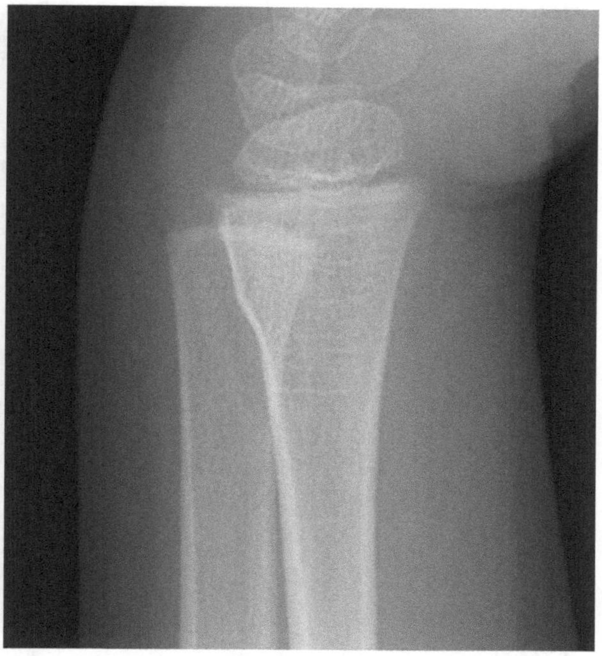

Fig. 19.36. Simple dorsal torus, or buckle fracture of the distal radial metaphysis

radiographs are usually all that are required for diagnosis, although care should be taken to look for associated injuries, particularly the Monteggia lesion. The peak incidence in boys is at age 12–14, and in girls at 10–12 (Kramhoft and Bodtker 1988). This age corresponds to the adolescent growth spurt, when the radial metaphysis is relatively weak. A typical fall on the outstretched hand results in forced dorsiflexion at the wrist. This may cause a simple torus or buckle fracture on the dorsal surface of the metaphysis (Fig. 19.36). More force produces a greenstick fracture (Fig. 19.37), or a complete fracture (Fig. 19.38). There is debate regarding the acceptable degree of angulation, with figures from 10 –35 degrees in patients under 5 quoted (Waters 2001). In general, more angulation can be allowed in younger children as they have the greater potential to remodel and the plane of the deformity is usually in the plane of the adjacent joint. Volar angulation (apex dorsal) is less common, and can remodel well (Zimmermann et al. 2004), but the deformity is more obvious because there is less soft tissue on the dorsum of the wrist. Complete displacement with overlapping of bone ends results in shortening with a bayonet configuration.

Torus (or buckle) fractures can be managed with either a padded bandage or a wrist splint. A cast is

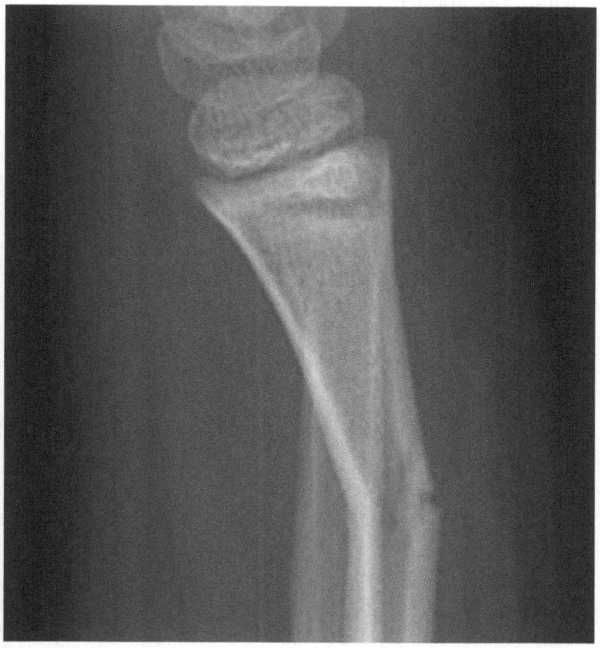

Fig. 19.37. Greenstick fracture of the distal radius, with volar angulation

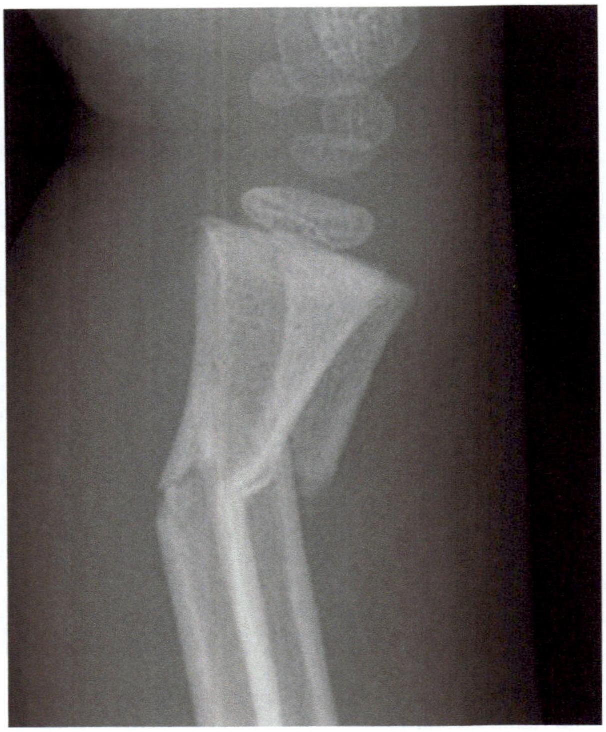

Fig. 19.38. Transverse fractures of the radius and ulnar with length maintained

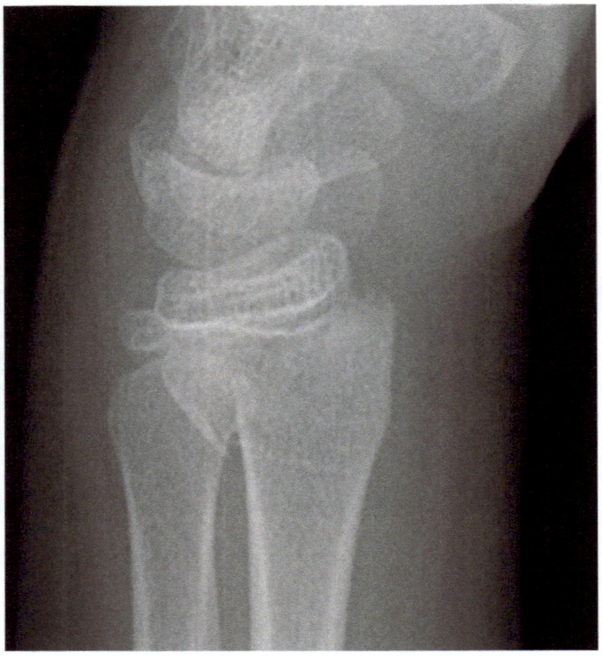

Fig. 19.39. Salter-Harris II fracture of the distal radius

unnecessary. Closed reduction and a plaster cast with meticulous moulding, is used for the majority of displaced or angulated distal radial fractures, with open reduction reserved for irreducible fractures or open fractures. Bayonet fractures will not reduce using longitudinal traction alone, as this tightens the residual intact periosteum. Increasing the dorsal tilting of the distal fragment relaxes the periosteum. Longitudinal traction will then allow the distal fragment to reduce. Pin fixation is used for unstable fractures, although some prefer routine pin fixation for all bayonet fractures.

19.7.2 Fractures Involving the Physis

The Salter-Harris classification is widely used to describe fractures affecting the physis, and type II predominate (Fig. 19.39) (Salter and Harris 1963). The radius is much more commonly affected than the ulna, and again the distal fragment is usually displaced dorsally (Mizuta et al. 1987). Further metaphyseal fracture types extending to the physis have been described, which may be associated with growth arrest (Peterson et al. 1994) (Fig. 19.40). Reduction of physeal fractures is usually straightforward. Longitudinal traction after increasing the deformity will reduce the fragment. Repeated attempts at reduction should be avoided for fear of iatrogenic growth plate damage. Anatomical reduction is preferred for Salter-Harris II injuries, but minor degrees of displacement can be accepted. Physeal injuries heal in 2–3 weeks and manipulation after 1 week may be difficult and risk injury to the physis.

19.7.3 Galeazzi Fractures and Equivalents

Galeazzi fracture patterns occur where there is a fracture of the distal radius associated with disruption of the distal radioulnar joint, and are relatively rare in children. More common is the Galeazzi equivalent lesion, where the radial fracture occurs with a distal ulnar physeal fracture (Fig. 19.41). Multiple subtypes have been classified (Letts and Rowhani 1993), most of which can be treated with closed manipulation and cast fixation. If the radial fracture is complete rather than greenstick, internal fixation will be required.

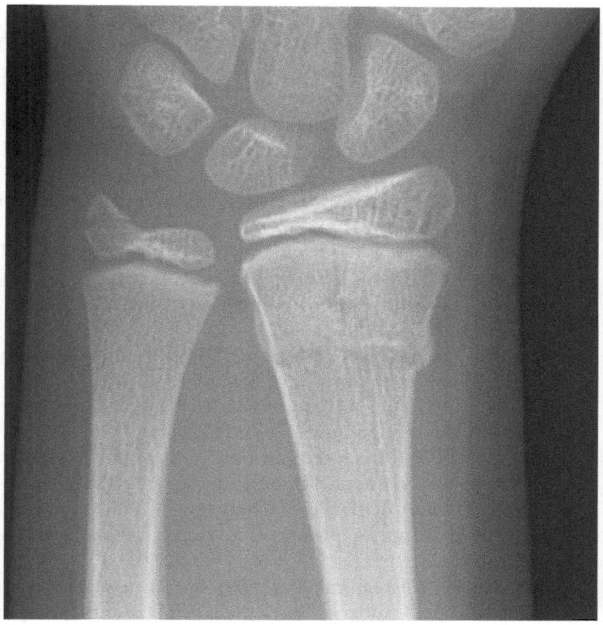

Fig. 19.40. Inverted 'T' shaped fracture of the distal radial metaphysis, extending to the physis

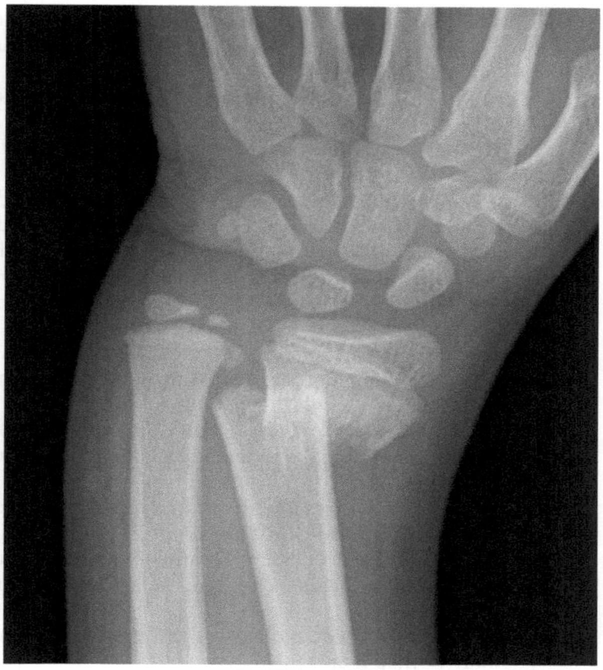

Fig. 19.41. Displaced fracture of the radius with associated Salter-Harris IV fracture of the ulna, a Galeazzi equivalent injury

References

Al Qattan MM (2001) Phalangeal neck fractures in children: classification and outcome in 66 cases. J Hand Surg [Br] 26:112–121

Al Qattan MM (2002) Juxta-epiphyseal fractures of the base of the proximal phalanx of the fingers in children and adolescents. J Hand Surg [Br] 27:24–30

Anderson WJ (1987) Simultaneous fracture of the scaphoid and capitate in a child. J Hand Surg [Am] 12:271–273

Barton NJ (1979) Fractures of the phalanges of the hand in children. Hand 11:134–143

Beatty E, Light TR, Belsole RJ, Ogden JA (1990) Wrist and hand skeletal injuries in children. Hand Clin 6:723–738

Beeres FJ, Hogervorst M, Hollander P, Rhemrev S (2005) Outcome of routine bone scintigraphy in suspected scaphoid fractures. Injury 36:1233–1236

Bhende MS, Dandrea LA, Davis HW (1993) Hand injuries in children presenting to a pediatric emergency department. Ann Emerg Med 22:1519–1523

Bohart PG, Gelberman RH, Vandell RF, Salamon PB (1982) Complex dislocations of the metacarpophalangeal joint. Clin Orthop Relat Res 208–210

Breitenseher MJ, Metz VM, Gilula LA, Gaebler C, Kukla C, Fleischmann D, Imhof H, Trattnig S (1997) Radiographically occult scaphoid fractures: value of MR imaging in detection. Radiology 203:245–250

Campbell RM Jr (1990) Operative treatment of fractures and dislocations of the hand and wrist region in children. Orthop Clin North Am 21:217–243

Christodoulou AG, Colton CL (1986) Scaphoid fractures in children. J Pediatr Orthop 6:37–39

Chung KC, Spilson SV (2001) The frequency and epidemiology of hand and forearm fractures in the United States. J Hand Surg [Am] 26:908–915

Cook PA, Yu JS, Wiand W, Cook AJ, Coleman CR, Cook AJ (1997) Suspected scaphoid fractures in skeletally immature patients: application of MRI. J Comput Assist Tomogr 21:511–515

Cornwall R (2006) Finger metacarpal fractures and dislocations in children. Hand Clin 22:1–10

Cornwall R, Ricchetti ET (2006) Pediatric phalanx fractures: unique challenges and pitfalls. Clin Orthop Relat Res 445:146–156

Currey JD, Butler G (1975) The mechanical properties of bone tissue in children. J Bone Joint Surg Am 57:810–814

Davies MB, Wright JE, Edwards MS (2002) True skier's thumb in childhood. Injury 33:186–187

Deibert MC, Aronsson DD, Johnson RJ, Ettlinger CF, Shealy JE (1998) Skiing injuries in children, adolescents, and adults. J Bone Joint Surg Am 80:25–32

Elson RA (1986) Rupture of the central slip of the extensor hood of the finger. A test for early diagnosis. J Bone Joint Surg Br 68:229–231

Fetter-Zarzeka A, Joseph MM (2002) Hand and fingertip injuries in children. Pediatr Emerg Care 18:341–345

Fischer MD, McElfresh EC (1994) Physeal and periphyseal injuries of the hand. Patterns of injury and results of treatment. Hand Clin 10:287–301

Giddins GE, Shaw DG (1994) Lunate subluxation associated with a Salter-Harris type 2 fracture of the distal radius. J Hand Surg [Br] 19:193–194
Goddard N (2005) Carpal fractures in children. Clin Orthop Relat Res 73–76
Grad JB (1986) Children's skeletal injuries. Orthop Clin North Am 17:437–449
Graham TJ, Waters PM (2001) Fractures and dislocations of the hand and carpus in children. In: Beaty JH, Kasser JR (eds) Rockwood and Wilkins' Fractures in children, 5th edn. Lippincott Williams and Wilkins, Philadelphia, pp 271–379
Hastings H, Simmons BP (1984) Hand fractures in children. A statistical analysis. Clin Orthop Relat Res 120–130
Johnson KJ, Haigh SF, Symonds KE (2000) MRI in the management of scaphoid fractures in skeletally immature patients. Pediatr Radiol 30:685–688
Kaplan EB (1957) Dorsal dislocation of the metacarpophalangeal joint of the index finger. J Bone Joint Surg Am 39–A:1081–1086
Kozin SH (2006) Fractures and dislocations along the pediatric thumb ray. Hand Clin 22:19–29
Kramhoft M, Bodtker S (1988) Epidemiology of distal forearm fractures in Danish children. Acta Orthop Scand 59:557–559
Landin LA (1997) Epidemiology of children's fractures. J Pediatr Orthop B 6:79–83
Letts M, Rowhani N (1993) Galeazzi-equivalent injuries of the wrist in children. J Pediatr Orthop 13:561–566
Light TR, Ogden JA (1987) Metacarpal epiphyseal fractures. J Hand Surg [Am] 12:460–464
Ljungberg E, Rosberg HE, Dahlin LB (2003) Hand injuries in young children. J Hand Surg [Br] 28:376–380
Mahabir RC, Kazemi AR, Cannon WG, Courtemanche DJ (2001) Pediatric hand fractures: a review. Pediatr Emerg Care 17:153–156
McElfresh EC, Dobyns JH (1983) Intra-articular metacarpal head fractures. J Hand Surg [Am] 8:383–393
Mizuta T, Benson WM, Foster BK, Paterson DC, Morris LL (1987) Statistical analysis of the incidence of physeal injuries. J Pediatr Orthop 7:518–523
Peterson HA, Madhok R, Benson JT, Ilstrup DM, Melton LJ III (1994) Physeal fractures: part 1. Epidemiology in Olmsted County, Minnesota, 1979–1988. J Pediatr Orthop 14:423–430
Rajesh A, Basu AK, Vaidhyanath R, Finlay D (2001) Hand fractures: a study of their site and type in childhood. Clin Radiol 56:667–669
Rang M (1983) Children's fractures, 2nd edn. JB Lippincott, Philadelphia, pp 221–232
Salazard B, Launay F, Desouches C, Samson P, Jouve JL, Magalon G (2004) Fingertip injuries in children: 81 cases with at least one year follow-up. Rev Chir Orthop Reparatrice Appar Mot 90:621–627
Salter RB, Harris WR (1963) Injuries involving the epiphyseal plate. J Bone Joint Surg Am 45-A:587–622
Sandzen SC (1973) Fracture of the fifth metacarpal resembling Bennett's fracture. Hand 5:49–51
Seymour N (1966) Juxta-epiphysial fracture of the terminal phalanx of the finger. J Bone Joint Surg Br 48:347–349
Vadivelu R, Dias JJ, Burke FD, Stanton J (2006) Hand injuries in children: a prospective study. J Pediatr Orthop 26:29–35
Vahvanen V, Westerlund M (1980) Fracture of the carpal scaphoid in children. A clinical and roentgenological study of 108 cases. Acta Orthop Scand 51:909–913
Valencia J, Leyva F, Gomez-Bajo GJ (2005) Pediatric hand trauma. Clin Orthop Relat Res (432):77–86
Waters PM (2001) Fractures and dislocations of the hand and carpus in children. In: Beaty JH, Kasser JR (eds) Rockwood and Wilkins' Fractures in children, 5th edn. Lippincott Williams and Wilkins, Philadelphia, pp 381–442
Weiss AP, Hastings H (1993) Distal unicondylar fractures of the proximal phalanx. J Hand Surg [Am] 18:594–599
Wyatt JP, Beattie TF (1995) Paediatric injuries on an artificial ski slope. Injury 26:87–88
Zimmermann R, Gschwentner M, Pechlaner S, Gabl M (2004) Remodeling capacity and functional outcome of palmarly versus dorsally displaced pediatric radius fractures in the distal one-third. Arch Orthop Trauma Surg 124:42–48

The Spine

20

Radhesh Krishna Lalam, Victor N. Cassar-Pullicino, and Prudencia N. M. Tyrrell

CONTENTS

20.1 Introduction

Paediatric spinal trauma is an uncommon form of injury. Spinal injuries in children and adolescents account for 1%–9% of total reported spinal injuries. Spinal fractures represent 1%–2% of all paediatric fractures and the cervical spine is the commonest region involved accounting for 60%–80% of paediatric spinal injuries (Kokoska et al. 2001). This in turn means that the average general radiologist and emergency physician is unlikely to see a significant number of paediatric spinal injuries and may there-

R. K. Lalam, MD
V. N. Cassar-Pullicino, MD
P. N. M. Tyrrell, MD
Department of Radiology, Robert Jones and Agnes Hunt Orthopaedic and District Hospital, Oswestry SY10 7AG, UK

fore have limited experience in dealing with these injuries. In the very young child, spinal injuries are usually a result of road traffic accidents or falls, while in the older child there are an increased proportion of injuries from sports related activities (Cirak et al. 2004; Kokoska et al. 2001). In one study involving cervical spine injuries, 75% were unrestrained or restrained using an inappropriate device (Brown et al. 2001). Therefore, satisfactory restraint of children in motor vehicles affords protection against cervical spine injuries. However, inappropriate lap belts used in children are associated with injuries to the thoracolumbar spine. The majority of deaths in children with spinal injury are due to associated brain injury (Kokoska et al. 2001). Careful attention should therefore be focussed for any associated brain or visceral injury.

Careful clinical evaluation is essential when evaluating a child with multiple injuries as spinal injuries can be overlooked. Tenderness, ecchymosis, swelling or a palpable defect posteriorly along spinous processes should alert the examiner to the possibility of spinal injury. A seatbelt mark or actual abdominal organ injury increases the likelihood of spinal injury.

Most children arrive in the emergency rooms after suspected spinal injury immobilised on a spinal board and in a cervical collar. As young children have a disproportionately large head, positioning on a spinal board leads to a flexed attitude of the C-spine, which can cause further anterior angulation and translation in the setting of an unstable spinal injury. Furthermore, the normal pseudo subluxation can be exaggerated in this situation and pose interpretation problems. Therefore, modifications must be made to the spinal board either in the form of creating a recess for the occiput to accommodate the large head or using a double mattress to raise the chest.

The stage reached in spinal growth at the time of injury has a bearing on both diagnosis and prognosis. Firstly, the interpretation of paediatric spine imaging can be difficult in the traumatic setting due to the complexity in development and ossification. In addition, the range of movements and biomechanics are different to adults. A clear anatomical knowledge is essential to avoid errors in interpretation. Areas of lucency seen on radiographs may be due to cartilaginous development. Epiphysis, apophysis and synchondrosis occur in predictable locations, have smooth well corticated margins and can usually be differentiated from traumatic lesions.

Secondly, injuries to the paediatric spine should be followed up over a long time as they demonstrate variable remodelling and may develop progressive deformity especially during the adolescent growth spurt (McPhee 1981; Pouliquen et al. 1997).

In this chapter, the anatomy, normal variants and injuries to the paediatric spine are discussed with emphasis on the role of imaging and the concept of stability.

20.2 Embryological Development, Anatomy and Normal Variants

The unique radiological anatomy of the paediatric spine can cause problems with interpretation in the setting of trauma. Knowledge of normal development, anatomy and variations is essential to avoid misinterpretation leading to either false positive or false negative conclusions.

20.2.1 Embryology

The vertebral column and the associated musculature develop from paraxial mesenchyme which is found lateral to the notochord and neural tube in early embryonal development. The paraxial mesenchyme on each side of the notochord initially undergoes segmentation and then somatogenesis. This occurs sequentially in a cranio-caudal direction and the duration is species specific. The ventro-medial aspect of the somite gives rise to the sclerotomal cells. Within each segment the sclerotomal cells are divided into cranial and caudal halves by the Von Ebner fissure. Each vertebra is formed by the combination of the caudal half of one bilateral pair of sclerotomes and the cranial halves of the sclerotomes below. This produces the blastemal centrum of each vertebra. The centrum thus encloses the notochord and lies ventral to the neural tube. The neural processes extend from the dorso-lateral angles of the centrum and curve to enclose the neural tube. This neural arch consists of paired bilateral pedicles (ventrolaterally) and laminae (dorsolaterally) which coalesce behind the neural tube to form the spinous processes. The definitive vertebral body is formed by the centrum and the expanding pedicle ends which fuse at the neurocentral synchondroses. The intervening notochord between vertebral bodies forms the nucleus pulposus while the mesenchyme surrounding the Von Ebner fissure forms the annulus fibrosis. The intervertebral discs have the same origins as the centrum.

The development of the occipitocervical junction varies from the rest of the vertebrae. The occiput is formed from four sclerotomes. The first of these disappears while the rest fuse to form the basiocciput. The first cervical vertebra is formed from the caudal portion of the 4th occipital somite and the cranial portion of the first cervical somite (5th somite). The centra from the 5th, 6th and 7th somites have a different fate to the rest of the vertebral column. The origin of the anterior arch of the atlas is unclear. It does not arise from the sclerotomes. The centra derived from the sclerotomes 5, 6 and 7 give rise to the tip of the dens, base of the dens and the centrum of the axis. The posterior arch of the atlas is formed from the neural processes of sclerotome 5. The posterior arch of the axis arises from sclerotome 6. The development of the upper cervical spine is therefore closely related to that of the basiocciput and anomalous development affects both regions.

20.2.2 Ossification

A typical vertebra is ossified from three primary centres, one in the centrum and one each for each half of the vertebral arch. Ossification centres appear as early as the ninth week of gestation. Generally, the arches unite posteriorly between 1 and 3 years of age while the centrum unites with the arches at the neurocentral synchondrosis between 3–6 years, usually earlier in the upper cervical spine than the lumbar spine.

Before fusion, the epiphyseal margins and synchondroses can be confused with fractures. Generally the epiphyseal margins are smooth, sclerotic and occur in predictable locations.

The upper two cervical vertebrae have unique ossification compared to the rest of the vertebrae.

C1 has three primary ossification centres, one for the anterior arch and one each for the neural arches (Fig. 20.1a,b). The anterior arch is only ossified in 20% of children at birth and becomes ossified by 1 year of age. The neural arches fuse between 3–6 years and the anterior arch fuses with the neural arches by 7 years of age. The ossification centre for the body of C1 may fail to appear. The neural arches in this instance may fail to fuse anteriorly resulting in a central cleft.

C2 has the most complex ossification of all vertebrae (Fig. 20.1a,b). There are four ossification centres at birth: one for each neural arch, one for the body and one for the odontoid process. The neural arches fuse with each other by 2–3 years of age and with the body between 3–6 years of age. The body of C2 fuses with the odontoid process by 3–6 years of age. This fusion line (sub-dental synchondroses) can be seen until about 11 years of age and can be confused with a fracture. A secondary ossification centre appears at the apex of the odontoid process (os terminale) between 3 and 6 years of age, which fuses by 12 years of age. This however, may not appear at all.

The C3–C7 vertebrae exhibit similar development with three primary ossification centres: one for the body and one each for each neural arch. The neural arches fuse posteriorly by 2–3 years of age

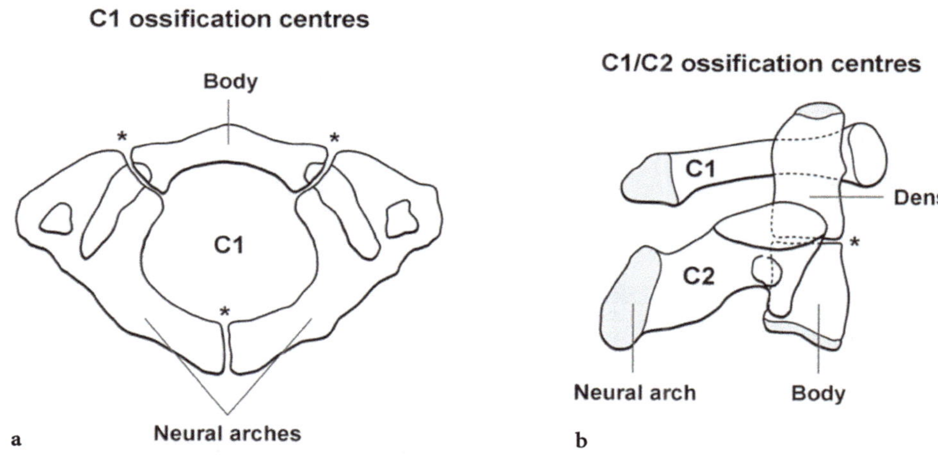

Fig. 20.1a,b. C1/C2 ossification centres as seen in the axial plane (**a**) and sagittal plane (**b**). The synchondroses are marked by an *asterisk*. The secondary centres of ossification are *shaded in grey*

and the body fuses with the neural arches between 3–6 years.

The thoracolumbar vertebrae have three primary ossification centres: one for the body and one each for the neural arches. The neural arches fuse between 1–3 years and the body fuses with the arches between 3–6 years.

At puberty five secondary centres appear, one for each transverse process, one for the spinous process and two ring apophyses for the circumferential parts of the upper and lower surfaces of the vertebral bodies. The hyaline cartilaginous endplate of early childhood at either surface of the vertebral body becomes thin centrally and thicker peripherally and becomes the *ring apophysis*. This is the secondary ossification centre of the end plate and is first seen at approximately 5 years of age. This is seen initially at the anterior inferior and anterior superior corners of the developing vertebral body as grooves and must not be mistaken as fractures. Calcification begins in this area at about 6–8 years of age in girls and 7–9 years of age in boys. These calcific foci unite around the vertebral body by 12 years of age to form the ring apophysis. The ring apophysis is parallel to the superior and inferior vertebral margins. These apophyses fuse with the rest of the vertebral body at about 17 years of age. The ring apophysis is the place where ligaments and discs attach and is an area of active growth. There are significant biomechanical forces acting on this area.

When tensile forces are applied to the spine, it is usually the physes that fail first. Partial or complete physeal separations can occur before the physes fuse. Therefore, before 6–8 years of age, the physes associated with the primary ossification centres may fail. After this age the physeal weakness exists at the apical odontoid physis, ring apophysis and the other secondary ossification centres.

20.2.3 Soft Tissues

There are multiple ligaments at the cranio-cervical junction which are important in injuries to this region (Fig. 20.2a,b). The anterior and posterior atlanto-occipital membranes extend from the anterior and posterior arches of C1 to the anterior and posterior margins of the foramen magnum. The tectorial membrane is a superior extension of the posterior longitudinal ligament and attaches to the anterolateral aspects of the foramen magnum. Anterior to the tectorial membrane is the cruciate ligament which has a vertical component extending superiorly to the occiput and a horizontal component, the transverse ligament. The transverse ligament extends from the tubercle on the inner aspect of one side to the atlas to the tubercle on the other side posterior to the odontoid process. The transverse ligament helps to control anterior movement of the atlas with respect to the axis. The apical ligament lies between the clivus and the apex of the dens. This ligament has an accompanying artery and vein. The vertical component of cruciate and the apical ligaments are weak ligaments and do not contribute significantly to atlanto-occipital stability. The alar ligament typically extends superiorly from the lateral aspect of the upper dens to the medial inferior aspect of the occipital condyles. The alar ligament limits the atlanto-axial rotation to the contra-lateral side. Alar ligament tear

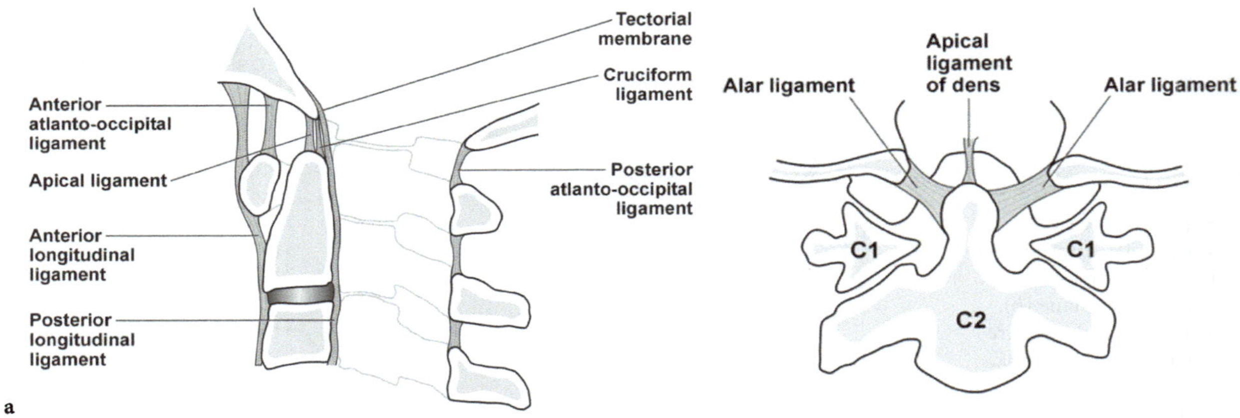

Fig. 20.2a,b. Ligaments at the cranio-cervical junction seen in the sagittal (**a**) and coronal (**b**) planes

can therefore result in a higher degree of contralateral rotation. The tectorial and alar ligaments are the main restrictors of atlanto-occipital extension. The anterior atlanto-axial ligament extends from the anterior mid portion of the dens to the inferior aspect of the anterior arch of C1.

The atlanto-dens interval (ADI) is the distance between the anterior aspect of the dens and the posterior aspect of the anterior ring of the atlas. While the normal ADI in adults is normally 3 mm, in children this can be up to 5 mm. An ADI of >5 mm in flexion and >4 mm in extension is abnormal. The distance is wider in children due to the lucent cartilage in the interval combined with the hyper mobility. The dens may be slightly posteriorly tilted in up to 4% of normal children and should be differentiated from acute fractures (Swischuk et al. 1979). The posterior tilting may result in a spuriously increased ADI in the cranial aspect due to a V shaped appearance to the joint. Normal ADI is noted at the caudal aspect of the joint in such cases.

The pre-vertebral soft tissue thickness is increased in children. A pre-vertebral space of less than 6 mm at C3 level is normal. Widening of the pre-vertebral space can be seen in expiration and in crying. A repeat radiograph in extension and inspiration would help to exclude this. The pre-vertebral space is unreliable in isolated posterior injuries to the spine.

20.2.4 Normal Variants

A number of normal variants are seen in the paediatric spine. These are usually due to variations in ossification and also due to hyper mobility of the spine. Consequently, these are more common in the upper cervical spine due to the hyper-mobility and complexity of ossification in this region.

20.2.4.1 Cervical Lordosis

The normal cervical lordosis may be reduced or absent in children up to 16 years of age with the neck in neutral position. The posterior inter-spinous distance is a good indicator of posterior ligamentous integrity and should not be more than 1.5 times the inter-spinous distance at either the immediately superior or inferior level (Naidich et al. 1977) and has been validated by Pennecot et al. (1984). Additionally, due to the tight ligamentous attachment between the occiput and C1, the C1–C2 inter-spinous distance can be increased on flexion which is a normal finding.

20.2.4.2 Pseudo Subluxation

Pseudo subluxation at the C2–3 level was seen in 46% of children under 8 years of age in one study on lateral flexion and extension radiographs. This can also be seen in about 14% of children at the C3–4 level to a lesser degree. Pseudo subluxation of up to 4 mm is acceptable in a child. Hyper-mobility of the paediatric spine, ligamentous laxity and a horizontal orientation of the articular surfaces in the upper cervical spine are thought to be responsible for this phenomenon. In some cases this can be so profound that it can be confused with a true injury. The posterior cervical line helps to differentiate this from true injury (Fig. 20.3a–d) (Swischuk 1977). The posterior cervical line is drawn from the anterior aspect of the spinous processes of C1 to the anterior aspect of the spinous process of C3. The anterior edge of the spinous process of C2 usually lies posterior to and within 1 mm of this line. However, it is important to note that, the posterior cervical line is only useful when there is malalignment of the C2 and C3 vertebral bodies and should not be used when the alignment is normal. If the anterior aspect of the C2 spinous process is posterior and more than 2 mm away from the posterior cervical line, a Hangman fracture is present. An abnormal posterior cervical line also occurs when the anterior aspect of the C2 spinous process lies anterior to the posterior cervical line indicating an injury to the facet joints and posterior ligament complex which promote a true C2/C3 subluxation. Further imaging is however warranted in children with persistent clinical symptoms, or with a strong clinical history even when pseudo subluxation is considered.

20.2.4.3 Pseudo Jefferson Fracture

Pseudo Jefferson fracture, or pseudo spread of the atlas on the axis, can be seen on the open mouth radiographs. The ossification of the lateral masses of C1 in young children often exceeds that of C2 .The lateral masses of the atlas therefore may overhang the axis by as much as 6 mm and is commonly seen in children less than 4 years of age and may be seen up to 7 years of age.

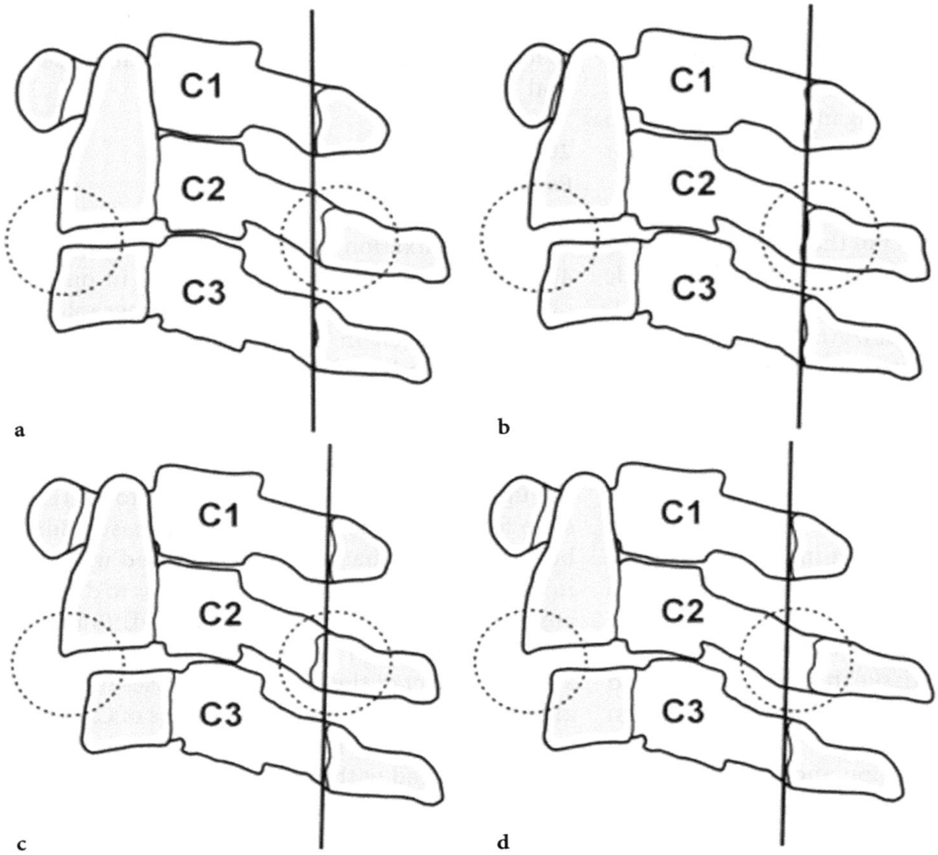

Fig. 20.3a–d. The posterior cervical line in the assessment of C2/C3 malalignment. **a** The spinolaminar junction of C2 normally lies posterior to and within 2 mm of the posterior cervical line. **b** In cases of pseudo subluxation, the spinolaminar junction of C2 can reach up to the posterior cervical line. **c** When the spinolaminar junction of C2 lies anterior to the posterior cervical line, true C2/C3 subluxation is present. **d** When the C2 spinolaminar junction lies 2 mm or more behind the posterior cervical line there is a hangman's fracture in the presence of C2/C3 subluxation

20.2.4.4 Pseudo Wedging

In early infancy vertebral bodies are ovoid in appearance. They become rectangular with advancing age. This is due to the fact that a radiograph demonstrates bony detail and therefore only the pattern of ossification rather than a true morphological appearance. Anterior wedging of vertebrae of up to 3 mm can be a normal variation and should not be confused with compression fractures. Some infants and children develop actual wedging of the ossification centres at C3 and rarely at C4 as shown by Swischuk et al. (1993). This wedging can be particularly prominent at the C3 level. This is thought to be due to the hyper-mobility of the paediatric cervical spine, resulting in an impaction of C2 on C3 in some children.

20.2.4.5 Bipartite Ossification Centres

Bipartite (anterior and posterior) ossification centres can be seen as a coronally cleft vertebral body which can be seen up to 4 years of age due to variation in endochondral ossification.

20.2.4.6 Anterior Ossification Centre

The ossification centre for the anterior arch of atlas usually appears in the first year but is present in 20% at birth. In a few cases, it may be absent resulting in a failure of anterior fusion leaving a cleft. The synchondrosis at the base of the odontoid with the C2 body fuses between 3–6 years of age but may be delayed. The vestigial outline of this fusion can be seen up to

11 years of age as a fine sclerotic line which must be differentiated from the lucent fracture line.

20.2.4.7 Congenital Spondylolysis

Congenital spondylolysis can be seen in the paediatric spine either during investigation for neck pain or for trauma. This is most commonly seen in the cervical spine at the C6 level. It can usually be clearly diagnosed from radiographs but CT can be performed for confirmation. The appearances include a spondylolytic defect with well corticated margins, hypoplastic posterior elements and an occult spina bifida. This can be difficult to detect on MR scan as the pedicle may not be clearly visualised but the diagnosis should be sought when there is an absent or hypoplastic spinous process on the sagittal sequences. A spondylolytic defect at C2 can be difficult to differentiate from a hangman's fracture.

20.2.4.8 Unfused Ring Apophysis

Unfused ring apophyses, ossification centres and secondary ossification centres can be confused with fractures. Understanding the normal anatomy and development should help in avoiding misinterpretation. Normal physeal plates are smooth, regular, have sclerotic margins and occur at predictable locations unlike acute fractures which are irregular, non-sclerotic and can occur at any location. The superior and inferior ring apophysis may not ossify simultaneously and should not be mistaken for fractures. The apical odontoid epiphysis can be seen in 26% of children between 6 and 8 years of age. The posterior ring of C1 can remain cartilaginous, become fibrous or absent though out the course of life.

20.2.4.9 Limbus Vertebrae

Limbus vertebrae occur at the anterosuperior or anteroinferior corners of single or multiple growing vertebral bodies. This is seen as a triangular radioopacity at the anterosuperior or anteroinferior margin of the vertebra frequently with adjacent indentation in the vertebral body. They can simulate fractures and although often included as "normal variants", are due to an intraosseous disc herniation usually in overuse which can be symptomatic. The bony fragment and the adjacent vertebra are well corticated with sharp margins (Fig. 20.4a–d).

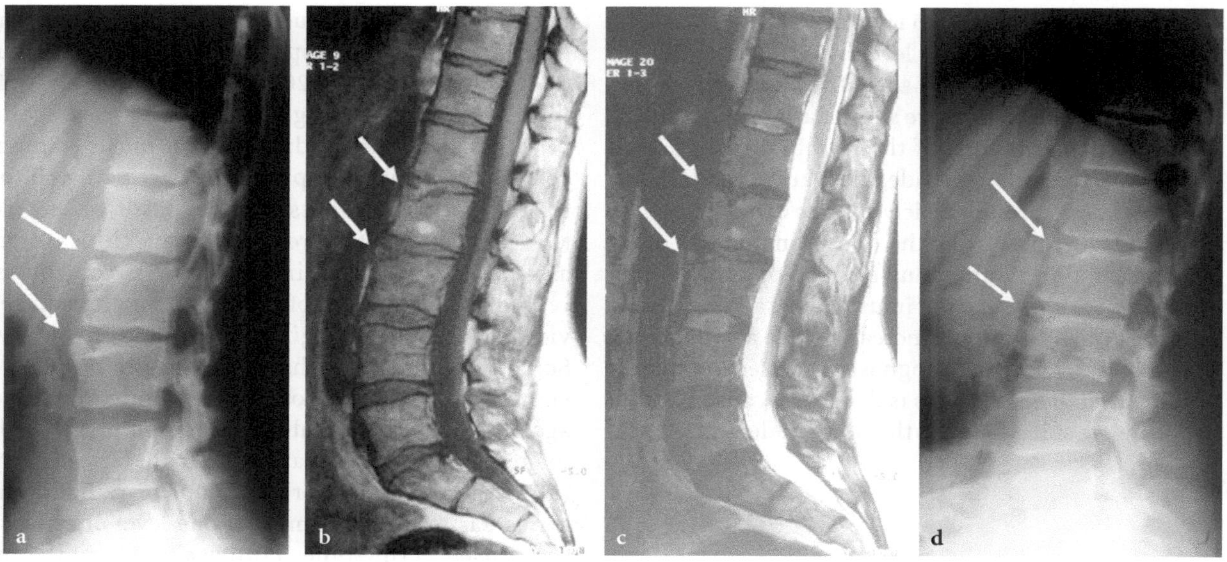

Fig. 20.4a–d. Initial lateral radiograph (**a**) in an adolescent girl shows limbus vertebrae (*white arrows*) at the L2 and L3 levels. Note the dense sclerosis and sharp margins of the triangular apophyseal fragment at the anterior superior corner with adjoining indentation of the vertebral body. The limbus fragments are nearly fused with the vertebral body on T1W (**b**) and T2W (**c**) sagittal MR images 20 years later. Lateral radiograph (**d**) performed at the same time as the MR scan demonstrates healing of these areas

20.3 Paediatric Versus Adult Spine Morphology

Injuries to the spine are rare in children but can contribute to significant morbidity and mortality. Mortality is usually due to associated injuries particularly to the cranium. Whilst cervical spine injury accounts for 30%–40% of all spinal injuries in adults, 60%–80% of all spinal injuries in children are in the cervical region (Rekate et al.1999).

The pattern of injuries to the spine in children varies from that of the adult due to a number of factors. The clinical examination may also be more challenging in children further adding to the difficulty in assessment.

The spinal column in children has an increased elasticity compared to adults and is therefore less susceptible to injury. However, the spinal cord does not share the same degree of elasticity and, therefore, spinal cord injury without radiographic abnormality (SCIWORA) is proportionally more common in children than in adults. The upper cervical spine is more susceptible to injury in young children because the fulcrum of movement of the C-spine is located in the upper C-spine in very young children due to the disproportionately large size of the head and the weak neck musculature. Previous studies have demonstrated that the maximum flexion in the cervical spine occurs at the C2/C3 level in infants, C3/C4 level by school age and C5/C6 level in adolescents (Athey 1991; Pang and Wilberger 1982). The cartilage endplates of the vertebrae are sites of attachment of ligaments at the margins of the vertebral bodies. Until fusion in the second decade, these are potential zones of weakness through which injuries can occur.

After 8 years of age, the bony components of the spinal column assume adult morphology and proportions, and the patterns of injury follow adult patterns. Whilst the mortality is increased with a younger age at injury, overall the prognosis is better in children compared to adults. This is due to the capacity of the paediatric spine for growth and remodelling.

20.4 Role of Imaging

The primary role of imaging in children with suspected spinal injury is the same as in adults. It involves identifying injury, assessing the extent and stability, identifying the cause of neurological deficit and demonstrating any concomitant injuries. Most missed spinal injuries are due to a combination of poor quality of radiographs and errors in interpretation. It is therefore essential that radiographic quality is not compromised and the imaged segment of the spine is completely visualised. Whilst interpretation skills can be developed by various means, the mere fact that most radiologists would only see a small number of paediatric spinal injuries in their professional career increases the risk of inaccurate diagnosis. Imaging is also needed to exclude injury to other areas including the viscera and brain. In particular, there is a frequent association of brain injury with cervical spine injury (Fig. 20.5a–d) and of abdominal visceral injury with lap-belt injury of the lumbar spine.

It can be more difficult to clinically assess an infant or young child than an adult and a multidisciplinary approach is indicated. A careful clinical evaluation is needed if there is a history of facial or head trauma, loss of consciousness, high speed motor vehicle accident, or birth trauma. A radiological examination should be undertaken in these circumstances and when there is an abnormality on neurological examination. The type of radiological investigation depends on the nature of injury and the clinical findings.

While the Nexus study included paediatric injuries, they had poor specificity in this age group (Hoffman et al. 1998, 2000; Viccellio et al. 2001). In the absence of clear guidelines, each case should be approached individually. The most common symptoms in cervical spine injury are pain and torticollis. Local tenderness, muscle spasm, or contracture and asymmetry are some of the clinical signs associated with spinal injury. There is controversy regarding the number of radiographic views in cervical spine injury ranging from one to five views. Some experts believe that the lateral radiograph is enough for evaluation of children under 5 years of age. Whilst the cross table radiograph picks up the majority of injuries, it has a significant false negative (21%) rate and therefore a complete radiographic series has to be performed. If one level of injury is recognised in the spine, a full evaluation of the rest of the spine should be performed to exclude injuries at other levels. The number of concomitant injuries identified in patients with spinal injury varies with imaging modality used. Studies using radiographs to evaluate the rest of the spine identified a 15% in-

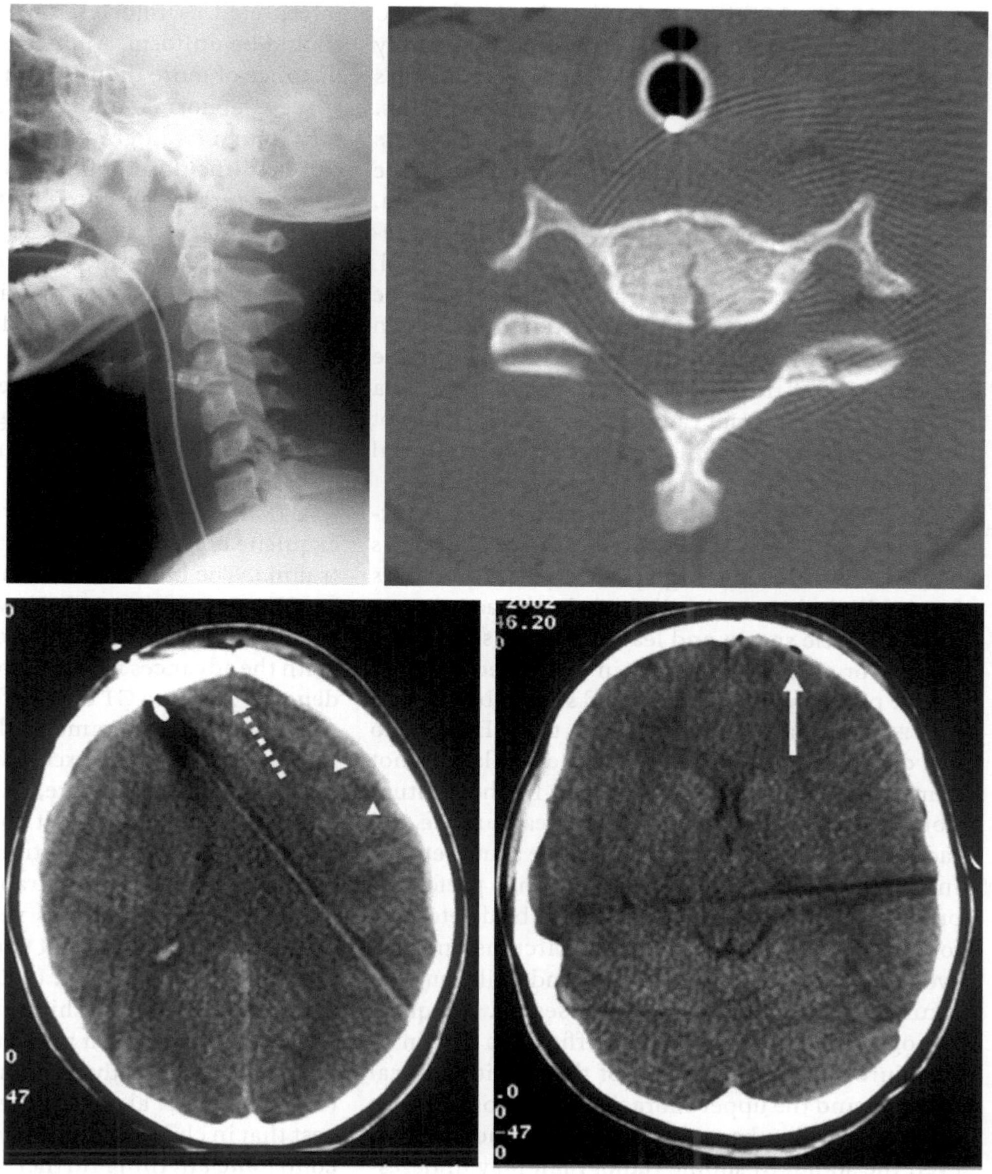

a b c d

Fig. 20.5a–d. A 14-year-old fell through a 15-ft skylight and presented with quadriparesis (C4 Frankel C). Lateral radiograph (**a**) and single axial CT section (**b**) show C5/6 three-column injuries with fractures involving the anterior, middle and posterior column. Also note the widened C5/C6 interspinous distance on the radiograph in keeping with posterior ligamentous injury. The GCS in this patient on admission was 10. Axial CT sections (**c,d**) of the cranium show a midline frontal fracture (*dashed white arrow*) and extra axial blood (*white arrowheads*) and air (*white arrows*). An intracranial pressure monitor is noted in the right frontal lobe. This case illustrates the frequent association of cervical spine and intracranial injury

cidence of concomitant injuries, while studies using MR imaging identified that 45% of patients had concomitant injuries (Henderson et al. 1991; Qaiyum et al. 2001). The clinical relevance of these additional injuries identified on MR imaging is still not clear.

The open mouth view is an area of controversy with some authors suggesting that it does not add further to evaluation and therefore can be abandoned. Obtaining the open mouth view in children can be difficult and frustrating. Some others have suggested that this view can be abandoned after two or three attempts if the lateral radiograph is entirely normal (Swischuk et al. 2000). However, Jefferson's fracture is best assessed on the open mouthed views. The Nexus study, which included children, suggests that the three view series is an appropriate first line of investigation for most patients with blunt trauma. The three view series has a 93% sensitivity for detecting cervical spine fractures (Streitwieser et al. 1983). Undisplaced posterior ring fractures may be missed by this approach. Hyperflexion injuries can be missed on initial radiographs and may only be picked up after the initial muscle spasm settles in a few days. So a normal radiographic series does not entirely exclude spinal injury and continued clinical suspicion warrants further imaging assessment.

Another area of controversy is the use of flexion/extension (F/E) views. While active F/E views have a role in evaluating spinal injuries to assess for stability, this can be difficult in the acute stage due to muscle spasm and lead to false assessments. Passive or forced F/E views in obtunded patients can be potentially hazardous and should be avoided (Griffiths et al. 2002). Moreover, the F/E views do not demonstrate a herniated disc and also do not demonstrate the state of the cord. In these situations, the F/E views may give a false reassurance. F/E radiographs should not be used in the acute setting. In most instances an MR examination is preferable prior to F/E views. The F/E views can be deleterious to the spinal cord and should in all circumstances be avoided in unconscious children and children who cannot be otherwise clinically assessed. Adequate radiographs, however, can be difficult to obtain in an injured patient especially of the cranio-cervical junction and the upper thoracic spine. Most injuries to the thoracolumbar spine produce kyphosis. However, the standard supine radiograph may underestimate the degree of kyphosis as it may be reduced in this position.

The radiographic assessment includes assessment for alignment. Lines drawn along the anterior vertebral margins, posterior vertebral margins and the spinolaminar junctions should normally curve gently. Any sudden steps in these lines should be carefully interrogated further. Some normal variations in alignment however occur in children and were discussed earlier in this chapter. The prevertebral soft tissue thickness is an important indicator of spinal injuries. It should be noted that radiographs only demonstrate the ossified elements and unossified normal cartilaginous elements may be misinterpreted as injuries. The interspinous distance should be uniform. An increase in the interspinous distance of more than 1.5 times the adjoining interspace is abnormal and suggests posterior ligamentous injury. Radiographs of the upper thoracic spine can be difficult to obtain. This area of the thoracic spine is further obscured by the overlap of the ribs and scapula. Fortunately, injuries in this area are uncommon. However, if there is clinical suspicion, further cross sectional imaging may be necessary. F/E radiographs are assessed for any acute change in the gentle curvature and for any displacement or widening of the joint spaces between the various vertebral levels. An acute angulation of more than 10 degrees at any level compared to the adjacent levels is abnormal.

CT with multiplanar reformatting demonstrates exquisite bone detail and has a crucial role in spinal trauma. The bony detail is far better demonstrated by CT compared to MR. Newer advances in multislice imaging allow isometric imaging in any axis. With the advances in technology, there is often a tendency to resort to CT even before radiographs. However, CT is not recommended for routine screening in children to avoid excessive and often unnecessary radiation. Therefore, clinical evaluation plays an important role. Whilst routine CT of the cervical spine included at the time of imaging the head with a CT scan for blunt trauma in adults has been proven to be effective in various studies (Barba et al. 2001), the same is not true in children. Furthermore, Hernandez et al. (2004) have demonstrated in their review of 606 children that CT only showed significant findings in patients where the abnormal findings were already seen on the initial radiograph (Hernandez et al. 2004). They went as far as to suggest that in children under 5 years of age, CT did not contribute anything further to the diagnosis of new spinal injuries. Studies in obtunded trauma patients utilising MDCT alone to assess cervical spine have found that no unstable injuries were missed (Hogan et al. 2005). However, ligaments and soft tissues are not adequately seen on CT. MR based studies demonstrate a higher incidence of ligamentous injuries than the CT based studies.

MR imaging is excellent at demonstrating soft tissue and cord injuries although radiography and CT scanning may show indirect signs of significant soft tissue injury like widening of the interspinous distance, widening of the disc space or divergence of articular processes. Radiographs and CT form the mainstay of imaging in the acute situation. MR imaging is most often used as a second line investigation mainly to exclude paediatric spinal injury in the absence of radiographic and CT abnormality but with persistent clinical suspicion, and also to further evaluate injuries already detected on initial imaging, particularly for assessing soft tissues and cord. MR is also performed to assess the cord prior to surgery and to evaluate for complications and sequelae. MR can be difficult to perform in the very young due to their inability to stay still during the examination and sedation may be necessary. MR can also be difficult to perform in the multiple injured patients in the acute setting due to the difficulty in monitoring the patient while in the scanner. MR should also be employed in cases of suspected soft tissue injury with normal radiographs before resorting to F/E views in children.

SCIWORA refers to spinal cord injury without radiographic abnormality. The term was first used to describe cord injury in the absence of plain radiographic abnormality by Pang and Wilberger (1982). With the evolution of imaging, two distinct definitions of SCIWORA can be identified in various publications. With the widespread use of CT along with radiographs in the initial assessment, the term is more commonly now used to describe cord injury (Fig. 20.6a–g) in the absence of radiographic or CT evidence of injury. A majority of these patients demonstrate abnormalities on MR imaging, with 6% of patients having SCIWORA by this definition in the review by Cirak et al. (2004). There is, however, a further group of patients in whom even the MR scan is normal despite definite clinical evidence of cord injury. With this definition, the incidence of SCIWORA in the review by Cirak et al. (2004) has reduced to 1%. SCIWORA is more common in children than in adults due to the variable elasticity of the cord and spinal column. SCIWORA makes up to 5%–55% of C-spine injuries in children. It is most common before 3 years of age. The main mechanisms of this type of injury are hyperextension, flexion, distraction and cord ischaemia. There is variable neurological deficit ranging from partial cord defects to complete transection. Various incomplete cord syndromes including central cord syndrome, Brown Sequard syndrome, anterior spinal cord artery syndrome and partial cord syndrome can occur depending on the site and mechanism of insult. Recurrent SCIWORA can occur if there is inadequate immobilisation or non compliance with advice regarding high risk activities. These children have an initial minor SCIWORA, but with a significant neurological deficit after the recurrent SCIWORA. Widespread use of MR imaging and careful immobilisation has reduced the incidence of recurrent SCIWORA. Nevertheless, due to the potential for persistent instability and re-injury in patients with soft tissue injuries, these patients often need long term follow-up and assessment of instability.

Whilst head imaging relies on CT and MR, spinal imaging is correctly still based on initial radiography, particularly in children. The reason for this is that the radiograph provides important information especially regarding stability. Whilst the Canadian C-spine rules provide guidelines for imaging in adults they do not apply for children. Although there are no guidelines as to a clear pathway for paediatric spine imaging, a few general principles apply. Initial imaging in suspected spinal injury includes a radiographic series depending on the level of injury. In an unconscious child after significant trauma, it is reasonable to evaluate the cervical spine at the time of a CT scan of the head. The imaging should be performed with thin slices of 1–2 mm to avoid missing subtle fractures. If there is persistent suspicion or neurological dysfunction after normal radiographs and/or CT, an MR scan should be performed. In the presence of a confirmed cervical injury, MR scan should include the whole of the spine. Sagittal TI and STIR sequences should be performed to identify non contiguous injuries. MR imaging should also be performed in all patients with neurological signs and also pre-operatively. F/E radiographs in the acute setting may be associated with both false positive and false negative results and should be avoided. In summary, unlike cranial trauma, it is unlikely that CT will replace radiographs in spinal trauma.

20.5 Upper Cervical Spine

The upper C-spine up to the C2/C3 disc space is a unique region of the paediatric spine. The development of this part of the C-spine is more related to the occiput than the rest of the spine as described earlier. The large size of the head changes the fulcrum of the neck motion to the upper cervical spine. Hypermobility of the spine secondary to ligamentous laxity and the horizontally orientated facets allow increased anterior translation.

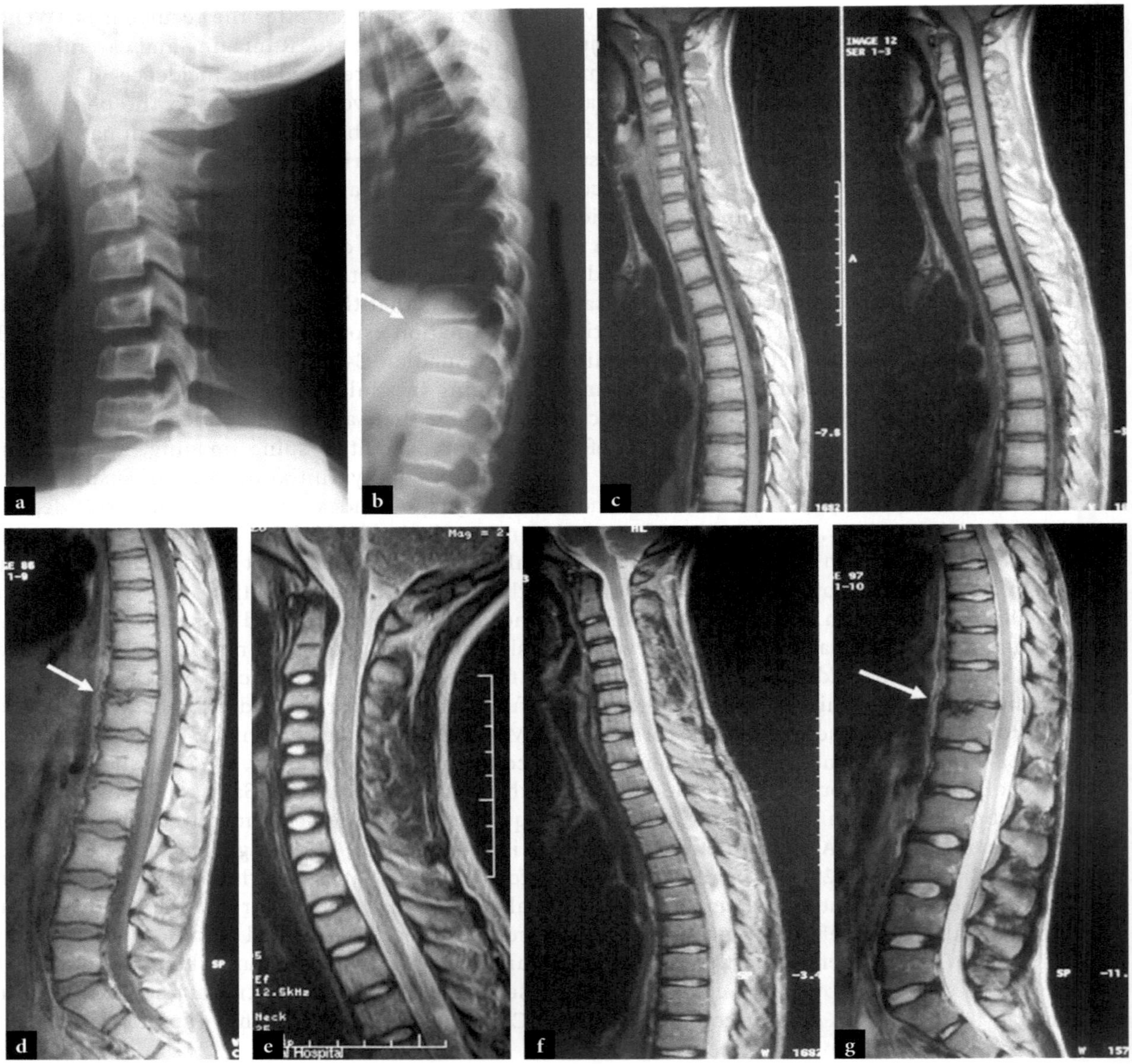

Fig. 20.6a–g. SCIWORA in a 12-year-old boy who fell off a 3-ft fence and presented with weakness in both lower limbs (T3 Frankel C paraplegia). Lateral radiographs of the cervical (**a**) and thoracic spine (**b**) shows no evidence of any significant injury. (**c–g**) T1W and T2W sagittal images representing the whole spine do not demonstrate any acute osteoligamentous injury or cord/neurological injury. Note the anterosuperior intraosseous disc herniation (*arrows*) at the T12 level with surrounding sclerosis on radiographs and absence of oedema in the adjacent vertebral body of T12 on the MR images in keeping with a chronic disc herniation. The patient demonstrated neurological recovery from T3 Frankel C to T4 Frankel D gradually. A normal MRI scan in SCIWORA is a good prognostic indicator

The younger the age of the child, the more common are the upper C-spine injuries. The upper c-spine injuries account for 70% of all C-spine injuries in children compared to 16% in adults (Sherk et al. 1976). Injuries from occiput to C4 accounted for all deaths which were solely by spinal injuries in one large study (Cirak et al. 2004).

20.5.1 Osseous Injury

20.5.1.1 Atlas Fractures

The Jefferson's fracture occurs as a result of axial compression injury on the vertex, either due to a fall or a blow to the head. The axial loading is transmitted through the occipital condyles onto the atlas. This results in a comminuted fracture of the atlas involving both the anterior and posterior arches. This should be differentiated from the pseudo Jefferson's fracture (pseudo spreading) which is a normal variant and also from developmental defects in the arches of the atlas. Jefferson's fracture is a rare injury while pseudo spreading is seen not uncommonly in children. Clinical history also helps to differentiate a true fracture from an anatomical variant. This fracture may sometimes pass through the normal synchondrosis, which is best appreciated on CT. Radiography demonstrates pre-vertebral soft tissue swelling. This, however, can be difficult to appreciate in young children due to the normal lymphoid tissue in the nasopharynx. The swelling may also be absent. The fracture line may be seen on the lateral view. Open mouth view demonstrates bilateral spreading of the lateral masses of C1 with respect to C2. Jefferson's fracture can be stable or unstable, depending on the integrity of the transverse ligament. The degree of lateral mass offset on the open mouthed view helps to differentiate stable from unstable injury. A bilateral combined offset of less than 7 mm is seen in a stable injury while a combined offset of more than 7 mm implies an unstable injury. A distance of 6 mm or more between the lateral mass of C1 and the odontoid process on the open mouthed view is also suggestive of transverse ligament disruption. There is also an increase in the atlanto-axial distance on the lateral view in the unstable injury. Isolated injuries of the anterior or posterior arch of atlas can also occur rarely.

20.5.1.2 C2 Fractures

The C2 vertebra has the most complex development and a problem with differentiation between developmental anomalies and a fracture can arise. The Hangman fracture is a fracture involving the pars interarticularis of the C2 usually caused by hyperextension injury. There may be intra-articular extension of the injury. Anterior subluxation of C2 on C3 due to intervertebral disc injury may be associated. Hangman's fracture has to be differentiated from congenital spondylolysis of C2. Spondylolysis of C2 has been reported previously but has been suggested to be a synchondrosis by some authors. However, posterior arch synchondrosis should not be visible on a true lateral radiograph and, therefore, any osseous defect seen on a lateral radiograph should be considered to be a fracture or a congenital defect. These congenital osseous defects can be seen in sclerosing dysplasias and pyknodysostosis. The presence of an osseous gap with smooth sclerotic margins in the pars interarticularis is in favour of a spondylolysis. The absence of pre vertebral soft tissue swelling and instability on F/E views also supports a spondylolytic defect against a fracture. In the presence of a significant history of trauma, any osseous defect should be considered to be due to the trauma itself and treated accordingly. Follow-up imaging may then help to make the definitive diagnosis.

20.5.1.3 Odontoid Fractures

Traumatic synchondrosis disruption injuries can occur at two locations at C2. The disruption can occur at either the dens/vertebral body synchondrosis or the vertebral body/posterior arch (neuro-central) synchondrosis. The odontoid process/C2 vertebral body synchondrosis injury results in an anterior slip of the odontoid process with respect to the C2 vertebral body. The cranial aspect of the odontoid will be tilted anteriorly (Fig 20.7a–d). This can be appreciated on a lateral radiograph. When there is no displacement, diagnosis can be difficult with radiography alone. On the other hand, as described earlier posterior angulation of the tip of the odontoid process can be seen in normal children. CT can demonstrate the disruption better. The odontoid injury is usually stable and can be reduced by gentle manipulation into extension. Neurological deficit is unlikely except when associated with more than 50% displacement.

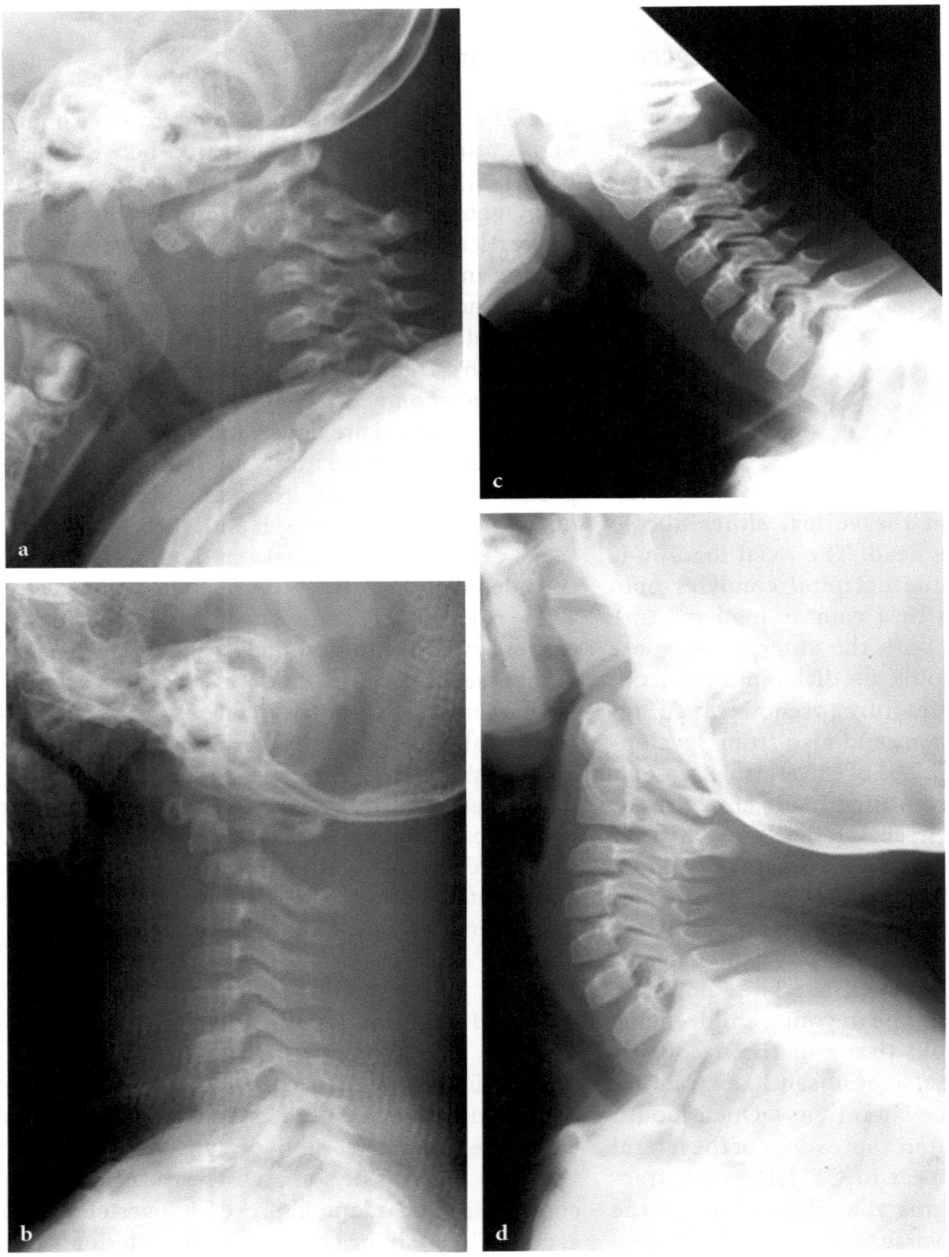

Fig. 20.7a–d. A 2-year-old back seat passenger involved in a head on collision. Initial radiograph (**a**) demonstrates a fracture through the basal synchondrosis of the C2 odontoid process with significant anterior displacement. Note the extensive soft tissue swelling anteriorly. Despite the dramatic appearances, the child was neurologically intact. This is not uncommon with this type of fracture due to the relatively capacious spinal canal at this level. Lateral radiograph obtained after initial traction and application of Minerva cast (**b**) shows a reasonable position. Flexion (**c**) and extension (**d**) radiographs 3 years later following conservative management demonstrate satisfactory healing with no instability

20.5.1.4 Os Odontoideum

The vascular supply to the dens is located above the synchondrosis and therefore, these fractures usually heal without any complications. In cases of non-union, the apical fragment continues to retain blood supply and forms a well defined rounded ossicle called the "os odontoideum". Trauma is thought to be responsible for os odontoideum rather than failure of fusion of ossification centres. It is seen on radiographs as a smooth well corticated ossicle separated from the hypoplastic dens by a variable gap. It can be either orthotopic when it is located at the normal position of the odontoid process or dystopic when it is located close to the base of the occiput close to the foramen magnum due to its attachment by to the alar ligament. Most patients have instability of the affected spinal segment. The os odontoideum can have a variable degree of movement and therefore can cause spinal cord impingement and compression in some cases. Neurological injury can occur even from minor trauma in these cases. MR imaging in F/E assesses the degree of instability.

20.5.2 Joint Injuries

20.5.2.1 Atlanto-occipital Dislocation (AOD)

Atlanto-occipital dislocation (AOD) is 2.5 times as common in children compared to adults. Young children are more susceptible to this injury due to the small occipital condyles and horizontally orientated articular surfaces. It is usually fatal due to the involvement of the brainstem, the upper cervical cord, upper cervical and lower cranial nerves. Lower cranial nerve injury is the most common neurological abnormality (WOODRING et al. 1981). This is caused by a sudden deceleration and deployment of air bags. The injury is associated with injury to the tectorial membrane and the alar ligaments. Anterior subluxation of the cranium relative to the cervical spine is typical but superior or posterior dislocation can also occur. Radiographic evaluation can be difficult due to rotation and superimposition of structures like the mastoid process in this region. CT with sagittal reconstructions is best for assessing this injury as this can be performed without moving the patient.

A significant pre-vertebral soft tissue swelling is usually associated with this injury. A gap of more than 5 mm between the occipital condyles and the condylar surface of the atlas is indicative of AOD. There is displacement of the basion with respect to the odontoid process or malalignment between the spino-laminar line of atlas and posterior lip of foramen magnum. The distance between the basion and the tip of the odontoid should normally be less than 12.5 mm (Fig. 20.8) (BULAS et al. 1993). Another method used is the Wachenheim clivus line, a line drawn along the posterior aspect of the clivus down towards the odontoid process. AOD should be suspected if this line does not intersect the odontoid process. The Powers ratio is useful in assessing for this injury and is based on a ratio rather than an absolute measurement, so that it is unaffected by patient size or film magnification (Fig. 20.8) (POWERS et al. 1979). The Powers ratio is a ratio between the distance from the anterior rim of foramen magnum to the spino-laminar junction of the atlas and the distance between the posterior rim of foramen magnum and the posterior aspect of the anterior arch of atlas. A ratio less than 1.0 is normal, while a ratio of greater than 1.0 is abnormal and suggestive of AOD. The ratio is useful in the common anterior AOD, but is not reliable in posterior AOD and when there are associated fractures of the atlas or congenital abnormalities. CT additionally shows haemorrhage in the region including extra-dural haemorrhage. MR can also demonstrate this injury and demonstrate ligamentous structures better. It can also demonstrate the state of the cord and medulla.

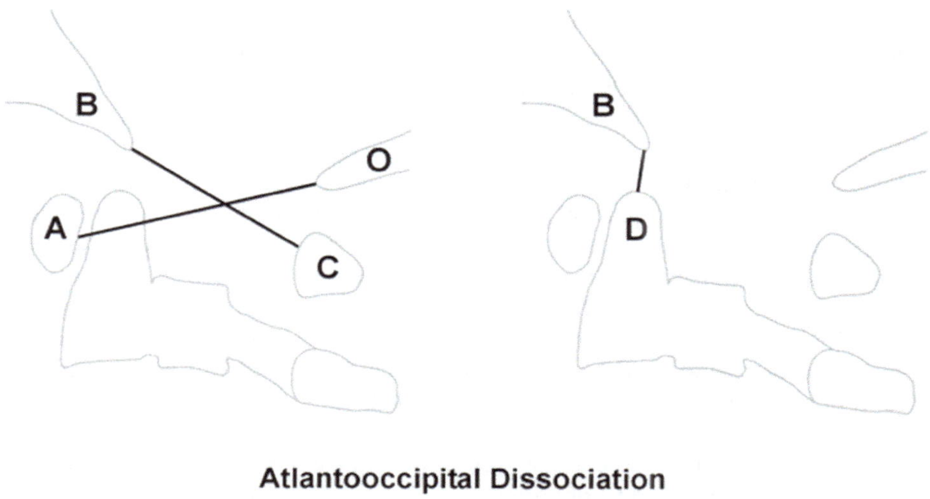

Fig. 20.8. The measurements used in assessment for atlanto-occipital dissociation. *B*, tip of basion; *C*, spinolaminar junction of atlas; *A*, posterior aspect of the anterior arch of atlas; *O*, posterior lip of foramen magnum; *D*, tip of dens. Powers ratio: BC/OA should normally be less than 1. The distance BD should normally be less than 12.5 mm

20.5.2.2
Traumatic Subluxation of C2 over C3

Traumatic subluxation of C2 over C3 can be difficult to differentiate from physiological subluxation seen in children. The clinical history of a hyperflexion injury, neck pain and specific tenderness at the spinous process of C2 are useful indicators of injury. Initial radiographs may not provide a definitive diagnosis without evidence of an abnormal posterior cervical line (Fig. 20.3a–d). However, serial radiographs may demonstrate the progressive subluxation and localised kyphosis. Mineralization may be seen adjacent to the C2 spinous process on follow-up radiographs as part of the healing of posterior soft tissues including supra-spinous ligament, inter-spinous ligament or paraspinal muscles. The mineralization may also be due to the avulsion of the secondary ossification centres from the spinous processes.

20.5.2.3
Atlantoaxial Dislocation

Atlantoaxial dislocation is a horizontal excessive motion between the odontoid and atlas of more than 5 mm due to rupture of the transverse ligament. The ligament is elastic and retracts once ruptured indicating an unstable injury. F/E radiographs demonstrate the increase in the distance between the anterior surface of the dens and the posterior surface of the anterior arch of atlas. This is an uncommon injury but can be associated with other cervical spine fractures in children. The incidence of this injury is increased in children with Down's syndrome, Klippel-Fiel deformity, skeletal dysplasias and inflammatory arthropathies. In children less than 7 years of age, the synchondrosis at the base of the dens is likely to fail before a rupture of the transverse ligament. The atlas usually displaces anteriorly with respect to the odontoid process. The atlanto-dens interval is increased and can reach up to 10 mm with isolated transverse ligament injuries. Further displacement usually requires alar and other ligament failure. Concomitant displacement of the C1 spino-laminar line with respect to C2 is seen and can be useful in children with incompletely ossified dens which makes radiographic detection difficult. Significant amount of displacement can be tolerated without cord damage at this level due to a capacious canal at this level. MR can be performed in flexion and extension to assess this injury. However, the head coil may prevent adequate flexion and extension to be obtained.

20.5.2.4
Atlanto-axial Rotatory Fixation

Atlanto-axial rotatory fixation is variously also referred to as atlanto-axial rotatory subluxation and atlanto-axial rotatory dislocation. However, atlanto-axial rotatory fixation (AARF) is the preferred term as rotatory fixation occurs within the normal range of rotation of the joint. It was previously thought that, in AARF, C1 and C2 must always be locked as one unit. However, patients with AARF have been shown to have some preservation of inter-segmental motion but manifest various degrees of pathological "stickiness" between C1 and C2. There is therefore abnormal rather than absent relative motion between the atlas and axis on rotation.

The normal range of cervical rotation is approximately 90 degrees to each side. Rotation is initiated at the atlanto-axial joint and half of the cervical spine rotation occurs at the atlanto-axial joints. This is facilitated by the horizontal orientation of the facets at this level. The dens acts as the pivot around which this rotation occurs. The multiple ligaments attached to the dens act as stabilising structures. The C1 rotation is almost complete before rotation of C2 and then rotation at the lower cervical vertebral levels begin. During normal rotation, C1 rotates alone in the first 23 degrees. From 24°–65° C1 and C2 move together but C1 always moves at a faster rate. From 65° onwards C1 and C2 move together in exact unison (Pang and Li 2004). The ipsilateral lateral mass of C1 rotates posteriorly into the spinal canal during rotation. This narrows the spinal canal but does not usually result in neurological dysfunction as the spinal canal is most capacious at this level. When rotation exceeds normal limits, the odontoid process can injure the cord and adjacent structures like the vertebral arteries. A wide range of normal rotation occurs at the atlanto-axial joints due to the horizontal orientation of the articular facets. This increased motion, however, comes at an expense of stability. Stability is provided by the transverse and alar ligaments which prevent anterior translation and excessive rotation, respectively.

AARF can be traumatic or more commonly atraumatic. The commonest cause is idiopathic. Other causes include trauma, infection, surgery to the head and neck region, inflammatory arthropathy and congenital anomalies of the cervical spine. Most cases resolve spontaneously. In a few cases AARF becomes fixed and irreducible. Fielding and Hawkins (1977) classified AARF into four types: (Fig. 20.9a–d)

- Type 1: Rotatory fixation without anterior displacement of the atlas. This is the most common type of AARF and occurs within the normal range of rotatory motion. The transverse ligament is intact and the atlanto-axial distance is normal.
- Type 2: rotatory fixation with anterior displacement of atlas of 3–5 mm. This is associated with deficiency of the transverse ligament and is the second most common type of AARF.
- Type 3: AARF with anterior displacement of the atlas of more than 5 mm. This is due to a deficiency of both the transverse and alar ligaments.
- Type 4: AARF with posterior displacement of the atlas and occurs with a deficiency of odontoid process. This is the least common type.

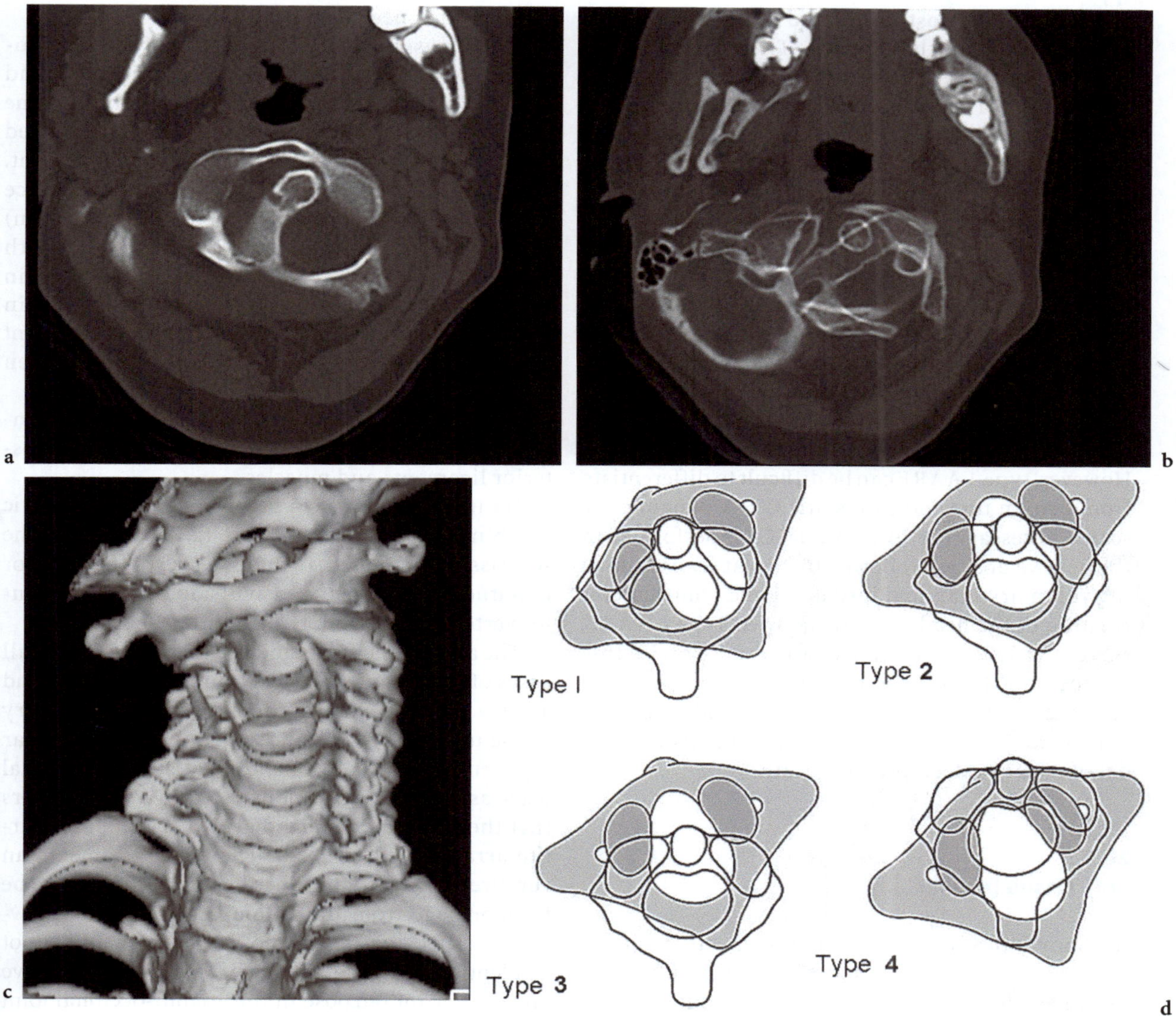

Fig. 20.9. a–c Atlanto-axial rotatory fixation (AARF) with composite axial CTs and 3D reconstruction showing a Type 2 AARF. **d** Diagrammatic representation of AARF Type 1, rotatory fixation without anterior displacement (occurs within normal range of motion). Type 2, rotatory fixation with atlas displacement of up to 5 mm. Type 3, anterior displacement of more than 5 mm. Type 4, posterior displacement. Image modified from Banit and Murrey (2005)

AARF presents with torticollis and a reduced range of neck rotation. The head is tilted to one side and rotated to the other side with a slight flexion. Types 2–4 are associated with spinal canal compromise and neurological signs. Vertebral artery compromise may occur with severe rotation. The assessment on radiographs is difficult as it is difficult to differentiate abnormal C1/C2 relationship in AARF from that seen in a normal child with head rotation. A normal C1/C2 relationship is not seen despite a well orientated lateral radiograph in AARF. On the open mouthed view, one lateral mass of C1 is rotated anteriorly and appears wider and closer to the midline while the other is rotated posteriorly and appears narrower and farther from the midline. These appearances may however be seen even in normal children with a rotated head. The odontoid/lateral mass asymmetry on open mouth views can also be seen incidentally. Dynamic fluoroscopy can demonstrate the fixed C1/C2 relationship. Spinous process deviation from the midline is also a good indicator of rotation at this level. These appearances on radiographs with a typical clinical picture should, however, arouse suspicion. Radiographs and fluoroscopy can be confusing and the patient may not be able to cooperate sufficiently. CT in the resting state and also with maximal rotation to the contralateral side is the best method for evaluation. Axial CT demonstrates the C1/C2 relationship well. Static CT is diagnostic for types 2–4 AARF. However, type 1 AARF can be difficult to differentiate from benign torticollis on static CT. A dynamic CT scan is necessary for this. An axial CT is performed in the neutral position followed by repeat scans following voluntary maximal ipsilateral and contralateral rotation of the head. In patients with Type 1 AARF, there is little or no rotation of atlas on axis with this manoeuvre. In transient torticollis, a reversal or reduction of rotation occurs. Although MR imaging may demonstrate the osseous relationship, osseous detail is not as clear as on CT scans.

20.5.3 Soft Tissue Injuries

All bony injuries are associated with soft tissue injuries. Sometimes, these soft tissue injuries may be severe enough to be the main cause of the patient's morbidity. Initial radiographs do not reveal the true extent of this soft tissue injury. This can, however, be deduced from the bony appearances and relationships. Radiological features of soft tissue and ligamentous injuries include widening of the interspinous distance, loss of parallelism of the articular facets, kyphosis at the disc space with opening up of the posterior disc space. Repeat follow-up radiographs may demonstrate secondary changes from soft tissue injuries like soft tissue mineralization and progressive instability. CT with reconstructions and more importantly, MR imaging is best to demonstrate soft tissue detail. Soft tissue injuries, unlike bony injuries may not heal completely even with prolonged conservative treatment. The injured soft tissues often do not regain full strength and are therefore susceptible to recurrent injury or persistent instability. Therefore, these injuries often need surgical treatment.

AOD is associated with rupture of the atlanto-occipital ligaments including the alar ligament and tectorial membrane along with capsular injury. The unstable variant of Jefferson's fracture is associated with rupture of the transverse atlantal ligament. This results in an increased atlanto-dens distance on the lateral radiograph and an increased (>7 mm) spread of the atlas over axis on the open mouth view. The transverse ligament is also ruptured in atlanto-axial dislocation. It can also be injured in forced flexion of the skull. The transverse ligament undergoes regressive changes with age and can then rupture more easily.

Subluxation of C2 over C3 is associated with inter-vertebral disc injury and also injury to the posterior ligaments and muscles.

Hangman's fracture involves a characteristic combination of bone and soft tissue injuries. The soft tissue component includes a tear of the anterior longitudinal ligament and avulsion of the C2/C3 inter vertebral disc from the adjoining endplates.

The alar ligaments are injured in up to a third of all cases of fatal cranio-cervical trauma (Saternus and Thrun 1987). In some of these cases, the only injury in the upper cervical spine was an injury to the alar ligament. The alar ligament can also suffer partial tears as it has been demonstrated by these authors that the alar ligament can have a variable multipartite arrangement of fibres. The apical ligament can rupture along with the other ligaments. There can be haemorrhage from the accompanying artery. However, isolated injuries to the apical ligament cannot be identified on imaging. The ligament does not serve any significant purpose in the atlanto-occipital joint although it bears physiological stresses with flexion and extension (Saternus and Thrun 1987).

Alar ligament and transverse ligament injuries are associated with AARF as discussed earlier. The tectorial membrane can be ruptured in flexion and extension injuries along with transverse ligament injury or odontoid fracture. This can result in epidural haematoma which is usually seen posteriorly in the cranio-cervical region from posterior ligamentous injuries. The flexion injury also results in tears in the soft tissues and muscles posteriorly.

Extension traction on the intervertebral disc can result in anterior separation of the annulus fibrosis from the vertebral endplate and is associated with rupture of the anterior longitudinal ligament. With axial loading the disc material can herniated through the endplates in older children resulting in acute 'Schmorl's node' lesions.

20.6 Lower C-Spine

The lower five cervical vertebrae are similar in development, morphology and injury patterns and differ from the upper two vertebrae. Lower C-spine injuries are more common in older children and adolescents and are usually due to sports or motor vehicle accidents.

20.6.1 Osseous Injuries

The typical fractures in the sub-axial cervical spine are usually compression fractures of the vertebral body and facet fractures.

20.6.1.1 Compression Fracture

The intervertebral disc in the paediatric spine has greater resistance to herniation. Therefore, there is a tendency to compression fracture with flexion and axial loading. Simple compression fractures are stable and heal satisfactorily. With severe axial loading, burst fractures can occur. The posterior vertebral line is a useful sign to assess this injury. There is retropulsion into the spinal canal which can be satisfactorily assessed on CT. MR imaging is optimal for the effects of the retropulsion on cord and nerve roots. Compression and burst fractures are discussed in detailed in Sections 20.7.1.2 and 20.7.1.4.

20.6.1.2 Spinous Process Fractures

C6 and C7 are particularly susceptible to spinous process injuries. Traction injuries occur in flexion and compression injuries occur in extension. In extension the spinous processes impact against each other. Clay-shoveler's fracture is an oblique fracture of the spinous process of the C6–T3 vertebrae due to avulsion by supra-spinous ligament injury. The juvenile form is referred to as Schmitt's disease. The avulsion may not be visible on initial radiographs in children due to unossified centre here. However, follow-up radiographs will show callus formation and ossification along the supra spinous ligament.

20.6.1.3 Physeal/Apophyseal Injury

Physeal injuries can occur anywhere in the spinal column but are most common in the lower cervical spine. The ossification at the ring apophysis starts at 6–8 years of age. Before this age, the physis are not radiographically visible and a physeal injury may be missed. Physeal injuries are seen radiographically as displacement of the ossified apophysis. There may be a widened fissure between the vertebral body and endplate. There may be widened inter vertebral space, which may be localised either anteriorly or more commonly, posteriorly. In the lower cervical spine these usually involve the inferior growth plate and can be multiple. The uncinate process provides a mechanical support against this injury of the vertebral bodies. The uncinate process is however underdeveloped in very young children and makes them susceptible to these injuries. These injuries may be radiologically inapparent. Aufdermaur (1974) has demonstrated in his necropsy studies that these injuries are more common than initially thought. In a series of 12 autopsies, he noted that only one endplate lesion was identified radiographically ante-mortem while all the patients had endplate injury on autopsy.

Although these physis are strictly apophysis/physis junctions, a Salter- Harris type epiphysis/physis junction injury classification has been proposed for these injuries. Radiographically, the clues to these injuries are the widening of the intervertebral space and displacement of the ossified fragments (Fig. 20.10a–d, 20.11a–d). In type I

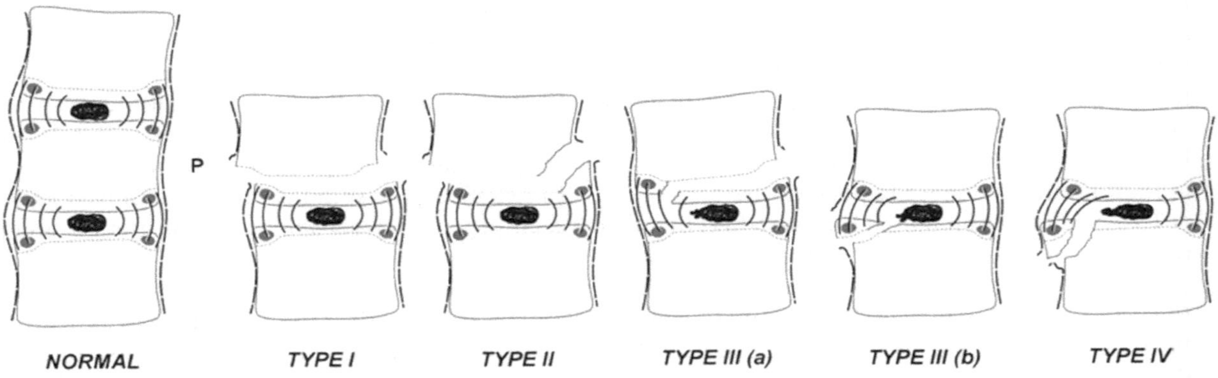

Fig. 20.10. Classification of growth plate injuries. Type I: There is complete separation of the physis from the underlying vertebral body. Associated tears of the anterior longitudinal ligament (ALL) and posterior longitudinal ligament (PLL) result in vertebral displacement. The intervertebral disc is intact in this type of injury. Type II: There is incomplete separation of the physis along with a corner flake of the vertebral body. The intervertebral disc is intact. Type III: This injury is a combination of physeal and intervertebral disc injury. In Type IIIA, the PLL is torn but the ALL is preserved. In Type IIIB, the ALL is torn but the PLL is intact. Type IV: There is a fracture of the vertebral body that traverses the physis and the intervertebral disc

injuries there is complete separation at the growth plate/vertebral body junction. There can be a significant displacement in this injury with return of the fragments together. This may then be missed on radiographs as the ossified physis are in a normal anatomical position at the time of radiography. Type III injuries are more common in the adolescent as the physis begin to close. There is a considerable underestimation of these injuries as the cartilaginous components of these injuries are not seen on radiographs. Even MR imaging may miss these injuries as it may not show displaced ossified fragments well. Furthermore, if the injury is completely through cartilage, MR imaging may not show any abnormality in the bones. Whilst types II and III may heal with conservative treatment due to the presence of bony injury, type I injuries frequently need surgery. The cervical ring apophyseal avulsion is at the superior apophysis in flexion injuries and at the inferior physis in extension injuries. Follow-up radiographs demonstrate new bone formation at the sites of these injuries. Apophyseal injury is seen as a partial separation of the ring apophysis and can occur anywhere along the vertebral outline. It is most common either anteriorly or posteriorly on the lateral radiograph. This is due to chronic overuse injury and results in a limbus vertebra. These can simulate acute fractures and can be diagnosed on radiographs but are best seen on CT and MR Imaging.

20.6.1.4
Tear-Drop Fracture

This is a fracture dislocation with a burst configuration consisting of a comminuted vertebral body fracture with a characteristic triangular or quadrilateral fragment from the anterior inferior margin of the vertebral body and is associated with a high incidence of cord injury (Fig. 20.12a–e). The seemingly innocuous small anterior inferior fragment is usually associated with a posterior dislocation of the remainder of the vertebral body associated with facet joint and posterior ligamentous disruption. There is usually a sagittal split in the vertebral body. This is also accompanied by fractures of the posterior neural arch.

In the immature spine, hyperextension injury can produce an avulsion of the anterior inferior ring apophysis. This is similar to a tear drop fracture seen in adults. This is however not associated with other osseous injury or neurological damage. Healing of the avulsed apophysis looks like a pronounced bony excrescence on follow-up radiographs.

20.6.1.5
Facet Fracture

These may be associated with facet joint dislocations. These result from extension rotation injuries. Unilateral fractures are more common than bilateral frac-

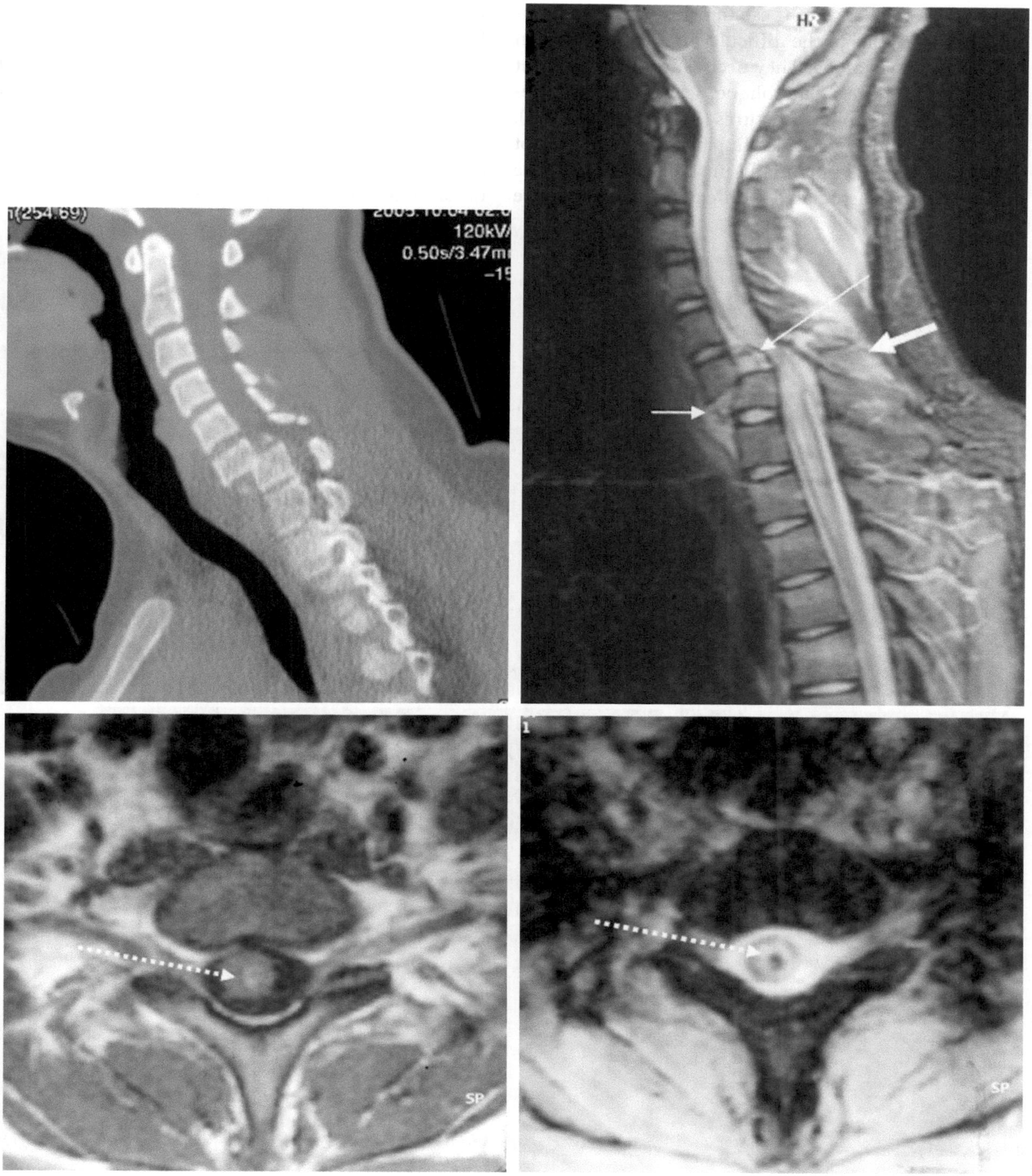

a b c d

Fig. 20.11a–d. A 16-year-old scooter rider involved in an RTA who presented with complete tetraplegia (C6 Frankel A). Sagittal CT reconstruction (**a**) and sagittal T2W MR (**b**) images show the severe fracture dislocation at C6/C7 level. The MR shows the associated soft tissue injuries including stripping of the anterior (*short white arrow*)and posterior (*long white arrow*) longitudinal ligaments, disruption of the posterior ligament complex (*wide arrow*) and prevertebral soft tissue swelling. There is cord compression and extensive cord signal change. Haemorrhage within the cord (*dashed white arrows*) is represented as low and high signal foci within the cord on the axial T2W (**c**) and T1W (**d**) images, respectively, and is suggestive of poor prognosis tures. The incidence of these injuries is probably underestimated due to the difficulty in identifying them on radiographs alone. They occur most commonly at the C6 and C7 levels. The oblique views are useful in detecting articular pillar fractures (McCall et al. 1973). However, oblique views needing head rotation are not preferable in this potentially unstable situation. The facet fractures associated with extension injuries are vertical against flexion fractures which are horizontal. Flexion injuries are associated with facet dislocations and usually involve the tip of the superior articular process of the inferior vertebra involved. These may not be appreciated on radiographs and need CT. Reconstructions of thin slices are essential to adequately assess facets on CT scanning due to the variable orientation of the facets to the scanning plane.

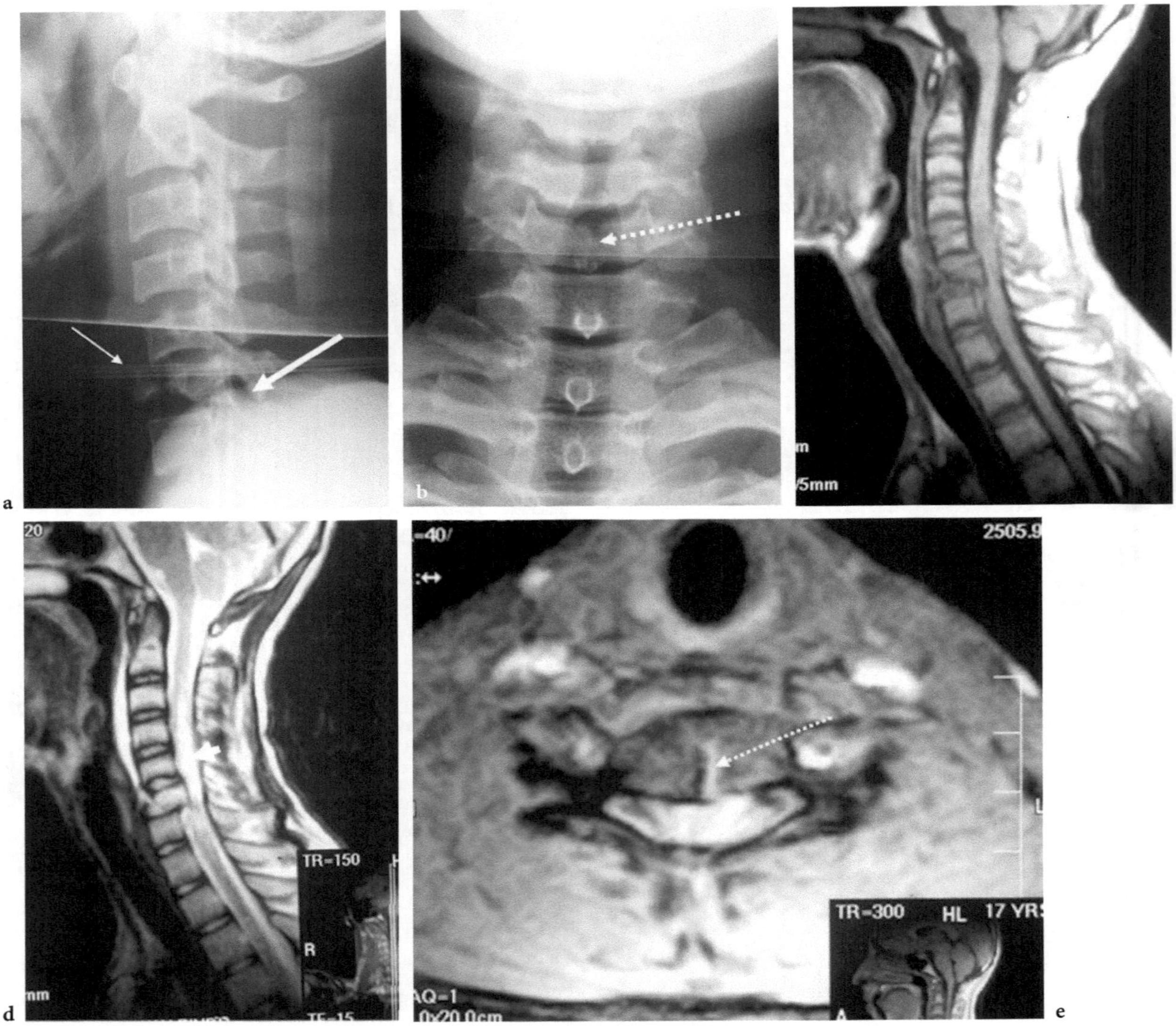

Fig. 20.12a–e. A 16-year-old fell 12 ft from a roof top and presented with complete tetraplegia (C5 Frankel A). Lateral radiograph (**a**) demonstrates a flexion tear drop (*thin white arrow*) fracture of the C6 vertebra. Note the posterior displacement of the rest of the vertebral body and the facet joint diastases (*thick white arrow*) in keeping with a significant three column injury. AP radiograph (**b**) shows the characteristic sagittal component (*dashed white arrow*) of the fracture involving the C6 vertebral body. Sagittal T1W (**c**), T2W (**d**) and axial T2W (**e**) images demonstrate the true extent of the injury with cord compression and extensive cord oedema/contusion (*white arrow head*). Note the extensive soft tissue injury including prevertebral soft tissue swelling, disc injury, elevation of the posterior longitudinal ligament from the posterior aspect of C7 vertebra and the posterior ligamentous complex injury

20.6.2
Joint Injuries

20.6.2.1
Facet Dislocation

This can be unilateral or bilateral. Bilateral facet dislocation can often result in significant spinal cord injury. Bilateral facet dislocations with locked facets can be seen with flexion injuries and are due to significant ligamentous disruption in the posterior and middle columns (Fig. 20.13a–e). On radiographs bilateral facet dislocation is seen as anterior displacement of one vertebra with respect to the adjacent vertebra of more than 50%. Facet dislocations may be associated with facet fractures. Again these injuries are best demonstrated by CT. Spondylolisthesis is seen in association with flexion injuries and usually denotes significant soft tissue injury. Similarly retrolisthesis can be seen in extension injuries.

20.6.3
Soft Tissue Injuries

20.6.3.1
Hyperflexion Injury

This is predominantly a soft tissue injury with disruption of ligaments of the posterior column and can extend to involve the posterior longitudinal ligament and the posterior portion of the disc. In children, hyperflexion usually involves the C2/C3 or C3/C4 level. The injured ligaments include supra-spinous ligament, inter-spinous ligament, ligamentum flava and facet joint capsule. If untreated, these injuries can lead to progressive kyphosis. Initial radiographs can be entirely normal. There can be widening of the interspinous distance or the facet joints. Localised kyphosis at the injured level is another feature on radiographs. There may be anterior narrowing and posterior widening of the disc space. Anterior displacement of the vertebra may be seen. F/E views may be useful but spasm may preclude adequate examination. In these cases, this should be repeated after the spasm settles.

20.6.3.2
Hyperextension Injury

This commonly affects the C5/C6 or C4/C5 level. This may be radiographically occult apart from a pre vertebral soft tissue thickening as the spine may return to normal alignment after the injury. There may be significant neurological deficit despite near normal radiographic findings. There is injury to the anterior longitudinal ligament and to the intervertebral disc. There may be retrolisthesis of the vertebra above the disc injury. F/E views may accentuate the radiographic appearances but have to be performed with care. MR is optimal at demonstrating both the soft tissue injuries and the state of the cord.

20.6.3.3
Posterior Ligamentous Injury

Conventional radiographs may or may not demonstrate posterior ligamentous injury. Delayed radiographs may demonstrate calcification in an area affected by previous ligamentous injury. MR imaging is the modality of choice for assessment of ligamentous injury. Significant posterior ligamentous injury requires surgical fusion. This is due to the fact that bones have a substantial potential for repair after injury. Soft tissues, on the other hand, do not have a similar potential for repair.

Ligamentum flavum injuries can occur along with spinous process fractures. However, these ligaments are strong and elastic and rarely tear. The injuries are usually avulsions at ligamentous insertions.

20.7
Thoracolumbar and Sacral Spine

Thoracolumbar spine injuries are less common than cervical spine injuries in children. The unique anatomy of the thoracic spine with its associated articulation with the ribs to form the thoracic cage provides additional resistance to injuries in this region. Therefore, the magnitude of force necessary to induce a thoracic spine injury is much greater than at other spinal levels. This, along with the smaller dimensions of the spinal canal, in turn account for the higher incidence and severity of neurological injury associated with thoracic injuries than at other levels. However, as the child grows, the spine assumes adult proportions at about 8–10 years of age and injury patterns follow adult type of injuries. In very young children thoracolumbar spine injuries

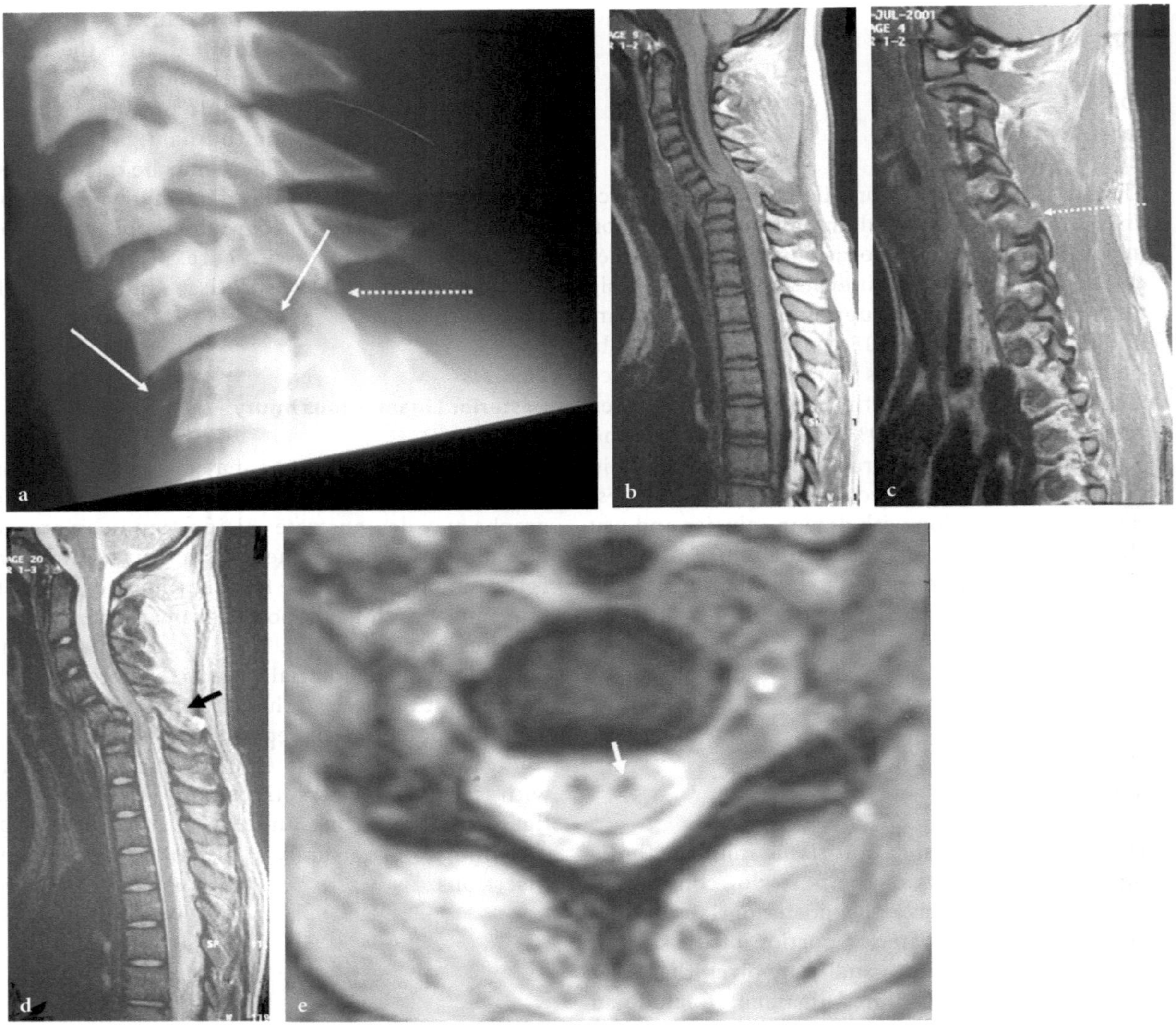

Fig. 20.13a–e. A 14-year-old involved in a trampolining accident presented with quadriparesis (C6 Frankel B). Bilateral C5/C6 facet dislocation. Lateral radiograph (**a**) shows the anterior displacement of the C5 vertebral body over C6 with widening of the interspinous distance. Associated intervertebral disc and physeal injury is suggested by the reduced disc height and the displaced apophyseal ossification centres (*white arrows*). T1W sagittal images (**b**,**c**), sagittal T2W (**d**) and axial T2W (**e**) show the extensive soft tissue injury associated with the facet dislocation. The dislocated facet joints (*dashed white arrows*) and the prevertebral soft tissue swelling are seen on both the radiographs and MR images. There is stripping of the anterior and posterior longitudinal ligaments, disruption of the posterior ligament complex (*short black arrow*). There is cord compression and extensive cord oedema/contusion. The axial MR image shows low signal foci (*short wide arrow*) within the cord in keeping with intramedullary haemorrhage

are associated with road traffic accidents or child abuse. In older children, these injuries commonly occur due to sporting activities. The upper four thoracic vertebrae are difficult to visualise on lateral radiographs. A modified swimmer's view can be performed to assess these vertebrae but needs movement of the arms.

There are a number of classification systems to categorise thoracolumbar injuries. A detailed description of all the classification is beyond the scope of this chapter. The most widely used is that proposed by Denis (1983), which classifies these injuries into four categories. The first type is the compression fracture, either anterior or lateral compression. These are associated with normal middle and posterior columns. The second type is the burst fracture, where there is failure of both the anterior and middle columns (Fig. 20.14a–h). The posterior column may be intact but fractures of the laminae and injuries to the facet joints can occur. The third type is the flexion/distraction or seat belt injury (Fig. 20.15a–e). In this injury, there is distraction injury to the middle and posterior columns due to tension and compression injury to the anterior column. The last category includes fracture/dislocations due to a combination of compression, rotation, tension and shearing forces (Fig. 20.16a–d). There is consequently significant translation or rotation at the fracture site. Other more elaborate classification systems have been proposed by others (Ferguson and Allen 1984; Magerl et al. 1994; McAfee et al. 1982). All these classification systems have considerable overlap. The common denominator in all classification systems is the importance of the failure of the middle column.

Lap belt injuries, also called "chance fractures", initially described by Chance (1948), are unique injuries in the very young child due to a sudden deceleration in the presence of a restraining lap belt. This injury is unlike cervical spinal injury which is more often caused by an absence of restraining devices. The lap belt is intended for adults, in whom it lies across the hips and pelvis. When worn by a child, this slides up and lies across the abdomen. Sudden deceleration leads to a flexion of the child across the lap belt which is also exaggerated by the higher centre of gravity in a child due to the large head size. This is a flexion distraction injury with an anterior fulcrum of movement. Due to flexion, there is failure of the middle and posterior columns and a degree of anterior compression. There is always a significant soft tissue injury with a variable bony involvement. There is often associated intra abdominal injury (30%–50% of cases) and superficial ecchymosis is a useful clue to this injury. The imaging features seen in lap belt injuries include disruption of the posterior elements of the spine, longitudinal separation of the disrupted posterior elements, minimal or no decrease in the anterior vertical height of the involved vertebral body, minimal or no forward displacement of the superior vertebral fragment or vertebra; and minimal or no lateral displacement. There is also an increase in the height of the middle column compared to the adjacent vertebra due to the distraction mechanism (Groves et al. 2005).

20.7.1 Osseous Injuries

20.7.1.1 Lap Belt Injury

These may be associated with a fracture of the spinous process, articular facets or pars interarticularis as part of the middle and posterior column injury. The usual level of injury is between L2 and L4 levels. Rumball and Jarvis (1992) described four different patterns of injury: Type A, with horizontal fracture through the spinous process and neural arch; Type B, inter-spinous ligamentous injury with facet joint dislocation; Type C, inter-spinous ligament injury extending anteriorly through a fracture of the articular process and into the posterior aspect of the vertebral body; Type D, inter-spinous ligament injury with articular process injury and anterior extension into the apophysis of the adjacent vertebral body. Type B were the most common. The middle column injury is usually through bone rather than posterior disc unlike that in adults. This can be a type I physeal injury through the growth plate. The middle column injury may be through the apophysis of the adjacent vertebral body. The anterior injury may include vertebral compression but usually less than 10% loss of height. The anterior and posterior column injury may involve multiple vertebral levels. The initial plain radiographs may only demonstrate this minor anterior compression but fail to demonstrate the posterior ligamentous injury. A high index of suspicion is necessary with appropriate history. A "sandwich" appearance on MR imaging has been described associated with the neural arch bony injury and consists of a linear or triangular layer of low signal intensity (hemorrhage) framed by two layers of high signal intensity (edema) on the T2-weighted images and STIR images on either side (Groves et al. 2005). Similar appearance with high signal intensity surrounded by low signal intensity can be seen on T1W images (Fig. 20.15a–e).

20.7.1.2 Compression Fractures

These are due to axial compression or flexion injuries and lead to a variable degree of loss of vertebral height. The majority of compression fractures in children occur in the thoracic spine (Vialle et al. 2006). These compressions are graded into mild, moderate or severe depending on the degree of compression.

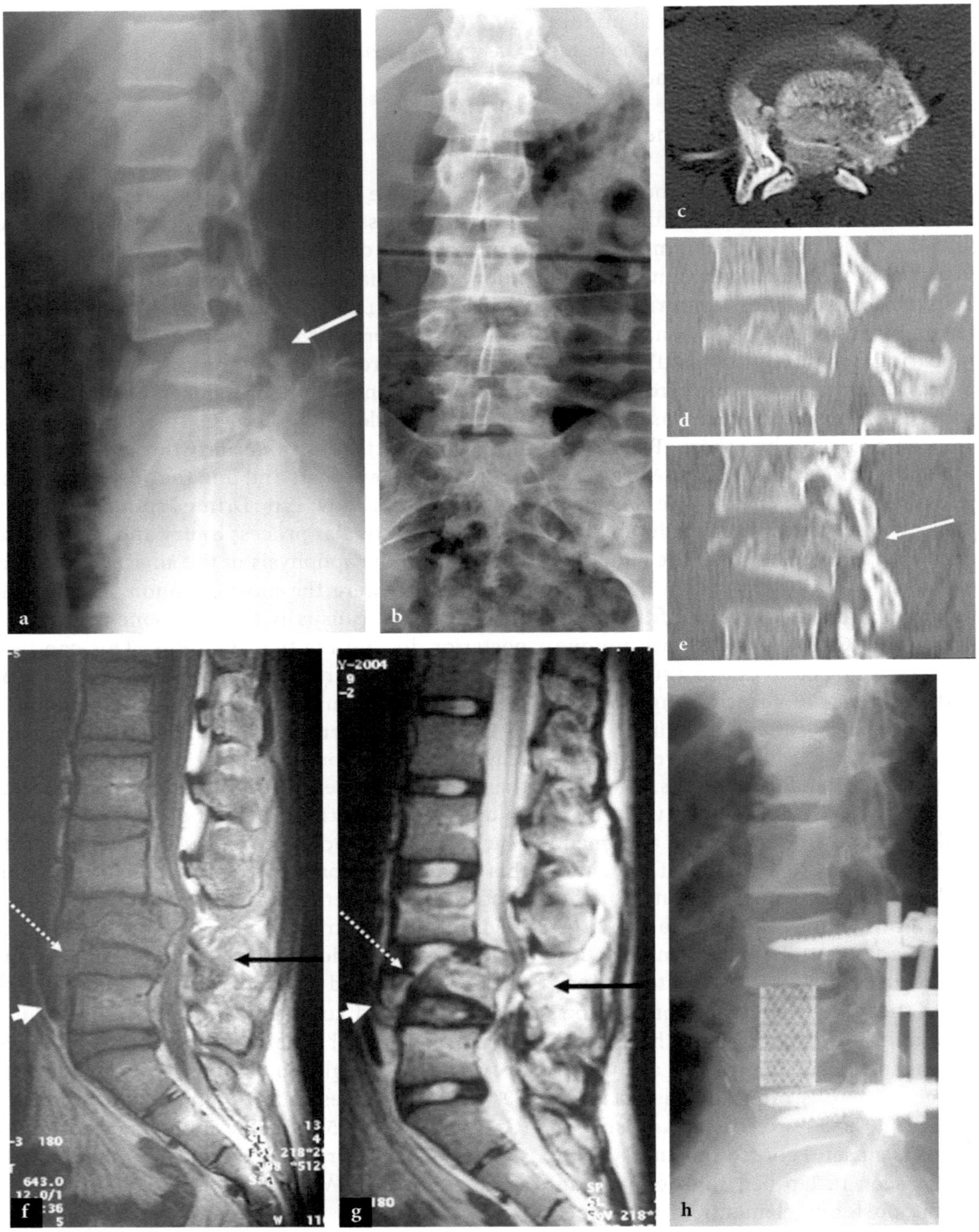

Fig. 20.14a–h. A 16-year-old after a horse riding accident presented with complete paraplegia. Lateral (**a**) and AP (**b**) radiographs of the lumbar spine show a severe burst fracture of L4 vertebra. The L4 vertebral outline is indistinct on the AP radiograph with increased interpediculate distance and deviated spinous processes of L4 and L5. There is, however, significant anterior displacement of L3 over L4 with facet joint dislocation (*long white arrows*). This therefore does not represent a pure burst fracture. Note the severe spinal canal compromise best depicted on the CT axial image(**c**) and sagittal reconstructions (**d**,**e**). The sagittal CT reconstructions also show the facet joint dislocation (*long white arrows*). Sagittal T1W (**f**) and T2W (**g**) images show the cauda equina compression. There is rupture of the anterior longitudinal ligament (*short white arrow*), intervertebral disc (*dashed white arrow*) and posterior ligament complex (*black arrow*). The patient was treated by a combined anterior and posterior decompression and stabilisation with vertebrectomy, cage insertion and pedicle screw fixation (**h**)

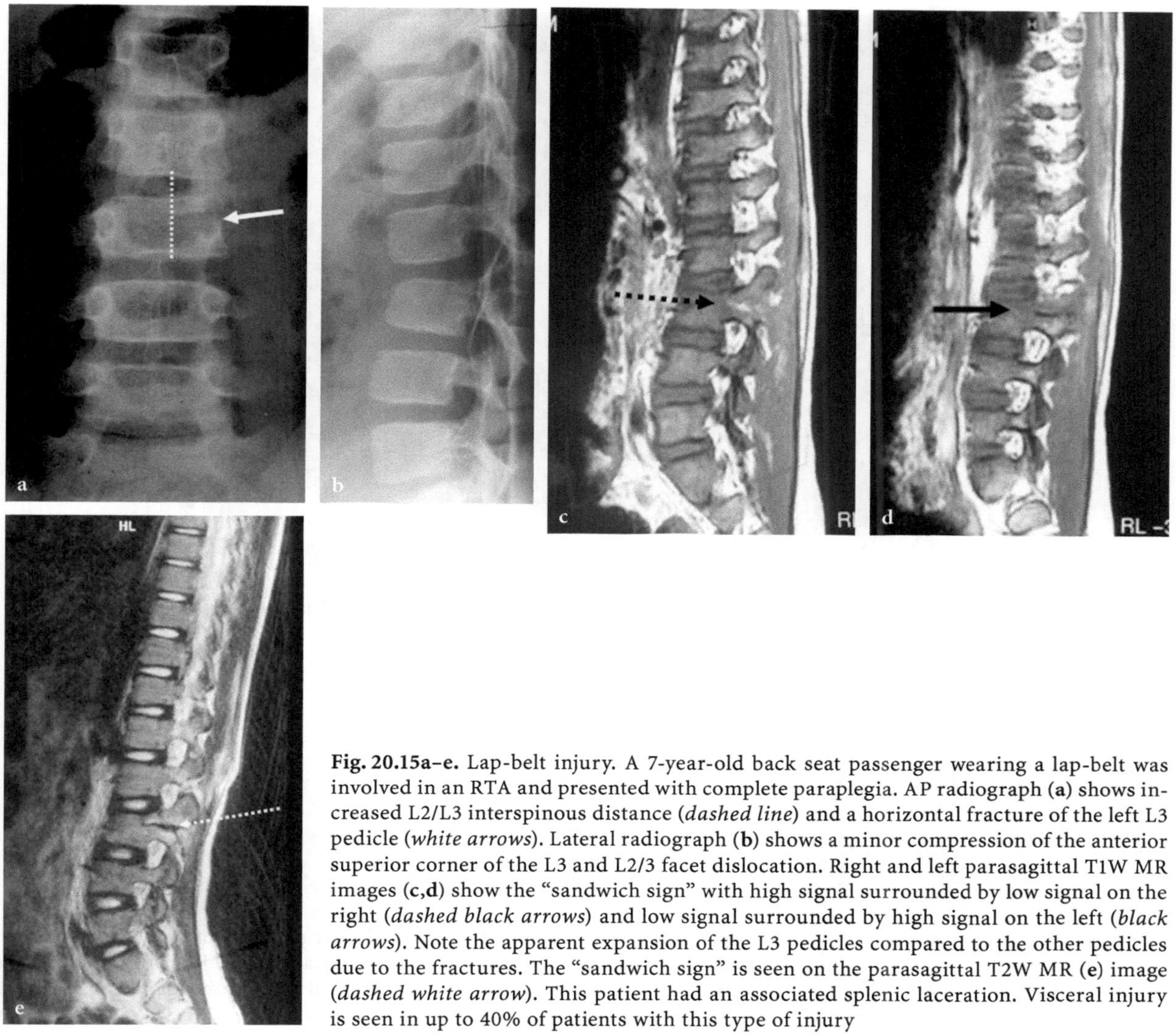

Fig. 20.15a–e. Lap-belt injury. A 7-year-old back seat passenger wearing a lap-belt was involved in an RTA and presented with complete paraplegia. AP radiograph (**a**) shows increased L2/L3 interspinous distance (*dashed line*) and a horizontal fracture of the left L3 pedicle (*white arrows*). Lateral radiograph (**b**) shows a minor compression of the anterior superior corner of the L3 and L2/3 facet dislocation. Right and left parasagittal T1W MR images (**c**,**d**) show the "sandwich sign" with high signal surrounded by low signal on the right (*dashed black arrows*) and low signal surrounded by high signal on the left (*black arrows*). Note the apparent expansion of the L3 pedicles compared to the other pedicles due to the fractures. The "sandwich sign" is seen on the parasagittal T2W MR (**e**) image (*dashed white arrow*). This patient had an associated splenic laceration. Visceral injury is seen in up to 40% of patients with this type of injury

Multilevel compressions are more common than single level injuries. If the compression is less than 10°, simple bed rest and gradual resumption of activities is recommended. Bracing and immobilisation in hyperextension may be needed for higher degree of compression. When compression is greater than 50° or when lateral compression is greater than 15°, surgical stabilisation is recommended (Pouliquen et al. 1997). Whilst most of these fractures will heal satisfactorily and regain height with growth, a small percentage of cases, especially those with growth plate injury, may demonstrate progressive kyphosis or scoliosis with adolescent growth spurt. In severe degrees of compression, there may be associated posterior ligamentous injury.

Radiographically, compression fractures are seen as a loss of vertebral height involving the anterior vertebral body. The posterior vertebral line is intact and there is no retropulsion. As the middle column is intact, these injuries are considered stable. There is a narrow zone of increased density parallel to the vertebral end plate caused by the impacted trabeculae. With minor injuries, the intervertebral disc is normal. However, if the compression is more vertically orientated, the disc material may protrude through the endplate into the vertebral body, resulting in a traumatic Schmorl's node. There is associated loss of the disc height. The compression usually involves the superior aspect of the vertebral body.

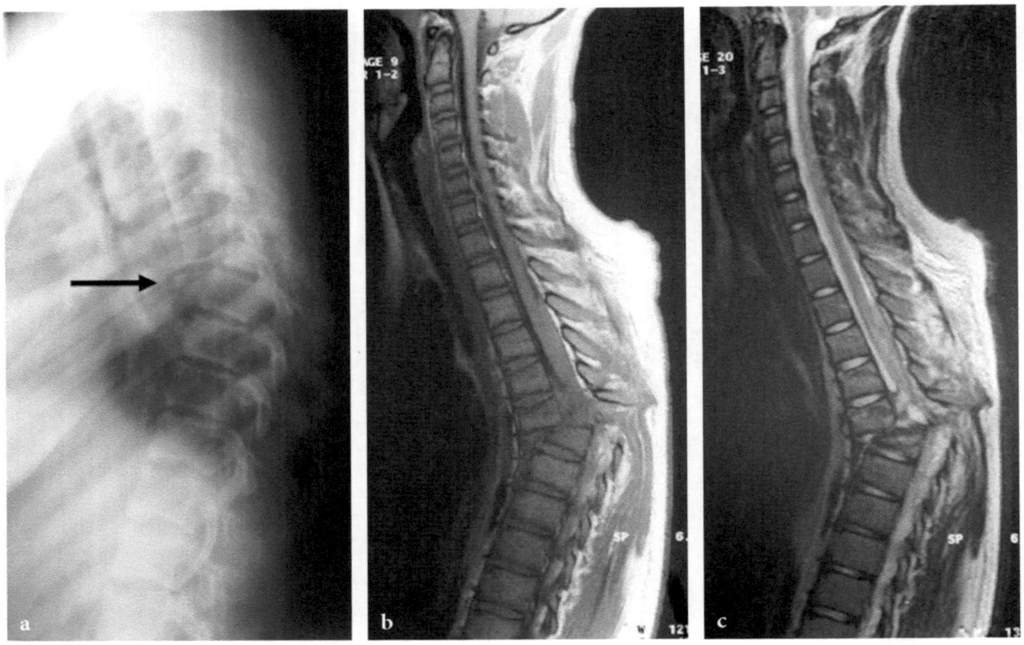

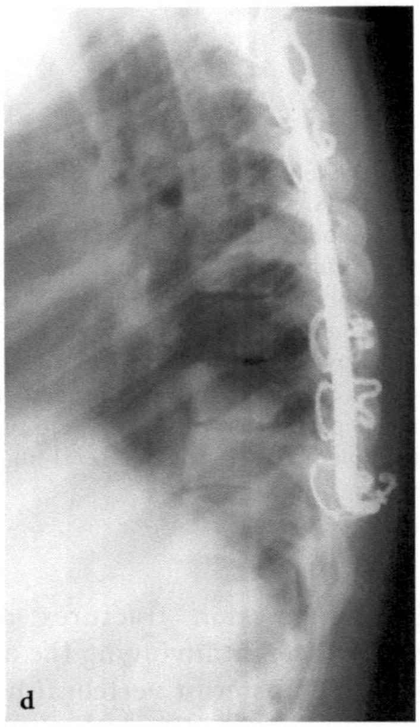

Fig. 20.16a–d. A 13-year-old who presented after a horse riding accident with complete paraplegia (D7 Frankel A). Fracture dislocation D6/7. Lateral radiograph (**a**), T1W (**b**) and T2W (**c**) MR images show the marked anterior translation of D6 over D7. Note the anterior superior ossified apophysis (*black arrow*) of D7 is displaced anteriorly with the D6 vertebra on the radiographs. There is complete cord transection with high signal extending superiorly in the cord up to the D3 level in keeping with cord oedema/contusion. All the soft tissues are injured including the anterior longitudinal ligament, posterior longitudinal ligament, intervertebral disc, and posterior ligament complex. The D5 and D4 vertebrae demonstrate high signal in keeping with concomitant injury to these vertebrae. Lateral radiograph (**d**) after posterior stabilisation performed in view of the extensive soft tissue injury shows satisfactory alignment

20.7.1.3 Kümmell's Disease

This is a form of delayed collapse of the vertebra after trauma and can occur weeks or months after injury (Brower and Downey 1981). This is presently thought to occur due to ischaemia induced at the time of trauma and delayed collapse due to osteonecrosis (Maldague et al. 1978). This condition demonstrates an intra-vertebral vacuum cleft in the collapsed vertebral body usually adjacent to the endplates on radiographs and CT. This vacuum cleft is exaggerated by extension and reduced by flexion. However, on MR imaging, this gas is replaced by fluid and demonstrates a high signal on T2W sequences in the centre of the vertebral body and is specific for vertebral osteonecrosis (Naul et al. 1989).

20.7.1.4
Burst Fracture

This is caused by axial loading. They are most common at the thoraco-lumbar junction (T11–L2).The integrity of the posterior vertebral line is a useful indicator of this injury on the lateral radiograph. The posterior vertebral line is seen as a single or bifid vertical line on the lateral radiograph. In the cervical region this line is continuous while there is a focal central interruption to this line in the thoraco-lumbar region for the entry of nutrient vessels. Disruption, displacement or rotation of this line is seen in a majority of burst fractures (Gehweiler et al. 1981). More importantly, this line is normal in simple compression fractures. In burst fractures, there is a variable degree of vertebral compression and a break in the posterior vertebral line. This should be differentiated from a simple compression fracture as the management varies due to the presence of retropulsed fragments in the spinal canal which can cause cord or cauda equina compromise and also due to the potential for instability with burst fractures. The retropulsed fragments usually arise from the postero-superior corner of the vertebral body. The sagittal and transverse dimensions of the injured vertebra are increased due to a centripetal force. There is increased interpedicular distance. There is an associated endplate fracture and there may be a sagittal fracture of the neural arch. The end plate fracture is usually through the inferior endplate while in simple compression fractures it is more commonly through the superior end plate. Posterior element fractures are seen in 50%–100% of burst fractures (Brant-Zawadzki et al. 1982; Cammisa et al. 1989). These include vertical fractures of the laminae and spinous processes. A wide interpedicular distance implies significant posterior injury. The posterior element fracture can be missed on plain radiographs. CT quantifies accurately the degree of bone retropulsion while MR imaging demonstrates the state of the cord and soft tissues. There is controversy as to whether all burst fractures are unstable. Denis (1983) considered all these injuries to be unstable, while others considered most burst fractures to be stable (McAfee et al. 1982). The features that indicate instability include progressive kyphosis, progressive neurological deficit, posterior element disruption, loss of more then 50% of vertebral height with facet joint subluxation and retropulsed bone fragments in the spinal canal. There is no clear correlation between the degree of retropulsion and severity of neurological compromise. This is probably because of the fact that at the time of imaging, the bone fragments are at a different position to their position at the time of maximal forces applied during the trauma. Previous studies have shown that the maximum canal compromise is 85% greater than that seen when assessed in hospital (Panjabi et al. 1995). The cord and neurological injury, therefore, occur at the time of impact. The imaging appearances only represent the final resting state. This is also the basis for conservative management of burst fractures advocated by many experts in the field now.

20.7.1.5
Physeal/Apophyseal Injuries

Growth plate fractures can occur in the thoraco-lumbar spine in the adolescent population. Clinically this presents like a herniated disc if it includes the posterior disco-vertebral junction. The patient may describe a pop after lifting, fall or twisting injury. Non-operative treatment is rarely successful and surgery is frequently needed. As described in earlier sections of this chapter, the apophysis consists of a ring of ossification at the edge of the cartilaginous growth plate. Before it fuses with the vertebral body, the ring of ossification is separated from the vertebral body by a layer of hyaline cartilage which represents a relative area of weakness. Posterior apophyseal ring fractures are usually seen in the lumbo-sacral region. They commonly involve the cephalad rim of the first sacral vertebra and the L4 and L5 vertebrae less frequently. Takata et al. (1988) have classified these injuries into three categories (Fig. 20.17a–d):

- Type I: Simple separation of the entire margin of the apophysis.
- Type II: Apophyseal injury including a portion of overlying cartilage of the annulus fibrosus.
- Type III: A more localised fracture but with a larger amount of vertebral body involved. There is a round defect in the bone adjoining the fracture in this type of fracture.

Epstein and associates (1989) have suggested a fourth type that involves a fracture of both the cephalad and caudad apophyses and involves the full length of the posterior margin of the vertebral body.

Type I fractures are commonly seen in children. These children present with symptoms suggestive of disc herniation. Whilst other authors have suggested that these fractures are due to trauma or strenuous activity (Handel et al. 1979), Takata et al. (1988) have not found major injuries associated with their patients. Instead they found irregularities of the end plates and suggested that fragility of the end plate is responsible for these fractures. These lesions can be difficult to see on conventional radiographs. Findings include disc space narrowing, irregularity of the posterior vertebral corner or an ossific defect displaced into the spinal canal. CT shows an arcuate fragment paralleling the posterior vertebral body outline. There is discontinuity or truncation of the normally convex posterior inferior vertebral margin on MR images, with elevation or disruption of the posterior longitudinal ligament.

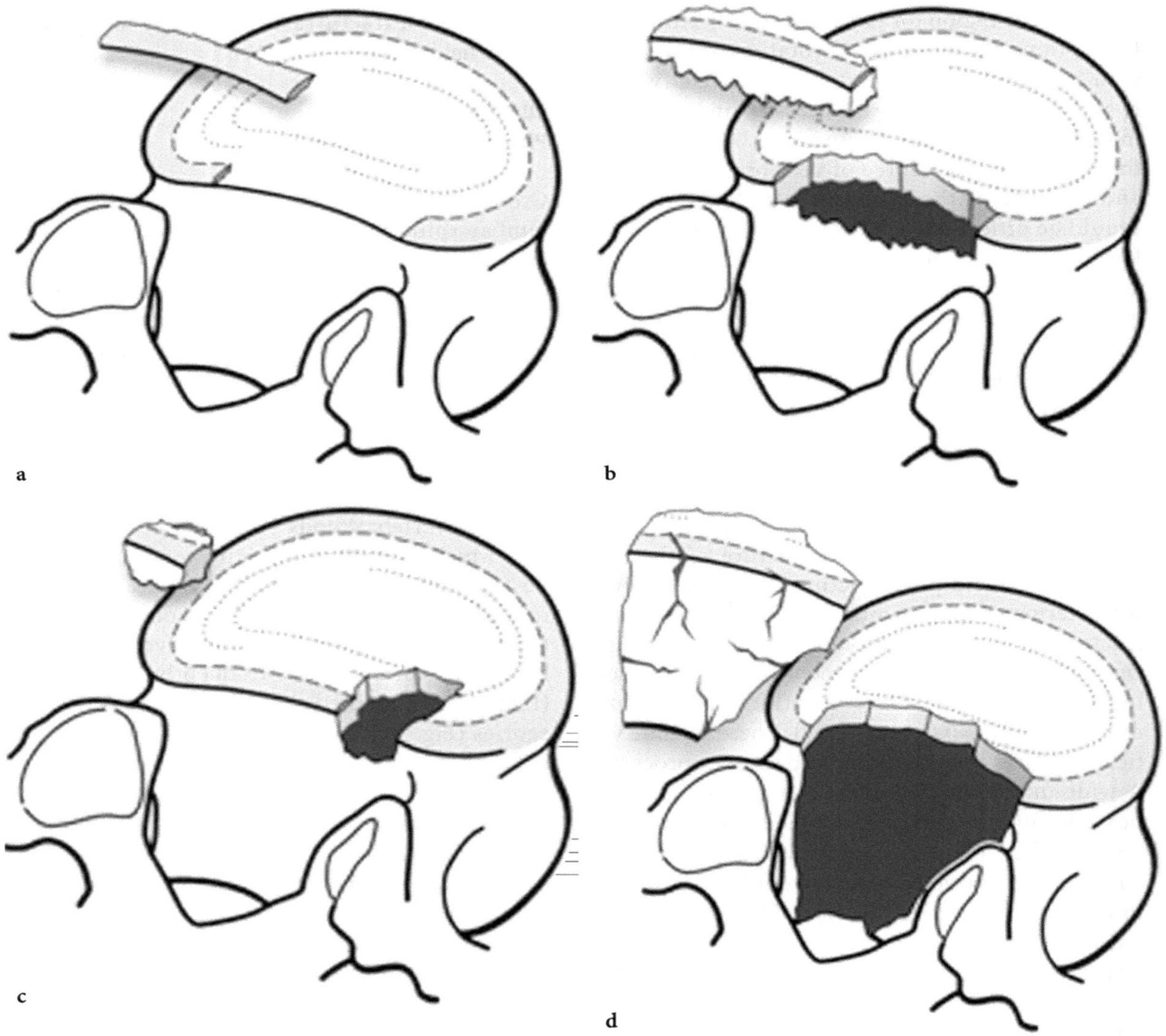

Fig. 20.17a–d. Classification of the posterior apophyseal ring fractures in the lumbosacral spine. In these diagrams, the fractured fragments of the vertebra are positioned away from the site of origin only for ease of understanding. **a** Type I: simple marginal separation of the apophysis. **b** Type II: apophyseal injury including a portion of overlying cartilage of the annulus fibrosis. **c** Type III: a more localised fracture but with a larger amount of vertebral body involved. There is a round defect in the bone adjoining the fracture in this type of fracture. **d** Type IV: fracture of both the cephalad and caudad apophyses and involving the full length of the posterior margin of the vertebral body

20.7.1.6
Physeal Fractures

These can also occur through the neuro-central synchondrosis and have been described in child abuse (Vialle et al. 2006). These can be suspected on antero-posterior radiographs where there is widening of the interpedicular distance. There is anterior or posterior displacement of the vertebral body on the lateral radiographs. The fracture line may be evident and there is varying degrees of kyphosis. With anterior displacement neurological injury is unlikely and the outcome is favourable, but the risk is increased with posterior displacement of the vertebral body. MR imaging is useful to assess cord and soft tissues but also to assess progress during healing and growth plate viability.

20.7.1.7
Spondylolysis

Spondylolysis, defined as a fracture or defect of the pars interarticularis, has been reported in up to 47% of adolescent athletes with low back pain and is associated with sports like gymnastics, weight lifting, rowing and cricket. However, spondylolysis may be seen in both symptomatic and asymptomatic individuals. Skeletally immature individuals are at increased risk of this injury during periods of rapid skeletal growth. There is a male preponderance with a male to female ratio of up to 3:1. Racial preponderance is seen with the highest incidence in Eskimos. There is association of spondylolysis with transitional lumbar vertebra, spina bifida occulta, Scheuermann's disease, osteogenesis imperfecta and osteopetrosis. It has been proposed that this injury results from repetitive trauma and develops in stages from stress related injury to complete spondylolysis. This most commonly occurs at the L5 level (85%) with 15% occurring at the L4 level. Other levels are only affected rarely. Spondylolysis can result in varying degrees of spondylolisthesis. Whilst lateral radiographs usually demonstrate the spondylolytic defect, 45° oblique radiographs demonstrate the pars interarticularis without overlap from the pars on the other side. Radiographs are insensitive to early stress reaction which can be seen on MR images as high signal change in the pars on T2 weighted images and is best seen with fat suppression techniques. CT may show sclerosis at this stage with no cortical interruption. A classification system has been proposed for MR staging of spondylolysis (Hollenberg et al. 2002): Grade 0 (normal) with no signal abnormality of the pars interarticularis. Grade 1 denotes patients with marrow oedema but no spondylolysis. Grade 2 was assigned to patients with T2 signal abnormalities and thinning, fragmentation, or irregularity of the pars. Grade 3 involved a visible unilateral or bilateral spondylolysis with abnormal T2 signal. Grade 4 involved complete spondylolysis without abnormal T2 signal. Hollenberg et al. (2002) demonstrated good intra- and inter-observer reliability with this classification system. CT scanning with reverse gantry orientation is reliable in assessing for spondylolytic defects and sometimes stress reactions. Reversing of the gantry is not necessary with the newer multislice scanners with isometric resolution in all three imaging planes. However, CT can potentially miss some patients with early stress reactions which can be seen on MR imaging and bone scintigraphy. Scintigraphy shows increased uptake in patients with stress response and active spondylolytic defects. However, chronic inactive spondylolytic defects may not be seen on scintigraphy. Moreover, it is difficult to be specific anatomically on routine scintigraphy. Single photon emission computed tomography (SPECT) is more sensitive. It is useful to identify an early stress reaction before spondylolysis occurs as treatment is more likely to be successful at this stage. Moreover, MR imaging demonstrates the associated disc degeneration and the effects on nerve roots. This will help to determine the operative approach should surgery be considered. Damage to the disc means that fusion between adjacent levels will be required rather than a repair of the defect itself.

Reports of rare sacral injuries in adolescents include a traumatic spondylolisthesis of S1, fracture dislocation of S1 (Novkov et al. 1996; Rodriguez-Fuentes 1993) and are associated with unusually excessive forces of injury.

Major fracture dislocations due to a combination of flexion, axial loading, rotational forces and shearing can cause complex injuries including adjacent vertebrae and all intervening soft tissues. The upper vertebra is subluxed anteriorly with respect to the inferior vertebra. Fractures of the laminae, facets and endplates are common. The bony components of this injury are best assessed by CT scan while an MR examination must be performed in all patients due to the significant associated soft tissue and cord injury.

20.7.2 Joint Injuries

The intervertebral disc is composed of a central nucleus pulposus with surrounding annulus fibrosis. The nucleus pulposus is composed of mucoid semifluid material and the annulus fibrosis consists of collagen fibres that surround the nucleus pulposus in concentric rings. The nucleus pulposus is in direct contact with the endplates superiorly and inferiorly. There are small areas of deficiency of underlying sub-chondral bone allowing for nutrition of the disc through diffusion. These areas, however, are areas of weakness through which the disc material could prolapse into the sub-chondral bone resulting in a Schmorl's node. The growth plate is susceptible to injury until the endplates ossify. These anterior endplate injuries are an important component of Scheuermann's disease. Whilst Scheuermann's disease definitely has genetic predisposition, mechanical factors involved in high energy sports have a significant role in its development. There is a classical variant seen in the lower thoracic spine from T7–T10, and a traumatic or atypical variant involving the thoraco-lumbar junction that is most susceptible to mechanical forces. These are seen with gymnastics, water sports, wrestling, young elite skiers and football. These abnormalities are most likely to be symptomatic during the acute phase of development of the abnormality. In the traumatic variant, there is a combination of anterior Schmorl's nodes, apophyseal ring abnormalities and usually involvement of only one or two vertebrae unlike classic Scheuermann's disease (Rachbauer et al. 2001). There is no correlation with back pain and these abnormalities in adult life. Therefore, serial radiographs are necessary to isolate these lesions during their developmental stage. MR imaging on the other hand can demonstrate the vertebral oedema associated with acute lesions and identify the symptomatic lesions. The role of trauma in disc degeneration is not clear.

There may be dislocation of the facet joints in lap belt injuries. This can be seen as widening, superior subluxation, perching or locking of the facets. Facet malalignment is best appreciated on CT reconstructions. Rotatory stability of the thoracolumbar spine is provided by the facet joints and these are injured in significant fracture dislocations caused by combined flexion and rotation. The major hallmark of fracture dislocation type of injuries is intervertebral subluxation or dislocation.

20.7.3 Soft Tissue Injuries

Fractures of the thoracic spine are associated with a paraspinal haematoma which is seen as a deviation of the paraspinal line. The paraspinal line represents the interface between the lung and the paraspinal soft tissues and is best appreciated on the left side. There is a deviation of this line in fractures of the thoracic spine representing a haematoma. This is however not specific to trauma and can be seen with infections, tumours and a variety of mediastinal disorders. Haematomas may track and form apical pleural capping or can be seen as an effusion. Other soft tissue signs associated with thoracic fractures include a widened mediastinum and a widened right paratracheal stripe (Dennis and Rogers 1989). However, these soft tissue signs can also be seen in serious mediastinal vascular injuries.

Isolated anterior column compression fractures do not result in neurological injury. Neurological injury in this setting should raise the suspicion of associated disc herniation. With compressions greater than 50 degrees, the middle column acts as a fulcrum and can lead to posterior ligamentous injuries.

Lap belt injuries may be due to an entirely soft tissue injury with failure of the posterior ligamentous structures including the interspinous ligaments and supra-spinous ligaments. This can be seen on radiographs as widening of the interspinous distance, increased height of inter-vertebral foramina. Anteriorly this may be associated with intervertebral disc injury. The ligamentous disruption is best appreciated on MR images. Disc injury associated with lap belt injury demonstrates high signal in the disc. The anterior longitudinal ligament is frequently intact and acts as a minor mechanical constraint to vertebral displacement. This may account for the lower rates of neurological injury associated with this injury.

Type 2 and 3 apophyseal injuries as described by Takata et al. (1988) may be associated with avulsion of the posterior longitudinal ligament.

The majority of patients with upper thoracic spine injuries sustain significant cord injury due to the excessive force necessary to cause this injury and the narrow spinal canal. A significant proportion of these patients develop complete paraplegia. With major fracture dislocations, there is injury to the interspinous ligaments and disc.

20.8 Stability

"Spinal stability" is poorly defined and variously interpreted. Spinal stability can be described as a condition in which there is no increased deformity or neurological deficit over time. So there are two broad factors: mechanical stability and neurological stability. Mechanical stability can be immediate or long term. This has therefore led to a number of classifications of spinal injury which are beyond the scope of this chapter. None of the available classification systems are perfect. They are either over-elaborate and are unusable, or they are over simplified and do not encompass the whole range of injury patterns. Moreover, the present classification systems do not incorporate MR findings. Suffice to say that it is important not to classify an injury very early in the assessment of an injured patient. Otherwise, there is a risk that inexperienced physicians may try to assign the injury to a particular class instead of documenting the extent of the whole injury (Fig. 20.14a–h). Most physicians use the Denis three-column concept. Denis (1983) has described the spine as consisting of three columns for the assessment of stability. In the sagittal plane, the anterior column extends from the anterior longitudinal ligament to the junction point of the middle and posterior third of the intervertebral disc. The middle column extends from this point to the posterior longitudinal ligament. The posterior column extends from the posterior longitudinal ligament to the supra-spinous ligament. He defined instability as any disruption involving two contiguous columns. The middle column appears to be the key element in instability. Gehweiler et al. (1981) described four radiographic features that indicate instability: vertebral displacement, widening of the inter-spinous distance, widening of the apophyseal joint and widening of the interpedicular distance. Assessment of the integrity of the posterior vertebral body line should be included in this as disruption of this line indicates middle column injury. However, this columnar assessment can be difficult in very young children where there is incomplete ossification and the actual bone margins may sometimes have to be deduced from other findings or conceptualised. Assessment of stability includes clinical assessment and radiological investigations including, where appropriate, F/E views. Biomechanical instability can cause further neurological injury. However, most vertebral fractures heal within 6–12 weeks of injury. Ligamentous injuries take longer to heal. The spine becomes biomechanically stable once healing occurs. Biomechanical instability is therefore time-related. There is also the concept of physiological instability of the injured cord due to various factors including loss of auto-regulatory mechanisms and disruptions of blood-brain barrier. This makes the patient vulnerable to further neurological injury from hypoxia, hypotension and sepsis.

The radiographic signs suggestive of instability are described in Table 20.1.

Table 20.1. Radiographic signs of instability

Vertebral Displacement
Interpediculate distance widening
Widened interspinous distance
Widened facet joints
Disruption of posterior vertebral body line
Compression >40%
Disc space narrowing
Mid sagittal canal narrowing
Posterior element fractures
Progressive kyphosis

20.9 Imaging in Chronic Spinal Cord Injury

Spinal cord injury has a wide and varied effect on all the systems of the body and can result in a multitude of complications. Due to a combination of altered sensation and autonomic function, localising the underlying cause in an unwell patient can be difficult. Any deterioration in neurological status in a patient with previous spinal injury even after a long period of time should be investigated further with follow-up MR scans. The deterioration may be due to a number of factors including post-traumatic myelomalacic myelopathy (PTMM), post-traumatic cystic myelopathy (PTCM), cord atrophy and syrinx formation (Fig. 20.18a–d). Persistent pain after spinal injury may be due to pseudoarthrosis formation and instability. Neuropathic spine (Charcot's spine) has also been described after thoracolumbar spinal injury due to denervation. Imaging features of neuropathic spine are similar to other neuropathic joints and include sclerosis, disorganisation, debris and extensive new bone formation.

Imaging surveillance is needed for the renal tract as these patients can develop calculi, reflux or obstruction. This is done by means of regular ultrasound and urodynamic assessment. Pressure sores may need contrast sinography or MR imaging to define the extent prior to surgery.

20.10 Conclusion

The paediatric spine can cause difficulties in image interpretation due to variable development, anatomical variations, ossification centres and biomechanics that are unique to this group of the population. Children also differ from adults with respect to mechanisms of injury, transportation methods after injury, diagnostic pathways and definitive treatment. Each case should be approached individually with attention to specific injury patterns to avoid misdiagnosis. SCIWORA is more common in children than adults and a lower threshold for further investigation in the presence of unexplained neurology is needed. Overall, spinal injuries are rare in children and spinal cord injury has a better prognosis than in adults. In cases of suspicion of injury, general radiologists should not refrain from seeking expert advice as these injuries are rarely seen in routine clinical practice and easily misinterpreted.

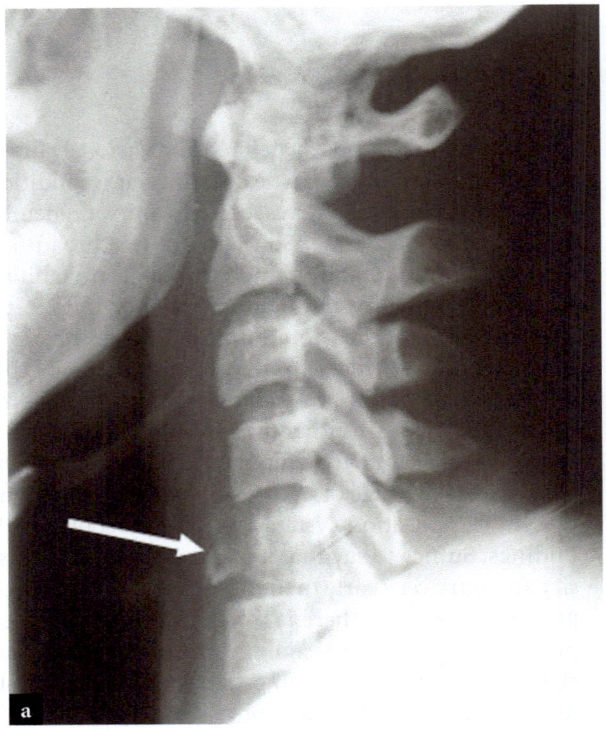

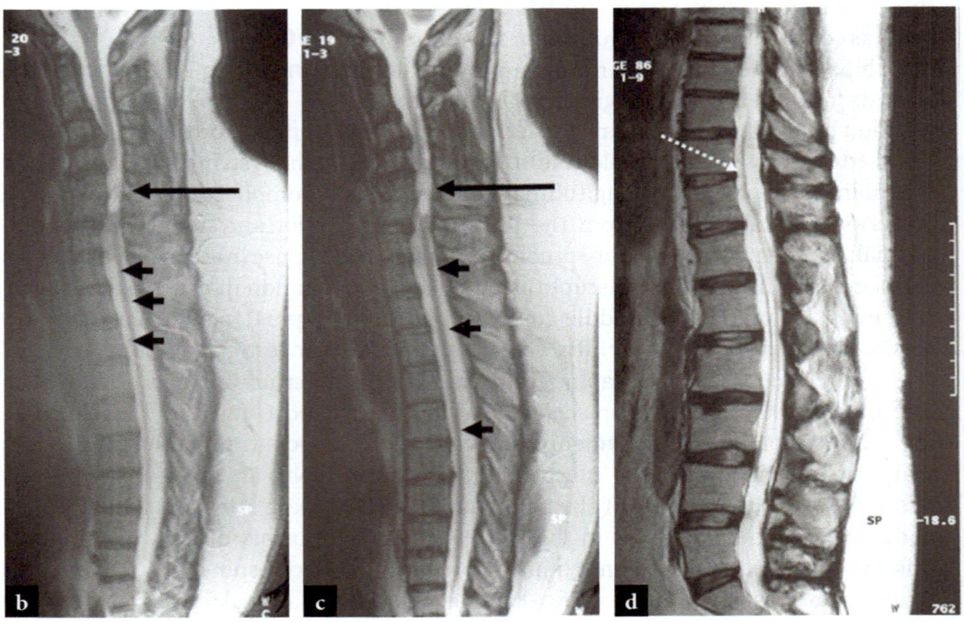

Fig. 20.18a–d. Chronic spinal cord injury. Lateral radiograph (**a**) immediately after spinal injury shows the flexion tear drop fracture (*long white arrows*) at C5/C6 level. T2W sagittal MR images (**b–d**) through the whole spine 20 years after initial injury show intramedullary cyst formation (*black arrows*) at the C5/C6 level. There is generalised cord atrophy (*black arrowhead*). A small syrinx (*dashed white arrow*) is noted at the distal cord and conus. Note the anterior fusion at the C5/C6 level

References

Athey AM (1991) A 3-year-old with spinal cord injury without radiographic abnormality (SCIWORA). J Emerg Nurs 17:380–384, discussion 385

Aufdermaur M (1974) Spinal injuries in juveniles. Necropsy findings in twelve cases. J Bone Joint Surg Br 56B:513–519

Banit D, Murrey SD (2005) Atlantoaxial Instability. http://www.emedicine.com

Barba CA, Taggert J, Morgan AS, et al. (2001) A new cervical spine clearance protocol using computed tomography. J Trauma 51:652–656; discussion 656–7

Brant-Zawadzki M, Jeffrey RB Jr, Minagi H, et al. (1982) High resolution CT of thoracolumbar fractures. AJR Am J Roentgenol 138:699–704

Brower AC, Downey EF Jr (1981) Kummell disease: report of a case with serial radiographs. Radiology 141:363–364

Brown RL, Brunn MA, Garcia VF (2001) Cervical spine injuries in children: a review of 103 patients treated consecutively at a level 1 pediatric trauma center. J Pediatr Surg 36:1107–1114

Bulas DI, Fitz CR, Johnson DL (1993) Traumatic atlanto-occipital dislocation in children. Radiology 188:155–158

Cammisa FP Jr, Eismont FJ, Green BA (1989) Dural laceration occurring with burst fractures and associated laminar fractures. J Bone Joint Surg Am 71:1044–1052

Chance G (1948) Note on a type of flexion fracture of the spine. Br J Radiol 21:452–453

Cirak B, Ziegfeld S, Knight VM, et al. (2004) Spinal injuries in children. J Pediatr Surg 39:607–612

Denis F (1983) The three column spine and its significance in the classification of acute thoracolumbar spinal injuries. Spine 8:817–831

Dennis LN, Rogers LF (1989) Superior mediastinal widening from spine fractures mimicking aortic rupture on chest radiographs. AJR Am J Roentgenol 152:27–30

Epstein NE, Epstein JA, Mauri T (1989) Treatment of fractures of the vertebral limbus and spinal stenosis in five adolescents and five adults. Neurosurgery 24:595–604

Ferguson RL, Allen BL Jr (1984) A mechanistic classification of thoracolumbar spine fractures. Clin Orthop Relat Res:77–88

Fielding JW, Hawkins RJ (1977) Atlanto-axial rotatory fixation. (Fixed rotatory subluxation of the atlanto-axial joint). J Bone Joint Surg Am 59:37–44

Gehweiler JA Jr, Daffner RH, Osborne RL Jr (1981) Relevant signs of stable and unstable thoracolumbar vertebral column trauma. Skeletal Radiol 7:179–183

Griffiths HJ, Wagner J, Anglen J, et al. (2002) The use of forced flexion/extension views in the obtunded trauma patient. Skeletal Radiol 31:587–591

Groves CJ, Cassar-Pullicino VN, Tins BJ, et al. (2005) Chance-type flexion-distraction injuries in the thoracolumbar spine: MR imaging characteristics. Radiology 236:601–608

Handel SF, Twiford TW Jr, Reigel DH, et al. (1979) Posterior lumbar apophyseal fractures. Radiology 130:629–633

Henderson RL, Reid DC, Saboe LA (1991) Multiple noncontiguous spine fractures. Spine 16:128–131

Hernandez JA, Chupik C, Swischuk LE (2004) Cervical spine trauma in children under 5 years: productivity of CT. Emerg Radiol 10:176–178

Hoffman JR, Mower WR, Wolfson AB, et al. (2000) Validity of a set of clinical criteria to rule out injury to the cervical spine in patients with blunt trauma. National Emergency X-Radiography Utilization Study Group. N Engl J Med 343:94–99

Hoffman JR, Wolfson AB, Todd K, et al. (1998) Selective cervical spine radiography in blunt trauma: methodology of the National Emergency X-Radiography Utilization Study (NEXUS). Ann Emerg Med 32:461–469

Hogan GJ, Mirvis SE, Shanmuganathan K, et al.(2005) Exclusion of unstable cervical spine injury in obtunded patients with blunt trauma: is MR imaging needed when multi-detector row CT findings are normal? Radiology 237:106–113

Hollenberg GM, Beattie PF, Meyers SP, et al. (2002) Stress reactions of the lumbar pars interarticularis: the development of a new MRI classification system. Spine 27:181–186

Kokoska ER, Keller MS, Rallo MC, et al. (2001) Characteristics of pediatric cervical spine injuries. J Pediatr Surg 36:100–105

Magerl F, Aebi M, Gertzbein SD, et al (1994) A comprehensive classification of thoracic and lumbar injuries. Eur Spine J 3:184–201

Maldague BE, Noel HM, Malghem JJ (1978) The intravertebral vacuum cleft: a sign of ischemic vertebral collapse. Radiology 129:23–29

McAfee PC, Yuan HA, Lasda NA (1982) The unstable burst fracture. Spine 7:365–373

McCall IW, Park WM, McSweeney T (1973) The radiological demonstration of acute lower cervical injury. Clin Radiol 24:235–240

McPhee IB (1981) Spinal fractures and dislocations in children and adolescents. Spine 6:533–537

Naidich JB, Naidich TP, Garfein C, et al. (1977) The widened interspinous distance: a useful sign of anterior cervical dislocation in the supine frontal projection. Radiology 123:113–116

Naul LG, Peet GJ, Maupin WB (1989) Avascular necrosis of the vertebral body: MR imaging. Radiology 172:219–222

Novkov HV, Tanchev PJ, Gyorev IS (1996) Severe fracture-dislocation of S1 in a 12-year-old boy. A case report. Spine 21:2500–2503

Palmieri F, Cassar-Pullicino VN, Dell'Atti C, et al. (2006) Uncovertebral joint injury in cervical facet dislocation: the headphones sign. Eur Radiol 16:1312–1315

Pang D, Li V (2004) Atlantoaxial rotatory fixation: Part 1 – Biomechanics of normal rotation at the atlantoaxial joint in children. Neurosurgery 55:614–625; discussion 625–626

Pang D, Wilberger JE Jr (1982) Spinal cord injury without radiographic abnormalities in children. J Neurosurg 57:114–129

Panjabi MM, Kifune M, Wen L, et al. (1995) Dynamic canal encroachment during thoracolumbar burst fractures. J Spinal Disord 8:39–48

Pennecot GF, Gouraud D, Hardy JR, et al. (1984) Roentgenographical study of the stability of the cervical spine in children. J Pediatr Orthop 4:346–352

Pouliquen JC, Kassis B, Glorion C, et al. (1997) Vertebral growth after thoracic or lumbar fracture of the spine in children. J Pediatr Orthop 17:115–120

Powers B, Miller MD, Kramer RS, et al. (1979) Traumatic anterior atlanto-occipital dislocation. Neurosurgery 4:12–17

Qaiyum, M, Tyrrell PN, McCall IW, et al. (2001) MRI detection of unsuspected vertebral injury in acute spinal trauma: incidence and significance. Skeletal Radiol 30:299–304

Rachbauer F, Sterzinger W, Eibl G (2001) Radiographic abnormalities in the thoracolumbar spine of young elite skiers. Am J Sports Med 29:446–449

Rekate HL, Theodore N, Sonntag VK, et al. (1999) Pediatric spine and spinal cord trauma. State of the art for the third millennium. Childs Nerv Syst 15:743–750

Rodriguez-Fuentes AE (1993) Traumatic sacrolisthesis S1–S2. Report of a case. Spine 18:768–771

Rumball K, Jarvis J (1992) Seat-belt injuries of the spine in young children. J Bone Joint Surg Br 74:571–574

Saternus KS, Thrun C (1987) [Traumatology of the alar ligaments]. Aktuelle Traumatol 17:214–218

Sherk HH, Schut L, Lane JM (1976) Fractures and dislocations of the cervical spine in children. Orthop Clin North Am 7:593–604

Streitwieser DR, Knopp R, Wales LR, et al. (1983) Accuracy of standard radiographic views in detecting cervical spine fractures. Ann Emerg Med 12:538–542

Swischuk LE (1977) Anterior displacement of C2 in children: physiologic or pathologic? Radiology 122:759–763

Swischuk LE, Hayden CK Jr, Sarwar M (1979) The posteriorly tilted dens. A normal variation mimicking a fractured dens. Pediatr Radiol 8:27–28

Swischuk LE, John SD, Hendrick EP (2000) Is the open-mouth odontoid view necessary in children under 5 years? Pediatr Radiol 30:186–189

Swischuk LE, Swischuk PN, John SD (1993) Wedging of C-3 in infants and children: usually a normal finding and not a fracture. Radiology 188:523–526

Takata K, Inoue S, Takahashi K, et al. (1988) Fracture of the posterior margin of a lumbar vertebral body. J Bone Joint Surg Am 70:589–594

Vialle R, Mary P, Schmider L, et al. (2006) Spinal fracture through the neurocentral synchondrosis in battered children: a report of three cases. Spine 31:E345–349

Viccellio P, Simon H, Pressman BD, et al. (2001) A prospective multicenter study of cervical spine injury in children. Pediatrics 108:E20

Woodring JH, Selke AC Jr, Duff DE (1981) Traumatic atlantooccipital dislocation with survival. AJR Am J Roentgenol 137:21–24

Pathological Fractures in the Immature Skeleton

21

A. Mark Davies

CONTENTS

A. M. Davies, MD
Consultant Radiologist, The MRI Centre, Royal Orthopaedic Hospital, Birmingham B31 2AP, UK

21.1 Introduction

A pathological fracture is defined as a fracture through diseased or abnormal bone, usually resulting from a force insufficient to produce a fracture in normal bone. They are infrequent in the paediatric population but can occur due to a large spectrum of different conditions. Pathological fractures may result from intrinsic or extrinsic processes (Dormans and Flynn 2001). Intrinsic processes include conditions such as osteogenesis imperfecta and bone tumours, whereas extrinsic processes include previous surgical intervention (biopsy, fixation etc.) and radiotherapy. Pathological fractures may be further classified as being due to pathology which is solitary, multifocal (polystotic), generalized to the whole skeletal system, or a generalized condition with skeletal involvement (Saraph and Linhart 2005). The diseases that may present with pathological fractures in children are listed in Table 21.1. This chapter will briefly review these conditions describing their salient imaging features. Although the epiphyseal fractures associated with the osteochondroses (e.g. Perthe's and Freiberg's disease) are due to the avascular disturbance and therefore strictly speaking "pathological" these are not covered in this chapter.

21.2 Biomechanics and Relative Incidence

Normal bone preskeletal fusion has greater plasticity than in the adult. A greater decrease of the mineral content or architecture may be required to generate a fracture than in an equivalent adult bone (Ortiz et al. 2005). In addition the thick periosteum found in children may contribute some stability to the fracture

(Bleck and Kleinman 1984). Pathological fractures in the child can present as a complete fracture or with repeated microfractures. The latter occurs in the trabecular bone such as in metaphyses of the long bones or vertebral body. In weight-bearing bones repetitive microfractures will result in progressive deformity such as the shepherd's crook deformity of the proximal femur typical of fibrous dysplasia (Fig. 21.1). Greater forces are required to produce a complete fracture and symptoms are similar to those of an acute fracture through normal bone (Ortiz et al. 2005). It is important to distinguish from the history a true acute fracture from a pathological fracture that may frequently present during physical activity with only a trivial injury. Many of the pathological fractures included in Table 21.1 can be considered insufficiency-type stress fractures in that they arise from normal physiological loading on abnormal bone.

It is difficult to estimate the true incidence of pathological fractures in children. Many factors may introduce bias when trying to assess the incidence. For example, in the developed world pathological fracture in osteomyelitis is unusual due to prompt diagnosis and management, whereas in the underdeveloped world it is much more common due to delayed diagnosis and frequently inadequate treatment. Geography may also play a role when looking at rare conditions whose prevalence may be much higher in a particular population, e.g. sickle cell disease and thalassaemia. In addition, referral bias may be a factor dependent on the particular specialist interest of the treating centre. It is to be expected that pathological fractures in renal osteodystrophy will tend to be seen in specialist renal units. Similarly, other rare conditions, such as Gaucher disease, are increasingly treated in tertiary referral centres thereby concentrating medical expertise and consequently affecting the incidence of a particular type of pathological fracture. Most paediatric pathological fractures through isolated bone lesions tend to be due to tumours or tumour-like lesions. A recent three-centre study identified a total of 88 cases collected over a period of 5 years. The commonest cause of fracture was a simple bone cyst (40%) followed by nonossifying fibroma (19%), fibrous dysplasia (16%), osteosarcoma (15%) and aneurysmal bone cyst (10%) (Ortiz et al. 2005). Scoring systems for assessing the risk of impending pathological fracture have been described but largely apply to metastases in the adult rather than primary bone tumours in the paediatric skeleton (Mirrels 1989; Damron et al. 2003; Van der Linden et al. 2004; Katagiri et al. 2005). The exception is several publications evaluating fracture risk in simple bone cyst (Kaelin and MacEwen 1989; Ahn and Park 1994) and nonossifying fibroma (Arata et al. 1981).

Table 21.1. Classification of musculoskeletal conditions that may present with pathological fractures in children. Several conditions could be included in more than one category. For example, sickle cell disease is both a congenital and developmental disorder as well as haematopoietic. For the sake of simplicity each disorder is only included once in the overall classification

Congenital and developmental
Osteogenesis imperfecta
Neurofibromatosis
Fibrous dysplasia
Osteopetrosis and pyknodysostosis
Tumour and tumour-like
Benign
Simple bone cyst
Aneurysmal bone cyst
Fibrous cortical defect/nonossifying fibroma
Enchondroma
Malignant
Osteosarcoma
Ewing sarcoma
Infection
Metabolic
Rickets
Hyperparathyroidism and chronic renal failure
Scurvy
Haematopoietic and marrow
Leukaemia
Sickle cell disease
Thalassaemia
Haemophilia
Gorham disease
Gaucher disease
Langerhans cell histiocytosis
Neuromuscular
Cerebral palsy
Spinal cord injury and spina bifida
Muscular dystrophy
Poliomyelitis
Iatrogenic
Radiotherapy
Biopsy/fixation/curettage
Drugs (steroids, chemotherapy)

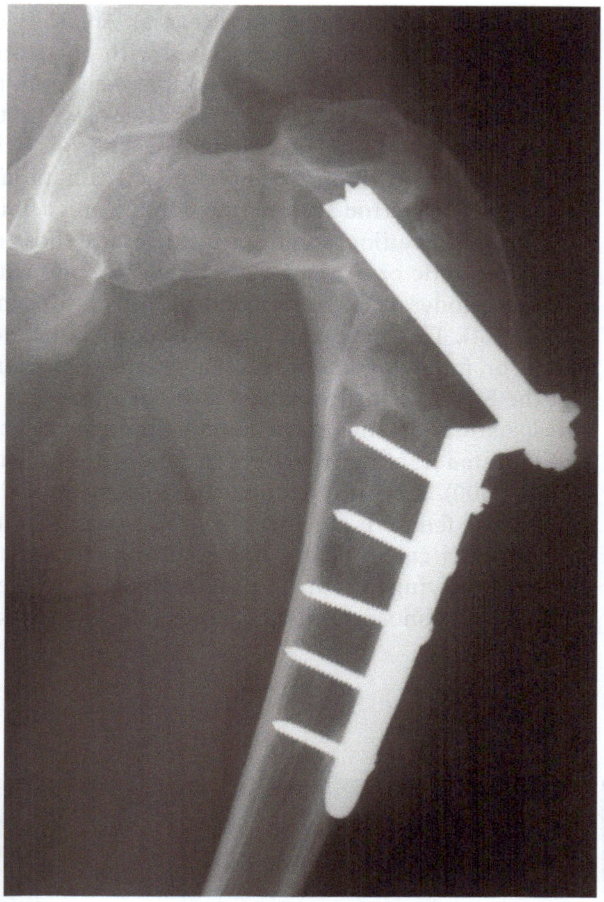

Fig. 21.1. Fibrous dysplasia. "Shepherd's crook deformity. The attempted internal fixation has failed

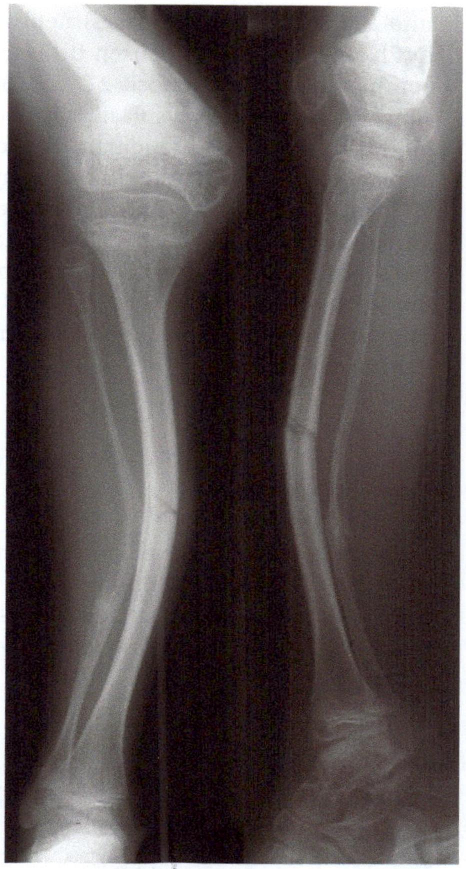

Fig. 21.2. Osteogenesis imperfecta. Gracile, osteopenic bones with malunion fracture distal femur and a more recent fracture of the tibial diaphysis

21.3 Congenital and Developmental Disorders

21.3.1 Osteogenesis Imperfecta

Osteogenesis imperfecta (OI) is an inherited disorder of collagen affecting the skeleton, ligaments, skin, sclera and dentin. The four major components of the disease are osteopenia with fragility of the skeleton, blue sclerae, premature osteosclerosis and dentinogenesis imperfecta. In the past OI has been classified as into two syndromes. The more severe 'congenita' form associated with a high infant mortality and a less severe 'tarda" form. In recognition of the variability of the disease now at least four types +/– subtypes are recognised (Sillence 1981). It is beyond the scope of this chapter to describe each type in detail; suffice it to say that Type 1 is the commonest and mildest phenotype estimated to occur in 1 of 30,000 births. The severity of the Type 1 disease can vary from multiple fractures and intracranial bleeding resulting in stillbirth or perinatal death to generalized osteopenia with gracile long bones, repeated fractures and bowing deformities (Fig. 21.2). Spinal fractures result in multiple level flattened or biconcave vertebral bodies. OI is a diagnosis frequently queried when a child is being investigated for suspected non-accidental injury.

21.3.2 Neurofibromatosis

Neurofibromatosis is one of the phakomatoses in which there are embryological abnormalities of all three germ layers. Although up to eight subtypes have been identified most texts classify the disorder into the common (90% cases) neurofibromatosis 1 (NF1 or Von Recklinghausen disease) and the less common neurofibromatosis 2 (NF2). Both types may show a mesodermal dysplasia with bowing, pathological fracture and pseudarthrosis formation. The latter typically affects the tibial diaphysis in infants and young children with delayed healing or persistent non-union (Fig. 21.3) (Murray and Lovell 1982). Less commonly the forearm bones and the fibula may be involved (Gregg et al. 1982). Interestingly, biopsy of the non-union shows no evidence of neurofibromatosis.

21.3.3 Fibrous Dysplasia

Fibrous dysplasia is a developmental anomaly of bone in which the normal medullary space is replaced by fibroosseous tissue (Smith and Kransdorf 2000). It may affect a single bone (monostotic – 75% cases) or multiple bone (polystotic – 25% cases). A variety of endocrinopathies can be associated with polystotic fibrous dysplasia. The classic example seen in up to one third of females with polystotic disease is McCune-Albright syndrome in which there is fibrous dysplasia (frequently mono- or hemimelic), café-au-lait spots and endocrine dysfunction notably precocious puberty. The radiographic appearances are those of a benign lytic or ground-glass lesion in bone with mild to moderate expansion and endosteal thinning (Fig. 21.4). This may result in small cortical infractions or, following minor trauma, complete fracture of the bone. Callus formation at the fracture site is dysplastic and patients are therefore prone to a cycle of repeated fractures resulting in deformity (Kumta et al. 2000). A typical feature of involvement of the proximal femur is an increasing varus deformity (shepherd's crook deformity) resulting from malunion following fracture or progressive bone modelling due to abnormal biomechanics (Fig. 21.1) (Jung et al. 2006).

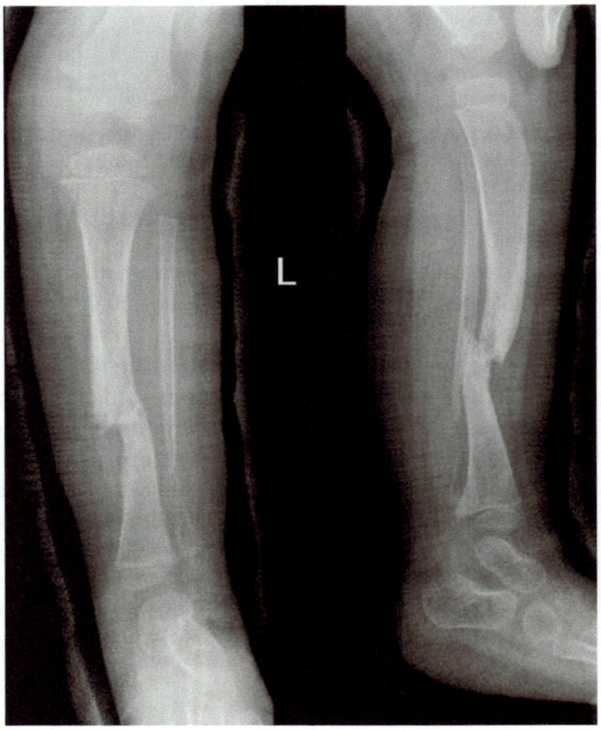

Fig. 21.3. Neurofibromatosis. Pseudarthrosis formation of both the tibial and fibular diaphyses. There has been resorption of the bone ends of the fibular lesion. (Case courtesy of Dr. K Johnson)

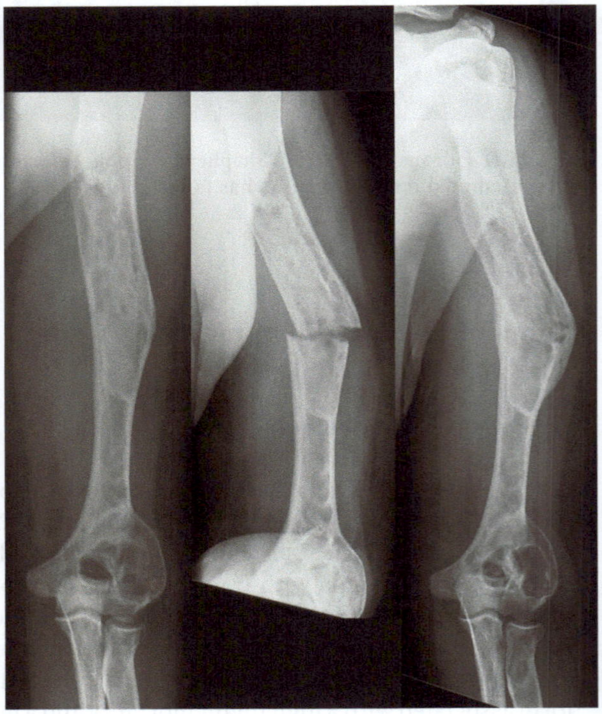

Fig. 21.4. Polystotic fibrous dysplasia prefracture, immediately postfracture and healed several months later with residual deformity

21.3.4 Osteopetrosis and Pyknodysostosis

There are two sclerosing bone dysplasias that are associated with an increased risk of fractures. Despite the sclerosis the bones are brittle and therefore susceptible to insufficiency type stress fractures (Fig. 21.5). There are four different forms of the dysplasia known as osteopetrosis. A relatively mild autosomal dominant 'benign/tarda' type (Albers-Schönberg disease) with sclerotic bones, 'bone-within-a-bone' appearance, 'rugger jersey' spine and insufficiency fractures. A severe autosomal recessive 'malignant/congenita' type manifesting in infancy with marrow failure and more severe osseous changes and complications together with modelling deformities (Erlenmeyer flask deformity). Affected patients frequently die in the first decade of life. There are two other autosomal recessive forms of osteopetrosis; an intermediate and a type associated with renal tubular acidosis. The other sclerosing dysplasia, also autosomal recessive, is pyknodysostosis in which there is generalized osteosclerosis, fractures and acroosteolysis (Fig. 21.6).

21.4 Tumour and Tumour-Like Lesions

21.4.1 Benign

A recent study showed that almost 70% of pathological fractures in children are due to benign tumours

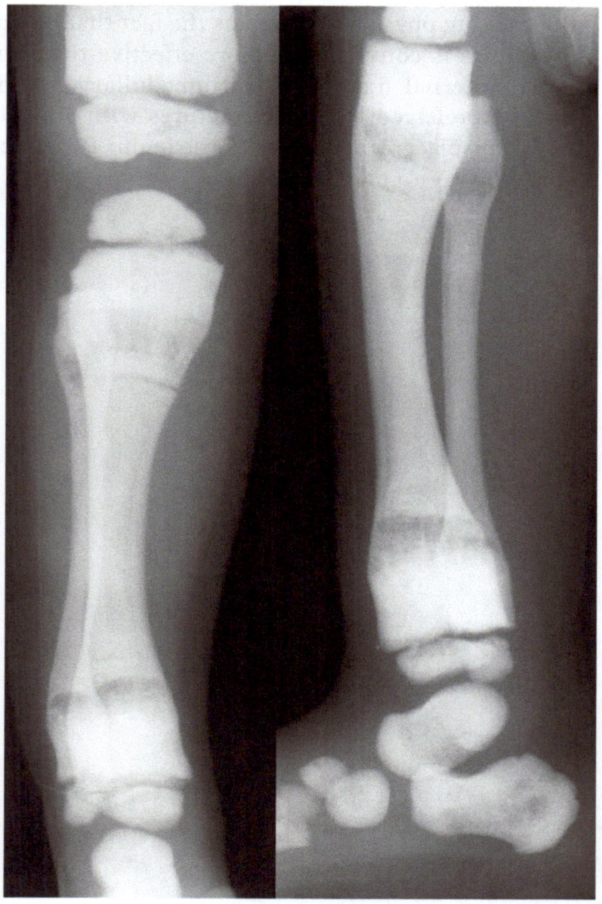

Fig. 21.5. Osteopetrosis. Osteosclerosis, modelling deformities (Erlenmeyer flask deformity distal femur) and an undisplaced insufficiency fracture of the proximal tibial diaphysis

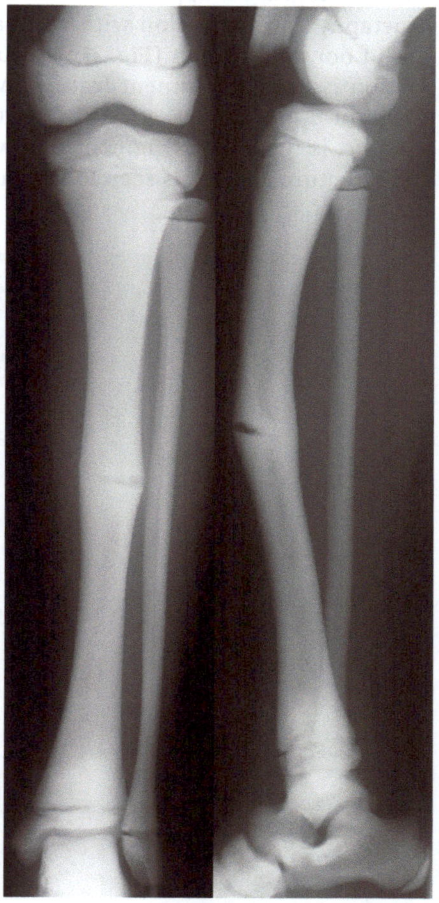

Fig. 21.6. Pyknodysostosis. Osteosclerosis with a chronic insufficiency fracture of the tibial diaphysis

or tumour-like lesions of bone (Ortiz et al. 2005). The four commonest causes are simple bone cyst, aneurysmal bone cyst, nonossifying fibroma and enchondroma.

21.4.1.1
Simple Bone Cyst

Simple bone cyst (SBC), also known as unicameral bone cyst, is a common nonneoplastic lesion of childhood with almost 95% cases occurring before the age of 20 years. Typical sites are the proximal humerus (50%) and the proximal femur 25% (Docquier and Delloye 2004). Clinically, the majority of SBCs are painless until minor trauma results in a pathological fracture. Over 75% cases therefore present with a fracture. In cases presenting without a fracture the fracture risk can be calculated using a scoring system (Kaelin and MacEwen 1989; Ahn and Park 1994). The radiographic appearances are those of a central metaphyseal lytic lesion with cortical thinning and mild bony expansion (Fig. 21.7). Septation/trabeculation is not a prominent feature. A typical feature seen in up to 20% cases of SBC, but not pathognomonic, is the 'fallen fragment sign' where a piece of the fractured cortex is seen to migrate to the dependent portion of the cyst (Fig. 21.7) (Reynolds 1969). With MR imaging the cyst contents appear mildly hypointense on T1-weighted and hyperintense on T2-weighted and STIR images. The thin cyst wall lining will show some minor enhancement with intravenous gadolinium. A fluid-fluid level may be seen in the presence of a recent fracture due to haemorrhage into the cyst. In time the SBC will grow away from the growth plate and, depending on the extent of healing, may mimic other lesions such as fibrous dysplasia. Complications include repeated fracture, healing with deformity and growth arrest of the adjacent physis resulting in limb shortening (Violas et al. 2004). Over the years numerous different treatments have been advocated for SBCs including curettage and bone grafting, percutaneous steroid injection, autologous bone marrow injection, Ethibloc injection and intramedullary nailing to mention only a few (Roposch et al. 2000). The wide variety of managements reflects the personal preference of the treating physician as well as the fact that no one procedure is convincingly more effective than any other. Internal fixation or intramedullary nailing may be preferred for those fractures with a bigger risk of displacement such as in the femur (Roposch et al. 2004; Vigler et al. 2006).

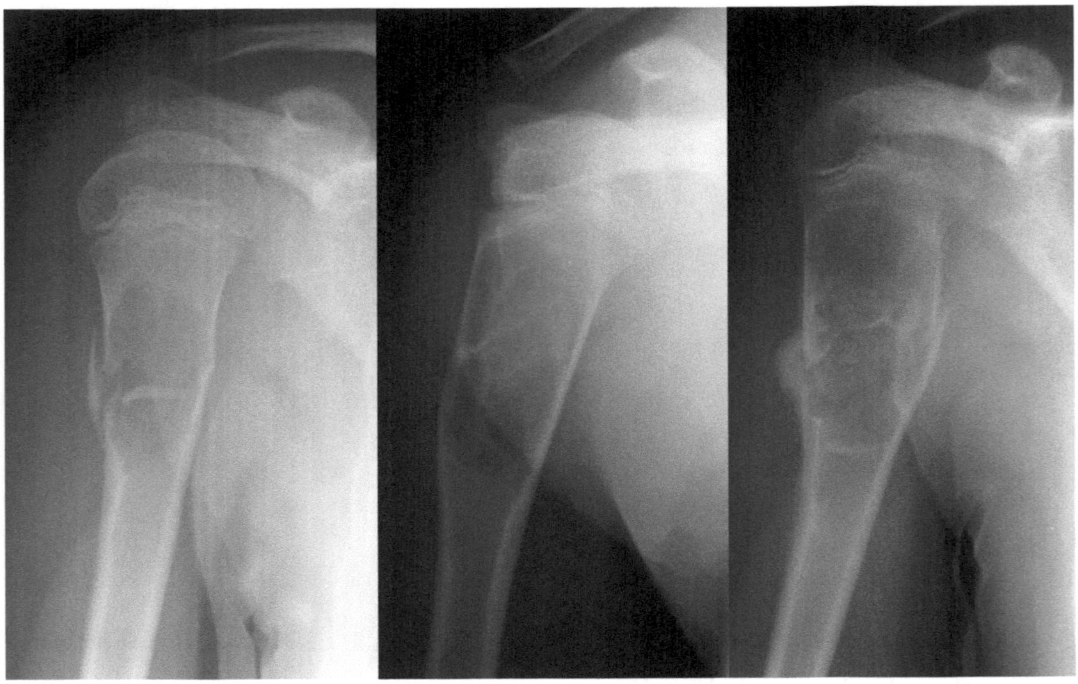

Fig. 21.7. Simple bone cyst. At presentation with a "fallen fragment" sign. Healed 6 months later and refracture with early callus formation at 12 months

21.4.1.2
Aneurysmal Bone Cyst

Aneurysmal bone cyst (ABC) is another benign lesion of bone with 80% cases occurring in patients under the age of 20 years. ABC occurs as either a primary bone lesion (70% cases) or as a secondary lesion in a pre-existing bone lesion (30% cases) (COTTALORDA and BOURELLE 2007). For a long time it has been considered a nonneoplastic lesion with numerous different theories as to its pathogenesis. Interestingly, recent genetic and immunohistochemical studies are suggesting that primary ABC is after all a true neoplasm and not a reactive lesion (LEITHNER et al. 2004; OLIVEIRA et al. 2004). Lesions predominate in the long bones (50% cases) and the spine particularly the posterior elements (20% cases). The radiographic appearances have been described as a progression through four stages (KRANSDORF and SWEET 1995). First, an initial phase when the lysis can mimic other benign bone lesions such as simple bone cyst and fibrous dysplasia (PARMAN and MURPHEY 2000). Second, an active or growth phase with marked expansion to give a "blown-out" appearance – most present in this phase with pathological fractures in 20% cases (Fig. 21.8a). Third and fourth, respectively, are stabilization and healing phases with progressive thickening of the peripheral shell of the tumour. In all, 85% cases arise within medullary bone and 15% in a cortical or subperiosteal location (MAIYA et al. 2002). Histologically ABCs comprise multiple blood filled cysts with intervening septae. Fluid-fluid levels due to the layering out of blood products within the cysts can be identified on CT and MRI (Fig. 21.8b). Fluid-fluid levels within bone and soft tissue lesions is a non-specific sign (VAN DYCK et al. 2006). However, the commonest cause of a bone lesion in a child showing multiple fluid-fluid levels is an ABC (DAVIES et al. 1992) and lesions comprising a proportion greater than 2/3 fluid-fluid levels are more likely to be primary or secondary ABC than a malignancy (O'DONNELL and SAIFUDDIN 2004). The modes of treatment of ABC advocated in the literature vary considerably including embolization, curettage, resection, Ethibloc injection and intralesional implantation of demineralised bone particles (COTTALORDA and BOURELLE 2006). Inactive lesions, once the diagnosis has been confirmed by biopsy, may be monitored with a 'watch-and-wait' policy.

21.4.1.3
Nonossifying Fibroma

The commonest fibrous lesion of bone is the fibrous cortical defect and the histologically identical but larger nonossifying fibroma. Both lesions are seen in childhood and adolescence, slightly more common in boys, with a predilection for the long bones around the knee. Fibrous cortical defects are seen in up to 30% of the normal population under the age of 15 years and

a

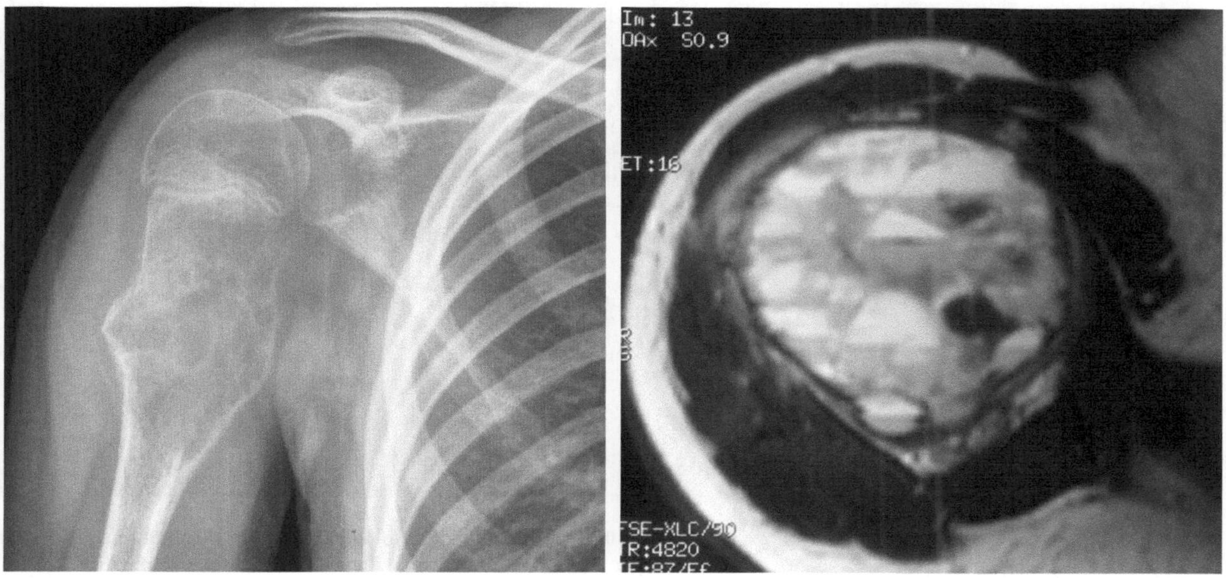

b

Fig. 21.8a,b. Aneurysmal bone cyst. Pathological fracture through the ABC in the proximal humerus in the active phase. The axial T2-weighted MR image shows multiple fluid-fluid levels are too small to present with a pathological fracture. The radiographic appearances are those of a well-defined lytic lesion arising eccentrically within the metaphysis of a long bone. Larger nonossifying fibromas can present with a pathological fracture (Fig. 21.9) (Drennan et al. 1974; Hase and Miki 2000). Arata and coworkers (1981) reported that if a nonossifying fibroma involves more than 50% of the transverse diameter of the bone or measures greater than 33 mm in length there is an increased risk of pathological fracture. A more recent series, however, showed that 59% cases of nonossifying fibromas exceeded these threshold measurements without fracturing (Easley and Kneisl 1997). Most cases of nonossifying fibroma, with or without fracture, can be satisfactorily managed with nonoperative treatment.

21.4.1.4
Enchondroma

Enchondroma is the second commonest benign tumour of bone after osteochondroma and is composed of mature hyaline cartilage arising within medullary bone. It comprises approximately 10% of all benign bone tumours and is the commonest tumour of the tubular bones of the hands and feet (Fig. 21.10). Many cases are an incidental finding on radiographs obtained for unrelated reasons or present with a pathological fracture following minor trauma. The main lesions appear lytic with minor expansion and varying degrees of cartilage mineralization described as flocculent, ring-and-arc or popcorn in appearance. The hands and feet are also a common site of involvement with the multiple forms of the tumour, Ollier disease and Maffucci's syndrome. Pathological fracture formation is no more of a problem in children than adults with enchondroma as shown by the absence of publications on this subject when conducting an electronic search of the paediatric literature. The most serious complication seen rarely in solitary enchondroma but more common in both Ollier disease and Maffucci's syndrome is malignant transformation to a central chondrosarcoma which may present with a patho-

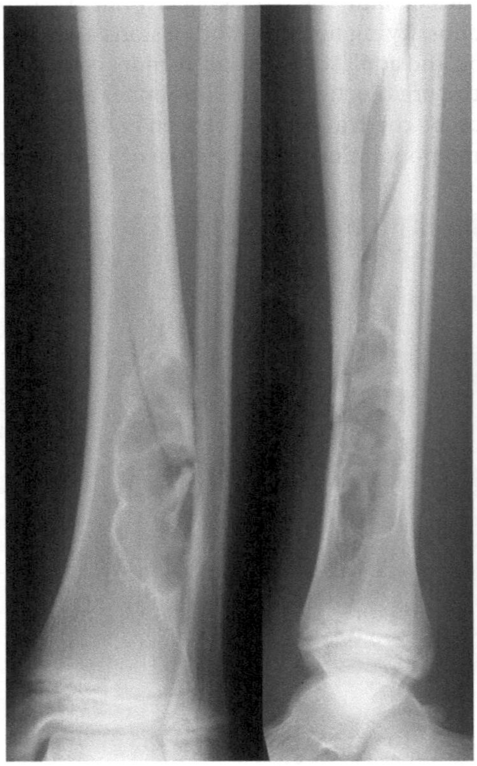

Fig. 21.9. Nonossifying fibroma. Well defined eccentric lytic lesion with a spiral fracture extending up the tibial diaphysis

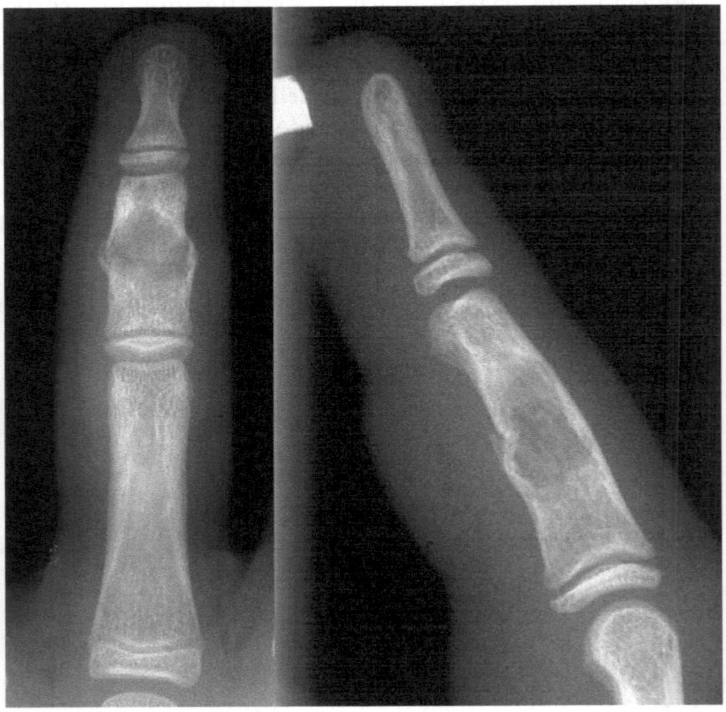

Fig. 21.10. Enchondroma. Pathological fracture through middle phalanx of finger. This case shows no evidence of cartilage calcification

logical fracture due to progressive bone destruction. Malignant change, however, is a complication really only seen in adults. Cellular atypia on histological examination, particularly in cartilage lesions in the hands and feet, should not be considered indicative of malignancy.

21.4.2 Malignant

Pathological fracture through an osteosarcoma as the presenting complaint or during preoperative treatment is seen in 5%–10% cases (Jaffe et al. 1987). They occur either spontaneously or as a result of minor trauma (Fig. 21.11). There is an increased risk in telangiectatic osteosarcoma as it is predominantly lytic (Huvos et al. 1982). It has been claimed that pathological fracture is associated with a poor outcome because of the dissemination of the tumour within the haematoma so that amputation is the preferred surgical treatment (Morris 1997; Scully et al. 2002). Some studies have suggested that limb-sparing surgery with adequate margins of excision can be achieved without compromising survival but may or may not have an increased risk of local recurrence (Abudu et al. 1996; Bacci et al. 2003; Natarajan et al. 2000). It is important when undertaking staging of the primary tumour with MR imaging that any haematoma is likely to be contaminated with tumour. Likewise if the fracture extends to an articular surface the joint should also be considered to be involved. Care should be taken in measuring longitudinal tumour dimensions in bone due to deformity and the concertina effect of overlapping fracture margins. The risk of pathological fracture as the presenting complaint or during preoperative treatment in Ewing sarcoma is similar to that in osteosarcoma (5%–10% cases) (Fig. 21.12) (Fuchs et al. 2003). The concerns regarding staging and the surgical options are also similar. Patients with treated sarcomas of bone are at an increased

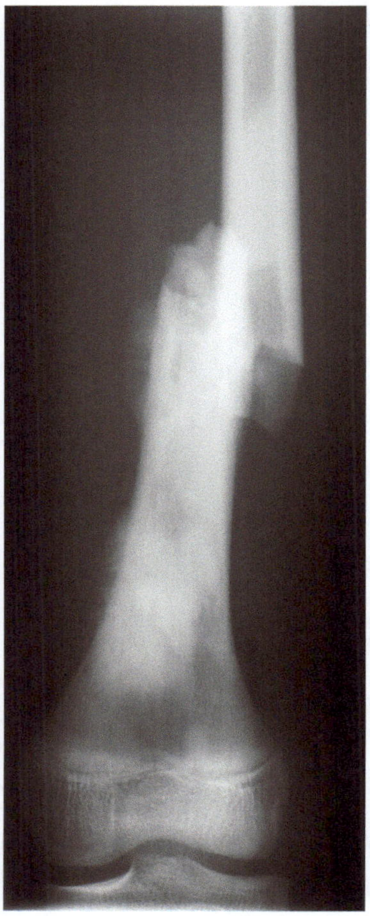

Fig. 21.11. Osteosarcoma. Pathological fracture through extensive sclerotic osteosarcoma of the femoral diaphysis

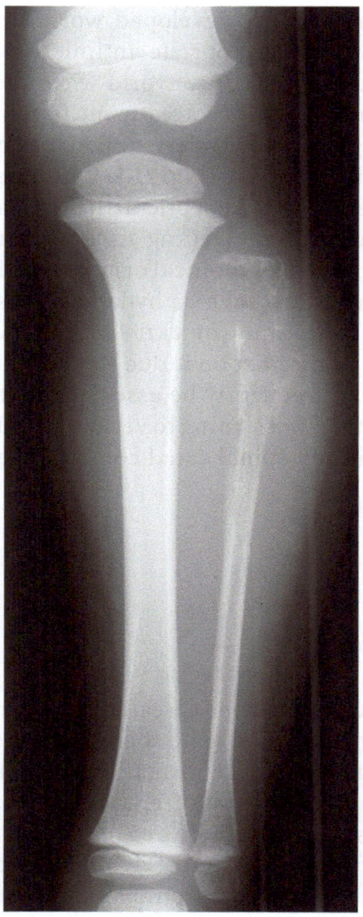

Fig. 21.12. Ewing sarcoma. Pathological fracture through an aggressive lesion in the proximal fibula

risk of insufficiency type fractures of the long bones due to prolonged immobilization, the effects on the bone of chemotherapy and radiation therapy.

Two modes of presentation of pathological fracture of sarcoma in children merit special mention. First, there are the cases where the underlying tumour is so subtle as to be overlooked on the initial radiographs (De Santos and Edeiken 1985; Ramo et al. 2006). Second, where the tumour is mistaken for a benign bone tumour. In both situations failure to recognize the underlying malignancy may lead to inappropriate internal fixation thereby potentially disseminating the tumour along the whole length of the bone that in turn makes curative limb-salvage surgery problematic.

21.5 Infection

Pathological fractures in association with osteomyelitis are uncommon in the developed world due to prompt diagnosis and appropriate antimicrobial treatment. In the underdeveloped world where delayed diagnosis and suboptimal treatment is commonplace then progressive bony destruction may be sufficient to result in a fracture (Fig. 21.13). Alternatively, an inadequately treated septic arthritis may spread to the adjacent bone leading to a fracture (Devnani 2002). Exotic geographical origins should suggest unusual infections such as hydatid disease and mycetoma (Kumar and Cornah 1983; Fahal et al. 1996). Spondylodiscitis, be it due to pyogenic infections or TB, can frequently be associated with major endplate destruction leading to vertebral body collapse with or without spinal canal compromise.

21.6 Metabolic Disorders

The spectrum of metabolic bone diseases will result in a generalized weakness of bone thereby predisposing to pathological fracture formation. In rickets, due to a dietary deficiency of vitamin D, this can manifest as insufficiency fractures in the pelvis and long bones of the lower limb (Fig. 21.14). Advances in the management of chronic renal failure have lessened the frequency and severity of renal osteodystrophy but skeletal problems may still be seen in children. These include lower limb deformities, osteonecrosis, epiphysiolysis -- notably slipped upper femoral epiphysis and insufficiency fractures (Fig. 21.15) (Barrett and Papadimitriou 1996). The fractures tend to develop at the apex of a long-standing bowing deformity (Mankin 1974a,b). In the past pathological fractures through the brown tumours of hyperparathyroidism were well recognised but tended to be seen in adults as the primary disease is rare in children (Morgan et al. 2002). Today, three quarters of cases of primary hyperparathyroidism are detected on biochemical assays well before there is any opportunity for radiographic evidence of the disease to develop. Scurvy, due to vitamin C deficiency, is another disease rarely seen these days. The classic radiographic appearances of scurvy are generalized osteopenia and the metaphyseal 'corner' or 'beak' sign of Pelkan due to small fractures around the margins of the metaphyses.

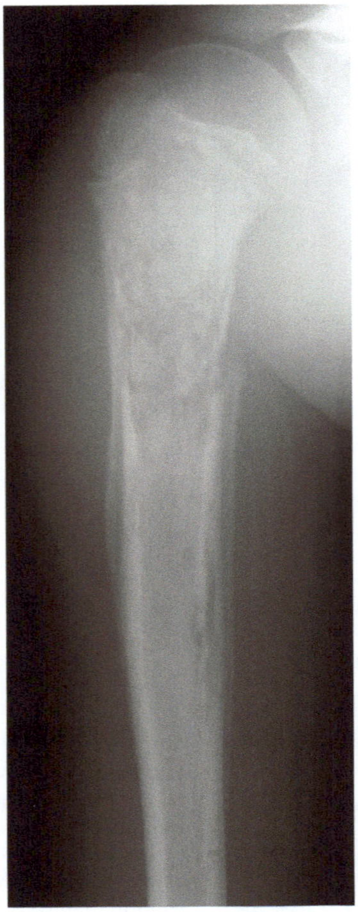

Fig. 21.13. Acute osteomyelitis. Pathological fracture through aggressive lesion indistinguishable from a primary sarcoma of bone

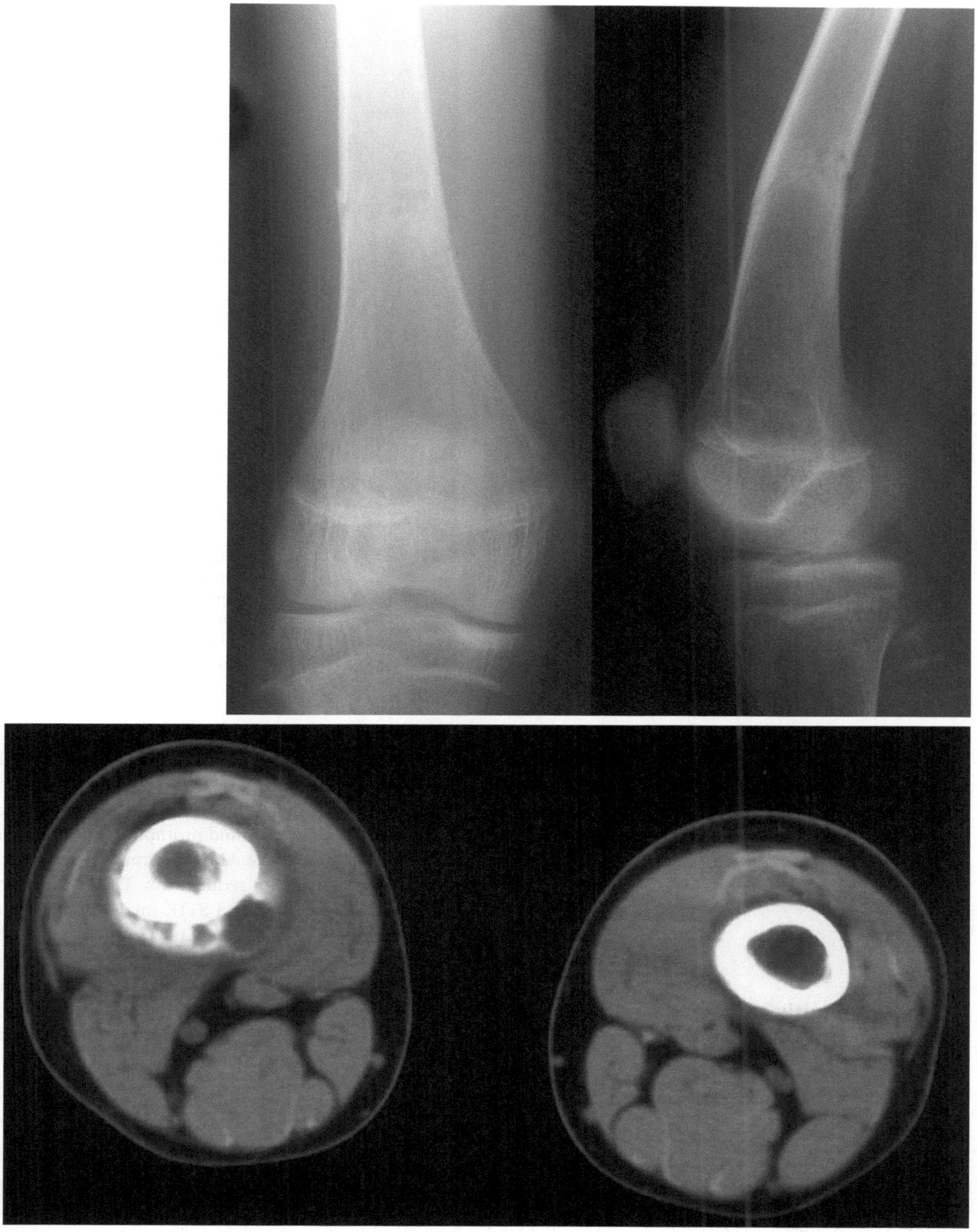

a

b

Fig. 21.14a,b. Rickets. Insufficiency fracture of the distal femoral diaphysis. The immature callus formation on the CT was originally misinterpreted as due to an osteosarcoma

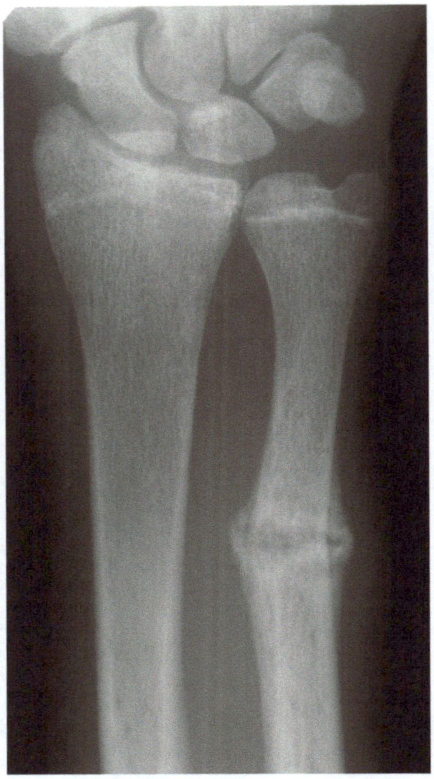

Fig. 21.15. Chronic renal failure. Looser's zone in the distal ulna extending to a full fracture

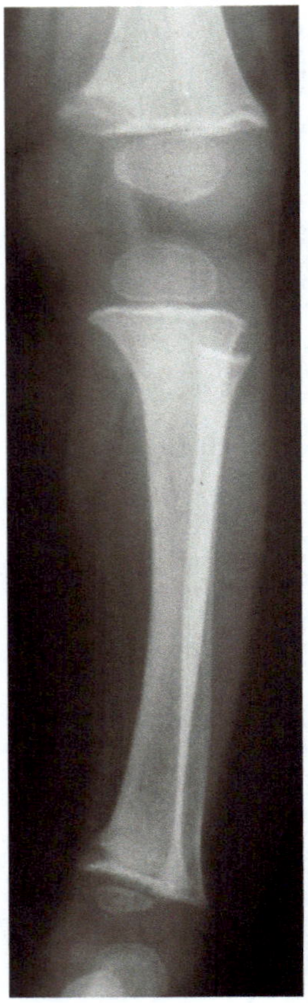

Fig. 21.16. Scurvy. Marginal metaphyseal fractures (Pelkan spurs) distal femur and distal tibia. The differential diagnosis includes non-accidental injury

These principally affect the long bones of the lower limb and anterior ends of the ribs (Fig. 21.16). Due to increased capillary fragility minor injury can also result in large subperiosteal haematomas that will ossify in time (McCann 1962).

21.7 Haematopoeitic and Other Marrow Disorders

21.7.1 Leukaemia

The leukaemias represent a group of diffuse malignancies of the bone marrow that frequently produce bony changes. The commonest form in children, particularly under 5 years of age, is acute lymphoblastic leukaemia (ALL). The radiographic features seen in up to three quarters of patients include diffuse osteopenia, radiolucent and radiodense metaphyseal bands, osteolytic lesions and periosteal new bone formation (Fig. 21.17). Identification of unexplained generalized osteopenia in a child should prompt urgent investigation to confirm/exclude ALL. MR imaging will reveal diffuse signal change, reduced on T1-weighted and raised on T2-weighted and STIR images, throughout the marrow (Thomsen et al. 1987). In the spine the presenting complaint may be vertebral body fractures with wedging and or collapse. The differential diagnosis of disseminated aggressive bone lesions in a young child should also include neuroblastoma metastases.

21.7.2 Sickle Cell Disease

Sickle cell disease is an autosomal dominant congenital haemoglobinopathy due to a defect in the protein component of haemoglobin. The abnormal haemoglobin S (HbS) causes the red blood cells to take on a sickle shape when deoxygenated or the blood pH

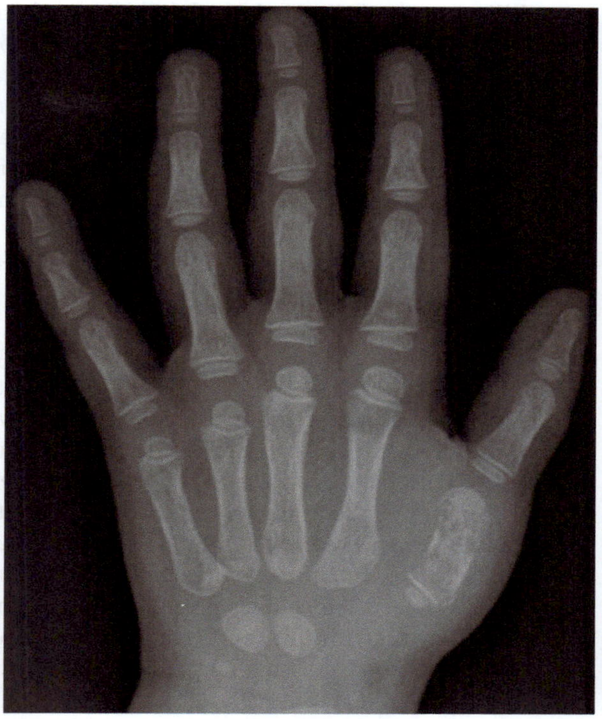

Fig. 21.17. Leukaemia. Pathological fracture developing through leukaemic deposit in the first metacarpal. The differential diagnosis would include dactylitis due to other causes. (Case courtesy of Dr. K Johnson)

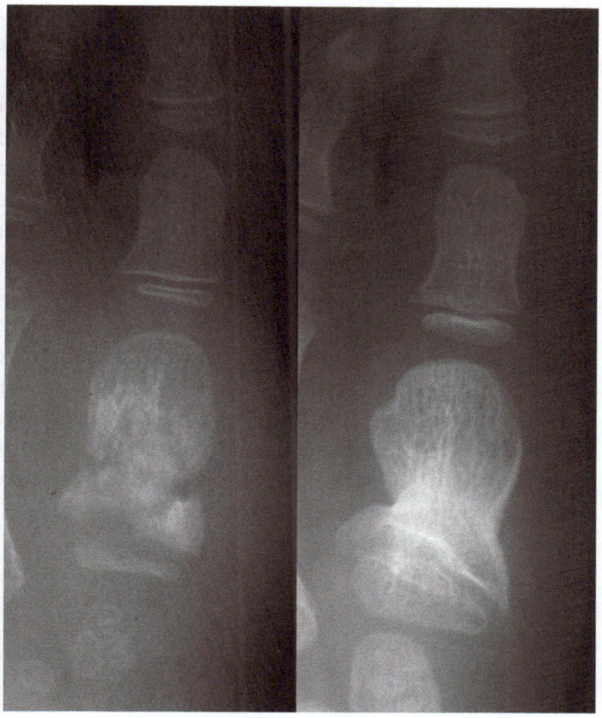

Fig. 21.18. Sickle cell disease – hand-foot syndrome. The initial radiograph shows a destructive dactylitis of the first metatarsal. At 14 months later this has healed with foreshortening

falls. This in turn causes increased blood viscosity that leads to thrombosis and infarction. The disease is most severe in the homozygote form (Hb SS) and milder in the heterozygote form (Hb AS – sickle cell trait). It is a disease of black Africans and also occurs wherever the black races have migrated, particularly in the US and Caribbean islands. Later migration from the Caribbean in the mid-twentieth century means that it is also frequently seen in the minority black population in the UK. The principal osseous changes of Hb SS are marrow hyperplasia due to the chronic haemolysis, osteonecrosis/infarction due to vascular occlusion and the complication of osteomyelitis. If bone infarction is particularly severe it can result in pathological fractures of the long bones and vertebral collapse. One well recognized form of massive infarction seen in young children is aseptic dactylitis of the hands and feet (hand-foot syndrome). It can affect one or more long bones and causes marked bony destruction and fractures (Fig. 21.18). Metaphyseal infarction in childhood can result in premature fusion of the growth plate leading to shortening of the affected bone (Cockshott 1963). The radiographic changes are frequently more pronounced in patients from underdeveloped countries not only because of inadequate treatment but the fact that the underlying anaemia may be exacerbated by coexistent parasitic infections. Osteomyelitis is a well-recognized complication of sickle cell disease but said to be 50 times less common than infarction (Lonergan et al. 2001). The commonest infective organisms are staphylococcus aureus and salmonella typhi. It can be difficult to distinguish osteomyelitis from infarction on clinical, laboratory and radiographic findings. Even with CT, MR imaging and different scintigraphic agents reliable and accurate differentiation of osteomyelitis from infarction can be problematic (Bonnerot et al. 1994; Frush et al. 1999).

21.7.3 Thalassaemia

Thalassaemia is an inherited group of disorders in which there is deficient globin production resulting in a severe haemolytic anaemia. It may affect the alpha chain synthesis in which case it can affect the foetus or the beta chain that tends to present in childhood. The severity of the disease will depend on whether it is inherited as the homozygous form (thalassaemia major) or heterozygous (thalassaemia minor). It is seen most commonly in the countries bordering the Mediterranean Sea of Greek and Italian origin hence the literal translation meaning anaemia of the sea. If untreated with blood transfusions the predominant radiographic feature is marrow hyperplasia with ostepenia, bone expansion, coarsening of the trabeculae and modelling deformities (Erlenmeyer flask deformity) (Tunaci et al. 1999). Multiple and recurrent fractures of the long bones and vertebral bodies are not uncommon due to the severe osteopenia (Fig. 21.19) (Finsterbush et al. 1985). These can be slow to heal with residual deformity.

21.7.4 Haemophilia

Recurrent haemorrhage into the soft tissues in patients with poorly controlled bleeding disorders such as haemophilia can result in erosion of the adjacent bone to produce the so-called haemophiliac pseudotumor. If left untreated these can progress to pathological fracture formation although this complication is more typically seen in adults than children (Ishiguro et al. 1998). In this day and age with better clinical management arthropathic complications are much more common in haemophilia than pseudotumors.

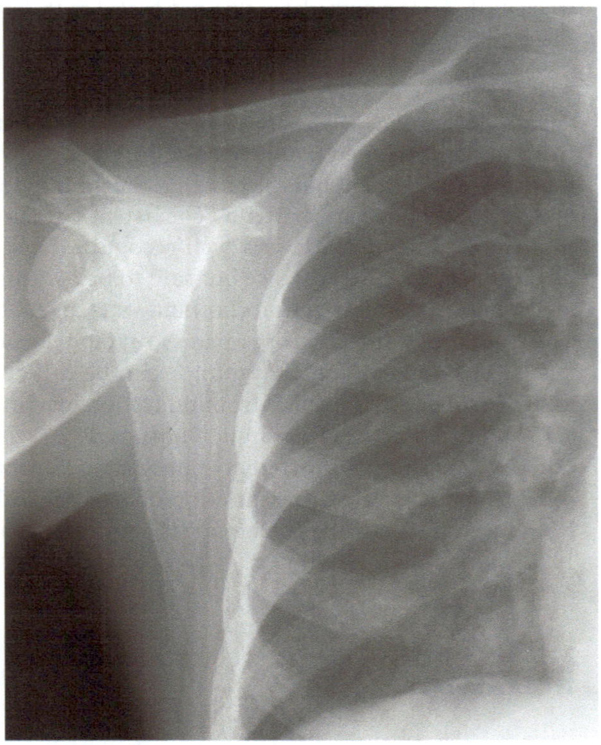

Fig. 21.19. Thalassaemia. Marrow hyperplasia with malunion of a fracture of the proximal humerus

21.7.5 Gorham Disease

Gorham disease is a rare bone disorder of unknown aetiology characterised by bone destruction, vascular and/or lymphatic proliferation with a lack of new bone formation. It is a non-familial condition with less than 200 cases reported in total (Moller et al. 1999). There is a wide range of age of onset from infants to the elderly. Most cases present in the second and third decades (Gorham and Stout 1955). Almost any bone can be affected with a predilection for the skull, thoracic cage, humerus and pelvis (Fig. 21.20). Single bone involvement is more common than multiple (Kai et al. 2006). The radiographic appearances have been classified into four stages (Chung et al. 1997; Yoo et al. 2002). The first stage, confined to bone, is typified by multiple ill-defined cortical and medullary lucencies. In the second stage the lucencies coalesce and the area of overall bone involvement increases. The third stage is characterised by cortical erosion and formation of a soft tissue mass. It is at this stage that patients may present with a pathological fracture (Sato et al. 1997). The bone is resorbed and replaced with fibrous tissue in the fourth and final stage. The tapered ends of the resorbed bone has been described as appearing like "sucked candy" (Moller et al. 1999). The MR imaging appearances are variable depending on the presence or absence of soft tissue extension and the relative proportion of fibrous tissue. Surgery with bone grafting is frequently unsuccessful due to resorption of the graft material. Radiation therapy can arrest the bone destruction and occasionally lead to some remineralization but the response is unpredictable (Yoo et al. 2002).

21.7.6 Gaucher Disease

Gaucher disease is a genetic deficiency in the lysosomal enzyme ß-glucocerebrosidase that causes excessive storage of glucocerebroside in macrophages and monocytes (Wenstrup et al. 2002). The resulting enlarged cells are known as Gaucher cells and their abnormal accumulation in the various organs, including the skeleton, gives rise to the various clinical manifestations of the disease. It is the commonest of the lysosomal storage disease and occurs in approximately one in every 500 Ashkenazic Jews and one of every 50,000 of the general population. Three basic clinical types of Gaucher disease have been identified. The commonest is the non-neuronopathic form referred to as Type 1. The remainder have the more severe acutely neuronopathic (Type 2) or the subacutely neuronopathic (Type 3) variants. Osteopenia with modelling abnormalities (Erlenmeyer flask deformity), osteonecrosis, osteosclerosis, bone crisis, chronic bone pain, pathological fracture and vertebral collapse are all associated with Gaucher disease (Fig. 21.21) (Li et al. 1988). Osteonecrosis may occasionally be complicated by osteomyelitis (Rademakers 1995). The severity of bone involvement and rate of disease progression vary considerably but in general the disease is more aggressive in patients who present in childhood (Maas et al. 2002). It is because of the intense osteopenia that there is an increased risk of pathological fractures. These fractures are associated with severe pain and disability particularly if involving the vertebrae. Decreased bone mineral density can be measured in these patients using dual-energy X-ray absorptiometry (DXA) (Pastores et al. 1999). Current management of Gaucher disease relies on enzyme replacement therapy and treatment of the complications of the disease as and when they

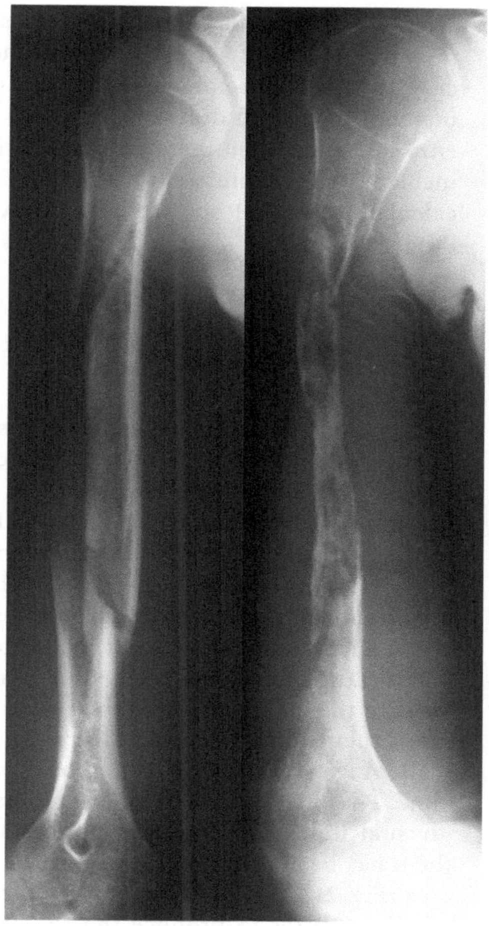

Fig. 21.20. Gorham disease. Two spiral fractures sustained following only minor trauma. Progressive lysis developed over the subsequent 12 months

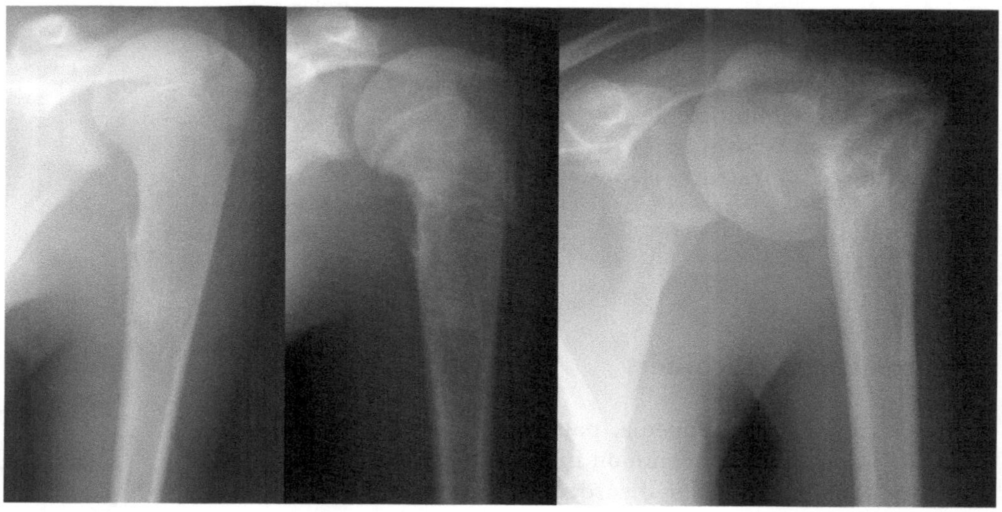

Fig. 21.21. Gaucher disease. Progression of fracture proximal humerus ending in malunion at 18 months

arise. MR imaging is currently being used to determine the extent of skeletal involvement with Gaucher disease. Both semiquantitative and quantitative methods have been described to assess response to enzyme replacement therapy. Quantitative methods include Dixon chemical shift imaging, T1-relaxation calculations and MR spectroscopy (Maas et al. 2002; Poll et al. 2002).

21.7.7 Langerhans Cell Histiocytosis

Langerhans cell histiocytosis (LCH) is a complex disease entity with three distinct clinical manifestations that all demonstrate identical histological features (Hoover et al. 2007). The most benign form of the disease is eosinophilic granuloma in which there is a solitary or multiple, but not disseminated, bone lesions. These appear as lytic lesions of flat bones such as the skull vault, mandible, ribs and pelvis (David et al. 1989; Kilborn et al. 2003). Lesions in the long bones tend to arise in the diaphyses of the femur, tibia and humerus with endosteal scalloping and overlying continuous periosteal new bone. Pathological fractures of the long bones are unusual unless the lesion is particularly large or there has been some minor trauma to the affected area (Fig. 21.22). More frequent in children are vertebral fractures to produce the so-called vertebra plana appearance due to symmetrical flattening of the body. This is not a pathognomonic sign of LCH and may be seen at this age in other conditions such a chronic recurrent multifocal osteomyelitis. The less common multisystem manifestations of LCH are the chronic form Hand-Schüller-Christian disease and the acute/aggressive Letterer-Siwe disease. The latter shows multiple destructive lesions of the skull vault and remainder of the skeleton with an increased risk of fractures (Hoover et al. 2007).

21.8 Neuromuscular Disorders

Bone atrophy and osteopenia, particularly affecting the lower limb, are common in patients with a variety of neuromuscular disorders including cerebral palsy, spina bifida and muscular dystrophy (Table 21.1) (Saraph and Linhart 2005). The deficient bone is susceptible to fractures without significant trauma. The major cause is long and fragile lever arms with stiffness in the major joints (Brunner and Doderlein 1996). An additional factor can be further exacerbation of the osteopenia following prolonged periods of postoperative immobilization. In severely handicapped patients the risk of fractures may be increased by coexistent vitamin D deficiency (Lee and Lyne 1990). In children with lower

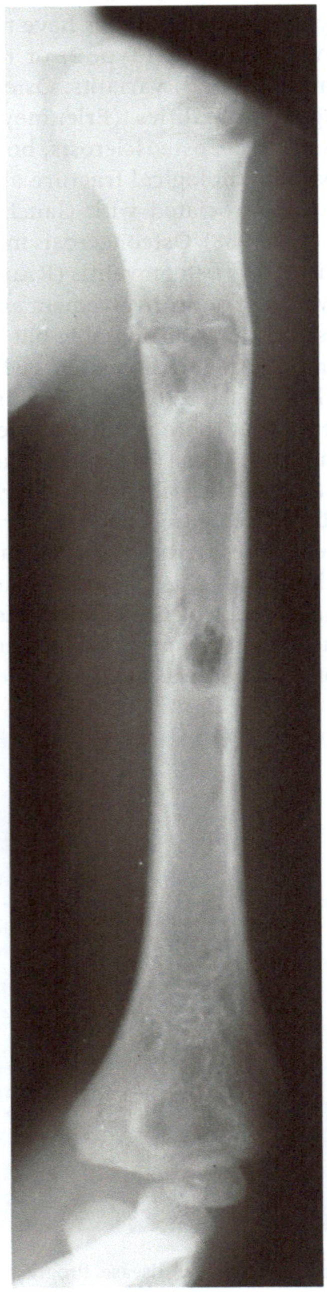

Fig. 21.22. Langerhans cell histiocytosis. Multiple lytic lesions with pathological fracture through the largest lesion

limb sensory loss, such as spina bifida, the fractures may be occult and delayed diagnosis not unusual (Fig. 21.23). In this situation unrestricted movement at the fracture site can lead to displacement, large subperiosteal haematoma and exuberant callus formation that can be mistaken on radiographs for a bone-forming tumour. Similar appearances may be seen with congenital insensitivity to pain although distal neuroarthropathic changes usually predominate.

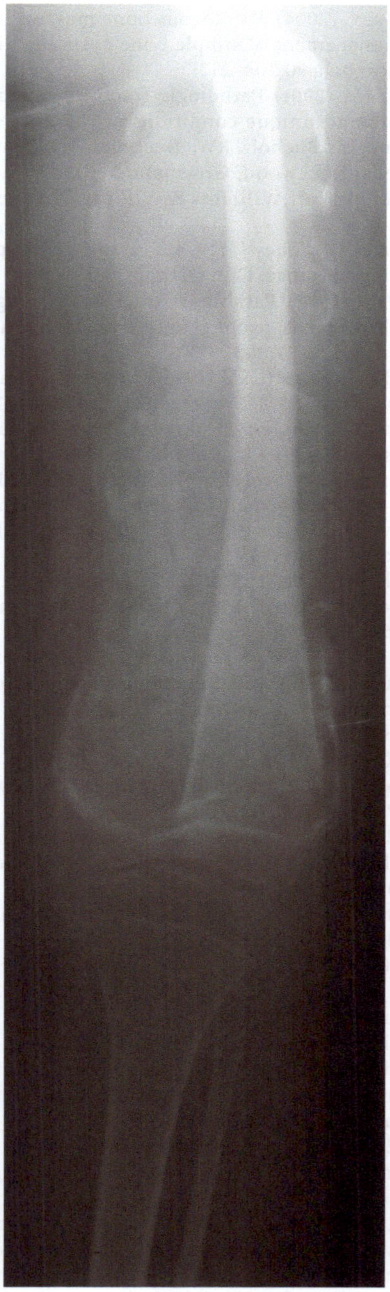

Fig. 21.23. Spina bifida. Chronic ununited fracture through the distal growth plate with a large calcifying subperiosteal haematoma

21.9 Iatrogenic Disorders

On occasion, the well-intentioned efforts of a physician may actually precipitate a pathological fracture or at the very least increase the risk. These include biopsy and curettage of bone lesions where the procedure may weaken the structural integrity of the bone resulting in a fracture. Prolonged immobilization following a surgical procedure will increase bone resorption causing osteopenia. Drug treatments including steroids and chemotherapy may stimulate bone resorption or reduce new bone formation (Fig. 21.24). Some patients may have the

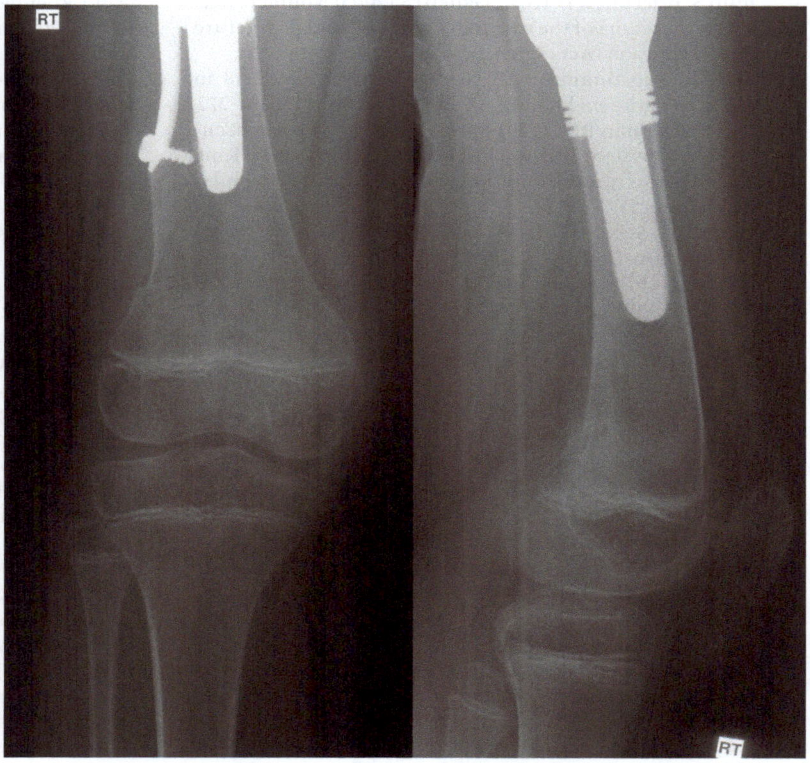

Fig. 21.24. Insufficiency fracture of the distal femoral metaphysis in a child treated for a sarcoma of the proximal femur. The osteopenia is due to a combination of disuse, immobilization and chemotherapy

misfortune to have a "double whammy" in which both the disease and therapy can reduce the strength of bone. Such an example would be juvenile inflammatory arthritis treated with steroids. As the prognosis for childhood malignancies improve patients are surviving longer and therefore may suffer complications from their treatment. This includes radiotherapy where there is a small risk of radionecrosis and after a latent period of at least 4 years a radiation-induced sarcoma.

References

Abudu A, Sferopoulos NK, Tillman RM, Carter SR, Grimer RJ (1996) The surgical treatment and outcome of pathological fractures in localised osteosarcoma. J Bone Joint Surg Br 78B:694–698

Ahn JI, Park JS (1994) Pathological fractures secondary to unicameral bone cysts. Int Orthop 18:20–22

Arata MA, Peterson HA, Dahlin DC (1981) Pathological fractures through nonossifying fibromas. J Bone Joint Surg Am 63A:980–988

Bacci G, Ferrari S, Longhi A, Donati D, Manfrini M, Giacomini S, Briccoli A, Forni C, Galletti S (2003) Nonmetastatic osteosarcoma of the extremity with pathologic fracture at presentation. Acta Orthop Scan 74:449–454

Barrett IR, Papadimitriou DG (1996) Skeletal disorders in children with renal failure. J Pediatric Orthop 16:264–272

Bleck EE, Kleiman RG (1984) Special injuries of the musculoskeletal system. In: Rockwood CA, Wilkins KE, King RE (eds) Fractures in children, vol 3. JB Lippincott, Philadelphia, pp 173–227

Bonnerot V, Sebag G, de Montalembert M et al (1994) Gadolinium-DOTA enhanced MRI of painful osseous crises in children with sickle cell anemia. Pediatr Radiol 24:92–95

Brunner R, Doderlein L (1996) Pathological fractures in patients with cerebral palsy. J Pediatr Orthop 5B:232–238

Chung C, Yu JS, Resnick D et al (1997) Gorham's syndrome of the thorax and cervical spine: CT and MRI findings. Skeletal Radiol 26:55–59

Cottalorda J, Bourelle S (2006) Current treatments of primary aneurysmal bone cyst. J Pediatr Orthop 15B:155–167

Cottalorda J, Bourelle S (2007) Modern concepts of primary aneurysmal bone cyst. Arch Orthop Trauma Surg 127:105–114

Cockshott WP (1963) Dactylitis and growth disorders. Br J Radiol 36:19–26

Damron TA, Morgan H, Prakash D, Grant W, Aronowitz J, Heiner J (2003) Critical evaluation of Mirrels' rating system for impending pathologic fractures. Clin Orthop 415: S201–S207

David R, Oria RA, Kumar R, Singleton EB, Lindell MM, Shirkhoda A et al (1989) Radiologic features of eosinophilic granuloma of bone. AJR Am J Roentgenol 153:1021–1026

Davies AM, Cassar-Pullicino VN, Grimer RJ (1992) The incidence and significance of fluid-fluid levels on computed tomography of osseous lesions. Br J Radiol 65:193–198

De Santos LA, Edeiken BS (1985) Subtle early osteosarcoma. Skeletal Radiol 13:44–48

Devnani AS (2002) Management of pathological fracture neck of femur following recent osteomyelitis in a child. Singapore Med J 43:205–207

Docquier PL, Delloye C (2004) Autologous bone marrow injection in the management of simple bone cysts in children. Acta Orthop Belg 70:204–213

Dormans JP, Flynn JM (2001) Pathologic fractures associated with tumors and unique conditions of the musculoskeletal system. In: Bucholz RW, Heckman JD, Beaty JH, Kasser JR (eds) Rockwood, Green and Wilkin's fractures, 5th edn. Lippincott Williams & Wilkins, Philadelphia, pp 139–240

Drennan DB, Maylahn DJ, Fahey JJ (1974) Fractures through large nonossifying fibromas. Clin Orthop 103:82–88

Easley ME, Kneisl JS (1997) Pathologic fractures through nonossifying fibromas: is prophylactic treatment warranted. J Pediatr Orthop 17:808–813

Fahal AH, Sheikh HE, El Hassan AM (1996) Pathological fracture in mycetoma. Trans RSM Trop Med & Hyg 90:675–676

Finsterbush A, Farber I, Mogle P et al (1985) Fracture patterns in Thalassaemia. Clin Orthop 192:132–136

Frush DP, Heyneman LE, Ware RE, Bissett GS (1999) MR features of soft-tissue abnormalities due to acute marrow infarction in five children with sickle cell disease. AJR Am J Roentgenol 173:989–993

Fuchs B, Valenzuela RG, Sim FH (2003) Pathologic fracture as a complication in the treatment of Ewing's sarcoma. Clin Orthop 415:25–30

Gorham LW, Stout AP (1955) Massive osteolysis (acute spontaneous absorption of bone, phantom bone, disappearing bone): its relationship to haemangiomatosis. J Bone Joint Surg Am 37A:985–1004

Gregg PJ, Price BA, Ellis HA et al (1982) Pseudarthrosis of the radius associated with neurofibromatosis. Clin Orthop 171:175–179

Hase T, Miki T (2000) Autogenous bone marrow graft to nonossifying fibroma with a pathologic fracture. Arch Orthop Trauma Surg 120:458–459

Hoover KB, Rosenthal DI, Mankin H (2007) Langerhans cell histiocytosis. Skeletal Radiol 36:95–104

Huvos AG, Rosen G, Bretsky SS, Butler A (1982) Telangiectatic osteogenic sarcoma: a clinicopathologic study of 124 patients. Cancer 49:1679–1689

Ishiguro N, Iwahori Y, Kato T, Ito T, Takamatsu J, Iwata H (1998) The surgical management of a haemophiliac pseudotumour in an extremity: a report of three cases with pathological fractures. Haemophilia 4:126–131

Jaffe N, Spears R, Eftekhari F et al (1987) Pathologic fracture in osteosarcoma: impact of chemotherapy on primary tumor and survival. Cancer 59:701–709

Jung ST, Chung JY, Seo HY, Bae BH, Lim KY (2006) Multiple osteotomies and intramedullary nailing with neck crosspinning for shepherd's crook deformity in polystotic fibrous dysplasia. Acta Orthop Scand 77:469–473

Kai B, Ryan A, Munk PL, Dunlop P (2006) Gorham disease of bone: three cases and review of radiological features. Clin Radiol 61:1058–1064

Kaelin AJ, MacEwen GD (1989) Unicameral bone cysts: natural history and the risk of fracture. Int Orthop 13:275–282
Katagiri H, Takahashi M, Wakai K, Sugiura H, Kataoka T, Nakanishi K (2005) Prognostic factors and a scoring system for patients with skeletal metastasis. J Bone Joint Surg Br 87B:698–703
Kilborn TN, Teh J, Goodman TR (2003) Paediatric manifestations of Langerhans cell histiocytosis: a review of clinical and radiological findings. Clin Radiol 58:269–278
Kransdorf MJ, Sweet DE (1995) Aneurysmal bone cyst: concept, controversy, clinical presentation, and imaging. AJR Am J Roentgenol 164:573–580
Kumar R, Cornah MS (1983) Hydatid disease – a rare cause of pathological fracture: a case report. Injury 15:284–285
Kumta SM, Leung PC, Griffith JF, Chow LTC (2000) Vascularised bone grafting for fibrous dysplasia of the upper limb. J Bone Joint Surg (Br) 82B:409–412
Lee JJK, Lyne ED (1990) Pathologic fractures in severely handicapped children and young adults. J Pediatr Orthop 10:497–500
Leithner A, Machacek F, Haas OA, Lang S, Ritschl P, Radl R, Windhager R (2004) Aneurysmal bone cyst: a hereditary disease? J Pediatr Orthop 13B:214–217
Li JKW, Birch PD, Davies AM (1988) Proximal humeral defects in Gaucher's disease. Br J Radiol 61:579–583
Lonergan GJ, Cline DB, Abbondanzo SL (2001) From the archives of the AFIP: sickle cell anemia. RadioGraphics 21:971–994
Maas M, Poll LW, Terk MR (2002) Imaging and quantifying skeletal involvement in Gaucher disease. Br J Radiol 75[Suppl 1]:A13–A24
McCann F (1962) The incidence and value of radiological signs of scurvy. Brit J Radiol 35:636–686
Maiya S, Davies AM, Evans N, Grimer RJ (2002) Surface aneurysmal bone cysts: a pictorial review. Eur Radiol 12:99–108
Mankin HJ (1974a) Rickets, osteomalacia and renal osteodystrophy. Part I. J Bone Joint Surg Am 56A:101–128
Mankin HJ (1974b) Rickets, osteomalacia and renal osteodystrophy. Part II. J Bone Joint Surg Am 56A:352–386
Mirrels H (1989) Metastatic disease in long bones: a proposed scoring system for diagnosing impending pathologic fractures. Clin Orthop 249:256–264
Moller G, Primel M, Amling M et al (1999) The Gorham-Stout syndrome (Gorham's massive osteolysis). J Bone Joint Surg Br 81B:501–506
Morgan G, Ganapathi M, Afzal S, Grant AJ (2002) Pathological fractures in primary hyperparathyroidism: a case report highlighting diagnostic difficulties. Injury 33:288–291
Morris HG (1997) Pathological fractures in bone sarcomas. Acta Orthop Scand 273S:106–107
Murray HH, Lovell WW (1982) Congenital pseudarthrosis of the tibia. Clin Orthop 166:14–20
Natarajan MV, Govardhan RH, Williams S, Gopal TSR (2000) Limb salvage surgery for pathological fractures in osteosarcoma. Int Orthop 24:170–172
O' Donnell, Saifuddin A (2004) The prevalence and diagnostic significance of fluid-fluid levels in focal lesions of bone. Skeletal Radiol 33:330–336
Oliveira AM, Perez-Atayde AR, Inwards CY, Medeiros F, Derr V, His BL, Gebhardt MC, Rosenberg AE, Fletcher JA (2004) USP6 and CDH11 oncogenes identify the neoplastic cell in primary aneurysmal bone cysts and are absent on so-called secondary aneurysmal bone cysts. Am J Pathol 165:1773–1780
Ortiz EJ, Isler MH, Navia JE, Canosa R (2005) Pathologic fractures in children. Clin Orthop 432:116–126
Parman LM, Murphey MD (2000) Alphabet soup: cystic lesions of bone. Semin Muscul Radiol 4:89–101
Pastores G, Wallenstein S, Desnick RJ, Luckey MM (1999) Bone density in Type 1 Gaucher disease. J Bone Min Res 11:1801–1807
Poll LW, Maas M, Terk MR, Roca-Espiau M, Bembi B, Ciana G, Weinreb NJ (2002) Response of Gaucher bone disease to enzyme replacement therapy. Br J Radiol 75[Suppl 1]:A25–A36
Radermakers RP (1995) Radiologic evaluation of Gaucher bone disease. Semin Hematol 32[Suppl 1]:14–19
Ramo BA, Kyriakos M, McDonald DJ (2006) Osteosarcoma without radiographic evidence of tumor: case report. Clin Orthop 442:267–272
Reynolds J (1969) The "fallen fragment sign" in the diagnosis of unicameral bone cyst. Radiology 92:949–953
Roposch A, Saraph V, Linhart WE (2000) Flexible intramedullary nailing for the treatment of unicameral bone cysts in long bones. J Bone Joint Surg Am 82A:1447–1453
Roposch A, Saraph V, Linhart WE (2004) Treatment of femoral neck and trochanteric simple bone cysts. Arch Orthop Trauma Surg 124:437–442
Saraph V, Linhart WE (2005) Modern treatment of pathological fractures in children. Injury 36:S-A64–S-A74
Sato K, Sugiura H, Yamamura S, Mieno T, Nagasaka T, Nakashima N (1997) Gorham massive osteolysis. Arch Orthop Trauma Surg 116:510–513
Scully SP, Ghert MA, Zurakowski D, Thompson RC, Gebhardt MC (2002) Pathologic fracture in osteosarcoma: prognostic importance and treatment implications. J Bone Joint Surg Am 84A:49–57
Sillence DO (1981) Osteogenesis imperfecta. An expanding panorama of variants. Clin Orthop 159:11–25
Smith SE, Kransdorf MJ (2000) Primary musculoskeletal tumors of fibrous origin. Semin Muscul Radiol 4:73–88
Thomsen C, Sorensen PG, Karle H et al (1987) Prolonged bone marrow T1-relaxation in acute leukaemia. Magn Reson Imaging 5:251–257
Tunaci M, Tunaci A, Engin G et al (1999) Imaging features of thalassaemia. Eur Radiol 9:1804–1809
Van der Linden YM, Dijkstra PDS, Kroon HM, Lok JJ, Noordijk EM, Leer JWH, Marjnen CAM (2004) Comparative analysis of risk factors for pathological fracture with femoral metastases. J Bone Joint Surg Br 86B:566–573
Van Dyck P, Vanhoenacker FM, Vogel J, Venstermans C, Kroon HM, Gielen J, Parizel PM, Bloem JL, De Schepper AMA (2006) Prevalence, extension and characteristics of fluid-fluid levels in bone and soft tissue tumors. Eur Radiol 16:2644–2651
Vigler M, Weigl D, Schwarz M, Ben-Itzhak I, Salai M, Bar-On E (2006) Subtrochanteric femoral fractures due to simple bone cysts in children. J Pediatric Orthop 15B:439–442
Violas P, Salmeron F, Chapuis M, de Gauzy JS, Bracq H, Cahuzac JP (2004) Simple bone cysts of the proximal humerus complicated with growth arrest. Acta Orthop Belg 70:166–170
Wenstrup RJ, Roca-Espiau M, weinreb NJ, Bembi B (2002) Skeletal aspects of Gaucher disease: a review. Br J Radiol 75[Suppl 1]:A2–A12
Yoo SY, Hong SH, Chung HY et al (2002) MRI of Gorham's disease: findings in two cases. Skeletal Radiol 31:301–306

Subject Index

H

I

J

K

L

M

S

T

U

V

List of Contributors

Edward Bache, FRCS (ortho)
Consultant Orthopaedic Surgeon
Birmingham Children Hospital
Steelhouse Lane
Birmingham B4 6NH
UK

Karen Bradshaw, MBChB, MRCP, FRCR
Department of Radiology
Withybush Hospital
Fishguard Road
Haverfordwest
Dyfed
UK

Victor N. Cassar-Pullicino, MD
Department of Radiology
Robert Jones & Agnes Hunt Orthopaedic Hospital
Oswestry
Shropshire SY10 7AG
UK

Stephen Chapman, MD
Consultant Paediatric Radiologist
Department of Radiology
Birmingham Children's Hospital
Steelhouse Lane
Birmingham B4 6NH
UK

A. Mark Davies, MD
Consultant Radiologist
The MRI Centre
Royal Orthopaedic Hospital
Birmingham B31 2AP
UK

Roderick Duncan
MB ChB, FRCSEd (Orth)
Consultant Paediatric Orthopaedic Surgeon
Department of Orthopaedic
Royal Hospital for Sick Children
Dalnair Street
Glasgow
Scotland G3 8SJ
UK

Katharine Foster, MD
Consultant Radiologist
Department of Radiology
Birmingham Children's Hospital
Steelhouse Lane
Birmingham B4 6NH
UK

Paul Gibbons, MBBS, FRCS (Orth), FRACS
Senior Staff Specialist
Clinical Senior Lecturer, Faculty of Medicine
University of Sidney
Department of Orthopaedic Surgery
The Children's Hospital at Westmead
Locked Bag 4001
Westmead NSW 2145
Australia

Phil Glithero, FRCSEd (Orth)
Consultant Paediatric Orthopaedic Surgeon
Birmingham Children's Hospital
Steelhouse Lane
Birmingham B4 6NH
UK

Angharad Harries, Msc.
Department of Radiology
Withybush Hospital
Fishguard Road
Haverfordwest
Dyfed
UK

Keith Hayward, FRCS
Orthopaedic Registrar
Birmingham Children Hospital
Birmingham BA 6NH
UK

David Horton, MD
Consultant Paediatric Radiologist
Hull Royal Infirmary
Anlapoy Road
Hull HU3 2JZ
UK

Greg John Irwin,
BMSc (Hons), MB ChB, FRCS (Edin), FRCR
Consultant Paediatric Radiologist
Diagnostic Imaging
Royal Hospital for Sick Children
Dalnair Street
Glasgow
Scotland G3 8SJ
UK

Karl J. Johnson, MD, MRCP, FRCR
Consultant Paediatric Radiologist
Birmingham Children's Hospital
Steelhouse Lane
Birmingham B4 6NH
UK

Raj Kanwar, MD
Orthopaedic Clinical Fellow
Birmingham
Birmingham Children's Hospital
Steelhouse Lane
Birmingham B4 6NH
UK

Radhesh Krishna Lalam, MD
Department of Radiology
Robert Jones & Agnes Hunt Orthopaedic and District Hospital
Oswestry, Shropshire SY10 7AG
UK

Caroline Lever, MD
Orthopaedic Specialist Registrar
Birmingham Children's Hospital
Steelhouse Lane
Birmingham B4 6NH
UK

James Metcalfe, FRCS (orth)
Consultant Orthopaedic Surgeon
Derriford Hospital
Plymouth, PL6 8DH
UK

Kate Parkes, MD
Superintendent Radiographer
Department of Radiology
Birmingham Children's Hospital
Steelhouse Lane
Birmingham B4 6NH
UK

Anne Paterson, MBBS, MRCP, FRCR
Consultant Paediatric Radiologist
Royal Belfast Hospital for Sick Children
180 Falls Road
Belfast BT12 6BE
UK

Alan Sprigg, MD
Consultant Paediatric Radiologist
Sheffield Children's Hospital
Western Bank
Sheffield S10 2TH
UK

Sean Symons, FRCS (Orth)
Orthopaedic Fellow
Orthopaedic Department
Royal Children's Hospital
Flemington Road
Parkville Vic. 3052
Australia

James Teh, BSc, MBBS, MRCP, FRCR
Consultant Musculoskeletal Radiologist
Radiology Department
Nuffield Orthopaedic Centre
Oxford OX3 7LD
UK

Prudencia N. M. Tyrrell, MD
Department of Radiology
Robert Jones & Agnes Hunt Orthopaedic Hospital
Oswestry, Shropshire SY10 7AG
UK

Helen Williams, MBChB, MRCP, FRCR
Department of Radiology
Birmingham Children's Hospital
Steelhouse Lane
Birmingham B4 6NH
UK

MEDICAL RADIOLOGY Diagnostic Imaging and Radiation Oncology

Titles in the series already published

DIAGNOSTIC IMAGING

Innovations in Diagnostic Imaging
Edited by J. H. Anderson

Radiology of the Upper Urinary Tract
Edited by E. K. Lang

The Thymus - Diagnostic Imaging, Functions, and Pathologic Anatomy
Edited by E. Walter, E. Willich, and W. R. Webb

Interventional Neuroradiology
Edited by A. Valavanis

Radiology of the Pancreas
Edited by A. L. Baert, co-edited by G. Delorme

Radiology of the Lower Urinary Tract
Edited by E. K. Lang

Magnetic Resonance Angiography
Edited by I. P. Arlart, G. M. Bongartz, and G. Marchal

Contrast-Enhanced MRI of the Breast
S. Heywang-Köbrunner and R. Beck

Spiral CT of the Chest
Edited by M. Rémy-Jardin and J. Rémy

Radiological Diagnosis of Breast Diseases
Edited by M. Friedrich and E.A. Sickles

Radiology of the Trauma
Edited by M. Heller and A. Fink

Biliary Tract Radiology
Edited by P. Rossi, co-edited by M. Brezi

Radiological Imaging of Sports Injuries
Edited by C. Masciocchi

Modern Imaging of the Alimentary Tube
Edited by A. R. Margulis

Diagnosis and Therapy of Spinal Tumors
Edited by P. R. Algra, J. Valk, and J. J. Heimans

Interventional Magnetic Resonance Imaging
Edited by J. F. Debatin and G. Adam

Abdominal and Pelvic MRI
Edited by A. Heuck and M. Reiser

Orthopedic Imaging
Techniques and Applications
Edited by A. M. Davies and H. Pettersson

Radiology of the Female Pelvic Organs
Edited by E. K.Lang

Magnetic Resonance of the Heart and Great Vessels
Clinical Applications
Edited by J. Bogaert, A.J. Duerinckx, and F. E. Rademakers

Modern Head and Neck Imaging
Edited by S. K. Mukherji and J. A. Castelijns

Radiological Imaging of Endocrine Diseases
Edited by J. N. Bruneton in collaboration with B. Padovani and M.-Y. Mourou

Trends in Contrast Media
Edited by H. S. Thomsen, R. N. Muller, and R. F. Mattrey

Functional MRI
Edited by C. T. W. Moonen and P. A. Bandettini

Radiology of the Pancreas
2nd Revised Edition
Edited by A. L. Baert. Co-edited by G. Delorme and L. Van Hoe

Emergency Pediatric Radiology
Edited by H. Carty

Spiral CT of the Abdomen
Edited by F. Terrier, M. Grossholz, and C. D. Becker

Liver Malignancies
Diagnostic and Interventional Radiology
Edited by C. Bartolozzi and R. Lencioni

Medical Imaging of the Spleen
Edited by A. M. De Schepper and F. Vanhoenacker

Radiology of Peripheral Vascular Diseases
Edited by E. Zeitler

Diagnostic Nuclear Medicine
Edited by C. Schiepers

Radiology of Blunt Trauma of the Chest
P. Schnyder and M. Wintermark

Portal Hypertension
Diagnostic Imaging-Guided Therapy
Edited by P. Rossi
Co-edited by P. Ricci and L. Broglia

Recent Advances in Diagnostic Neuroradiology
Edited by Ph. Demaerel

Virtual Endoscopy and Related 3D Techniques
Edited by P. Rogalla, J. Terwisscha Van Scheltinga, and B. Hamm

Multislice CT
Edited by M. F. Reiser, M. Takahashi, M. Modic, and R. Bruening

Pediatric Uroradiology
Edited by R. Fotter

Transfontanellar Doppler Imaging in Neonates
A. Couture and C. Veyrac

Radiology of AIDS
A Practical Approach
Edited by J.W.A.J. Reeders and P.C. Goodman

CT of the Peritoneum
Armando Rossi and Giorgio Rossi

Magnetic Resonance Angiography
2nd Revised Edition
Edited by I. P. Arlart, G. M. Bongratz, and G. Marchal

Pediatric Chest Imaging
Edited by Javier Lucaya and Janet L. Strife

Applications of Sonography in Head and Neck Pathology
Edited by J. N. Bruneton in collaboration with C. Raffaelli and O. Dassonville

Imaging of the Larynx
Edited by R. Hermans

3D Image Processing
Techniques and Clinical Applications
Edited by D. Caramella and C. Bartolozzi

Imaging of Orbital and Visual Pathway Pathology
Edited by W. S. Müller-Forell

Pediatric ENT Radiology
Edited by S. J. King and A. E. Boothroyd

Radiological Imaging of the Small Intestine
Edited by N. C. Gourtsoyiannis

Imaging of the Knee
Techniques and Applications
Edited by A. M. Davies and V. N. Cassar-Pullicino

Perinatal Imaging
From Ultrasound to MR Imaging
Edited by Fred E. Avni

Radiological Imaging of the Neonatal Chest
Edited by V. Donoghue

Diagnostic and Interventional Radiology in Liver Transplantation
Edited by E. Bücheler, V. Nicolas, C. E. Broelsch, X. Rogiers, and G. Krupski

Radiology of Osteoporosis
Edited by S. Grampp

Imaging Pelvic Floor Disorders
Edited by C. I. Bartram and J. O. L. DeLancey
Associate Editors: S. Halligan, F. M. Kelvin, and J. Stoker

Imaging of the Pancreas
Cystic and Rare Tumors
Edited by C. Procacci and A. J. Megibow

High Resolution Sonography of the Peripheral Nervous System
Edited by S. Peer and G. Bodner

Imaging of the Foot and Ankle
Techniques and Applications
Edited by A. M. Davies, R. W. Whitehouse, and J. P. R. Jenkins

Radiology Imaging of the Ureter
Edited by F. Joffre, Ph. Otal, and M. Soulie

Imaging of the Shoulder
Techniques and Applications
Edited by A. M. Davies and J. Hodler

Radiology of the Petrous Bone
Edited by M. Lemmerling and S. S. Kollias

Interventional Radiology in Cancer
Edited by A. Adam, R. F. Dondelinger, and P. R. Mueller

Duplex and Color Doppler Imaging of the Venous System
Edited by G. H. Mostbeck

Multidetector-Row CT of the Thorax
Edited by U. J. Schoepf

Functional Imaging of the Chest
Edited by H.-U. Kauczor

Radiology of the Pharynx and the Esophagus
Edited by O. Ekberg

Radiological Imaging in Hematological Malignancies
Edited by A. Guermazi

Imaging and Intervention in Abdominal Trauma
Edited by R. F. Dondelinger

Multislice CT
2nd Revised Edition
Edited by M. F. Reiser, M. Takahashi, M. Modic, and C. R. Becker

Intracranial Vascular Malformations and Aneurysms
From Diagnostic Work-Up to Endovascular Therapy
Edited by M. Forsting

Radiology and Imaging of the Colon
Edited by A. H. Chapman

Coronary Radiology
Edited by M. Oudkerk

Dynamic Contrast-Enhanced Magnetic Resonance Imaging in Oncology
Edited by A. Jackson, D. L. Buckley, and G. J. M. Parker

Imaging in Treatment Planning for Sinonasal Diseases
Edited by R. Maroldi and P. Nicolai

Clinical Cardiac MRI
With Interactive CD-ROM
Edited by J. Bogaert, S. Dymarkowski, and A. M. Taylor

Focal Liver Lesions
Detection, Characterization, Ablation
Edited by R. Lencioni, D. Cioni, and C. Bartolozzi

Multidetector-Row CT Angiography
Edited by C. Catalano and R. Passariello

Paediatric Musculoskeletal Diseases
With an Emphasis on Ultrasound
Edited by D. Wilson

Contrast Media in Ultrasonography
Basic Principles and Clinical Applications
Edited by Emilio Quaia

MR Imaging in White Matter Diseases of the Brain and Spinal Cord
Edited by M. Filippi, N. De Stefano, V. Dousset, and J. C. McGowan

Diagnostic Nuclear Medicine
2nd Revised Edition
Edited by C. Schiepers

Imaging of the Kidney Cancer
Edited by A. Guermazi

Magnetic Resonance Imaging in Ischemic Stroke
Edited by R. von Kummer and T. Back

Imaging of the Hip & Bony Pelvis
Techniques and Applications
Edited by A. M. Davies, K. J. Johnson, and R. W. Whitehouse

Imaging of Occupational and Environmental Disorders of the Chest
Edited by P. A. Gevenois and P. De Vuyst

Contrast Media
Safety Issues and ESUR Guidelines
Edited by H. S. Thomsen

Virtual Colonoscopy
A Practical Guide
Edited by P. Lefere and S. Gryspeerdt

Vascular Embolotherapy
A Comprehensive Approach
Volume 1: *General Principles, Chest, Abdomen, and Great Vessels*
Edited by J. Golzarian. Co-edited by S. Sun and M. J. Sharafuddin

Vascular Embolotherapy
A Comprehensive Approach
Volume 2: *Oncology, Trauma, Gene Therapy, Vascular Malformations, and Neck*
Edited by J. Golzarian. Co-edited by S. Sun and M. J. Sharafuddin

Head and Neck Cancer Imaging
Edited by R. Hermans

Vascular Interventional Radiology
Current Evidence in Endovascular Surgery
Edited by M. G. Cowling

Ultrasound of the Gastrointestinal Tract
Edited by G. Maconi and G. Bianchi Porro

Imaging of Orthopedic Sports Injuries
Edited by F. M. Vanhoenacker, M. Maas, J. L. M. A. Gielen

Parallel Imaging in Clinical MR Applications
Edited by S. O. Schoenberg, O. Dietrich, and M. F. Reiser

MRI and CT of the Female Pelvis
Edited by B. Hamm and R. Forstner

Ultrasound of the Musculoskeletal System
S. Bianchi and C. Martinoli

Spinal Imaging
Diagnostic Imaging of the Spine and Spinal Cord
Edited by J. W. M. Van Goethem, L. van den Hauwe, and P. M. Parizel

Radiation Dose from Adult and Pediatric Multidetector Computed Tomography
Edited by D. Tack and P. A. Gevenois

Computed Tomography of the Lung
A Pattern Approach
J. A. Verschakelen and W. De Wever

Clinical Functional MRI
Presurgical Functional Neuroimaging
Edited bei C. Stippich

Imaging in Transplantation
Edited by A. A. Bankier

Radiological Imaging of the Digestive System in Infants and Children
Edited by A. S. Devos and J. G. Blickman

Pediatric Chest Imaging
Chest Imaging in Infants and Children
2nd Revised Edition
Edited by J. Lucaya and J. L. Strife

Radiological Imaging of the Neonatal Chest
2nd Revised Edition
Edited by V. Donoghue

Radiology of the Stomach and Duodenum
Edited by A. H. Freeman and E. Sala

Imaging in Pediatric Skeletal Trauma
Techniques and Applications
Edited by K. J. Johnson and E. Bache

Percutaneous Tumor Ablation in Medical Radiology
Edited by T. J. Vogl, T. K. Helmberger, M. G. Mack, and M. F. Reiser

Screening and Preventive Diagnosis with Radiological Imaging
Edited by M. F. Reiser, G. van Kaick, C. Fink, and S. O. Schoenberg

Color Doppler US of the Penis
Edited by M. Bertolotto

Image Processing in Radiology
Current Applications
Edited by E. Neri, D. Caramella, and C. Bartolozzi

Springer

MEDICAL RADIOLOGY Diagnostic Imaging and Radiation Oncology

Titles in the series already published

RADIATION ONCOLOGY

Lung Cancer
Edited by C.W. Scarantino

Innovations in Radiation Oncology
Edited by H. R. Withers and L. J. Peters

Radiation Therapy of Head and Neck Cancer
Edited by G. E. Laramore

Gastrointestinal Cancer – Radiation Therapy
Edited by R.R. Dobelbower, Jr.

Radiation Exposure and Occupational Risks
Edited by E. Scherer, C. Streffer, and K.-R. Trott

Radiation Therapy of Benign Diseases
A Clinical Guide
S. E. Order and S. S. Donaldson

Interventional Radiation Therapy Techniques – Brachytherapy
Edited by R. Sauer

Radiopathology of Organs and Tissues
Edited by E. Scherer, C. Streffer, and K.-R. Trott

Concomitant Continuous Infusion Chemotherapy and Radiation
Edited by M. Rotman and C. J. Rosenthal

Intraoperative Radiotherapy – Clinical Experiences and Results
Edited by F. A. Calvo, M. Santos, and L.W. Brady

Radiotherapy of Intraocular and Orbital Tumors
Edited by W. E. Alberti and R. H. Sagerman

Interstitial and Intracavitary Thermoradiotherapy
Edited by M. H. Seegenschmiedt and R. Sauer

Non-Disseminated Breast Cancer
Controversial Issues in Management
Edited by G. H. Fletcher and S.H. Levitt

Current Topics in Clinical Radiobiology of Tumors
Edited by H.-P. Beck-Bornholdt

Practical Approaches to Cancer Invasion and Metastases
A Compendium of Radiation Oncologists' Responses to 40 Histories
Edited by A. R. Kagan with the Assistance of R. J. Steckel

Radiation Therapy in Pediatric Oncology
Edited by J. R. Cassady

Radiation Therapy Physics
Edited by A. R. Smith

Late Sequelae in Oncology
Edited by J. Dunst and R. Sauer

Mediastinal Tumors. Update 1995
Edited by D. E. Wood and C. R. Thomas, Jr.

Thermoradiotherapy and Thermochemotherapy
Volume 1:
Biology, Physiology, and Physics
Volume 2:
Clinical Applications
Edited by M.H. Seegenschmiedt, P. Fessenden, and C.C. Vernon

Carcinoma of the Prostate
Innovations in Management
Edited by Z. Petrovich, L. Baert, and L.W. Brady

Radiation Oncology of Gynecological Cancers
Edited by H.W. Vahrson

Carcinoma of the Bladder
Innovations in Management
Edited by Z. Petrovich, L. Baert, and L.W. Brady

Blood Perfusion and Microenvironment of Human Tumors
Implications for Clinical Radiooncology
Edited by M. Molls and P. Vaupel

Radiation Therapy of Benign Diseases
A Clinical Guide
2nd Revised Edition
S. E. Order and S. S. Donaldson

Carcinoma of the Kidney and Testis, and Rare Urologic Malignancies
Innovations in Management
Edited by Z. Petrovich, L. Baert, and L.W. Brady

Progress and Perspectives in the Treatment of Lung Cancer
Edited by P. Van Houtte, J. Klastersky, and P. Rocmans

Combined Modality Therapy of Central Nervous System Tumors
Edited by Z. Petrovich, L. W. Brady, M. L. Apuzzo, and M. Bamberg

Age-Related Macular Degeneration
Current Treatment Concepts
Edited by W. A. Alberti, G. Richard, and R. H. Sagerman

Radiotherapy of Intraocular and Orbital Tumors
2nd Revised Edition
Edited by R. H. Sagerman, and W. E. Alberti

Modification of Radiation Response
Cytokines, Growth Factors, and Other Biolgical Targets
Edited by C. Nieder, L. Milas, and K. K. Ang

Radiation Oncology for Cure and Palliation
R. G. Parker, N. A. Janjan, and M. T. Selch

Clinical Target Volumes in Conformal and Intensity Modulated Radiation Therapy
A Clinical Guide to Cancer Treatment
Edited by V. Grégoire, P. Scalliet, and K. K. Ang

Advances in Radiation Oncology in Lung Cancer
Edited by Branislav Jeremić

New Technologies in Radiation Oncology
Edited by W. Schlegel, T. Bortfeld, and A.-L. Grosu

Technical Basis of Radiation Therapy
4th Revised Edition
Edited by S. H. Levitt, J. A. Purdy, C. A. Perez, and S. Vijayakumar

CURED I • LENT
Late Effects of Cancer Treatment on Normal Tissues
Edited by P. Rubin, L. S. Constine, L. B. Marks, and P. Okunieff

Clinical Practice of Radiation Therapy for Benign Diseases
Contemporary Concepts and Clinical Results
Edited by M. H. Seegenschmiedt, H.-B. Makoski, K.-R. Trott, and L. W. Brady

Springer

MIX
Papier aus verantwortungsvollen Quellen
Paper from responsible sources
FSC® C105338

If you have any concerns about our products,
you can contact us on
ProductSafety@springernature.com

In case Publisher is established outside the EU,
the EU authorized representative is:
Springer Nature Customer Service Center GmbH
Europaplatz 3, 69115 Heidelberg, Germany

Printed by Libri Plureos GmbH
in Hamburg, Germany